RC458.S94
Collected wo
046000079923
S0-AKF-702

The COLLECTED WORKS *of* HARRY STACK SULLIVAN, M.D.

VOLUME I

The Interpersonal Theory of Psychiatry
Conceptions of Modern Psychiatry
The Psychiatric Interview

W. W. NORTON & COMPANY, INC. · NEW YORK

Printed in the United States of America

D IN THE UNITED STATES OF AMERICA
PUBLISHERS BY THE VAIL-BALLOU PRESS
1 2 3 4 5 6 7 8 9

HARRY STACK SULLIVAN, M.D.

THE Interpersonal Theory of Psychiatry

Edited

HELEN SWICK PERRY

With an Introduction by

PRINT
FOR THE

W·W·NORT

1

Contents

▾

Editors' Preface

IN THE preparation of this first book from the unpublished lectures of Harry Stack Sullivan, the initial problem was one of selection from the wealth of material which Sullivan left. The most detailed statements of his later conceptual framework are found in five series of unpublished lectures which he gave in the Washington School of Psychiatry, and the William Alanson White Institute of Psychiatry, Psychoanalysis, and Psychology, in New York; the sixth series was terminated by his death in 1949. Fortunately, these lectures were recorded, and he also left behind two Notebooks outlining them, the first prepared in 1944–1945, and a revision dated 1946–1947. At the suggestion of David Mc Kenzie Rioch, M.D., a friend and colleague of Sullivan's, the present book has been limited mainly to a series of lectures which Sullivan gave in the Washington School of Psychiatry in the winter of 1946–1947, since this series represents the last complete statement which Sullivan made of his conceptions of psychiatry.

Sullivan's conceptions were not static; his lectures changed from year to year as his own ideas and formulations unfolded and developed. Yet each series which he gave presented a carefully organized approach to psychiatry via the developmental route—that is, he traced from earliest infancy to adulthood the development of the person, from this study arriving at certain conclusions as to mental disorder in later life. Thus, while the general framework of his thinking remained the same, in each series certain ideas were discarded and certain new ideas were woven in, often intricately. It is for this reason that it has seemed desirable to use his last complete statement as the basis for this book.

A few exceptions have been made, however. We have found it possible, mainly through the use of bracketed footnotes, to incorporate most of the new material which appeared in the unfinished lecture series which he began in 1948. In addition, we have occasionally relied on lectures from earlier years to clarify obscure passages or to enrich sections where the limitations of lecture time had obliged him to refer only hurriedly to ideas which he had elsewhere discussed in detail. We have also had to rely on earlier series to supply a few sections which were lacking because of mechanical failures of recording equipment. But in all such incorporations from other series, we have been guided by the outline in his last Notebook, since we did not wish to include formulations which he had, by 1946–1947, revised or abandoned, nor did we wish to change the emphasis of his own plan of presentation. All major incorporations of this kind are indicated in footnotes.

There is some difference in style between the earlier and later parts of the book. The chapters which deal with infancy represent, not primarily observations on the human infant, but hypotheses as to what must have occurred in the life of every person during these early months, in view of the given psychobiological equipment of the infant, the order of maturation of abilities, the inevitable impact of the culture, and the data of later life. For these lectures, in which he was often presenting inference rather than observation, Sullivan made full and careful notes, precisely wording many of the postulates which he wished to present; in lecturing, he often read from his Notebook, expanding and explaining it. But in the later lectures, when he was dealing with material that could be supported by observation and might be within the recall of his hearers, he spoke extemporaneously, from only outlined notes. Thus much of the material in the earlier chapters reflects Sullivan's writing style, which was at times complex; in the later lectures, Sullivan spoke in a more easy and colloquial vein. In editing the book, we have avoided any change of those statements which have been fully worded by Sullivan in writing. We have, however, had to do more stringent editing and reorganization in those places where Sullivan spoke extemporaneously, for the meaning and emphasis of his spoken statements did not always carry over in written form.

Many students have commented on the importance of Sullivan's Notebooks. In this series of lectures, Sullivan included, usually in the same wording, most of the statements which appear in his last Notebook. Where a formulation in this Notebook did not appear in the corresponding lecture, we have usually included it at the appropriate place, provided its omission seemed not to have been intentional. The titles of the Parts and Chapters of this book also conform, with very few changes, to Sullivan's Notebook headings. His use of quotation marks has not usually been changed in passages taken from his Notebook; his use of single quotation marks, to indicate special fringes of meaning which he attached to certain words or phrases, is particularly characteristic of all his writings.

One omission has been made in preparing this book: Sullivan devoted three lectures, following Part II, to a discussion of the work of the psychiatrist—in particular, the psychiatric interview. Since these overlap a separate lecture series on this specific topic, which will be published in another book, they have been omitted here.

The preparation of this book has represented collaboration in what Sullivan would have called the syntaxic mode, for many people have contributed generously of their time, money, and thought. The Sullivan papers were turned over to the Foundation, in which Sullivan worked and which is made up of his students and colleagues, by James I. Sullivan, who has been unfailingly helpful in the project of assembling the papers for publication. In order to finance the initial phases of the work of cataloguing and editing the papers, a $15,000 fund was set up by ninety-three of Sullivan's students and colleagues. Without this very practical demonstration, by those who knew Sullivan's work best, of their interest in seeing that it reached a wider audience, this book could not have been published.

In the editing of this book, Mabel Blake Cohen, M.D., has acted as psychiatric consultant, and she has been our chief adviser at all stages of the work. All of the members of the Committee on Publication of Sullivan's Writings have read the manuscript, approved its content, and offered criticisms.

At the time the Foundation came into possession of the Sullivan papers, it was Patrick Mullahy and Otto Allen Will, Jr., M.D., who first read through much of the material and impressed the Foundation with its richness and the importance of publishing it. And Mr. Mullahy has also read the final manuscript of this book and made many splendid suggestions regarding it. Many other students and colleagues of Sullivan's helped in the initial planning for the publication of the papers and contributed encouragement and momentum, notably Alfred H. Stanton, M.D. In the days when Sullivan was still lecturing, Mary Julian White, M.D., personally supervised the recording and transcribing of the lecture series on which this book is based; because of her planning, this is one of the finest and most complete sets of lectures available to the Foundation.

Among those who have read all or part of this book and made excellent suggestions are Robert A. Cohen, M.D., Philip A. Holman, and Stewart E. Perry. And finally, we are profoundly grateful to Katherine Barnard, Editor for Norton, who skillfully added the finishing touches to the book.

Grateful acknowledgment is made for permission to quote from the following published works: To the American Psychological Association for P. W. Bridgman's "Some General Principles of Operational Analysis" (*Psychological Review*, 1945, 52:246–249). To Beacon House, Inc., for Leonard Cottrell and Ruth Gallagher's *Developments in Social Psychology, 1930–1940* (1941). To the Thomas Y. Crowell Company for Seba Eldridge's *The Organization of Life* (1925). To Harcourt, Brace and Company, Inc., for Edward Sapir's *Language: An Introduction to the Study of Speech* (1921). To Hermitage House, Inc., for Patrick Mullahy's *Oedipus: Myth and Complex* (1948). To the Houghton Mifflin Company for Ruth Benedict's *Patterns of Culture* (1934). To the McGraw-Hill Book Company, Inc., for Kurt Lewin's *A Dynamic Theory of Personality* (1935). To Macmillan & Company, Ltd. (London), for Charles Spearman's *The Nature of 'Intelligence' and the Principles of Cognition* (1923). To The Macmillan Company (New York) for Bronislaw Malinowski's "Culture" and T. V. Smith's "Mead, George Herbert" (in the *Encyclopedia of the Social Sciences*). To the University of Illinois Press for Harry Stack Sullivan's "Tensions Interpersonal and International" (in *Tensions That Cause Wars*, edited by Hadley Cantril; 1950).

Helen Swick Perry
Mary Ladd Gawel

Introduction

That the field of theoretical psychiatry is today in a state of healthy flux is due in large part to the impact of Sullivan's thinking. And his thinking was, in no small part, a product of his ability to see the relatedness of the social sciences. His use of an operational approach and field-theory concepts, his recognition that the psychiatrist is not merely an observer but quite specifically a *participant* observer, and his utilization of concepts derived from the anthropologist's analyses of other cultures—all these have introduced a more dynamic character into psychiatric practice and theory. And, conversely, the contributions of Sullivan's thinking to the social psychologist's frame of reference have influenced the latter to alter his concept of "normal" behavior in order to take account of some of the forces and influences from the past which had hitherto been the province only of abnormal behavior.

This book embodies Sullivan's latest conceptions. The most appropriate introduction to it is an attempt to identify and perhaps put somewhat into historical perspective those concepts which represent his most unique and valuable contributions to the field of psychiatry.

Looking back on the development of Sullivan's theories, I find it significant that one of his very early concerns was with the problem of communication. His association with Edward Sapir, an anthropologist primarily interested in linguistics and communication, forwarded and enriched Sullivan's own investigations in this field. His treatment of language, symbols, and communication in the present book is one of the most useful for psychiatrists that I have ever seen. Sullivan's interest gradually broadened from a consideration of communication between two or a few persons to include problems of communication between larger aggregates of people, and thus to include also problems of disturbed behavior in the social scene at large. And the UNESCO Tensions Project bears witness to Sullivan's interest in the application of his theory of personality to problems between nations.

This interest in communication is not a side branch but is basically related to the core of Sullivan's work. This core can be described as the psychiatry of interpersonal relations, or as the study of communication between persons, or as the operational approach to psychiatry in which the psychiatrist plays the role of participant observer. It rests on the propositions that: (1) a large part of mental disorder results from and is perpetuated by inadequate communication, the communicative processes being interfered with by anxiety; and (2) each person in any two-person relationship is involved as a portion of an interpersonal field, rather than as a separate entity, in processes which affect and are affected by the field.

Sullivan has not been alone in his interest in interactional psychiatry and the study of behavior in terms of field theory. He has been very much in step with the times. Modern social science, no less than modern physics, now considers field processes rather than isolating out single and separate units to study. Such scientists as George Mead, John Dewey, Ruth Benedict, Edward Sapir, Leonard Cottrell, Kurt Lewin, and Karen Horney have also been aware of the significance of the cultural setting in influencing personal development, and have recognized that what is studied is a field of interaction.

Sullivan's primary discipline was that of psychiatry rather than that of social psychology, and he has brought a psychiatrist's thinking and clinical experience to bear upon the problems of field psychology. His major work consisted of clinical investigation, which for him was inseparably connected with the therapeutic approach to patients. His broad theoretical structure began to take form only after he had spent almost twenty years in such clinical investigation. Approximately the first ten years of clinical work were spent in the intensive investigation of schizophrenia; his first paper on this subject appeared in 1924, and the publication of numerous other papers on schizophrenia reflected his continuing study. Beginning in 1931, when he entered private practice, he spent approximately ten years in the equally intense investigation of neurotic processes. Toward the end of this period the theoretical structure for which he is now best known began to emerge. At the same time, he began to turn his interest increasingly to the communication of his concepts to others, and the Washington School of Psychiatry began giving instruction under his leadership. In 1938 the journal *Psychiatry* was founded with Sullivan as coeditor, and in 1939 he delivered the series of lectures which were published in the following year as *Conceptions of Modern Psychiatry*. The present book reflects the further elaboration and refinement of his theory after that time.

What school of psychiatric thought does Sullivan belong to? The old controversy as to whether Sullivanian psychiatric theory is or is not psychoanalytic has, in my opinion, no validity. Sullivan was trained in the psychoanalytic school; he developed serious theoretical differences with some of Freud's original hypotheses; he accepted others, which are included in his own formulation, such as concepts of conscious and unconscious processes. In this he has been no different from the other major workers since Freud in the field of theoretical psychiatry (and under that general term I include psychoanalysis). The ongoing development of any science requires the refinement and alteration of old concepts and assumptions in the light of new findings. An unfortunate tendency to cultism, both in certain of Freud's students and in certain of Sullivan's, has created a picture of two watertight, competing theories of personality. A careful examination of Sullivan's work will reveal, first, that he did not interest himself in some of the phenomena that Freud studied, such as infantile sexual behavior or the detailed phenomena of hysterical processes; and, second, that Sullivan has observed and theorized about certain phenomena which were relatively neglected by Freud. The most important of these areas which were relatively neglected by Freud has to do with the particular patterns of interaction which occur between particular people. Sullivan's formulation is in contrast to Freud's earlier one, which located the person in a generalized environment in which he manifests generalized and predetermined biological needs rather than specific patterns of interaction. Thus Sullivanian psychiatry brings to the whole field of psychiatric theory a particular point of view and a set of observations which can be and should be integrated with what was known before, and which then should be used in the true scientific spirit for further development, rather than preserved intact in the spirit of discipleship.

In attempting to delineate some of Sullivan's major contributions to psychiatric theory, one might mention first his formulation of infantile and childhood experience. In order to develop successfully into a predictive science, psychiatry must know what the effects will be of a specific constellation of parental and other forces acting upon the constitutional matrix of a specific child. The dynamic patterns of interaction must be known both specifically and also generally, in terms of types or categories of pattern. Sullivan has contributed to progress in this direction in two main ways. First, he has attempted to conceptualize in a systematic way the nature of experience. Much of what is experienced by the infant prior to the development of language must be inferred, although some direct observations can be made on the child-mother relationship in the early months of life, by trained workers with special opportunities. Sullivan's conclusions are based in part on inference and in part on his clinical observations, especially of schizophrenics, since much of their psychotic experience partakes of the nature of experience in early infancy. Observation of infants such as that done by Margaret Ribble, David Levy, and others has tended to confirm the conclusions arrived at by Sullivan. In Sullivan's conceptualization, experience occurs in three modes, which he has called prototaxic, parataxic, and syntaxic. The lines of demarcation between the modes point up the crucial role of language in human experience: prototaxic refers to experience occurring before symbols are used; parataxic refers to experience characterized by symbols used in a private or autistic way; and syntaxic is used for experience which one person can communicate to another, for it is conceptualized in symbols which are defined alike by each. Each of these modes of experience is discussed and elaborated on in considerable detail in this book.

Sullivan's second important contribution to a theory of child development is the concept of dynamism. He defines dynamisms as "the relatively enduring patterns of energy transformation which recurrently characterize the interpersonal relations . . . which make up the distinctively human sort of being." In this context, pattern is defined as the envelope of insignificant particular differences. Each organism develops a variety of interwoven and overlapping patterns, in relation to the important zones of interaction with the environment (such as the oral and anal zones), and also in relation to the important needs (such as hunger and lust). These dynamisms are developed and patterned from early interpersonal experience and are then carried by the person into his subsequent interpersonal experience.

The interpersonal field, then, is made up of the interaction of a variety of dynamisms of two or more organisms. Some of these dynamisms are *conjunctive* (for example, the need for intimacy) and lead to an integration of a situation, with a resolution or reduction of tension; others, which involve anxiety, are *disjunctive* and lead to disintegration of the situation; sometimes a dynamism can be nonoperative, since there is no corresponding dynamism brought to the situation by the other person. The patterns of interaction are those established in earlier living; and to the extent that anxiety processes have entered into the formation of these patterns, they will be inappropriate and inadequate. One of the dynamisms complicated by anxiety is the "malevolent transformation," in which the need for tenderness has, under the impact of anxiety, been replaced by malevolent behavior. Sullivan has made a number of generalizations which are stated in the form of theorems; to some extent, these have a predictive value. To illustrate: the theorem of tenderness states that "the observed activity of the infant arising from the tension of needs induces tension in the mothering one, which tension is experienced as tenderness and as an impulsion to activities toward the relief of the infant's needs." The use of this type of generalization avoids the pitfalls of instinct theory, yet has the merit of bringing a wide variety of individual responses together into a meaningful category. However, Sullivan has by no means achieved a complete classification and systematization of the dynamic patterns of interaction, and there is no doubt that this point of view, if it proves sufficiently useful, will require expansion.

Much of what has been said so far has included by implication the fact that Sullivan made use of the concept of anxiety as the chief disruptive force in interpersonal relations and the main factor in the development of serious difficulties in living. Anxiety too has been defined operationally. Sullivan has made no attempt to say what anxiety *is*—he describes it in terms of its effects. Certainly it has its origins in the conditions of prolonged and complete human dependency in infancy: the urgency of the biological needs, and the fact that the efforts of a mothering person are necessary for their satisfaction.

"Now, in discussing anxiety, I have come to something that has nothing whatever to do with the physicochemical needs of the living young. The tension called anxiety primarily appertains to the infant's, as also to the mother's, communal existence with a *personal* environment, in utter contradistinction to the physicochemical environment." The need for relief of anxiety is called the need for interpersonal security. The tension called anxiety, in early experience, is differentiated from all other reductions in euphoria by the absence of anything specific, and consequently there is in the infant no capacity for action toward the relief of anxiety. "Therefore, there is, from the very earliest evidence of the empathic linkage, this peculiar distinction that anxiety is not manageable. Anxiety is a tension in opposition to the tensions of needs and to action appropriate to their relief. . . . Of all experience of the present, the experience of anxiety is the sort least clearly interpenetrated by elements of the past and the future; it is the least interpretable and productive of foresight."

The question of the method of communication of anxiety from mother to child has been left largely unanswered by Sullivan. He lumped such communicative experiences under the category of "empathy"; but by empathy he did not mean anything resembling extrasensory perception. He meant rather that the sensory pathways of communication from mother to child are, as yet, uninvestigated, and therefore cannot be adequately described.

A summing up of Sullivan's major contributions to psychiatry would not be complete if one omitted his clinical work itself. It was in the actual treatment of patients that his theory grew, with a constant return to the therapeutic situation for verification and further development. In fact, it is natural for one who knew and worked with Sullivan to think of him primarily as a clinician, since the teaching of the art and science of psychotherapy was one of his greatest skills. In supervising the work of a student psychiatrist, he would, after listening for an hour or so to a student's stumbling report on a patient, have a grasp of the patient as a person which was astonishing and clarifying. To cite but one example of the application of his theory to the practice of psychotherapy: in working with a patient, Sullivan always listened to the data with the question in mind, "Where is the flow of communication being interfered with by the threat of anxiety?" Such a point could be identified by noting where the patient shifted from a presumably significant subject; where the security operations of the patient began to intensify; or where various somatic accompaniments of anxiety began to appear. Having identified such a point of change, a therapist is then in a position to recall, or to inquire about, what was going on just prior to the shift. This technique, when grasped and correctly used, gives a precise and reliable method for identifying and investigating patterns of difficulty in living.

In the present book, the mental disorders per se are touched on but briefly, and principles of therapy only by implication. While later books in this posthumous group of Sullivan's writings will be concerned specifically with these topics, here the main concern is with the developmental approach to the understanding of human personality. However, the three chapters on mental disorders in Part III merit careful consideration, since they present in very condensed fashion many of Sullivan's ideas on the psychoses and on obsessional states. It is hardly necessary to mention that his contribution to the psychopathology and therapy of these conditions was outstanding. In the discussion published here, he has used the central theme of dissociation in presenting the psychoses. Thus, in acute schizophrenia, "not-me" processes are actually present in awareness; other conditions, such as paranoid states, represent a variety of methods for disposing of dissociated systems which have erupted into awareness, and therefore in a sense represent unfortunate outcomes of efforts at reintegration. Sullivan tentatively proposes that the severely obsessional person be thought of as showing evidence of the presence of serious dissociation: "the obsessional substitutions which make up such conspicuous and troublesome aspects of [the lives of severely obsessional people] are simply all-encompassing attenuations of contact which protect them from their abnormal vulnerability to anxiety."

And finally, it should be pointed out that Sullivan's psychiatric theory and his psychotherapeutic techniques were alike predicated on the assumption that human behavior is positively directed toward goals of collaboration and of mutual satisfaction and security, unless interfered with by anxiety. He never ceased to admire the marvelous capacity of the human being, and to use, implicitly or explicitly, as his frame of reference the idea that "we are all much more simply human than otherwise, be we happy and successful, contented and detached, miserable and mentally disordered, or whatever."

Mabel Blake Cohen, M.D.

PART I

Introductory Concepts

CHAPTER
1

The Meaning of the Developmental Approach

AFTER A good many years of effort at teaching psychiatry I have concluded that either certain appraisals of myself as a good teacher are entirely unfounded or the teaching of psychiatry is extremely difficult; and I think quite possibly both are the case. But the fabulous difficulty of teaching psychiatry, as I have seen it over the years, is that it is quite easy to learn certain things—that is, to get so you can talk about them—but it is extremely difficult to get any two people to mean just the same thing when they talk about what they have supposedly learned.

This difficulty is a result of the fact that psychiatry deals with living and that everybody has a great deal of experience in living. But no one lives in anything like the highest style of the art; and it is very disconcerting to notice how badly one lives in the sense of the extent to which fatigue and other discomforts are connected with one's most important dealings with other people. So it is not very easy to develop that type of objectivity about the subject matter of psychiatry which one can acquire about the works of a clock or the principles of physics or even the phenomena of *quantum meruit* in law.

We interpret everything that we hear in this field of psychiatry on a double basis and, unhappily, neither of the bases is very helpful: first, on the basis of what one presumes the data mean in terms of what one knows already, or half-knows; and secondly, on the basis of how this can be interpreted so that it does not increase one's feeling of discomfort and inadequacy in living—one's ***anxiety***, an extremely important term which I shall later define.

Some psychiatrists have had a great deal of training in the area in which psychiatry can perhaps be most easily taught; namely, in the area of describing, as if they were museum pieces, those people who have such great difficulties in living that their situation would be apparent to all. This is the psychiatry of mental disorders; and what one learns about mental disorders by way of descriptive psychiatry is not very meaningful. It does of course provide the psychiatrist with justification for making a living; and he has a feeling of being worth while because he knows a good deal about what these un-understood beings are apt to look like for a long time to come. If the patients manage to change for the better, everybody is so pleased that no one wastes much time condemning the psychiatrist for his mistakes in prognosis.

But the kind of psychiatry I am talking about attempts to *explain* serious mental disorders; and it also is of some use in living in general. How to communicate this particular theory of psychiatry has puzzled and harassed me for a great many years, and I have finally come to the decision that the only approach is by the developmental route. In other words, if we go with almost microscopic care over how everybody comes to be what he is at chronologic adulthood, then perhaps we can learn a good deal of what is highly probable about living and difficulties in living. The success of this kind of teaching has not been impressively great. It has taken the collaborative work of a group of extraordinarily gifted people, including some of my most distinguished colleagues in the Washington and New York areas, to arrive at something of a consensus about one of the central theoretical formulations in the type of psychiatry that I am attempting to teach.

In understanding what I am trying to say you will have to discard the notion that it is something you have known all the time, which just happened to get well formulated or peculiarly formulated by me. We are really up against one of the most difficult of human performances—organizing thought about oneself and others, not on the basis of the unique individual *me* that is perhaps one's most valuable possession, but on the basis of one's common humanity.

Briefly, I shall proceed by examining one hypothesis after another, selecting those which seem to be the best theoretical formulations now available as to how, from birth onward, a very capable animal becomes a person—something very different from an animal; and as to how this transformation of a very gifted animal—who is always there but who cannot be defined because he is constantly being transformed—is brought about, step by step, from very, very early in life, through the influence of other people, and solely for the purpose of living with other people in some sort of social organization.

No matter what kind of social organization there is, everyone who is born into it will, in certain ways, be adapted or adjusted to living in it. If the person is very fortunate, he will be pretty well adapted to living in that social organization. If he is extremely fortunate, he may come to know almost by intuition, you might say—which simply means that it isn't clearly formulated—so much about living itself that he can move into a quite different social organization; and fairly rapidly—but by no means immediately—he may learn to live quite successfully in this new social organization. That sort of transfer is practically out of the question for a great many of the people that psychiatrists see as patients. They are not quite able to live adequately as people in the social organization that they have been trained to live in.

To repeat, no very simple explanation is adequate to communicate some of the instrumentalities that might be useful for improving one's own life and the life of others. The only way that has occurred to me of providing something more useful is by this careful following of that which is possible and probable from birth onward. When psychiatry is approached that way it does not become simple—far from it. Since we have six or seven, or even more, extremely refined channels of contact with events around us, our experience of various combinations of the functions of these channels becomes pretty complicated. And since most of human life is not by any means concerned merely with events in the physicochemical universe, but is concerned also with matters of cultural definition—values, prejudices, beliefs, and so on—the actual complexity of the field becomes mathematically rather overwhelming. The best that I can hope to present are dependable frames of reference as a guide in exploring this complex field, and the conviction that I have had personally for many years, that the great capabilities of the human animal do not fail to make sense when given an adequate chance.

I would like to say—I think with no material fear of extravagance—that I don't believe many psychiatrists have a very good theoretic framework for thinking about difficulties in living, their origin, their dependable manifestations, or their fairly certain improvements. I do not mean to imply that most psychiatrists are not useful to people. But I am stressing the need for a genuinely scientific approach to cope with the rapidly multiplying inefficiencies, inadequacies, misfortunes, and miscarriages of life which come to the attention of the psychiatrist. When I talk about a scientific approach I mean something about as far from empiricism as the mind will go—something precise, something capable of formulation, with a varying range of probability. So far as I know, most of the ways in which one goes about being a human being could be very different from anything we have ever heard of. In other words, the human organism is so extraordinarily adaptive that not only could the most fantastic social rules and regulations be lived up to, if they were properly inculcated in the young, but they would seem very natural and proper ways of life and would be almost beyond study. In other words, before speech is learned, every human being, even those in the lower imbecile class, has learned certain gross patterns of relationship with a parent, or with someone who mothers him. Those gross patterns become the utterly buried but quite firm foundations on which a great deal more is superimposed or built.

Sometimes these foundations are so askew from what I would describe as good foundations for living in a particular society that the subsequent development of the person is markedly twisted from conventional development—that is, from the average in the purely statistical sense, from the way in which most people live. In those circumstances we recognize the results as psychoneuroses or psychoses. But to make anything useful in the way of thought about these psychoneuroses and psychoses and to develop any certainly helpful technique for dealing with these 'warped' people, your thinking has to reach very much further back than the presenting situation. The great difficulty is that in this reach-back you find that a large part of the person's living is not particularly different from yours. And this apparent identity between your living and his living confuses the fact that this living, while outwardly identical, may not be at all identical in meaning to you and to him. And so you cannot ignore those aspects of his living that seem quite natural or normal to you.

In attempting to formulate and teach a theoretic framework for psychiatry over the years it has seemed to me necessary to avoid as far as possible psychiatric neologisms. Of course, every science has to have its technical language. But since this is the study of living and since it has the difficulties which I have already stressed, why add to the certainty of confusion and the Tower-of-Babel phenomena by putting in a lot of trick words? For these trick words, so far as I can discover, merely make one a member of a somewhat esoteric union made up of people who certainly can't talk to anybody outside the union and who only have the illusion that they are talking to one another. Any experiment in the definition of most of the technical terms that have crept into psychiatry shows an extraordinary fringe of difference in meaning. For that reason, I think we should try to pick a word in common usage in talking about living and clarify just what we mean by that word, rather than to set about diligently creating new words by carpentry of Greek and Sanskrit roots.

If I succeed then in communicating my ideas—and to the extent that I succeed—I hope that psychiatrists may derive some benefit in formulating their professional and other dealings with people in rather general terms; such general terms will, I believe, permit further exploration in the direction of getting highly probable statements. There are people who want certainties; they want to be able to distinguish certainly between correct and incorrect propositions. That is a perfectly foredoomed goal in psychiatry. You see, we are not that simple. We have so much spare adjustive equipment that we really live for the most part with only shockingly poor approximations to what might be correct or incorrect.

All of us are afflicted by the fact that long before we can remember, certainly long before we can make brilliant intellectual formulations, we catch on to a good deal which is presented to us, first, by the mothering one and, then, by other people who have to do with keeping us alive through the period of our utter dependence. Before anyone can remember, except under the most extraordinary circumstances, there appears in every human being a capacity to undergo a very unpleasant experience. This experience is utilized by all cultures, by some a little and by some a great deal, in training the human animal to become a person, more or less according to the prescriptions of the particular culture. The unpleasant experience to which I am referring I call anxiety. And here I am making the first of a long series of references to the basic conception of anxiety, which incidentally I have set forth briefly in my paper, "The Meaning of Anxiety in Psychiatry and in Life."[1]

In discussing the concept of anxiety, I am not attempting to give you the last word; it may, within ten years, be demonstrated that this concept is quite inadequate, and a better one will take its place. But this concept of anxiety is absolutely fundamental to your understanding what I shall be trying to lay before you. I want to repeat that, because I don't know that I can depend on words really to convey the importance of what I am trying to say: Insofar as you grasp the concept of anxiety as I shall be struggling to lay it before you, I believe you will be able to follow, with reasonable success, the rest of this system of psychiatry. Insofar as I fail to get across to you the meaning of anxiety, insofar as you presume that I mean just what you now think anxiety is, I shall have failed to communicate my ideas.

Because a great many phenomena in the whole biological field are easier to understand if you trace them from their beginnings to their most complex manifestations, I would like to describe how I think anxiety begins in the infant. I do not know how early in life anxiety first manifests itself. It is not exactly a field that you can get mothers and children to cooperate in exploring. I have no doubt that as a great many other things vary from person to

1 [Harry Stack Sullivan, "The Meaning of Anxiety in Psychiatry and in Life," *Psychiatry* (1948) 11:1–13. Also, see "Towards a Psychiatry of Peoples," *Psychiatry* (1948) 11:105–116. And "The Theory of Anxiety and the Nature of Psychotherapy," *Psychiatry* (1949) 12:3–12.]

person, so the precise data which have to do with being anxious vary from infant to infant. It is demonstrable that the human young in the first months of life—and I think it is true of some other young, but it is very conspicuous in the human young—exhibits disturbed performance when the mothering one has an 'emotional disturbance'—I am using that term quite loosely to mean anything that you think it means. Whatever the infant was doing at the time will be interrupted or handicapped—that is, it will either stop, or it will not progress as efficiently as before anxiety appeared.

Thus anxiety is called out by emotional disturbances of certain types in the significant person—that is, the person with whom the infant is doing something. A classical instance is disturbance of feeding; but all the performances of the infant are equally vulnerable to being arrested or impeded, in direct chronological and otherwise specific relationship to the emotional disturbance of the significant other person. I cannot tell you what anxiety feels like to the infant, but I can make an inference which I believe has very high probability of accuracy—that there is no difference between anxiety and fear so far as the vague mental state of the infant is concerned. Some of you may feel inclined to say, "Well, do infants have fear?" And that, of course, becomes a matter of, "Well what do you mean by fear?" But I would like to point out that if an infant is exposed to a sudden loud noise, he is pretty much upset; certain other experiences of that kind which impinge on his zones of connection with the outside world cause the same kind of upset. Almost anybody watching the infant during these upsets would agree that it didn't seem to be fun; the infant didn't enjoy it. There is no doubt that this—whatever you call it—develops, with no break, into manifestations which we in ourselves call fear, and identify in others as fear. I have reason to suppose, then, that a fearlike state can be induced in an infant under two circumstances: one is by the rather violent disturbance of his zones of contact with circumambient reality; and the other is by certain types of emotional disturbance within the mothering one. From the latter grows the whole exceedingly important structure of anxiety, and performances that can be understood only by reference to the conception of anxiety.

In this connection, I will venture to say that the sort of experience which the infant probably has as primitive anxiety, or primitive fear, reappears much later in life under very special circumstances—perhaps in everyone, but certainly in some people. These circumstances are fairly frequent in the earlier stages of what we call the schizophrenic disorders of living. In quite a number of people, they are not too infrequent in so-called dreams at disturbed times of life, perhaps more specifically in the adolescent era. In these circumstances, anything from a hint to perhaps a fairly full-scale revival of the most primitive type of anxiety arouses *uncanny emotion.*

By uncanny emotion—which is just a trick term, since it hasn't any divine warranties for existing—I refer to an indeterminately large group of feelings of which the most commonly experienced is *awe*. Perhaps some of you have experienced it on first hearing a huge pipe organ. Many people experience great awe on their first glimpse into the Grand Canyon. Everybody has had some experiences of awe. I couldn't begin to name all the different sorts of circumstances in which most people experience awe. The rest of the named uncanny emotions are less well known. I would number them as *dread*—dread in far more than the purely conversational sense—*horror*, and *loathing*. All of these uncanny emotions have a sort of shuddery, not-of-this-earth component which is, I believe, a curious survival from very early emotional experience, all of which can be thus characterized. If you think of an occasion in your own early life when you really experienced one of these uncanny feelings, of which, as I say, awe is much the most common, you will realize that it is as if the world were in some way different. If you try to analyze the experience, you may talk about your skin crawling, or this or that; at any rate, you know that it was very curious. I think any of you who recall an awe-inspiring incident will realize it could easily have been terribly unpleasant. True, many of you, perhaps, have never experienced awe to that extent; awe is certainly the mildest of the uncanny emotions. But if there were a great deal more of such emotion, you would be very far from a going concern as long as you had it. That is the nearest I can come to hinting at what I surmise infants undergo when they are severely anxious.

In attempting to outline this whole system of psychiatry, I want to stress from the very beginning the paralyzing power of anxiety. I believe that it is fairly safe to say that anybody and everybody devotes much of his lifetime, a great deal of his energy—talking loosely—and a good part of his effort in dealing with others, to avoiding more anxiety than he already has and, if possible, to getting rid of this anxiety. Many things which seem to be independent entities, processes, or what not, are seen to be, from the standpoint of the theory of anxiety, various techniques for minimizing or avoiding anxiety in living.

For years and years psychiatrists have been struggling to cure this-and-that distortion of living as it came up in patients. Some of these distortions have proven extraordinarily resistant. I am inclined to say, when I don't feel that too many people are hanging on my words, that some of the cures have probably just been the result of mutual exhaustion. And why has this been so? Well, the present indication is very strongly in the direction of the wrong thing having been tackled. There was nothing particularly wrong with that which was allegedly to be cured. It was a pretty remarkable manifestation of human dexterity in living.

Then what was the trouble? Was it susceptibility, vulnerability to anxiety which called out this alleged symptom? When you begin to look for the anxiety or the vulnerability to anxiety—which from the standpoint of this theory explains the occurrence of the symptoms—then the picture becomes quite different. Much more can be accomplished—much more has been accomplished—from this standpoint.

And here let me say that I would not dare to speak in this way on the basis of my own experience alone. The same things that make psychiatry slippery for others make it slippery for me; it is awfully easy to be deceived. But a much more practical psychotherapy seems to be possible when one seeks to find the basic vulnerabilities to anxiety in interpersonal relations, rather than to deal with symptoms called out by anxiety or to avoid anxiety. I would not state this so positively had it not been tested by a considerable number of my colleagues in their work over the years. Although the results have been quite impressive, this does not mean that psychiatry is getting so easy that we can do it for recreation. I will probably be an utterly forgotten myth long before psychiatry gets to be remotely like an easy job for anyone. But I think that a grasp of the concept of anxiety—and seeing where it fits into the development of a person's living—will save a great deal of psychiatric effort if one is a therapist, and prevent a great many commonplace stupidities if one chooses to use psychiatry in other ways.

CHAPTER
2

Definitions

Psychiatry as Interpersonal Theory

I THINK that there is no other field of scientific endeavor in which the worker's preconceptions are as troublesome as in psychiatry. To illustrate this I will give three definitions of psychiatry. The first and broadest definition would run something like this: Psychiatry is the preoccupation of psychiatrists; it is all that confounding conglomerate of ideas and impressions, of magic, mysticism, and information, of conceits and vagaries, of conceptions and misconceptions, and of empty verbalisms. That is the broadest definition of psychiatry and, so far as I know, a good many people are very far advanced students of that field.

Now there is a second definition which I was moved to make a good many years ago when I was attempting to find out what, if anything, I thought about psychiatry; and this is a polite definition for psychiatry of the prescientific era. This second definition sets up psychiatry as an art, namely, the art of observing and perhaps influencing the course of mental disorders.

The third definition of psychiatry, which is the one relevant here, may be approached by considering it as an expanding science concerned with the kinds of events or processes in which the psychiatrist participates while being an observant psychiatrist. The knowledge which is organized in psychiatry as a science is not derived from anything special about the data with which the psychiatrist deals. It arises not from a special kind of data but from the characteristic actions or operations in which the psychiatrist participates. The actions or operations from which psychiatric information is derived are events in interpersonal fields which include the psychiatrist. The events which contribute information for the development of psychiatry and psychiatric theory are events in which the psychiatrist participates; they are not events that he looks at from atop ivory towers. But of all the actions or operations in which the psychiatrist participates as a psychiatrist, the ones which are scientifically important are those which are accompanied by conceptual schematizations or intelligent formulations which are communicable. These, in turn, are those actions or operations which are relatively precise and explicit—with nothing significant left equivocal or ambiguous.

With the coming of the operational view, at least in the realm of physics, a certain interest has developed in whether there could be an operational approach to the field of psychology. A very interesting symposium, which includes a discussion of operationalism in psychology, is to be found in the *Psychological Review* for September 1945.[1] To this symposium, a very restrained contribution was made by the eminent philosopher and physicist, P. W. Bridgman. "A term," says Bridgman, "is defined when the conditions are stated under which I may use the term and when I may infer from the use of the term by my neighbor that the same conditions prevailed." I have found myself somewhat entertained by this very exact statement. I am going to define terms, you see, but I won't have succeeded, according to Bridgman. All I can certainly do is state what I intend by a term, but long experience has taught me that your intention in using that term may not necessarily be the same. That, if anything, shows how far psychiatry is from being scientific. In a great many of the discourses that I have heard as a psychiatrist, the speaker has not defined his terms, nor have I provided him with any basis for guessing the conditions which covered my use of those terms. Thus when I use some particular word with a rather heavy freight of conditions as to its usability, I hope that you will at least hear me out and see whether you can come to a similar use of that term, so that you will gradually understand

1 ["Symposium on Operationism," *Psychological Review* (1945) 52:241-294. See especially P. W. Bridgman, "Some General Principles of Operational Analysis," pp. 246–249. (By permission of the American Psychological Association.)]

fairly well what I have to say. If you do not pay some attention to the way in which I take a word that you are thoroughly accustomed to and tuck it into a particular meaning—instead of a whole dictionary of meanings—then shortly we will be parting company for quite dissimilar goals.

Let me quote Bridgman further. "Terms used in a scientific context must be subject to the presuppositions of scientific enterprise. One of the most important of these is the possibility of checking or verifying the correctness of any statement . . . [and] for all essential purposes the definition may be specified in terms of the checking operations [by which one determines that this condition is satisfied]." In other words, it is important that the statements which are used can be checked as to their validity, not, needless to say, merely by the person who uses them, but by the person who hears them. Psychiatry as a scientific enterprise should consist of a great body of statements, the correctness of which could be thus checked. It does not come anywhere near that ideal yet. Many statements which will be made in the course of this formulation leave a good deal to be desired when viewed from this precise standpoint formulated by Bridgman. Yet if one is occupied not merely with taking exceptions, with misunderstanding, and so forth, but with studying the actual basis for these statements, it will be found that while many of them do not get past all the requirements of Bridgman's definition, they need but fairly simple operations and inference to come very close to it. In other words, they are not yet satisfactory statements, but they are not awfully far from satisfactory statements; and there are very real difficulties about making entirely satisfactory scientific statements in this particular area. That happens to be the case in practically all statements about, for instance, covert operations; it has to be the case with certain statements regarding the very early stages of personality development. And in these instances you might apply yourself to considering the probable correctness of the inference incorporated in the statement.

The history of this field includes two tributaries which I am inclined to mention at this point in an attempt to set up as precisely as possible the reason for the interpersonal approach. Needless to say, behind all this phase of psychiatry are the discoveries of Sigmund Freud.

The first tributary is the psychobiology of Adolf Meyer. Both the Freudian discoveries and the formulae of Meyer center their attention emphatically on the individual person, as the central unit of study. Some of you may be well acquainted with the system of psychiatry which Adolf Meyer developed and to which he applied the term psychobiology. By this organization of thought, Meyer made, in my opinion, a very important contribution to the understanding of living. Before Meyer's contribution, the grand divisions of knowledge included—in the upper reaches beyond biology—psychology and sociology; and psychology was something which pertained to the mind but with the clear implication that the mind rested on concomitant physiological substrates. So psychology was a purely scientific discipline that studied something that rested on something else.

Psychobiology—and I will abstract the definition, or lack of definition, of the field provided by Meyer—is the study of man as the highest embodiment of mentally integrated life. In other words, it is a more-or-less conscious integration, which makes use of symbols and meanings. This embodiment of mentally integrated life includes the peculiar phenomenon of subject organization by which one is able to think of oneself as if objectively. While certain statements of psychobiology may seem somewhat uncertain, Meyer has stated specifically and succinctly that psychobiology is concerned with the individual human organism as a primary entity. He says that although he likes to speak of persons and groups, the person is the agent of contact. The individual has to do the choosing of his interpersonal material. The person is an object with subject capacity.

In the days when psychobiology was coming into being as a very important member of the hierarchy of knowledge—to my way of thinking a vast improvement on psychology—another discipline was being born called social psychology, which was the second tributary to the interpersonal approach. Under provocation of some very original thinking by Charles H. Cooley, George Herbert Mead, at the University of Chicago, developed a formula of social psychology which included the development of the self—not too far removed from what I discuss as the *self-system*—on the basis of reflected appraisals from others and the learning of roles which one undertook to live or "which live one"—to use a not very closely related statement of Georg Groddeck. The social psychology of Mead was much less vividly and utterly centered on the unique individual person. It showed very clearly that the unique individual person was a complex derivative of many others. It did not quite serve for the purpose of psychiatry as here defined, because there was, you might say, no source of energy presented to account for shifts in roles, the energy expended in playing roles, and so on.

I want to refer now to a very condensed comment on the significant work of Mead in founding social psychology:

> Although Mead's interests were wide and touched fruitfully the history and significance of science, the role of religion, the basis of politics and the claims of metaphysics, his central preoccupation was with the genesis of the self and the nature of mind. Mead took more seriously than most philosophers the task bequeathed to speculative thinkers by Darwin: the elaboration of a purely natural history of the psyche. He early enunciated the thesis . . . that the psychical is a temporary characteristic of the empirical interaction of organism and environment concomitant with the interruption of that interaction.
>
> He thus set for himself the task of explaining the development of this discontinuous characteristic of a continuing process into a functional mind or self. The essentially active nature of the organism furnishes the basis for this achievement. The capacity of the human organism to play the parts of others (inadequately described, he thought, as imitation) is the basic condition of the genesis of the self. In playing the parts of others we react to our playing as well. When the organism comes to respond to its own role assumptions as it responds to others it has become a self. From roles assumed successively and simultaneously there arises gradually a sort of "generalized other," whose role may also be assumed. One's response to this generalized role is his individual self.[2]

Thus one can see a certain very striking convergence of thought in the psychobiology of Meyer and the social psychology of Mead, which is concerned with the evolution of the self.

There is another field which is very powerfully tributary to the

[2] [T. V. Smith, "Mead, George Herbert," *Encyclopaedia of the Social Sciences;* 10:241–242. (By permission of The Macmillan Company.)]

development of this theory, cultural anthropology, which is concerned with the study of the social heritage of man. I should like to refer, in this connection, to Malinowski; the briefest statement of his extremely helpful views appears in the *Encyclopaedia of the Social Sciences*. While I would like to say a good deal on this subject, I shall confine myself to one short quotation from Malinowski:[3] "In every organized activity . . . human beings are bound together by their connection with a definite portion of environment, by their association with a common shelter and by the fact that they carry out certain tasks in common. The concerted character of their behavior is the result of social rules, that is, customs, either sanctioned by explicit measures or working in an apparently automatic way." Among the latter type of customs are moral values, "by which man is driven to definite behavior by inner compulsion," to quote Malinowski again. Without considerable help from the student of cultural anthropology on such massive questions as language, for example, I believe that it is impossible at all readily to pass from the field of psychobiology and social psychology, as defined, to that of psychiatry as here defined.

And finally, I believe that there is also an absolutely necessary convergence of social psychology as the study of interpersonal interaction, and of psychiatry as the study of interpersonal interaction—a tautology which I hope you will forgive me. As a psychiatrist, I had come to feel over the years that there was an acute need for a discipline which was determined to study not the individual human organism or the social heritage, but the interpersonal situations through which persons manifest mental health or mental disorder. Approaching it from another viewpoint, Leonard Cottrell,[4] who has, I think, carried social psychology a long way,

[3] [Bronislaw Malinowski, "Culture," *Encyclopaedia of the Social Sciences;* 4:621–645; p. 622. (By permission of The Macmillan Company.)]

[4] [Leonard Cottrell and Ruth Gallagher, *Developments in Social Psychology, 1930–1940;* New York, Beacon House, Inc., 1941. See also Cottrell, "The Analysis of Situational Fields in Social Psychology," *Amer. Sociological Rev.* (1942) 7:370–387. In the former, Cottrell and Gallagher have this to say on Sullivan's amendment to Mead's work (see pp. 23–24): "In a brilliantly organized theory of personality development, Sullivan attempts to show the influences within a given culture which channelize awareness, the disciplines which actually repress the child's interest in certain objects and activities, and the cultural omissions which serve to blind him to certain meanings by

came to the conclusion that investigations in social psychology had to be made within the frame of reference of interpersonal situations.

In my attempt to outline such a field, I discovered that it seemed to be the field in which the activity—the actions and the operations—of a psychiatrist could be given communicable conceptual schematization, and, therefore, seekable scientific meaning.

It is, I believe, perfectly correct to say with Bridgman ". . . I act in two modes . . . . my public mode . . . and in the private mode, [in which] I feel my inviolable isolation from my fellows. . . ." [8] Psychiatry studies, as I see it, activity in the public mode and also that part of activity in the private mode which is not in any sense inviolably isolated. Let me say that insofar as you are interested in your unique individuality, in contradistinction to the interpersonal activities which you or someone else can observe, to that extent you are interested in the really private mode in which you live—in which I have no interest whatever. The fact is that for any scientific inquiry, in the sense that psychiatry should be, we cannot be concerned with that which is inviolably private. The setting up of the psychiatric field as a study of interpersonal relations is certainly necessary if psychiatry is to be scientific; furthermore, by this simple expedient of so defining psychiatry, we weed out from the serious psychiatric problems a great number of pseudo-problems—which, since they are pseudo-problems, are not susceptible of solution, attempts at their solution being, in

withholding the tools of awareness. These objects of the child's perception, but not his apperception, enter to complicate the patterns of verbal response which he learns along the way. When the discrepancy between his verbal self-other patterns and these 'parataxic' or dissociated elements becomes so great as to cause serious anxiety, we have all the symptoms of a neurosis. . . .

"If we accept Mead's analysis of the way in which meaning emerges from an incorporated verbal structure of rights and duties, Sullivan's work suggests an important amendment. The meaning that is borne by verbal interchange in interpersonal relations can be completely distorted by the dissociated elements which are at work to set the tone and color of the situation. It is impossible to know the intentions of another fully; but it becomes easier to approximate this understanding when you are aware of the subverbal reaction tendencies in your own behavior which you would otherwise unwittingly project on the situation, and when, at the same time, you are aware of the meaning of certain tensions and irrelevant motions which are complicating the verbal response of the other."]

[8] [Work cited.]

fact, only ways of passing a lifetime pleasantly. Let me repeat that psychiatry as a science cannot be concerned with anything which is immutably private; it must be concerned only with the human living which is in, or can be converted into, the public mode.

Thus as psychobiology seeks to study the individual human being, and as cultural anthropology, which has been a powerful tributary to social science, seeks to study the social heritage shown in the concerted behavior of people making up a group, so psychiatry—and its convergent, social psychology—seeks to study the biologically and culturally conditioned, but *sui generis*, interpersonal processes occurring in the interpersonal situations in which the observant psychiatrist does his work.

Man the Animal and Human Experience

Man is born an animal. Man, the animal, is known only as newborn. The processes which convert man, the animal, into something else begin to become effective in a very short time after birth. It is safe to infer that man, the animal, if he continued to exist as such, would be found to be an exceedingly gifted member of the biological series, and especially gifted in the evolution of his central integrative apparatus, which has provided unique capabilities of three sorts: (1) in the interrelation of vision and the prehensile hands—the greatest tools of interrelation other than the mouth; (2) in the interrelation of hearing and the voice-producing apparatus, which is so exquisitely refined as to permit that fantastic evolutionary development, language; and (3) in the interrelation of these and all other receptor-effector systems in an exceedingly complicated forebrain, which permits operating with many kinds of abstracts of experience.

There is abundant evidence that the human animal is not able to look after himself for a long time after birth; and that the abilities that characterize him are matured serially over a term of no less than ten to twenty years. The human animal is utterly dependent at birth and, diminishingly but still greatly, dependent on the tender cooperation of the human environment for five or six years after birth. The human animal is furthermore characterized by a remarkably long period during which various biological capabilities mature in turn.

It is likewise clear that the inborn potentialities which thus mature over a term of years are remarkably labile, subject to relatively durable change by experience, and antithetic to the comparatively stable patterns to which the biological concept of *instinct* applies. The idea of 'human instincts' in anything like the proper rigid meaning of maturing patterns of behavior which are not labile is completely preposterous. Therefore, all discussions of 'human instincts' are apt to be very misleading and very much a block to correct thinking, unless the term *instinct*, modified by the adjective *human*, is so broadened in its meaning that there is no particular sense in using the term at all.

Excluding the outcomes of hereditary or developmental disasters to which the term, idiot, is correctly applied, the individual differences in inborn endowment of human animals are relatively unimportant in comparison with the differences of the human animal from any other species of animal—however spectacular the differences between humans may seem against the background of life histories in any particular culture area. This problem of human differences is basic to a simply delusional interest in personality and the uniqueness of personality; because this is so troublesome, so preoccupying to some otherwise very capable students of so-called human nature, I wish to put plenty of emphasis on whatever individual differences there are. At the same time, I want to warn you that in psychiatry as a study of interpersonal relations, all these individual differences are much less important than are the lack of differences, the similarities in the arts for instance, the parallels in the manifestation of human life wherever it is found.

If we exclude instances of identical twins, we may assume that each human animal is somewhat different from every other one, with respect to matters of organization as a living creature, and with respect to functional activities concerned with living in the biologically necessary environment. I need scarcely remind you of such differences as hair color and texture and its distribution over the body surface; in the color of the iris; in skin pigmentation; in blood group and type; and in size and shape of sundry items such as fingers, nose, and ears. I could go on almost indefinitely on the differences, which may be described as varying from the obvious to the recondite, between one particular biological organization and another.

Rather more impressive for the student of interpersonal relations are the hereditary or at least inborn differences in function of (1) the visual receptor with respect to light frequencies; (2) the hearing receptor with respect to sound frequencies; (3) anatomical differences reflected in the possibilities of sundry dexterities, including speech; and (4) differences in the complex of factors underlying the activities which are measured by the Binet type of 'intelligence tests.'

It is commonly but quite erroneously supposed by those not really informed in the field that man shows a typical response to light waves of frequencies within the so-called visible spectrum. Although it is true, statistically, that one can apply the visual sensitivity or color sensitivity curve of a thousand people to the next hundred thousand, one finds that the color sensitivity of a particular retina, when it is mapped with great care, does not precisely approximate the statistical curve. So there are differences—and for all we know there may be rather notable differences, particularly, for example, in the Chinese. I don't know whether their added kink in the occipital zone does affect vision, but I surmise it does. Most likely it does not affect vision in the area of color sensitivity; yet it may do so even there—we are not too sure.

Besides this, there are great individual differences in response to light intensity—for instance, the particular time when the rods take over in dim illumination—and those differences are particularly impressive in that they vary with the health, nutrition, and other conditions of the person concerned; such variations may be quite significant in certain special circumstances affecting the survival of the person concerned, as, for example, in night flying and even in night driving of an automobile.

These variations in the distance receptor for light are trifling compared with the differences in the auditory receptor for air waves. Here too we have a fairly typical curve of sensitivity arrived at by statistical method and this curve applies to a great many data of individual hearing. Individual variation from these statistical curves is very much greater than is that in the field of color vision. As a matter of fact, hearing is a fairly simple function of age: in most people the curve changes at perhaps an imperceptible velocity up to a certain age; and then there is a more or less steady diminution with time in acuity of hearing. Differences here can be more readily observed so that we know that the heard word is quite notably different for some people than it is for others. Moreover, there are pathological variations, due to early disease and injury, which are much more frequent than is the case in the visual receptor area, and have much more insidious effects on the world as experienced. Dexterity, too, is notoriously variable among different people; we are all aware, for example, of the utility of long fingers if one is to be a pianist, or the handicap of a cleft palate if one wants to be an orator.

But the differences that have been most talked about over the past two decades, sometimes with great enthusiasm, are the remarkable range of intelligence factors, intellectual endowments, and so on, which vary, as you well know, from the low-grade imbecile to the genius, if genius can be considered a function of intelligence; by genius I mean those people who have really outstanding ability to see the relatedness of events, which seems to be the ultimate of the measurable intelligence factors. We all know that it is much easier to explain things to some people than it is to others; and all too many of us are very free in classifying people as to whether they are bright or dull, clever or stupid. Enough of an indeterminately great number of inborn factors have already been discovered to justify one in feeling that one's own animal substrate is certainly uniquely individual. Moreover, we already know something of the durable effects that may arise from defects of interchange with the optimum physicochemical environment, as in the case of the deficiency diseases.

Another field of difference, which is of even more interest to the psychiatrist, is the differences, the presumably inborn differences, in the rate of maturation of one's capabilities. Then there are differences arising from factors of the character of health, accidental injury, and diseases, already indicated in the case of hearing, but needless to say, applying in many other fields.

All these differences which I have so far mentioned are differences in inborn potentialities and individual development histories of human animals as underlying human beings. Now I would like to consider differences in nongenetic factors, elements, circumstances, or influences that determine human career-lines in terms of satisfaction or frustration of needs, and the enhancement or depreciation of self-regard. One of these factors is language. And while I shall not at the moment discuss language as determining differences in human career-lines, I should like to provide some background for later consideration of this by quoting from Edward Sapir's *Language:* •

> [Language is a] purely human and noninstinctive method of communicating ideas, emotions, and desires by means of a system of voluntarily produced symbols . . . [which] are, in the first instance, auditory and . . . produced by the so-called "organs of speech." . . . the essence of language consists in the assigning of conventional, voluntarily articulated, sounds, or of their equivalents, to the diverse elements of experience. . . . The elements of language, the symbols that ticket off experience, must . . . be associated with whole groups, delimited classes, of experience rather than with the single experiences themselves. Only so is communication possible, for the single experience lodges in an individual consciousness and is, strictly speaking, incommunicable. To be communicated it needs to be referred to a class which is tacitly accepted by the community as an identity. . . .
>
> [This field of language includes much more than the basic] cycle of speech, [which] in so far as we may look upon it as a purely external instrument, begins and ends in the realm of sounds. . . . the typical course of this process may undergo endless modifications or transfers into equivalent systems without thereby losing its essential formal characteristics.
>
> The most important of these modifications is the abbreviation of the speech process involved in thinking. This has doubtless many forms . . . . it is well known what excellent use deaf-mutes can make of "reading from the lips" as a subsidiary method of apprehending speech. The most important of all visual speech symbolisms is, of course, that of the written or printed word . . . [in which] each element (letter or written word) in the system corresponds to a specific element (sound or sound-group or spoken word) in the primary system.

There are still more complex transfers, of which Sapir mentions the Morse telegraphic code and the different gesture languages such as those "developed for the use of deaf-mutes, of Trappist monks vowed to perpetual silence, or of communicating parties

• [*Language, An Introduction to the Study of Speech;* New York, Harcourt, Brace and Co., 1921; see pp. 7–23.]

that are within seeing distance of each other but are out of earshot," as, for example, the flag language used in the Signal Corps. Sapir continues:

> There is no more striking general fact about language than its universality . . . . we know of no people that is not possessed of a fully developed language. . . . The fundamental groundwork of language—the development of a clear-cut phonetic system, the specific association of speech elements with concepts, and the delicate provision for the formal expression of all manner of relations—all this meets us rigidly perfected and systematized in every language known to us. . . .
>
> Scarcely less impressive than the universality of speech is its almost incredible diversity. . . . [This universality and diversity of speech force us] to believe that language is an immensely ancient heritage of the human race. . . . It is doubtful if any other cultural asset of man, be it the art of drilling for fire or of chipping stone, may lay claim to a greater age. I am inclined to believe that it antedated even the lowliest developments of material culture, that these developments, in fact, were not strictly possible until language, the tool of significant expression, had itself taken shape.

Here then is a field not biologically given, or the result of accidents to biologically given equipment, but of human transmission. This transmission is from other people and takes place by other than biological genetic processes or by disturbances of the physicochemical transfer which makes up the basic life processes. This is, as Sapir says, a field almost infinitely diversified, and is a symbolic way of referring to all the classes of experience and all the relationships which man under sundry circumstances has come into contact with.

There are also differences which lie in the general field of culture more or less exterior to language, which is perhaps the most important field of culture, but is by no means the exclusive field of culture. I have mentioned the extremely helpful work of Malinowski. I should also like to refer to the work of Ruth Benedict who has this to say about the nature of culture and its place in living:

> . . . The inner workings of our own brains we feel to be uniquely worthy of investigation, but custom, we have a way of thinking, is behaviour at its most commonplace. As a matter of fact, it is the other way around. Traditional custom, taken the world over, is a mass of detailed behaviour more astonishing than what any one person can ever evolve in individual actions, no matter how aberrant. Yet that is

a rather trivial aspect of the matter. The fact of first-rate importance is the predominant rôle that custom plays in experience and in belief, and the very great varieties it may manifest.

No man ever looks at the world with pristine eyes. He sees it edited by a definite set of customs and institutions and ways of thinking. . . . John Dewey has said in all seriousness that the part played by custom in shaping the behaviour of the individual as over against any way in which he can affect traditional custom, is as the proportion of the total vocabulary of his mother tongue over against those words of his own baby talk that are taken up into the vernacular of his family. . . . The life history of the individual is first and foremost an accommodation to the patterns and standards traditionally handed down in his community. From the moment of his birth the customs into which he is born shape his experience and behaviour. By the time he can talk, he is the little creature of his culture, and by the time he is grown and able to take part in its activities, its habits are his habits, its beliefs his beliefs, its impossibilities his impossibilities. Every child that is born into his group will share them with him, and no child born into one on the opposite side of the globe can ever achieve the thousandth part. There is no social problem it is more incumbent upon us to understand than this of the rôle of custom. Until we are intelligent as to its laws and varieties, the main complicating facts of human life must remain unintelligible.[7]

From my discussion of all these varied factors of human difference, one might think, at first glance, that these differences should be the subject of our study. We will attempt, however, to study human similarities. And we will not study people as such, but what they do, and what can be fairly safely inferred as to why they do it.

One of the most inclusive biological and psychobiological terms with which we have already had several contacts is *experience*, for which I shall offer the following defining statement:

Experience is anything lived, undergone, or the like. Experience is the inner component of events in which a living organism participates as such—that is, as an organized entity. The limiting characteristics of experience depend on the kind of organism, as well as on the kind of event experienced.

Experience is not the same as the event in which the organism

[7] [Ruth Benedict, *Patterns of Culture;* Boston: Houghton Mifflin Co., 1934; pp. 2–3.]

participates; when I look at and see a frog, my experience of the frog—my perception of the frog—is not the frog. The frog, if he is a 'real' frog—which is by no means necessary—has reflected a particular pattern of light which then existed; my eyes have undergone the impinging of this particular pattern of light; sundry different 'internal changes' have ensued, including the identification of the 'inner' data with the concept, frog.

In other words, there is a relatively 'outer' object, giving rise to something which 'puts me in contact with' it, as we say; and there is a very complex, relatively private or 'inner' bundle of changes of state here or there, to which I may refer as the act of perceiving, which results in the *percept.* Nothing in the present state of our acquaintance with the universe suggests any necessary correspondence between the perceived characteristics of a course of events like the frog as frog and the ultimate 'real' characteristics of this course of events.

Failure to take into account the interpolated act of perception leads to a multiplicity of pseudo-facts and pseudo-problems, as witness the fact that even a competent philosopher—I think it was Charles Morris—in setting up a theory of signs, comments on the fact that we wink, close the eye, before an approaching object strikes the cornea. This is quite typical of a wide variety of approximations in common speech—however allegedly scientific this common speech is—which literally mislead one quite gravely. Actually, of course, a pattern of reduced illumination, moving in a certain fashion which has already been interpreted by previous experience, touches the cornea.

Charles Spearman used the word *sentience* to refer to the primary data out of which we come to have information.[8] I should

[8] [*Editors' note:* See, for instance, Charles Spearman's discussion of sentience and experience in *The Nature of 'Intelligence' and the Principles of Cognition* (London: Macmillan and Co., 1923; in particular, pp. 36–47): ". . . All knowing inevitably begins with sensory experience. . . . Between the material thing and the perceptual experience there has intervened a long, complicated, and often loosely linked chain of events that are extremely unlike either the conscious percept at their near end or the material thing disappearing at the far end. . . . Percepts, by the time they have become amenable to ordinary introspection, are already far removed from what is here mainly at issue, namely, the *initial* effect of sensory stimulation upon consciousness; they have already behind them an eventful history, not only

like to offer here a theory of sentience and any other primary data of experience—and of the phenomenology of memory—as being the totality of significant states of the organism related to the impinging of events.

In my example about the frog, I have tried to emphasize the importance of the act of perceiving, which is interpolated between whatever outside reality is and what we have in our minds. What we have in our minds begins in experience, and experience for the purpose of this theory is held to occur in three modes which I shall set up, one of which is usually, but by no means certainly, restricted to human beings. These modes are: the *prototaxic*, the *parataxic*, and the *syntaxic*.[9] I shall offer the thesis that these modes

on previous occasions in the person's life, but even on *the very occasion itself*. . . . The initial (and for the most part unintrospectable) mental effect of sensory stimulation will be taken by us to be indeed sensation in the strict meaning of a state . . . . for which, perhaps, 'sentience' is a better term. . . ."]

[9] [*Editors' note:* We are indebted to Patrick Mullahy for permission to quote his definition of Sullivan's three modes of experience (Patrick Mullahy, *Oedipus, Myth and Complex;* New York: Hermitage Press, Inc., 1948; pp. 286–291):

"All experience occurs in one or more of three 'modes'—the prototaxic, parataxic, and syntaxic. As the Greek roots of this horrendous term indicate, the *prototaxic mode* refers to the first kind of experience the infant has and the order or arrangement in which it occurs. . . . According to Sullivan's hypothesis all that the infant 'knows' are momentary states, the distinction of before and after being a later acquirement. The infant vaguely feels or 'prehends' earlier and later states without realizing any serial connection between them. . . He has no awareness of himself as an entity separate from the rest of the world. In other words, his felt experience is all of a piece, undifferentiated, without definite limits. It is as if his experiences were 'cosmic.' . . .

"As the infant develops and maturation proceeds, the original undifferentiated wholeness of experience is broken. However, the 'parts,' the diverse aspects, the various kinds of experience are not related or connected in a logical fashion. They 'just happen' together, or they do not, depending on circumstances. In other words, various experiences are felt as concomitant, not recognized as connected in an orderly way. The child cannot yet relate them to one another or make logical distinctions among them. What is experienced is assumed to be the 'natural' way of such occurrences, without reflection and comparison. Since no connections or relations are established, there is no logical movement of 'thought' from one idea to the next. The *parataxic mode* is not a step by step process. Experience is undergone as momentary, unconnected states of being.

". . . The child gradually learns the 'consensually validated' meaning of

are primarily matters of 'inner' elaboration of events. The mode which is easiest to discuss is relatively uncommon—experience in the syntaxic mode; the one about which something can be known, but which is somewhat harder to discuss, is experience in the parataxic mode; and the one which is ordinarily incapable of any formulation, and therefore of any discussion, is experience in the prototaxic or primitive mode. The difference in these modes lies in the extent and the character of the elaboration that one's contact with events has undergone.

The prototaxic mode, which seems to be the rough basis of memory, is the crudest—shall I say—the simplest, the earliest, and possibly the most abundant mode of experience. Sentience, in the experimental sense, presumably relates to much of what I mean by the prototaxic mode. The prototaxic, at least in the very early months of life, may be regarded as the discrete series of momentary states of the sensitive organism, with special reference to the zones of interaction with the environment. By the term, sensitive, I attempt to bring into your conception all those channels for being aware of significant events—from the tactile organs in, say, my buttocks, which are apprising me that this is a chair and I have sat on it about long enough, to all sorts of internunciatory sensitivities which have been developed in meeting my needs in the process of living. It is as if everything that is sensitive and centrally represented were an indefinite, but very greatly abundant, luminous switchboard; and the pattern of light which would show on that switchboard in any discrete experience is the basic prototaxic experience itself, if you follow me. This hint may suggest to you that I presume from the beginning until the end of life we undergo a succession of discrete patterns of the momentary state of the organism, which implies not that other organisms are impinging on it, but certainly that the events of other organisms are moving toward or actually effecting a change in this momentary state.

The full implication of these and many other terms cannot

---

language—in the widest sense of language. These meanings have been acquired from group activities, interpersonal activities, social experience. Consensually validated symbol activity involves an appeal to principles which are accepted as true by the hearer. And when this happens, the youngster has acquired or learned the *syntaxic mode* of experience."]

appear until I have sketched a series of phases gone through by the newborn human being—in my language, a potentially mature person. I shall therefore shortly begin to trace the developmental history of personality, which, as you will see, is actually the developmental history of possibilities of interpersonal relations.

CHAPTER 3

Postulates

Three Principles Borrowed from Biology

I WANT at this point to mention three principles which are a part of my logical philosophy or theory and are woven into my system of thought. These three principles, which I have borrowed from the biology of Seba Eldridge,[1] are the principle of communal existence, the principle of functional activity, and the principle of organization. It is by dealing with applications of these principles that all basic phenomenology of life can, at the biological level, be thrown into meaningful reference. The principle of communal existence refers to the fact that the living cannot live when separated from what may be described as their necessary environment. While this is not as vividly apparent at some of the higher levels of life as it is at the lowest, because storage capacities somewhat disguise the utter dependence on interchange in the higher organisms, the fact is that the living maintain constant exchange through their bordering membranes with certain elements in the physicochemical universe around them; and the interruption of this exchange is tantamount to death of the organism. Thus by the principle of communal existence I mean that all organisms live in continuous, communal existence with their necessary environment. I will not develop the principle of organization, since it scarcely needs any particular emphasis; and the principle of func-

[1] The first time that I encountered these principles succinctly stated was in a book by Eldridge entitled *The Organization of Life* [New York: Thomas Y. Crowell Company, 1925], and it is from this source that I have borrowed them. Although this book sets up some excellent general considerations, it goes on to more or less vitalize a particular doctrine of life which at least is not popular at this time.

tional activity is, of course, the most general term for the processes which literally make up living.[2]

From a consideration of these three principles, it is possible to think of man as distinguished from plants and animals by the fact that human life—in a very real and not only a purely literary or imaginary sense—requires interchange with an environment which includes culture. When I say that man is distinguished very conspicuously from other members of the biological universe by requiring interchange with a universe of culture, this means, in actual fact, since culture is an abstraction pertaining to people, that man requires interpersonal relationships, or interchange with others. While there are apparent exceptions, which I shall later mention, it is a rare person who can cut himself off from mediate and immediate relations with others for long spaces of time without undergoing a deterioration in personality. In other words, being thus cut off is perhaps not as fatal as for an animal to be cut off from all sources of oxygen; but the lethal aspect of it is nonetheless well within the realm of correct referential speech, and is not merely a figure of speech or an allegory.

The One-Genus Postulate

I now want to present what I used to call the one-genus hypothesis, or postulate. This hypothesis I word as follows: We shall assume that *everyone is much more simply human than otherwise*, and that anomalous interpersonal situations, insofar as they do not arise from differences in language or custom, are a function

[2] [*Editors' note:* The other two principles were described by Eldridge as follows: "At every stage of the interaction between organism and environment . . . a complicated set of responses comes into play. . . . These processes of interaction between the organism and the environment, including the interactions between component parts of the organism and *their* environments, constitute what is termed functional, or physiological, activity. . . . A third property of the organism is that of organization itself. The term connotes not only the structure of the organism statically regarded, but the variability of this structure, both in the individual and in the race. . . . This property might also be conceived as the organization, in matter, of the physiological processes, together with the tendency of this organization to vary. Or, to vary our terms again, it is the morphological property in vital activity, the property which has manifested itself in countless forms of life in the past, and is destined to take countless other forms in the future" (p. 2).]

of differences in relative maturity of the persons concerned. In other words, the differences between any two instances of human personality—from the lowest-grade imbecile to the highest-grade genius—are much less striking than the differences between the least-gifted human being and a member of the nearest other biological genus. Man—however undistinguished biologically—as long as he is entitled to the term, human personality, will be very much more like every other instance of human personality than he is like anything else in the world. As I have tried to hint before, it is to some extent on this basis that I have become occupied with the science, not of individual differences, but of human identities, or parallels, one might say. In other words, I try to study the degrees and patterns of things which I assume to be ubiquitously human.

Heuristic Stages in Development

I would like at this point to set up a heuristic classification of personality development which is very convenient for the organization of thought. These heuristic stages are: infancy, childhood, the juvenile era, preadolescence, early adolescence, late adolescence, and adulthood or maturity.

Infancy extends from a few minutes after birth to the appearance of articulate speech, however uncommunicative or meaningless. *Childhood* extends from the appearance of the ability to utter articulate sounds of or pertaining to speech, to the appearance of the need for playmates—that is, companions, cooperative beings of approximately one's own status in all sorts of respects. This ushers in the *juvenile era*, which extends through most of the grammar-school years to the eruption, due to maturation, of a need for an intimate relation with another person of comparable status. This, in turn, ushers in the era that we call *preadolescence*, an exceedingly important but chronologically rather brief period that ordinarily ends with the eruption of genital sexuality and puberty, but psychologically or psychiatrically ends with the movement of strong interest from a person of one's own sex to a person of the other sex. These phenomena mark the beginning of *adolescence*, which in this culture (it varies, however, from culture to culture) continues until one has patterned some type of performance which satisfies one's lust, one's genital drives. Such patterning ushers in *late adolescence*, which in turn continues as an era of personality until any partially developed aspects of personality fall into their proper relationship to their time partition; and one is able, at *adulthood*, to establish relationships of love for some other person, in which relationship the other person is as significant, or nearly as significant, as one's self. This really highly developed intimacy with another is not the principal business of life, but is, perhaps, the principal source of satisfactions in life; and one goes on developing in depth of interest or in scope of interest, or in both depth and scope, from that time until unhappy retrogressive changes in the organism lead to old age.[8]

I shall try to outline my theory by exhausting the easily conceivable possibilities of each of these stages of development, showing the beginnings of things wherever they are either observable or fairly safely inferable, beginning at birth and moving toward at least chronological adulthood.

Euphoria and Tension

In our thinking we need, besides biological or human postulates, certain concepts that are borrowed from other fields of human activity, including a few from the field of mathematics. The one I particularly want to mention at this time is the idea of limits, and the notion of the absolute. I use absolute constructs every now and then in thinking about interpersonal relations. That is, I attempt to define something I know does not exist by extrapolation from extreme instances of something that does exist. These ideal constructs or polar constructs are useful for clear discussion of phenomena which fall more or less near one of these polar absolutes.

The two absolutes that I want to present at the moment are absolute *euphoria* and absolute *tension*. Absolute euphoria can be defined as a state of utter well-being. The nearest approach to anything like it that there is any reason for believing one can observe might occur when a very young infant is in a state of deep sleep.

[8] [*Editors' note:* The definitions of these heuristic stages have been incorporated here from another of Sullivan's lectures, given in 1945, on *The Psychiatric Interview.*]

Absolute tension might be defined as the maximum possible deviation from absolute euphoria. The nearest approach to absolute tension that one observes is the rather uncommon, and always relatively transient, state of terror.

Now, it is a peculiarity of life that the level of euphoria and the level of tension are in reciprocal relation; that is, the level of euphoria varies inversely with the level of tension. And now I am going to make—partly, I suppose, for my own amusement—a frank and wholehearted reference to mathematics. This reciprocal relation may be expressed by saying that y is a function of x, and the relationship is $y = 1/x$.

Those of you who remember the conversion of the mathematical formula $y = 1/x$ into numerical representation will perhaps recall that y has a boundless limit when x equals zero and that, however much the value of x is increased, y never reaches zero. That is, the limits—zero for the one and infinity for the other—are never actually observed. This is just another way of saying that absolute euphoria and absolute tension are constructs which are useful in thought but which do not occur in nature. These absolutes are approached at times, but almost all of living is perhaps rather near the middle of the trail; that is, there is some tension, and to that extent the level of euphoria is not as high as it could be.

While euphoria need not trouble us very much, tensions are a very important part of our thinking.[4] On this matter of tensions, I should like to include here an excerpt from an article of mine:

In any discussion about personality considered as an entity, we must use the term *experience*. Whatever else may be said about experience, it is in final analysis experience of *tensions* and experience of *energy transformations*. I use these two terms in exactly the same sense as I would in talking about physics; there is no need to add adjectives such

[4] I would refer anyone who is deeply interested in the philosophical justification of the concept of tension to a paper by Albert Dunham ["The Concept of Tension in Philosophy," *Psychiatry* (1938) 1:79–120], in which he discusses the philosophy of the concept of tension, and also to the works of Kurt Lewin, who set up the earliest, I think, systematic treatment of the concept of tension in explaining human behavior. [See Kurt Lewin, *A Dynamic Theory of Personality*, translated by Donald K. Adams and Karl E. Zener; New York: McGraw-Hill, 1935.] However, Kurt Lewin's conceptions are by no means identical with those that I am about to unwind.

as 'mental'—however 'mental' experience itself may be conceived to be.

In the realm of personality and culture, tensions may be considered to have two important aspects: that of tension as a potentiality for action, for the transformation of energy; and that of a *felt* or wittingly noted state of being. The former is intrinsic; the latter is not. In other words, tension *is* potentiality for action, and tension *may* have a felt or representational component. There is no reason for doubting that this contingent rather than intrinsic factor is a function of experience rather than of tension *per se*, for it applies in the same way to energy transformations. They, too, *may* have felt or representational components, or transpire without any witting awareness.[5]

EXPERIENCE is of { tensions / energy transformations }

occurs in 3 modes { prototaxic / parataxic / syntaxic }

TENSIONS are those of { needs { general / zonal } / anxiety }

ENERGY TRANSFORMATIONS are { overt / covert }

Yet the undergoing of tensions and of energy transformations, however free the events may have been from any representative component, is never exterior to the sum total of *living* and in many instances not beyond the possibility of some kind of *recall*—indication as of the dynamically surviving, actual past, with detectable influence on the character of the foreseen and dynamically significant neighboring future.[6]

[5] When I mention felt components of tension or energy transformation, I am talking about experience in the later two modes—the parataxic and the syntaxic—because, as I have insisted repeatedly, it is practically impossible to get anything into consciousness for discussion about experience in the prototaxic mode; for all I know, when a tension exists in a person and is wholly unnoted, that may merely mean that it is felt in the prototaxic mode. But this doesn't make very much difference because there is no way of demonstrating that it is so; it is purely for theoretical perfectionism, if you please, that I bring this to your attention.

[6] [Statement by Sullivan, in *Culture and Personality*, edited by S. Stansfeld Sargent and Marian W. Smith (Proceedings of an Interdisciplinary Conference held under auspices of The Viking Fund, Nov. 7 and 8, 1947); New York: The Viking Fund, Inc., 1947.]

Returning now to my account of the development of the human animal in becoming a person, I have suggested that euphoria may be equated to a total equilibrium of the organism, which we know never exists, but which is approached in those time intervals or instants when tension is at its minimum. In the very young infant these intervals occur when the breathing cycle has started on its lifelong course; when there is no deficiency of body temperature, of water supply, and of food supply (in the stomach usually); and when no noxious events are impinging on the so-called periphery of what will later be called awareness.

The Tension of Needs

The tensions that episodically or recurrently lower the level of the infant's euphoria and effect the biologic disequilibration of his being are *needs* primarily appertaining to his communal existence with the physicochemical universe. Now very early in life we need assume nothing except a communal existence with the physicochemical universe; but when we make that assumption we must be very clear in realizing that the infant is not himself adequately equipped to maintain that absolutely necessary communal existence. There has to be a mothering one; while I know no inherent difficulty about this being a wolf or an ape, as the historic myths have it, the brute fact is that we have no authentic or verifiable account of anyone who has been raised by wolves, apes, or the like —if we did have, we might know a little more about the human animal.

The relaxations of these episodic or recurrent tensions which disturb the equilibrium of the infant's being are, of course, equilibrations with specific respect to the source of disequilibrium, whether it be lack of oxygen, lack of sugar, lack of water, or lack of adequate body temperature. And the relaxation of the tensions called out by lacks of this kind I call *satisfaction* of the specific need which was concerned.

I will mention at this time—and the immediate relevance of this will gradually appear—that satisfactions can be defined by noting the biological disequilibration which actions, that is, energy transformations, of the infant have served to remedy. In other words, a need, while it is in a broad biological sense disequilibrium, acquires its meaning from the actions or energy transformations which result in its satisfaction.

When I speak of the actions or energy transformations of the infant which serve to remedy biological disequilibration or to satisfy needs, it may be fairly easy to see how the infant's breathing movements serve to remedy his oxygen needs and how sucking movements serve to remedy his sugar and water needs. It may not be quite so evident how any activity of the infant serves his need for maintaining body temperature, for example. But those who have dealt with newborn infants know that they are quite audible, once they are going concerns, if they are not covered with insulating material that reduces heat loss. The outcry is the initial action of the infant which is directed toward the remedy of the need for reduced heat loss; and the reduction of the heat loss, the experience of adequate internal temperature, is a satisfaction of that need.

The alternation of need and satisfaction gives rise to experience or, if you will, *is* experience—needless to say, in the prototaxic mode. The need—that is, the felt discomfort of the disequilibrium, the specific tensional reduction in euphoria—begins to be differentiated in terms of the direction toward its relief, which amounts to increasingly clear foresight of relief by appropriate action. It need scarcely be said that this foresight is the experience of the neighboring future—and this experience, too, must occur in the prototaxic mode in very early infancy, because there is no other basis for experience. What I am saying in essence is that the first successful activity of an infant—such as breathing to relieve anoxia—begins to define the nature of the need for oxygen, which, before that, is undifferentiated, and also begins to define the nature of extreme tension, or almost complete absence of euphoria. Thus beginning with the first activities of the infant, the first transformations of energy that are associated with the diminution of need and its ultimate extinction for the time being, the personality develops what is later clearly identifiable as the foresight function. A great many truths, which will gradually appear, are wrapped up in that statement, but the one that I wish to note now is that this does imply something of the neighboring future.

By and large any experience that can be discussed—that is, any experience in the syntaxic or parataxic mode—is always interpenetrated by elements of the near past, sometimes even the distant past, and by elements of the near future—anticipation, expectation, and so on. These elements are powerfully influential in determining the way that tensions are transformed into activity—that is, the way in which potentiality in the tension becomes action.

The comparatively great influence of foresight is one of the striking characteristics of human living in contrast to all other living. The whole philosophical doctrine of representation might, if one wished, be wrapped up in this statement that successful action creates or is identified with—I might use any number of vague words that don't quite convey what I mean here—foreseen relief.

I want to quote next a section by Kurt Lewin on environmental structure and needs:

> The life-space of the infant is extremely small and undifferentiated. This is just as true of its perceptual as of its effective space. With the gradual extension and differentiation of the child's life-space, a larger environment and essentially different facts acquire psychological existence, and this is true also with respect to dynamic factors. The child learns in increasing degree to control the environment. At the same time—and no less important—it becomes psychologically dependent upon a growing circle of environmental events. . . . For the investigation of dynamic problems we are forced to start from the psychologically real environment of the child. In the "objective" sense, the existence of a social bond is a necessary condition of the viability of an infant not yet able itself to satisfy its biologically important needs. This is usually a social bond with the mother in which, functionally, the needs of the baby have primacy.[1]

From recasting similar considerations concerning the relationship of the very young human and the necessary environment, it becomes possible to draw out a general principle which I used to call a theorem. This principle or theorem is designed to be an especially compact and meaningful way of expressing one of the basic derivatives from this approach.

My theorem is this: *The observed activity of the infant arising from the tension of needs induces tension in the mothering one, which tension is experienced as tenderness and as an impulsion to activities toward the relief of the infant's needs.* In other words,

[1] [Work cited; pp. 74–75.]

however manifest the increasing tension of needs in an infant may be—and we will study a very important manifestation of that tension in the energy transformations of the cry—the observation of these tensions or of the activity which manifests their presence calls out, in the mothering one, a certain tension, which may be described as that of tenderness, which is a potentiality for or an impulsion to activities suited to—or more or less suited to—the relief of the infant's needs. This, in its way, is a definition of tenderness—a very important conception, very different indeed from the miscellaneous and, in general, meaningless term 'love,' which confuses so many issues in our current day and age.

The manifest activity by the mothering one toward the relief of the infant's needs will presently be experienced by the infant as the undergoing of tender behavior; and these needs, the relaxation of which require cooperation of another, thereon take on the character of a general *need for tenderness.*

To sum up: The tension called out in the mothering one by the manifest needs of the infant we call *tenderness*, and a generic group of tensions in the infant, the relief of which requires cooperation by the person who acts in the mothering role, can be called *need for tenderness.* As I have said, I regard the first needs that fall into the genus of the need for tenderness as needs arising in the necessary communal existence of the infant and the physicochemical universe.[8]

Even though the needs which I include when I speak of the generic need for tenderness are direct derivatives of disequilibrium arising in the physicochemical universe inside and outside the infant—that is, making up the infant and the necessary environment—nonetheless these generic needs all require cooperation from another; thus, the need for tenderness is ingrained from the very beginning of things as an interpersonal need. And the complemen-

[8] The only nonphysicochemically induced need that is probably somewhere near demonstrable during very early infancy and which certainly becomes very conspicuous not much later than this, is the *need for contact*, by which I mean just about what the word ordinarily means. The very young seem to have very genuine beginnings of purely human or interpersonal needs in the sense of requiring manipulations by and peripheral contact with the living, such as lying-against, and so on. But, when I talk as I do now of the first weeks and months of infancy, this can only be a speculation which need keep no one awake nights worrying over whether it is justified.

tary need of the mothering one is a need to manifest appropriate activity, which may be called a general need to give tenderness, or to behave tenderly; and this, whatever tensions and energy transformations may be mixed up in it, is again interpersonal in kind, if not in all details.

So far I am saying—in what may seem a very complicated way—that because the infant is practically absolutely dependent on the intervention of others, or a particular other, for survival and for the maintenance of the necessary interchange, the mother behaves tenderly and helps in the relieving of sundry recurrent disequilibria. There is a reason for the complexity of the explanation, if only to emphasize that this is not merely a business of the nourishing of the young as if by a good incubator.

The Tension of Anxiety

But now I pass to another broadly important statement, where there is much less chance for confusion over whether things are interpersonal or impersonal. This again I call a theorem: *The tension of anxiety, when present in the mothering one, induces anxiety in the infant.* The rationale of this induction—that is, *how* anxiety in the mother induces anxiety in the infant—is thoroughly obscure. This gap, this failure of our grasp on reality, has given rise to some beautifully plausible and perhaps correct explanations of how the anxiety of the mother causes anxiety in the infant; I bridge the gap simply by referring to it as a manifestation of an indefinite—that is, not yet defined—interpersonal process to which I apply the term *empathy*. I have had a good deal of trouble at times with people of a certain type of educational history; since they cannot refer empathy to vision, hearing, or some other special sense receptor, and since they do not know whether it is transmitted by the ether waves or air waves or what not, they find it hard to accept the idea of empathy. But whether the doctrine of empathy is accepted or not, the fact remains that the tension of anxiety when present in the mothering one induces anxiety in the infant; that theorem can be proved, I believe, and those who have had pediatric experience or mothering experience actually have data which can be interpreted on no other equally simple hypothetical basis. So although empathy may sound mysterious, remember that there is much that sounds mysterious in the universe, only you have got used to it; and perhaps you will get used to empathy.

Everything that I have discussed before coming to anxiety is a function of the biologically necessary communal existence of the infant, barring only the hint I have given of a need for contact with the living. Now, in discussing anxiety, I have come to something that has nothing whatever to do with the physicochemical needs of the living young. The tension called anxiety primarily appertains to the infant's, as also to the mother's, communal existence with a *personal* environment, in utter contradistinction to the physicochemical environment. For reasons presently to appear, I distinguish this tension from the sundry tensions already called needs by saying that the relaxation of the tension of anxiety, the re-equilibration of being in this specific respect, is the experience, not of satisfaction, but of interpersonal *security*.

The tension called anxiety, as early experienced in the prototaxic mode, is differentiated from all other reductions in euphoria by the *absence* of anything specific—you will recall that, when speaking of tensions of needs, I referred to *specific* sources of disequilibration, such as the lack of oxygen, water, or sugar. Because of the absence of anything so specific in anxiety, there is a consequent lack of differentiation in terms of the direction toward its relief by appropriate action. There is in the infant no capacity for action toward the relief of anxiety. While needs, as already suggested, begin to be, as it were, recognized or experientially represented in terms of the first of the infant's actions associated with their relief, the relief of anxiety has none of that aspect. No action of the infant is consistently and frequently associated with the relief of anxiety; and therefore the need for security, or freedom from anxiety, is highly significantly distinguished from all other needs from its very first hypothetical appearance.

Perhaps I should expand this idea somewhat so that its meaning becomes less obscure. At an indeterminately early age the tensions which appear in the infant connected with his relationship to the physicochemical environment tend to be relatively localized and marked with the prototype of what later we call emotional experience. Thus the experience connected with the need for water, or the tension associated with this need, begins to take on specific character. The same is true of the need for heat, the need for sugar, and, as I will develop at very considerable length presently, the need for oxygen. This more or less specific character of the connected experience, this mark, if you please, which characterizes the experience, permits the differentiation of activity suited to or appropriate to the relief of these needs. To leap a great many years of development, as an adult you *know*, for example, when you are hungry; that is, you can differentiate the experience connected with tensions due to your need for food, or due to the liver's resistance to giving up food until it has a new supply in prospect. You, by the mark of this particular experience, think, "I am hungry," and seek a restaurant or consider sponging a meal off of someone. This is the differentiation of appropriate action for the relief of a tension on the basis of the specific character of the experience that you are having.

Now my point is that anxiety, in contradistinction to these other tensions, has nothing specific about it; it does not gradually get itself related to hypothetical but reasonably probable contractions in the stomach, or dryness of the throat, or what have you. It does not have any specific characteristics of that kind, and consequently there is no basis in the experience of early anxiety for any differentiation, or clarification, of action appropriate to the avoidance or relief of anxiety. Therefore, I say that the infant has no capacity for action toward the relief of anxiety.

As I have said, human beings manifest needs for sundry more or less specific satisfactions. Converted into this language, the need for interpersonal security might be said to be the need to be rid of anxiety. But anxiety is not manageable: It comes by induction from another person; the infant's capacity for manipulating another person is confined, at the very start, to the sole capacity to call out tenderness by manifesting needs; and the person who would respond to manifest need in the situation in which the infant is anxious is relatively incapable of that response because it is the parental anxiety which induces the infant's anxiety—and as I shall explain shortly, anxiety always interferes with any other tensions with which it coincides. Therefore, there is, from the very earliest evidence of the empathic linkage, this peculiar distinction that anxiety is not manageable.

Anxiety is a tension in opposition to the tensions of needs and to action appropriate to their relief. It is in opposition to the tension of tenderness in the mothering one. It interferes with infantile behavior sequences—that is, with the infant's growing effectiveness in his communal existence with the physicochemical environment. It interferes, for example, with his sucking activity and doubtless with his swallowing. In fact, one may say flatly that anxiety opposes the satisfaction of needs. Of all experience of the present, the experience of anxiety is the sort least clearly interpenetrated by elements of the past and the future; it is the least interpretable and productive of foresight. In other words, because of the factors that I have been discussing and various others, the explanatory identifying elements of the past and the foresight of relief in the future, which are so important in accounting for activities or energy transformations in any particular situation, are, in this realm of anxiety, the easiest to overlook and the hardest to find.

Everywhere else the differentiation, however fantastic, of needs and the choosing of appropriate actions directed toward their relief—or even very inappropriate actions but allegedly, you might say, directed toward their relief—show the effect of the past and, even at a very early stage, the element of anticipation of the near future. In anxiety, however, because there is no lever with which to begin such differentiation, it is hard to get experience of anxiety in the past to fit into interpreting present instances of it, and anxiety can almost be said to cut off foresight. Now that is very loosely expressed. But at least one can say that the more anxious one is, the less the distinguished human function of foresight is free to work effectively in the choice, as we call it, of action appropriate to the tensions that one is experiencing.

The capacity to experience anxiety is not an exclusively human capacity, but the role of anxiety in interpersonal relations is so profoundly important that its differentiation from all other tensions is vital. I shall, therefore, next review the probabilities as to the infant's tensional history up to and including the occurrence of the earliest experiences of anxiety. In this process I shall touch particularly upon the seeming, and perhaps very real, relationship of terror and anxiety. But this will be with the earnest hope that no one will think that I am saying that anxiety is terror. What I am instead attempting to say is that of all the experiences which are differentiated on the basis of specific marking, the only one that comes within gunshot of the experience of primitive anxiety is terror, which, I have already hinted, is the closest approach to absolute tension that one can imagine.

PART II

The Developmental Epochs

CHAPTER
4

Infancy: Beginnings

Ways of Dealing with the Tension of Fear

THE FIRST great danger to the newborn is that of anoxia, deprivation of oxygen in contact with the tissues. This danger becomes acute with the separation of the newborn infant from the maternal circulation and continues, intensifying very swiftly thereafter, until the successful institution of the breathing cycle by which air flows in and out from thenceforth. Recurrence of this danger of anoxia at any time in life is accompanied by an extraordinary form of fear to which we refer as terror. Occasions of danger other than the failure of oxygen supply may call out terror, but from very early in extrauterine life any interference with freedom of the bodily movements which are concerned with the cyclic alternation of negative and positive pressure in the lungs calls out general activity of the infant or older person which is suggestive in appearance of what we later in life would unquestionably call rage behavior. However, when I speak of activity of the infant which is suggestive of what we later see in people who are enraged, I am not, like the old behaviorists, asking you to picture rage as one of the primitive emotions. I am suggesting that the most certain way of terrifying anybody at any time in his life is to interfere rather quickly with his supply of air. Choking, submersion in carbon dioxide or other oxygen-free gases, and so on, are extremely terrifying experiences. A peculiarity of the danger of anoxia is that not only does anything which impedes breathing tend to call out severe fear which rapidly becomes terror and this sort of behavior which is seen in the infant as screaming and kicking and so on, but, if the oxygen starvation progresses, the organism is so built that there will be general convulsions, convulsive releases of undifferentiated motor impulses, before death actually happens.

Fear, from its mildest to its most extreme form, that of terror, is to be considered to be the felt aspect of tension arising from danger to the existence or biological integrity of the organism. Such dangers are, in general, those of anoxia—oxygen starvation, which I have just been discussing; of thirst—water starvation; of starvation for carbohydrates and other chemical foodstuffs; of subcooling; of molar injury to the body—that is, massive injury to the body; and of impairment or failure of sundry vital factors. Circulatory failure is probably the same old danger of anoxia and, if at all rapidly deepening, is very apt to be accompanied by terror.

If you think of fear from a rather adult standpoint, you will notice that there are four generic patterns for dealing with or relaxing the tension of fear. And if you will forget infancy entirely for the moment and think of yourself in a fear-provoking situation, such as being threatened by an oncoming enemy in a warfare situation, you will realize that one of the patterns for dealing with fear is to remove or destroy the fear-provoking circumstances. Another is to escape from the fear-provoking circumstances. A third, not so immediately self-evident, is to neutralize the fear-provoking circumstances. To describe the fourth generic pattern I shall use a word which is rather misleading: the fourth pattern is to *ignore* the fear-provoking circumstances. If you consider even the ordinary risks to our somatic organization, such as traffic hazards and other hazards of transportation, you will immediately realize that when I speak of *ignoring* the danger, I am referring to pretty complicated processes. For example, even if a person knows that the risk incurred in crossing busy streets is fully as great as the risk incurred in traveling in airplanes, it is obvious that he must ignore a great deal of this risk inherent in crossing streets when he is going about his daily business; yet actually to say that the risk is ignored implies, as I say, something pretty complicated.

As to the other patterns for dealing with fear, removing or destroying the source of a danger is fairly evident. The classical way of handling fear is to get away from that which is feared, to escape it. In certain circumstances one can neutralize fear. Thus, for example, if you are dealing with a person who is given to violence, you can neutralize the danger of his violence if you can impress him with the equal probability of your successful use of violence; and another way, of course, is to ignore him.

The vigorous motor activity which is called out by restraint of the infant's freedom of respiratory movements may be effective in removing or escaping from the restraining circumstances. This effectiveness may be direct, or it may be mediate by way of calling out mothering activity. Now some people have doubts as to the propriety of using so-called teleological arguments in which the goal is supposed to cause, in a certain curious fashion, the phenomena discussed. And so I shall defer, as long as I can, any attempt to make use of so-called teleological explanations. In a great many ways, many of the details of the equipment of the human animal can readily be discussed from this teleological standpoint, but they can also be considered as the result of evolutionary change controlled by survival value. Thus if you will think, not of a human infant, but of a kitten or a puppy, you will realize that one of the encompassing risks to this infant dog or cat is that, when it is under the mother for purposes of reducing heat loss, it will be cut off from communal existence with the atmosphere by the body of the mother. When this happens, the sort of vigorous movement which is called out fairly early in oxygen privation serves to apprise the mother of the danger to the puppy or kitten. In the same way, if a human infant is threatened with anoxia because a blanket is cutting off his oxygen supply, here again vigorous movements, which may ultimately become convulsive discharges, will have a very strong likelihood of calling out mothering activity, of displacing this obstruction, or of displacing the infant to the point where contact with the air can be renewed. Since we store less oxygen than we do water and sugar, very extensive provisions for insuring a practically continuous contact with the circumambient atmosphere have had great survival value for the human animal and in fact for all the higher animals.

As I have said, the vigorous movements which are called out by oxygen hunger, and which look like performances of older children in rage, are effective in escaping from the restraining influences or circumstances bearing on the oxygen supply, either directly—in the example I have spoken of, by getting out from under a blanket—or mediately, by way of calling out mothering activity. The audible vibratory air movements which accompany the institution of the breathing cycle—the birth cry—are the first instance of infantile activity which evokes the tensions of generic tenderness in the mothering one. Crying remains for some time the most effective infantile behavior appropriate to the relief of fear. To the extent that the tender acts of the mothering one are correctly addressed to removing the disturbing circumstances, this crying, which is heard by the infant, is experienced as adequate and appropriate action. In many other instances, while it may not bring immediate relief of the danger causing the tension of fear, it at least brings tenderness in the course of what might be described as random efforts on the part of the mothering one, which are closely, or reasonably closely, identified with the relief of the fear-evoking danger.

Since I want to forestall, as far as I can, any possible reservations to these thoughts, I shall here take up the question of the hearing of the infant's crying by the infant. The middle ear and the Eustachian tube are filled with fluid, at least in many infants, for a little while after birth, and under those circumstances it might be quite difficult to demonstrate that an infant can hear someone playing a piano ten feet away. But while air is a comparatively elastic medium which carries sound waves quite nicely, water, saline solution, and so on are relatively inelastic media which carry vibrations still better. Now since vibration occurs in the neighborhood of the larynx, as in crying, and is reflected and refined in the neighborhood of the opening of the Eustachian tube well back in the throat, the only question about an infant's hearing his own crying is whether the auditory division of the appropriate nerve is functionally adequate at birth. Since it can be demonstrated that that nerve is functionally adequate before birth, it seems to me perfectly possible to speak of even the birth cry as being heard by the infant; certainly very soon after the institution of the breathing cycle, the infant hears himself cry. Thus you will realize that, since we are talking about a very primitive type of experience, it is quite as credible to talk about the experience of the newborn infant as it is, for example, to talk about the experience of an amoeba—and the experience of an amoeba is something that can safely be set up as an hypothesis to account for certain observable facts.

From the standpoint of the infant's prototaxic experience, this crying, insofar as it evokes appropriate tender behavior by the mothering one, is adequate and appropriate action by the infant to remove or escape fear-provoking dangers. Crying thus comes to be differentiated as action appropriate to accomplish the foreseen relief of fear.

Anxiety as a Threat to the Organism

Let us now consider the case of the anxious infant—the infant suffering anxiety induced by anxiety on the part of the mother. Anxiety does not arise from danger to the communal physicochemical interchange or to the organization of the infant's body. It arises by induction from the anxiety of the mother. It is a function of the necessary interpersonal communality with someone mature enough to cooperate in the complex activities needed for the relief of the infant's physicochemical needs. I would like to repeat that dangers calling out fear can be handled in four ways, at least by adults. But if you will now think of anxiety, which is originally induced by anxiety in the mothering one, you will immediately see that, not only in infancy but for the rest of life, the circumstances conducive to anxiety cannot be removed, nor destroyed, nor escaped. Some of you may think that an adult can remove or destroy the source of anxiety by killing the person who makes him anxious, or escape it by leaving town; but later on in my discussion it will become apparent that the source of anxiety is not so easily handled. Certainly there is no possibility of the infant's doing anything to remove or destroy the source of the infantile anxiety, nor is there any escaping it.

Crying in relation to infantile anxiety is often ineffectual or worse. It often increases the anxiety of the mothering one, and thereby increases the anxiety of the infant. This is partly because of the direct induction of more anxiety in the infant when anxiety increases in the mother, and partly because the anxiety of the mother interferes with her competence to manifest tenderness and particularly with her competence to do the right thing, you might say, to cooperate in the infant's escaping dangers, and so on. There isn't any right thing to do with infantile anxiety except for the mother to cease to be anxious. Anxiety interferes with both the mother's cooperation and the infant's behavior patterns for the relief of his need, which calls out fear when it is not relieved; thus if the infant has some need at the same time that he becomes anxious, there is then in the infant a double handicap, because not only is he anxious, but also a need is being left unresolved and is, therefore, presumably increasing. The act of crying itself—that is, the production of the audible vibrations which make up the cry—is a reductive modification of freedom of expiring breath, and, in fact, as the crying becomes violent, may also represent an interference with inspiring breath. Thus any intensification of crying, such as one would expect when the crying reflects both the danger of need and infantile anxiety induced by the mother's anxiety, may incur the danger of interference with the oxygen exchange. And this, added to everything else, rapidly aggravates fear in the direction of terror. Now as I have said before, this particular type of restraint in the communal existence of the infant—marked interference with breathing—calls out a vigorous type of molar activity on the part of the infant which suggests what is later quite properly called rage behavior. It is an actual fact of pediatric experience that sometimes this combination of unsatisfied need, anxiety in the infant, and succeeding threat to the respiratory freedom progresses to the point that the infant is blue, cyanotic, which means that there is nothing like enough oxygen in the circulating blood, and also progresses into general convulsions called spasms by most people, I believe. Now here is a picture, which, I trust, clearly shows the relative inappropriateness and inadequacy of the infantile behavior for the relief of anxiety. For the source of the anxiety is, at this stage of development, solely anxiety in the mothering one—that is, in the significant, relatively adult personality whose cooperation is necessary to keep the infant alive.

This picture may seem to suggest that when this coincidence of needs and anxiety occurs, things rapidly progress in a fashion which becomes thoroughly dangerous for the survival of the infant. To a certain extent that is true, but if this were the whole story, there would probably be no extant specimens of our particular species. I can perhaps best suggest what happens by describing the way the heart is protected from any dangerous or fatal activities of the apparatus which slows and regulates—that is, evens—the cardiac rhythm. This is the so-called vagus influence, which not only slows the heart, but can actually stop the heart from beating—a fatal performance if it were prolonged. In order to prevent this, an apparatus manifests itself which enables the heart to escape from inhibition. Thus while the vagus influence may stop the heart for a little while, the heart then escapes and hurries to make up for lost time in circulating oxygen and foodstuffs. Similarly in the development of terror connected with infantile anxiety, we have dynamisms (I shall use this word instead of apparatus) which protect the infant from the otherwise extremely dangerous kind of coincidence I have described. The exact meaning of dynamism I shall exemplify later when we have more to work on.

The Dynamisms of Apathy and Somnolent Detachment

There are dynamisms which are called out by these emergency situations both in very early life and in later life. In the infant, one of these dynamisms manifests itself particularly in saving the infant from this geometrical progression, so to speak, of disaster called out by unsatisfied need, anxiety, and the resulting interference with breathing which provokes terror, the maximum state of tension. The dynamism which intervenes in the type of situation that I have described—which is quite often aggravated continuously by the mounting anxiety of the mothering one—is part of the adaptive capabilities of man and of some, at least, of the higher animals. It is the possibility of becoming apathetic, of manifesting under certain circumstances the condition which we call *apathy*. In apathy all the tensions of needs are markedly attenuated. You will remember that I have previously set up a discrimination between two tensions: the tension of needs, which can be satisfied, and which can be experienced as fear of a danger of the need; and the tension of anxiety, which is brought about by the interpersonal situation. The latter can be said to be the need for interpersonal security, and it is very distinct from the need for interchange with the physicochemical environment—for preserving the integrity of the bodily organization and the smooth working of its vital processes. I have now said that in the state called apathy the tension of all needs is markedly attenuated. I am not too sure about the relationship of apathy and anxiety. It is a recondite problem, and I shall tell you almost at once how I have, at least provisionally, resolved it.

But first I want you to consider the anxious and terrified infant, who may be described as a shrieking, kicking infant, and to consider how apathy intervenes to markedly attenuate the infant's tensions—that is, not actually to obliterate them, but to greatly reduce them. Let us say that the tensions were, in this particular example, first, a need for food, then, because feeding was impaired by the mother's anxiety, ultimately a need for both food and oxygen. Apathy reduces the tension of these needs; in states of apathy, however, the needs are not abolished, but are merely markedly attenuated, and there is usually enough of the tension of needs to maintain organic life. That is, apathy does not ordinarily so attenuate needs that one will calmly or apathetically starve to death, die of thirst, undergo devastating injury, or the like. But this is true only in the absence of any extraordinary danger in the physico-chemico-biological sphere; as long as apathy prevails, there is no possibility of an adequate tensional response to an acute or extreme danger. I am adding this not because it pertains immediately to our discussion of the infant, but because I want you to realize that apathy as an escape from this pyramiding of tension, which culminates in terror—an extremely expensive state—is not nearly as charmingly efficient and safe as is the apparatus for the escape of the heart from inhibition. In the latter, the apparatus always works if the person is well enough to survive the stoppage of the heart, as is almost invariably the case; but in the case of the infant, terror when mixed with anxiety might easily lead to death. Thus the vulnerability of the infant in this process of getting to be a person is somewhat greater than is the vulnerability of the heart in the example which I have cited.

To get back to my resolution of the problem of the relationship between apathy and anxiety, I would like to set up provisionally the term *somnolent detachment* as the protective dynamism called out by prolonged severe anxiety, in contradistinction to apathy as the protective dynamism called out by unfulfilled needs. I do not know whether the dynamism of somnolent detachment is manifested early in infancy—and it is impossible, so far as I have yet been able to find, to devise any procedure which would settle that question—but certainly later in life something corresponding to apathy intervenes in anxiety if it is severe and prolonged. The difference in actual appearance between the young when apathetic and the young involved in somnolent detachment is nil. There is no objective difference. But since a good deal of our speculation and inference about the very early stages of life comes from following backward from later clearly discriminable states to their first manifestations, we are, I think, entirely justified in saying that from the beginning these escape or safety devices are entitled to different names. Apathy is called out by unsatisfied, extremely aggravated needs; somnolent detachment is called out by inescapable and prolonged anxiety. That is, somnolent detachment, since anxiety is induced by interpersonal situations, is the safety device which attenuates the susceptibility to the interpersonally induced tension of anxiety. It suffices, at this stage of our consideration of developmental history, to observe that the intervention of these, as it were, safety dynamisms attenuates the infant's disturbed condition to a point at which a very important change of state of awareness occurs, and the infant sleeps.

Tension of the Need for Sleep

I have spoken several times of awareness without defining it. Let me say that the state of awareness has to be inferred about the infant; presently we will have some data which will make awareness more than just a "given." But one can safely say that from practically the first hour of extrauterine life, there are two phases of existence: one, awareness, which anyone should be able to accept provisionally, and the other, the state of sleep.

Now sleep as a phase of living is quite as important, and in some ways just as intricate, as is waking. In man and in the higher animals, at least, the *phasic* variation of living between waking and sleep is necessary for the continuation of life. Apathy and somnolent detachment may from this standpoint be regarded as dynamisms that insure life despite grave interference with the ability to fall asleep. Most of the life of the infant is spent in the phase of sleep. Roughly the division of life between sleeping and waking varies inversely with developmental age. But this reciprocal relationship (remember that inverse variation is a reciprocal relationship) is a complex function which is by no means as simple as my former example of the inverse relationship between tension and euphoria. We may say, however, that no other significant factor being concerned, the portion of the life of the infant spent in sleep varies inversely with the developmental age of the infant. It should be noted that at the start of extrauterine life, the developmental age and the chronological age are nearly or very nearly equivalent. But this one-to-one relationship disappears quite early in life; in fact, every day the infant lives, there is a less close correspondence between developmental age and chronological age as measured by a calendar or a clock.

This whole topic of needs, anxiety, and sleep will come up again and again and will be developed more as we go on. But since I am still trying to set forth a consideration of the developmental epoch of infancy, I shall, after making a few more remarks, defer any further development of the subject of sleep.

I have already pointed out that living has two phasic variations, sleeping and waking. But living in the phase of sleep is not a state of tensionless euphoria. The more one 'needs sleep,' the more intense becomes the particular tension state which is the disequilibrium of being that is relaxed or remedied by sleeping; so sleep has the relation to this particular tensional state that satisfaction, let us say, of the need for sugar has to the need for sugar. By this statement, which I trust has been adequate, I have brought you to the third and last of the great genera of tensions which pertain to human living: In addition to the tensions of needs and the tensions which we call anxiety, induced by disturbance of interpersonal relations, we have here the tensions concerned with the phasic state of living which is called sleep. We shall presently discover that the tensions of needs and of anxiety are oppositional to the tensions of sleeping. None of these tensions are of the same genus; they are very significantly different.

I have discussed at some length the differences, which appear very early in the infant, in the tension of anxiety as compared with the tension of needs. The handicaps of language being what they are, I would like to review what I have been saying. I have chosen to use one word, *needs*, to refer to tensions primarily connected with the physicochemical requirements of life, with the avoiding of injury, and with the maintenance of internal, if you please, functional activities of various kinds. I have labeled all these *tensions of needs* and discriminated them from the *tension of anxiety*, which does not directly pertain to the physicochemical universe, but pertains instead to the relationship of the infant with the relatively adult person whose cooperation is necessary for the survival of the infant. And finally I would say that there is a third great type of *tensions which pertain to sleeping* in contrast with waking. While, as I have said, a certain amount of sleep in a certain span of time is necessary for the survival of man and some, at least, of the higher animals, this necessity is distinctly different from the needs for oxygen, sugar, water, heat, and so on; and it is certainly different from the extremely disturbing tensions of anxiety. So it is that when I use the locution *need for satisfaction*, I shall be using *need* as a technical term, because a need in the technical sense can be satisfied. When I talk about the *need for interpersonal security*, I shall be talking about anxiety; and when I talk about the *need for sleep*, I shall be talking about a third genus of tension not readily to be related to the other two grand divisions of tension. I am reviewing these points so that we will be secure in our use of language.

At this stage of our consideration of the first year of developmental history, infancy, I have, I trust, shown that the infant has physicochemically conditioned recurrent needs, the satisfaction of which—aside from breathing—requires interpersonal cooperation, which cooperation can be called tenderness. The manifestation of this tender cooperation for the relief of the infant's needs is disturbed, interfered with, by anxiety in the mothering one. This anxiety in the mothering one not only interferes with her tender cooperation with the infant, but also induces anxiety in the infant. That anxiety in the infant interferes, in turn, with his part of the cooperation for the satisfaction of his needs, such as sucking, swallowing, and so on. Now the continuing tension of these unsatisfied needs, along with the tension of anxiety itself, interferes in turn with the biologically necessary sleeping which the infant must do an extraordinarily large part of the time or else die. But this phasic change from waking to sleeping is protected from the piling up of needs and anxiety by the infant's ability to become apathetic.

Now, clearly, I have not quite solved the problem of anxiety, but in my discussion of the anxious infant you observed that it was the appearance of terror, or the movement toward terror, that made the situation extremely aggravated. The dynamism of apathy attenuates fear to the point that it does not interfere with going to sleep. I realize that I am leaving the matter of anxiety somewhat at loose ends here. In general, we can say, however, that after a mothering one has had the experience of an infant going into what looks like rage behavior—perhaps becoming cyanotic from screaming, perhaps having spasms—the maternal anxiety is enormously relieved once the infant begins to quiet down and goes to sleep. Since the maternal anxiety has diminished, it is difficult to say anything concrete about the relief of the infant's anxiety. The probability is that even a mother who was made intensely anxious, for example, by a telegram bringing bad news portending most unpleasant consequences for the future, will be so distracted from the threat of mere future trouble by an infant in a condition resembling rage that when apathy spreads over the infant and he becomes quieter and moves toward sleep, the anxiety of the mother provoked by the so-called rage behavior of the infant naturally diminishes quite rapidly.

Now there is one more thing I want to touch on briefly here. The physicochemical growth rate—the rate of organizing physicochemical-biological structures—is very high in the earlier phases of extrauterine life, as illustrated by the very rapid relative increase in weight of the infant, which means that physicochemical substances have been built into the infant from the outer world. Since this rate is very high in the earlier phases of extrauterine life, any considerable period of lifetime spent in the state of apathy is of grave moment. In this connection, I should like to call attention to the work of Margaret Ribble,[1] who has done some excellent observational work on underprivileged infants and whose data I respect very highly. She has described the syndrome of infantile apathy which, once it is well established, provides a very unfavorable outlook for the infant's survival. In other words, if the circumstances of interpersonal collaboration or cooperation which keep an infant alive are so much disturbed that the infant has to have recourse to apathy during quite a large part of his waking life, then the infant perishes.[2] Thus apathy, while it is lifesaving, as I hope I have shown, is something which, if it is used very much, literally starves the infant in all ways, and the infant perishes.

[1] [Margaret A. Ribble, "Clinical Studies of Instinctive Reactions in New Born Babies," *Amer. J. Psychiatry* (1938) 95:149–158.]

[2] This outcome of apathy is not nearly so likely later on; the way in which apathy can make people perish later in life is by making them unable to escape sudden or rapidly oncoming dangers.

CHAPTER

5

Infancy: The Concept of Dynamism—Part 1

Zones of Interaction

I AM NOW beginning to lead up rather directly to the very important concept of dynamism, although I shall not reach that goal for a while yet. In the meantime, we will learn something more about the concept of anxiety and all that is implied in this concept, which is quite basic to this whole way of looking at psychiatry, and also about the prototaxic, parataxic, and syntaxic modes of experience.

We have seen that, from the very beginning of the breathing cycle, the infant has a whole list of needs, activities, and satisfactions, and that delays in satisfactions constitute dangers to early infantile survival and as such are sources of augmented tension to which we refer as fear. Throughout all this list, crying is adequate and appropriate action toward the relief of the fear, because it brings into being the circumstances necessary for the satisfaction of the particular need which is involved. So far as the infant is concerned, in these very early weeks of life, the cry effects (1) the relief of anoxia by starting the breathing cycle; (2) the relief of thirst and hunger by 'producing,' in a certain sense, the nipple in the infant's lips, from which the infant sucks relief-giving substance which is swallowed; (3) the relief of subcooling by preventing excessive heat loss; and (4) the removal of noxious physical circumstances, such as a restraint of bodily freedom of movement, painful local pressures, and the like. The cry is functional activity of the infant, principally appertaining to (besides the breathing cycle) the head end of the alimentary tract. The infant's part in relief of thirst and hunger also centers here, in the sucking and swallowing activity.

The receptor-effector organ complex which is here concerned —that is, the audible-sound-producing and hearing apparatus, the nipple-investing, nipple-holding, and sucking apparatus, and the neuro-glandular-muscular complexes concerned in breathing, crying, and the transporting of foodstuffs—all this is an instance of what we call a *zone of interaction* in the communal existence which is necessary for the survival of the infant. It is evident that the actual interchange of oxygen and carbon dioxide occurs in the pulmonary respiratory epithelium, and that the actual interchange of water and foodstuffs occurs far from the mouth; in other words, the tissues actually concerned in communal existence with the physicochemical environment, only begin in what we shall call the *oral zone*—or, in the case of oxygen, only begin and end in the oral zone. But, physiologically considered, the oral zone is a remarkable organization which can be divided for purposes of discussion into three types of apparatus: (1) receptor apparatus, which I have already touched on—organization of special sense apparatus, such as sight, special tactile sensitivities, gustatory or taste sensitivities, and olfactory or smell sensitivities; (2) eductors, of which I have not yet spoken; and (3) effectors, which are ordinarily muscles and glands. Now what are the eductors? The eductors, a word borrowed from Spearman,[1] are the elaborate apparatus, a large part of it in the brain, which pertains to the central and other nervous systems, and which—in a sensible and use-

[1] [*Editors' note:* Spearman uses the word *eduction* in an endeavor to reduce cognitive events to a set of ultimate laws. Sullivan uses the word as the mid-process between the receptors and effectors. According to Spearman, "an item in thought or perception is said to be 'educed' from other items there when derived from these by their very essence or nature" (Charles E. Spearman, *Creative Mind;* London: Nisbet and Co. Ltd., Cambridge Univ. Press, 1930, p. 34). Spearman discriminates between eduction and *apprehension of experience;* for example, "I-see-red" would represent apprehension of experience, in Spearman's terms. But while knowing, according to Spearman, must begin in such actually occurring experience, it extends further, for relations and correlates are *educed* from the bare presenting experience. (*The Nature of 'Intelligence' and the Principles of Cognition;* London: Macmillan and Co., 1923. See Chapters IV, V. VII, and XXI.)]

ful fashion, as it were—connects what impinges on the receptors with the activity of the effectors.

Now in all the zones of interaction that I shall discuss, it will be possible, from the standpoint of physiology—that is, from the standpoint of the effective functional activity of the organized creature—to observe the functioning of the receptors, the eductors, and the effectors, the eductors making what is received useful for life.

The oral zone is a remarkable organization of these three different kinds of apparatus; these apparatuses are concerned with the maintenance of the breathing cycle, the acquiring or rejecting of fluids and solids, and the utterance of those audible sounds basically important in interactions in the interpersonal field. The zone of interaction may then be considered to be the end station in the necessary varieties of communal existence with the physicochemical world, the world of the infrahuman living, and the personal world.

Processes in and pertaining to these zones of interaction must have a great deal to do with the occurrence of experience, with the perduring evidence, in other words, of living. So far as experience is, or effects, useful durable change in the functional activities of the living organism, it must relate backward and forward—that is, in phenomena of recall and foresight—to the zone of interaction to which it is primarily related, however much more widespread its relationship may actually be or become. Here is a discrimination of what *must* be the case from what *may* be the case.

As I have said several times, there is a good deal of evidence to show that all the way down to the level of the amoeba there is actually favorable—that is, profitable—durable change from experience. It must be that experience is related to the particular part of our communal existence and functional activity with the necessary environment from which the experience rose. If experience were not so necessarily related, it would not, needless to say, produce durable and favorable change in the particular functional activity. So I say that experience either *is* the useful durable change, or that it *brings about* the useful durable change in the function of the living organism.

From the data of later life, I hold that experience takes special color from, or is especially marked with reference to, the zone of interaction which is primarily concerned in its occurrence; and I believe that there is no necessity to make any particular change in this general statement when a very young infant is concerned in contradistinction to a grown person. In other words, the zone of interaction which is involved in a particular course of events gives a particular kind of mark, or color, to the experience which the living creature undergoes. For example, if I put salt in my mouth, or, to say it another way, if sodium chloride impinges upon me at the right place—namely, in my mouth—it tastes salt, and former experiences with salt are recalled to the extent of my identifying this as a salty taste; if there seems to be a good deal of that which tastes salt, I can foresee that I shall presently be thirsty, and therefore take steps to provide water with which to wash it down and otherwise make it useful instead of harmful when it is inside me. Now salt applied to an open wound is an experience, I assure you, but it has no marks in any sense relating it to the oral zone. Therefore, although sodium chloride is still the thing which has impinged upon me, because it has impinged upon a different zone of interaction with the environment, the experience of sodium chloride impinging upon me is an extraordinarily different thing; and instead of my having the experience of the ingestion of an absolutely necessary foodstuff which is identified as such, I have the experience of very severe pain due to a particular problem of fluid distribution, hypertonic solution, and so on, in my wound.

I make this rather obvious digression to illustrate what I really mean when I say that experience as experience, whatever else it may be, has color-reference back to, you might say, or some special type of marking which refers it to, a zone of interaction. Now the place where the real interaction between sodium chloride and my organism takes place is a long way from the place where the sodium chloride impinges significantly upon my organism. Thus even in this simple example you see that the oral zone in connection with sodium chloride, common salt, has much significance for me, although the point at which sodium chloride is of the most vital and absolute necessity for my continued survival begins several feet from there—and exists throughout all the tissues of the body, salt being an imperative necessity for the carrying on of the complex physicochemical arrangements by which we live. So the zone of interaction, the end station of a particular type of communal existence, has striking psychiatric importance, that is, striking importance for the human organism in a large and total sense.

While experience is experience of the living of the organism, and is total rather than local or partial in character, it is primarily the experience of particular events impinging upon one or more of the zones of interaction, which are end stations of the living organism. Note that the zone of interaction is not to be equated with any particular fixed tissue organization; it is not quite as static as the mouth, nose, pharynx, and larynx are in the anatomical person. Thus not alone in man, but well down the biological series, if because of a misfortune in genetic constitution, or an injury or misfortune in development, a creature is born with an unusual defect, or comes to suffer the destruction of part of the apparatus of a zone of interaction with the necessary environment, then quite frequently other apparatus can be modified—chiefly the eductor apparatus, the central nervous system. And so the zone of interaction, defined from the standpoint of that which impinges upon it, becomes functional again, although the biological apparatus, the histological apparatus, if you please, is very different. An internationally famous instance of this is the development in Helen Keller of quite adequate zones of interaction with personal environment, despite very grave and extensive destruction of apparatus which, if you think of zones of interaction in terms of apparatus, you might expect would destroy completely the possibilities for such interaction.

The Role of Anxiety in the Beginning Differentiation of Experience

Crying, as I have said, is adequate and appropriate action of the hungry infant in that it frequently 'produces' the nipple-lips experience and its satisfaction-giving consequents of sucking, swallowing, and so on. Now crying is adequate and appropriate action for the relief of the infant's hunger, not because it *invariably* gets him fed, but because it *frequently*, so far as he is concerned, leads to that change which is the nipple between his lips, which is the instituting or initiating step in the procedure of sucking and swallowing, which in the end relieves or at least diminishes the hunger. This lips-nipple experience, which we are sure the infant has, generally produces the fluid sucked and swallowed, the arrival of which is closely related to the relaxation or reduction of the tension of need for water and food.

Now one of the things I most detest in the German language is the production of words that take a printed line, by compounding other words. Unhappily, in trying to throw some light on the essentially simply inferable living of the infant, I have had to resort to compound hyphenated words. The one which provokes my distress at the moment is crying-when-hungry. Crying-when-hungry has no necessary relatedness, in the infant's experience, with crying-when-cold, crying-when-pained, or crying-under-any-other-circumstances. If crying-when-hungry frequently initiates the necessary circumstances for the relief of hunger and thirst, it comes to mean, in a primitive, prototaxic way, something like what I may suggest by the word sequence: "Come, nipple, into my mouth." It is a vocal gesture with reasonably dependable power of so manipulating what will later be called reality that the nipple complies. In other words, crying-when-hungry, so far as infantile experience can go, has power to manipulate quite ungraspable aspects of something-or-other, later lumped as reality, so that the nipple dutifully appears.

The most refined study of the sound waves which make up crying-when-hungry need show no 'objective difference' whatever from the sound waves making up crying-when-cold, for example. The two may not only sound alike, but in the physical acoustic sense may be the same, may have a one-to-one correspondence in every measurable sense; that is, the pattern of progression of sound waves, if duly recorded on a cathode-ray oscillograph, may be absolutely identical in every characteristic that can be measured through such a device. And yet, from the infantile standpoint, crying-when-hungry and crying-when-cold will not be in any sense the same thing.

The same kind of physical acoustic correspondence often appears when one says *whole* and *hole*. The so-called objective facts do not have significance with respect to the meaning, to the speaking person, of the (as we say) two different words. He may never have discovered that his two words are homonyms or homophones. We may say, under these circumstances, that he has not differentiated the homophonous character of the two words. As long as the use of either of these two homophones generally proves adequate to his needs, it is of no great importance to his living to discover that the two words, very different in dictionary meaning, sound alike—that is, are experienced by the hearer as quite exactly the same. Until something has called for such differentiation, our person may well believe that he "sounds different," as he might put it, when he utters "hole" from the way he sounds when he says "whole." In general, the matter will never have occurred to him, never have been the subject of what I shall later discuss as *observation, identifying,* and *valid formulation* of two different, but acoustically identical, verbal acts. I trust that I have illustrated, by this discussion of two homonymous or homophonous words, how, from the standpoint of the physics of sound, or from the study of linguistic process in actual operation, two very different words are utterly the same. Their difference, which comes out nicely when written words are substituted for them (remember that written words are symbols for spoken words) is a difference in the use to which they are put—that is, their usefulness as tools, their meaning to the user, what they are good for.

In the same way, the infant's crying-when-hungry, however utterly indistinguishable outside, you might say, it is from crying-when-cold, is an entirely different performance so far as the infant and his experience go. Thus one's actions, however they may impress the observer, are most importantly defined by what they are 'intended' for—that is, they are determined by the general pattern of motivation that is involved, by what is significant to the person concerned, quite irrespective of any impressions an observer may have.

A great many mistakes are made in psychiatry as a result of overlooking this fact. Some of these mistakes are very devastating indeed, such as the ancient superstition that the performances of the schizophrenic are essentially unpsychological. Few more sad combinations of words could be spouted. The truth is that however the performance of a Javanese head-hunter might look to a clerk in a Wall Street financial institution, the clerk's opinions would have only recreational or conversational value; they would be of exceedingly little importance with respect to head-hunters in Java.

The infant's experience of crying-when-hungry comes very early to relate backward and forward—that is, as recall and as foresight—to the 'producing' of the lips-nipple experience with its desired consequents of sucking and swallowing. I have said that crying-when-hungry *frequently* produces the nipple and the possibilities of relief. I want now to discuss two special instances in which this very early magical potency of vocal behavior goes wrong, as it were. Before I do that, I wish that you could rid yourself of any preconceptions about magic. I would like to suggest that when we speak of *magical potency* we are likely to mean—I think it may be adequately stated this way—that we have an exceedingly inadequate grasp on all that is actually happening. When you do something that works, it is like turning on the electric lights by flipping a switch. The lights come on magically because you flipped the switch—that is, if you don't know anything in particular about electricity and electric circuits, it seems magical; if the lights don't come on, that's extraordinary, indicating that something must be wrong somewhere. But if you know enough to guess *where* something may be wrong, you are pretty well acquainted with reality. I might add—perhaps slightly to parallel the relationship of the infant's crying-when-hungry and getting food—that even though sometimes when you flip a switch the lights don't come on, the fact that they generally have will probably lead you to flip switches in the future when you want light; and you will remain convinced that there is considerable potency in flipping a switch when you want light, even though it hasn't always worked. And so it is with a great deal in life.

I want particularly now to discuss very early experience of this sort of *infrequent* event. The first is the failure of the crying-when-hungry, arising from (as we see it) the absence of the necessary, more adult person who actually (in our sense) is the provider of the nipple. To digress for a moment, it is well to remember that the very young infant has no grasp on those phases of reality which we call independent persons, with or without nipples, and with or without milk to run through those nipples; this is utterly exterior to any reasonable supposition about very young infants. Now let us assume that the infant happens to be surrounded only by male persons—perhaps the mother is out doing some shopping or whatever. Crying-when-hungry therefore does not produce, in its usual magical fashion, the nipple in the mouth, which is the initiatory stage of infantile activity which satisfies hunger and thirst. In this case crying-when-hungry is continued until the nipple is produced, or until mounting fear has called out apathy and the infant finally sleeps. Crying-when-hungry then recurs as soon as the infant awakens. Now this is the beginning of a very important train of events with which we have dealings throughout life.

The other special instance which I wish to discuss is that in which anxiety is a complicating factor. We shall take a case in which the crying-when-hungry has produced the nipple, but this success, preliminary to sucking and the satisfaction of hunger and thirst, is complicated by the interference of the anxiety which has been induced in the infant because of or by anxiety in or pertaining to the person who carries the nipple in actuality. The satisfaction-giving consequents on the production of the nipple under these circumstances do not follow. Investing the nipple with the lips, sucking, swallowing, or any or all of these and other parts of the accessory behavior of nursing may be disordered by the coincidence of anxiety in the infant, induced by the mothering one's anxiety, with the infant's crying-when-hungry. The infant may produce the nipple in the magical fashion that has become frequent enough to be the normal expectation, as you might describe it—the proof of the power of crying-when-hungry—but this time something is very wrong.

The first of the special instances which I have mentioned—that is, crying-when-hungry when there is nobody to rally around tenderly—is a very early experience of the occasional inadequacy or powerlessness of otherwise generally appropriate and adequate behavior for the manipulation of what later will be called reality. The infant cries when hungry, and nothing happens except the development of processes in the infant which culminate finally in apathy and sleep, with the recurrence of crying on awakening. As I have said, this is a very early instance of a type of situation which recurs more or less frequently throughout life, in which a generally appropriate and adequate series of acts—that is, behavior—proves to be inadequate, and proves to have no power to bring about that which this behavior is ordinarily entirely sufficient to produce. This sort of experience, the experience of unexpected powerlessness, as we may call it, is an event infrequent enough to be quite exterior to expectation; in other words, it is an exception to something to which we are accustomed, an exception to the many times we have done something and the right result has come of it.

The accompaniments of these experiences of powerlessness are various. The significance of such experiences of powerlessness probably increases for some time after birth, until one has developed adequate ways of handling such experiences, and by adequate I mean personally adequate in the sense of avoiding very unpleasant emotion. The very early experiences would, if they continued long enough, unquestionably produce very marked effects on the developing personality of the infant, but here the intervention of the dynamism of apathy tones off, as it were, these instances of powerlessness, somewhat after the fashion that the old magic lanterns produced vignettes—you remember, something would fade out gradually, and later something would gradually come in. And so the intervention of the apathy processes, to which I have already referred, prevents a serious complicating effect from the relatively infrequent instances of the infant's powerlessness to produce the nipple by the cry.

I hope that I have made it clear that, even very early in life, frequent success has a very powerful influence in determining the character of foresight. I believe that I will not mislead you if I talk quite loosely and say that, given a pressing need which is increasing, it is not strange that the extremely young infant does not accumulate negative instances; and in any case the accumulation of negative instances is less apt to be significant because apathy has a sort of fade-out effect on things, and the chances of success upon the resumption of crying after sleep are pretty fair. Thus the relatively frequent, rather consistent success stamps in the magical power of the cry; and the occasional failures, due to the absence of the mother, and so on, do not greatly impair this growing conviction of what we would much later call a cause-and-effect relationship, which could be expressed—putting a great many words into the mouth of a very early infant—as, "I cry when I suffer a certain distress, and that produces something different which is connected with the relief of the distress."

This relief need not absolutely always occur for such convictions of relationship in the universe to become firmly entrenched in the infant. If this seems doubtful, let me say that one of the most conspicuous things we see, in the intensive study of personality, is the fantastic ease with which unnumbered negative instances can be overlooked for years in the area of one's more acute personal problems. It may even be that under certain circumstances, although not in very early infancy, a success which is purely an accident—that is, which is so exceedingly complex that it may be regarded as pure chance—may give rise to firm conviction that there is a vital causal relationship involved, and that if one could only do the right thing again it would produce the desirable result with which it was originally associated only by the merest and most terribly complex chance. So the erasing effect of negative experience is not very impressive, even from extremely early in life.[2]

Now what I have said thus far concerns the first of the special instances in which the infant's crying-when-hungry fails—the instance in which the provider of the nipple is absent. The second of the special instances, on the other hand, the case where anxiety is induced in the infant along with the showing up of the nipple, is to the infant an utterly different sort of experience. The ade-

[2] [*Editors' note:* The preceding three paragraphs are taken from Sullivan's 1948 lecture series, which was interrupted by his death. Earlier he had discussed these experiences of powerlessness as belonging generically to the field of the uncanny emotions—awe, dread, loathing, and horror. Sullivan remarked in his 1948 lecture, "Since this lecture series was originally prepared, I have changed my mind about uncanny emotion, about which I have done some fairly active thinking in the recent past. . . . It used to be very depressing to discover that I didn't agree with myself from one year to another, but ultimately I have found it rather encouraging. At least it gives me a chance to re-emphasize to you that psychiatry is a developing field, in which, perhaps, it is not to one's vast discredit that one does not become entirely and rigidly crystallized in the defense of what is an archaic idea. . . ."]

quate and appropriate crying-when-hungry has produced the nipple, but in the process has evoked anxiety; I am talking entirely from the standpoint of the infant, who is unable to discriminate anxiety as induced by the mother's anxiety—in fact, all of this is exterior to the clear understanding of the infant. But as mother draws near with her nipple—in other words, as from the infantile standpoint this mighty power of crying-when-hungry is about to bring results—lo, there comes the very severe drop in euphoria, in the general feeling of well-being, which is anxiety. Thus in this instance, while crying-when-hungry has produced the first step in the business, the nipple in the mouth, it has also brought anxiety—very severe tension which interferes with behavior activity in satisfaction of the need for water and food. What this must be like in infantile experience is suggested when I say that under these circumstances crying-when-hungry has produced a *different* nipple; the nipple now produced is not the same nipple, so far as the infant is concerned. The lips-nipple configuration is something new, and is anything but the satisfying lips-nipple configuration ordinarily produced; in fact, it is one that will not work, that is anything but relieving. It is, to use an exceedingly broad term in one of its exceedingly early relevancies, an evil eventuality which has arisen in connection with the oral zone of interaction, although we, in contradistinction to the infant, know that the anxiety has no primary or necessary relationship to the oral zone. On the contrary, the first time anything like this happens, it is perfectly certain that the anxiety in the mother which induced anxiety in the infant did not have any relation to the infant's taking nourishment. Afterward her anxiety may have something to do with the difficulties about feeding that characterized the first time she was anxious with her infant. But this is utterly outside the experience of the infant, and a matter of no consequence whatever in thinking about his experience, because the infant cannot differentiate the source of the anxiety. The anxiety is just there, and is extremely unpleasant; nothing that generally went right *does* go right, and the experience which unquestionably occurs—that is, the conjunction of nipple and lips—may actually be so clearly different that the infant rejects this particular nipple, will not hold it in his mouth, and therefore does not suck it.

Anxiety relates to the whole field of interpersonal interaction; that is, anxiety about *anything* in the mother induces anxiety in the infant. It doesn't need to have anything to do with the infant or the nursing situation. For example, as I mentioned before, a telegram announcing something of very serious moment to the prestige or peace of mind of the mother may induce a state of anxiety in her which induces anxiety in the infant; the infant's anxiety shows, so far as she is concerned, in this unexpected and exceedingly unsatisfactory difficulty in getting the infant to nurse. Now looking at it from the infant's standpoint, we can infer with certainty only that in this particular circumstance the outcome of ordinarily appropriate and adequate behavior when hungry—namely, crying-when-hungry—has produced the wrong nipple, a very evil situation with very unpleasant and unsatisfactory consequences.

Now oral rejection, in which the infant will not invest and hang on to the nipple, is not an appropriate and adequate way to deal with this particular evil or bad nipple. It does not in any way diminish or favorably affect the anxiety, which is induced by the mother's anxiety. In fact, if the mother is capable of noticing what's going on, and observes that the infant now rejects the nipple, avoids it, and will not hold and suck it, this will probably aggravate the mother's anxiety, adding a new anxiety, which will tend to aggravate the infant's anxiety. So mere rejection (you will remember that when first I spoke of the oral zone, I suggested that it accepted and rejected certain things) of this bad or anxiety-toned nipple is not adequate or appropriate: it doesn't reduce the anxiety, it certainly doesn't satisfy the need for food, and therefore it is a very perduring instance of the relationship of anxiety to living.

Now let me invite your attention briefly to something which I hope to express better later on. Even though anxiety is experience, and, as such, is total, and even though it has no necessary relationship to any particular zone of interaction, anxiety can be, as we put it, erroneously associated with a particular zone of interaction. For example, it may be erroneously associated with the mother's nipple, and consequently with the oral zone, since the nipple is significant to the infant only in connection with the oral zone at this very early stage—the infant has no interest in nipples except the nipple in the mouth or in the immediate proximity of the mouth. If the circumstances are something like those I have just discussed in my example of the mother made anxious by a telegram, there is no possibility of the infant's discriminating the irrelevance of his behavior in the oral zone of interaction, in rejecting the nipple, from something quite properly related to that zone of interaction as profitable experience—that is, extending backward and forward as recall and foresight. Now if you begin to grasp this aspect of anxiety-laden, or anxiety-colored, details of behavior, you will begin to have a hint of what a devastating complication of development frequent experiences of anxiety can be.

Here we have inferred what I believe perfect logical necessity requires: beginning discrimination by the infant of an actual nipple as two very different nipples, one conventional and desirable, the other evil and connected with, you might almost say, unending trouble. The more I talk about anxiety, the more you will see that this first appearance of anxiety which I have discussed is not so very different from an enormous number of the very troublesome results of anxiety in human living.

Signs, Signals, and Symbols in Early Experience

As I continue to build up data on which to support the statement of the concept of dynamism, we shall find the infant beginning to move out of the prototaxic and into the parataxic mode of experience, and perhaps the meaning of these modes may become more clear.

We have seen that recurrent physicochemical needs in the communal existence of the infant cause tension, the felt aspect of which later will be called the experience of, say, hunger and thirst. The experience of hunger includes the recall and the foresight of experiencing the satisfaction of hunger through adequate and appropriate behavior pertaining to one or more zones of interaction. This satisfactory, satisfaction-giving, adequate, and appropriate behavior *can be said* [3] to achieve a foreseen goal. The fore-

[3] By this I mean that it is perfectly appropriate to think in those terms if one has first thought in more valid terms before plunging into, for instance, the matter of "goal-directed behavior." Whenever I use these locu-

seen goal in this particular case is the satisfaction of hunger by means of crying-when-hungry and by means of the nursing behavior sequence which follows when crying-when-hungry has produced the nipple. The felt tension of hunger calls for crying-when-hungry. The nipple thus frequently evoked comes to be differentiated as the first significant step in satisfaction—the nipple comes to *mean* foreseen satisfaction. The tactile and thermal sentience arising from it in the region of the oral zone of interaction, and presently the organization of visual sentience about the nipple, comes to be a *sign* that satisfaction of hunger will follow. The novel terms I have introduced here are *goal* (which idea will not be developed for the present), *meaning*, and *sign*. The nipple is a *sign* that satisfaction of hunger will follow except when crying has evoked the evil or bad nipple with its aura of anxiety; and this latter eventuality, which we know is the case when the mother is anxious, comes to mean foreseen increasing distress.

At this point I wish to mention the term *prehension*, which I have used for a good many years. By prehension I mean what might be called the most rudimentary form of perception; in other words, the infant prehends the nipple-in-lips experience well in advance of his perceiving the nipple as something existing and durable and relatively independent of the lips. Prehension, in this sense of the very most rudimentary sort of perception, is a word that I like to use to remind you always that that which is prehended is important to the prehender, but is not, in any sense, the sort of full-blown experience that we ordinarily mean when we speak of *perceiving* something. Perception grows out of prehension, one might say, and, for all I know, this rudimentary process is always present behind perception; but as I go on with this idea, you will begin to see why I want a word that is less rich in meaning than is perception.

Thus the oral-tactile and the oral-thermal prehension, the visual

---

tions—such as *in a way of speaking*, or *it can be said*—I am suggesting that what I have previously attempted to communicate is more generally valid than the particular term that follows. There are a great many things that can be said which are all right in the particular universe or subuniverse of discourse in which they occur; but we are attempting to build up from more or less definitely indisputable evidence a particular referential language, so I shall attempt to indicate when I am not being exact in my language.

prehension, and the increasingly general tension associated with, or coincident with, the evocation of the bad nipple constitute a sign that evil consequences will follow. This sign and meaning aspect of experience is an exceedingly important one; from the study of this aspect of early experience we shall arrive presently in the exceedingly important field of language behavior. A sign is a particular pattern in the experience of events which is differentiated from or within the general flux of experience (at this stage of life, prototaxic experience); and this differentiation occurs in terms of recall and foresight of a particular frequent sequence of satisfaction or of increasing distress. The sign, as a pattern of experience, is a differentiation of frequently coincident elements in prototaxic experience of recurrent needs and satisfactions, and of recurrent anxiety or fear. A not uncommon eventuality in the infant's nursing behavior is the escape of the nipple from investiture by the lips—the incidents when the infant 'loses hold of' the nipple. Experience of the abrupt cessation of oral-tactile sentience arising from the presence of the nipple in the lips comes very early to be the signal for cessation of the sucking behavior; and it is the signal for the appearance of behavior which we can call searching for the nipple, with or without a resumption of crying-when-hungry. Here I have spoken of an abrupt cessation of certain inflowing 'stuff of sensation,' becoming or being a signal for a change of behavior. And let me say at this point that signals are a particular kind of signs. We will later discover that there are two major kinds of signs, of which the first, the one we have just discussed, is the signal.

At this point it is necessary for me to make rather a long digression on various matters which may be in your mind, to the confusion of or confounding of what I am attempting to communicate. And so at this point I invite you to notice that we are discussing prototaxic experience, not behavior as a nonrepresented aspect of neuro-muscular-glandular organization of the infant. I am not talking about the biology of nursing or neurophysiology when I speak of the abrupt cessation of influx over the afferent channels being a signal for a change in musculoglandular action. Of course, the neuro-muscular-glandular organization and the degree of its functional maturation at a particular time set limits to the possibility of experience. Such processes involving 'outer' and 'inner' factors are the raw materials out of which is made up the living of the living organism—the momentary states and the succession of momentary states of the organism which are the prototaxic experience of the organism; and the prototaxic experience includes the ultimate elements of all reference to the past and the neighboring future. Of course there are afferent impulses carried over sensory nerves, and the central integrating nervous system, and motor and secretory nerves going out to the mouth, and so on; but if you will realize that in addition to all that, there is *experience* and that we are dealing with experience, then perhaps you will understand what seemed to necessitate this digression.

Survival value may be a useful concept for accounting for the biological equipment of the infant. This sort of thinking, however, is exterior to our interest. Our concern is the formulation of psychiatrically significant aspects of human life, to which end we are now considering the processes by which the newborn human animal becomes a person. Our concern is not with the patterns of excitation in the central nervous system, and the abrupt or gradual changes in these patterns; rather we are concerned with an all-inclusive aspect of the dynamic organism-environment complex —the enduring influence of the tensional history of the organism's living on the present and the near-future living of the organism, to which we refer as more-or-less elaborated experience. The series of significant states of the organism-environment complex, all but the first elements of which include factors of the past and future—factors of history and potentiality, as it were, which make up the mnemic series—includes also secondary elements which are the organization or the elaboration of experience. The sign is such an organization or elaboration of experience; but, as such, it is also a part of living, so that signs, and behavior conditioned by signs, are experience. In the same way, that out of which they were elaborated, from which, we might say, they were evolved, is more primitive, or less elaborated experience. An experience is always the experience of an organism. Signs exist 'in' experience and not "outside in objective 'reality.' "

The comment which I have made—namely, that signs exist 'in'

experience and not somewhere else—may seem to be saying that the sign is a subjective rather than an objective "reality." In this and in much that I have said thus far it may seem that I am expressing, however obscurely, the 'philosophy' of "idealism," in contrast or as opposed to the 'philosophy' of "realism." I suggest that these and all other tangential issues be held in abeyance for the present and that you observe only that the meaning intended to be conveyed by the term, sign, is all that is immediately relevant. I believe that you will ultimately discover that discriminations of the nature of subjective versus objective, ideal versus real, and so on, are all quite irrelevant to an understanding of the theory which I am here attempting to set up.

Now, returning to our nursing infant, let us consider another frequent eventuality, the 'failure to get milk out of' a particular nipple—that is, failure to produce or to continue the experience of milk-to-be-swallowed by sucking a particular nipple or nipplelike object. This eventuality is a signal for relaxing the 'hold' on the nipple and searching for a different nipple, perhaps with crying-when-hungry. If the same nipple, now unproductive of milk, is 'found,' it is invested, sucked, but quickly relinquished. There is in this eventuality experience of the kind which will lead to the differentiation of a third class of nipples. So far we have had good and bad nipples, the bad one being the nipple of an anxious mother. The third class of nipples is that of nipples neither good nor bad, but *wrong,* in the sense of incorrect, in the further sense of unsuitable and useless in the satisfaction of hunger.

In the nursing behavior of very young offspring of some of the mammals with more than one pair of teats, such as dogs, cats, cows, and mares, we observe clearly another set of facts which is sometimes indicated in human nursing and occasionally very clearly observable—namely, the differentiation of preferred nipples, doubtless dependent on experience factors which are related to ease or difficulty of investing and 'holding,' or on factors of productivity in terms of returns on the effort of sucking. These are teats good and correct, but better or worse in terms of the oral experience in the satisfaction of hunger and thirst. This is so striking in some instances that, although along with multiple teats there usually go multiple births and there are as many puppies as there are mother's teats, or close to the same number, some of the teats will be large and blunt, or obtuse, and they will be so neglected that those breasts actually are in danger of caking. Clearly they give milk—as a matter of fact, not uncommonly they are more productive than some of the others; but, to talk in adult objective language, they are hard to hold, they slide out of the puppy's mouth very readily, and probably they take up so much space in the mouth that they make sucking somewhat more difficult than when only a small area of the lip surface is used in investing the nipples.

These sundry experiences with the nipple or teat may be listed as encounters with

(A-1) the good and satisfactory nipple-in-lips which is the signal—the uncomplicated signal—for nursing, and

(A-2) the good but unsatisfactory nipple-in-lips which is a signal for rejection until the need of hunger is great enough to make this good but unsatisfactory nipple acceptable.

(B) the wrong nipple-in-lips—that is, one that does not give milk any longer—which is a signal for rejection and search for another nipple, and

(C) the evil nipple, the nipple of an anxious mother which, so far as the infant is concerned, is a nipple preceded by the aura of extremely disagreeable tension—anxiety—which is a signal for avoidance, often even the avoidance of investing the nipple with the lips at all. So the signal might be converted into rather adult words by saying it is a signal for not-that-nipple-in-my-lips.

Groups A and B—encounters with good satisfactory and good unsatisfactory, and with wrong nipples—are experiences primarily of the oral zone of interaction; group C, on the other hand—the encounter with the anxiety-invested nipple—is experience of anxiety as an evil which has been evoked by the oral-zone behavior of crying-when-hungry. When one keeps in mind the delayed functional competence of the human visual apparatus and the condition of mammalian young which are "born blind"—that is, without the eyelids being opened—it is evident that experience in groups A and B is built out of the following types of sentience: vibratory and aural sentience arising from the crying-when-hungry; tactile, thermal, and kinesthetic sentience from the lips area; kinesthetic sentience from the sucking and swallowing performances; and tactile and gustatory sentience from the transportation of the milk across the tongue and through the pharyngeal passage. This is the sort of influx from the impinging events of which the nipple-in-lips is the prehension. As visual sentience is added to these experiences, and permits clear visual experience of something more than moving patterns of light and shade, nipples good and satisfactory can often be distinguished at a distance from nipples good but unsatisfactory. But there is no visually discriminable difference between the bad nipple of anxiety and the objectively identical nipple which on another occasion is good.

Discriminating differentiation of good and satisfactory, good and unsatisfactory, and wrong—that is, useless—nipples, is the first of an exceedingly important field of useful additions to behavior—in this case, behavior in the relief of hunger and thirst. It is peculiarly significant in the elaboration of behavior more appropriate and dependably adequate than the initial magically appropriate and adequate crying-when-hungry. The important idea to be grasped here is that the infant is beginning to acquire useful additions to his behavior, and that these useful additions are those which are more appropriate because they are less 'magical' and more dependably adequate than the preceding behavior which in the beginning was crying-when-hungry. And the elaboration of this more useful behavior comes about by the *identifying of differences* in what we call perceived objects. The extremely useful improvements of behavior in nursing which we are now discussing have as their raw material the discrimination of these sundry kinds of nipples, including the very awkwardly identical—that is, so far as visual sentience can go—good nipple and nipple of anxiety. From our standpoint, which has nothing to do with the infant, it is the same nipple, but carried in one case by a tender mother and in the other case by an anxious one. To repeat, the useful additions to the infant's behavior arise by identifying the difference in what we call perceived objects—that is, important, more-or-less independent aspects of the infant-environment complex—whether objectively of the infant or of the environment. It is necessary in thinking about this stage of human development to realize that while toes, fingers, and so on, can be identified even to the point where one finger is distinguished from another—actually the thumbs are the things that come in for special attention—still these are, to the infant, independent perceptual objects. Even though they, from our adult standpoint, 'belong to' the infant, the probability is that toes, and particularly big toes, are just as independent to the infant as mothers and nipples for some time after the infant's visual receptor has combined its activities with other receptors concerned in the oral zone.

If I may digress again for a moment, I would like to comment on the fact that there are some rather startling coincidences in the make-up of the central nervous system, although I do think that biological and neurophysiological terms are utterly inadequate for studying everything in life. The most astonishing example that I can think of offhand is the coincidence in a receptor area of the afferent inflowing impulse nerves from around the middle of the lips in immediate juxtaposition to afferent nerve endings from the thumbs and also the neighboring side of the index finger. Now there is a day coming doubtless, long after we will all have been embalmed in history, when it will be possible in some fashion to translate these interesting and exciting coincidences in, say, the realm of neuroanatomy into some of what we have to learn in a quite different universe of discourse—namely, psychology, so-called psychobiology, and psychiatry. Although it is important to remember that that which is 'given' in structure sets limits to what may be possible in behavior and, even more broadly, in experience, we actually will very seldom be discussing structurally given things. When we are, I will make particular effort to invite attention to the fact that here does seem to be a correlation of 'somatic' organization with psychiatrically important phenomena. I hope that you will not try to build up in your thinking correlations that are either purely imaginary or relatively unproven, which may give you the idea that you are in a solid, reliable field in contrast to one which is curiously intangible; such a feeling of reliability is, I think, an illusion born out of the failure to recognize that what we know comes to us through our *experiencing* events, and is therefore always separated from anything really formed or transcendentally real by the limited channels through which we contact what we presume to be the perduring, unknown universe. So if a person really thinks that his thoughts about nerves and synapses and the rest have a higher order of merit than his thoughts about signs and symbols, all I can say is, Heaven help him.

I shall now return to my discussion of the independent aspects of the infant-environment complex, which are identified as similar perceived objects, but among which differences come to be identified. This identifying of differences among perceived objects is the precursor, in two senses, of any *re*-cognition: it is a precursor in the sense that it invariably antecedes recognition; and it is a precursor in all acts of recognition, because the differences evoke references to the past, in the process of which the experience of similar differences is effective in causing what we lump under the term *I recognize.*

The infant's identifying eventually progresses to the point where he is able to generalize experience that is marked with the characteristics of several zones of interaction as experience pertaining to *one* recurrent pattern of sentience from the distance receptors, which pattern is frequently evoked by the infant's crying (whether it be crying-when-hungry, crying-when-cold, or whatever). When he has progressed to this point, he has begun to experience living in an elaboration which is beyond the prototaxic mode. We might say that he is experiencing the good mother in the parataxic mode. Generalizing, then, is a particular development in the identifying of differences; it is, we might say, what is left of things that are similar when the differences have been identified. In other words, the forms of experience are generalized so that things in common in them, as well as all their sundry differences, are in perception as useful experience. These influxes of experience are marked by any one of several zones of interaction. Perhaps I can make all this clear by putting it in another way. We know from our ivory tower that the same mothering one, the *same* mother, produces, for instance, a nipple when the infant is hungry, produces blankets when the infant is cold, produces dexterous manipulation when the infant is on a safety pin that is open, and, needless to say, changes the diapers when that is a most suitable and timely activity. Although we, from our objective superiority, know that the *same mother* does all this, it is necessary to study what can be inferred with some certainty as to what goes on in the infant: Originally all these needs which the mother cooperates in meeting are marked or colored by the zone of interaction with the environment in which the sentience related to the need and its satisfaction had its origin; thus, we have already set up the difference, objectively invisible and indetectable, between crying-when-hungry, crying-when-cold, and so on. Now we come to the infant's ability to generalize, to detect the factors in *common* in the 'cooperating' person (who, needless to say, is not perceived in that elaborate fashion); all of this is generalized experience arising from, and distinguished by, more than one zone of interaction. Furthermore, this experience is generalized as pertaining to one recurrent pattern of sentience of the eyes and ears, the distance receptors, which is frequently evoked by crying-when-hungry, by crying-when-cold, and so forth, which in turn is generalized as *crying*. Thus the infant is generalizing also about crying, progressing from all these different kinds of perhaps identical-sounding crying, to crying as a generalization of what is identical or what is *not different* in these various vocal operations of crying. We might speak of this as analytic synthesis because it eliminates differences and finds that which is common to very important aspects of the infant-environment complex which are necessary for life. When we come, in living, to the point where this sort of synthesis is taking place, we encounter a degree of elaboration of experience which is removed from what I have thus far discussed—namely, experience in the prototaxic or earliest mode, in which one, as it were, 'lives one's living.'

The identifying of differences can make very useful contributions to behavior in the satisfaction of needs; and the generalizing of experience so that the significant common factors mixed in with the differences are identified or connected with one recurrent pattern of experience, primarily mediated by the distance receptors, elevates the complexity or elaboration of experience from the prototaxic to the parataxic mode of experience. I hope that it begins to be clear why I have set up these modes of experience—the prototaxic, the parataxic, and the syntaxic. The prototaxic mode, as I have suggested, is a very early form of, and presently a very strikingly odd form of, living as a living being.

On any given occasion, the experience of vision by and large takes place before there is contact with tactile, thermal, kinesthetic, gustatory, or olfactory end organs; the auditory experience takes place in the same way, as soon as the infant develops and hears sounds other than his own crying. In the same way, experience with anxiety, like experience through the distance receptors, begins before there is contact with any of the contact receptors—that is, begins before the anxious mother and her nipple reach the infant's mouth—but not, you remember, before light waves reach the infant's eyes or sound waves reach the infant's ears from the mother. Since anxiety has in common with the function of these distance receptors the fact that it begins before there is any contact with a nipple, any 'profiting' by the experience with the nipple of anxiety *must be* by wave discriminations, primarily referable to the functional activity of the auditory and visual distance receptors, a process which is more inclusive than seeing the nipple and its immediate adnexa. The nipple and the breast and the arrangement of clothing, and so on, of an anxious mother need be in no physically discriminable sense at all different from those of the tender nonanxious mother. And so, if there is to be any *useful* addition to behavior with respect to anxiety, it must arise by discriminating something not pertaining to that which really matters at this stage—namely, the nipple, nursing, and so on. Yet the functional activity of the distance receptors, hearing and sight, gives no gross clues to success or failure of crying-when-hungry in bringing to the infant the carrier of the good nipple, the good mother, in contrast to the most unpleasant experience of bringing to the infant the carrier of the nipple of anxiety, the bad mother, with her foreshadowing aura of anxiety.

Differentiation of the 'appearance'—that is, of distance receptor data—of the bad mother from that of the good mother is a complex refinement of visual and auditory perception which is called into being under the driving force of what we may call a desire to avoid anxiety, an inhering 'preference' for relative euphoria. To give a little hint of what I am talking about here, it may be useful for me to refer to my bitch and her puppies. While it is unfortunately true that dogs are so organized and so reared that they suffer anxiety provoked by anxious or tense people around them, still, by and large, the experience of the evil nipple or the nipple of anxiety by puppies is rare. But there comes a time in the life of the puppy, which in many respects I think is importantly connected with the development of his teeth, when nursing does not seem to be quite the right thing to encourage, and the mother then provokes in the puppies puppy-anxiety; I surmise that this includes very real elements of fear, since the mother has no hesitancy in inflicting pain in discouraging further nursing behavior.

I mention this to stress the statement previously made, which I would now like to repeat. Differentiation of the 'appearance' (and I hope you will notice that appearance is not the exact word here because it includes distance reception by the ear) of the bad mother from that of the good mother is a complex refinement—a visual and auditory perception which is called into being by the driving necessity of protecting one's euphoria, one's feeling of well-being, from anxiety, so far as one can. And since there is no gross perceptible difference, this differentiation can only be accomplished by a refinement. Thus there comes into being the first instance of another class of signs of which the current instance is the discrimination of what we may call *forbidding gestures*, presently to be referred to the perceived mothering one who has been fused into one, by this generalizing process, out of the earlier, separate, perceived objects, the good mother and the bad mother. This matter of the infant's refined discrimination of what we call forbidding gestures first applies to the mother and thereafter applies throughout life to practically all significant people—that is, those people who come to have an important place in his living, in other words, his interpersonal relationships. The discrimination of heard differences in the mother's vocalization and seen differences in the postural tensions [4] of the mother's face, and perhaps later of differences in speed and rhythm of her gross bodily movements in coming toward the infant, presenting the bottle, chang-

[4] Of course, postural tensions are not seen—the skin is seen—but I am talking about the configuration of the face, the appearance of the face as determined by the postural tensions of the so-called expressive muscles of the head.

ing the diapers, or what not—all these rather refined discriminations by the distance receptors of vision and hearing are organized as indices frequently associated with the unpleasant experience of anxiety, including the nipple of anxiety instead of the good nipple. As such indices, these discriminations, the organization of the data of these discriminations, become *signs of signs*—signs for other signs of avoidance, such as the nipple when the mother is anxious. So these discriminations by the distance receptors become signs of categories of signs, one might say, which so frequently follow that it suffices for the establishment of this relation. And signs of signs we call symbols. Thus while signals are rather simply related to behavior, symbols are more complexly related, in that they refer to sundry signals which affect behavior. And those symbols which we call forbidding gestures mean anxiety interfering with behavior in the satisfaction of a need.

To the mothering one, the heard crying of the infant is a sign that the infant is experiencing a need or is anxious. It signalizes the infant's generic need for tenderness, for some one or more of the sundry procedures required as cooperation in the satisfaction of the infant's needs or for the relief of his anxiety. The audible components of a whole series of different magic acts of the infant, his crying-when-hungry, crying-when-cold, and the like, evoke tender behavior of the mothering one and mean to her the infant's need for tenderness of one kind or another.

To be more exact about what the infant's crying is and does, one may say that his heard crying is physically a special pattern of sound waves which are emitted by his mouth and received by the mother's ears, and that this crying communicates the infant's need by, as we may say, being thus *interpreted* by the mother. The single generic meaning which might be phrased as 'baby needs tenderness' exists not 'in' the infant but 'in' the mother. This illustrates the relationship of a sign and its interpreter. In the language of Charles Morris, "any organism for which something is a sign will be called an *interpreter*." [5] The expression "organism

[5] [Charles Morris, *Signs, Language and Behavior;* New York: Prentice-Hall, Inc., 1946, p. 17.

Editors' note: At this point in the lecture, Sullivan added: "Incidentally, in my old age it is my unhappy fate that I can refer to nothing in the way of elaborate statements of views and ideas with which I find myself perfectly

for which" would be more suitably expressed, from my standpoint, as *organism 'in' which*. The sign interpretation evoked by experiencing the sign is educed by the experiencing organism from the present or actual encounter with the sign, on the basis of past and foreseen experience. Living with road signs, red and green lights, telephone bells, and the like makes it easy to overlook the absolute dependence of signs, as significant details of human experience, on the persons who thus interpret their encounters with the corresponding nonsignatory physical events.

Thus I would like to wean you somewhat from the very easy idea that a sign can exist irrespective of any organism to, for, or in which it is a sign. That is all right if you are trying to arrange automobile traffic on a chart, or by means of laws and statutes. But in developing a theory of personality you must remember that signs *are* signs only when there is an interpreter to attach meaning to a body of otherwise physical phenomena.

The infant acts to relieve a particular need, and the audible component of his act is experienced by the mother as a sign that he needs tender cooperation in satisfying some need, or for the relief of anxiety. Now as the infant's ability to prehend visible aspects of his surroundings grows, he comes to differentiate two signs in this connection: the sign of impending satisfaction (the appearance of and approach of the good mother), and the sign of trouble (the appearance of and approach of the bad mother). As the organization of his experience progresses, the infant comes to foresee that by his crying *in general* he will accomplish the appearance, approach, and satisfying cooperation of the good mother, or the appearance and distressing approach of the bad mother, in which latter eventuality, he will then cry to be rid of her and of her attendant anxiety.

Now here I am discussing how *any* crying of the very young infant is a sign to the mother, if she hears it, that the infant needs tenderness. From the infant's standpoint, as he gets his visual and auditory receptors into good working order by developmental

in harmony. I should have mentioned this before in quoting from my greatly esteemed late friend Sapir, as well as Cottrell and Benedict and others. I believe that many of you will find Morris' book very valuable in clarifying thought, although I have already expressed considerable difference with its beginning presentation."]

process in his organization, he begins to differentiate two signs of what is about to happen, namely, success or disaster; and as this progresses a little further he cannot fail—from mere frequency of instances, or absence of frequent negative instances—to notice that any crying he does brings either the sign of forthcoming satisfaction or relief, or the sign of the disaster of anxiety. So his crying can in a way now take on sign aspects, in that he is using it in, or it is fitting into, a pattern of adequate and appropriate behavior, which he observes. His own heard crying is coming to mean that he is experiencing a need and is acting to evoke the sign that satisfaction will follow, or perhaps the unwelcome sign of anxiety and increasing distress which calls for a different act of crying—crying to be rid of the bad mother. To the infant, the prehended—that is, primitively perceived—good mother is the symbol of forthcoming satisfaction; and the prehended bad mother is the symbol of anxiety and increasing distress. Generically, tender cooperation is meant by the good mother; urgently increased need for tenderness is meant by the bad mother and by the forbidding gestures which are gradually differentiated as her distinguishing perceived characteristics.

I have already attempted to indicate that there is no visual difference between a good and satisfactory nipple on the mother's breast and the same nipple when the mother is anxious. But so far as the infant's experience is concerned, these nipples are extremely different and call for entirely different treatment or behavior; and because they cannot readily be distinguished by vision, as in the case with some other things, there is, owing to the particular evolutionary history of the human animal, a distinct need to find some clues by which one can be oriented. Now I am using very adult language. If, to speak now of my puppies, their mother has one teat which is very large and also has a lot of black on it, whereas some nice handy teats are just pink, that makes it doubly simple for a puppy, when he can see, to recognize the unsatisfactory character of this large nipple, which is hard to hold although it is otherwise good. We are very strongly oriented by vision, when we can use it, that being a characteristic of the human animal beyond doubt. Where the visual sentience is grossly the same—but the objects concerned are terribly different, in that the one is a good thing and gives satisfaction, while the other is a minor disaster and must be avoided—under those circumstances, other clues are looked for. As I have said before, all this discussion of nipples applies, of course, a little later to the carriers of the nipple, the good and the bad mother, who, however, again are visually grossly identical. More refined discrimination is called for and becomes possible, including the discrimination of differences in the audible aspects of the good and the bad mother, as well as discriminations in the facial expression—that is, the results of postural tensions in the face—of the good and the bad mother. Now speaking objectively, which is charmingly simple and very apt to be misleading, we would say that the mother sounds and looks different when she is anxious from the way she sounds and looks when she is not anxious. These differences are the possible distance clues, we might say, to whether one has got what one wants or whether one has got the wrong thing, namely, the bad mother. This discrimination of good and bad mothers, like the discrimination of good and bad nipples, is, at this particular developmental period, just as real as is your discrimination of a person sitting next to you.*

* [*Editors' note:* In his 1948 lecture series, Sullivan developed this idea somewhat differently:

"Initially nothing like an extended visual grasp of the mother exists, although it unfolds fairly rapidly. So far as gross visual data are concerned, there is no particular difference between the good mother and the bad mother as a visual percept. There are, however, certain refined differences, but even before these become significant, other aspects of the distance contact with the mother have shown in all likelihood quite material refinements. Those that are associated with the good mother require no vast attention, but anything that gives warning of, or differentiates the bad mother—the source of anxiety—will, because of the extremely disagreeable nature of anxiety, get as much attention as can be given it. And the distance data in that field are heard data, vocal and tonal details, and so on.

"In particular, restrictions on the tonal scope of the voice probably are the first forbidding gestures that are built into the separate personification of the bad mother in contrast to her physically identical counterpart, the good mother. It is clear in dealing with domesticated animals, and it is certainly very clear in later phases of human life after infancy, that a great deal of what might be called 'the way the wind blows' is conveyed tonally; it has nothing in particular to do with verbal content, but is instead a matter of how verbal content is expressed, and the like. So the first forbidding gestures, and among the world's most dependable forbidding gestures that human beings ever differentiate in the interest of avoiding anxiety and pain,

I particularly want to note here that the forbidding gestures are, so to speak, pared or peeled off from the bad mother, and become occasional characteristics of an unspecified mother at a later stage of development; by that time these forbidding gestures, these audible and visible differences in the mother, are becoming signs in themselves of impending anxiety. This is a hint of how entities originally quite different to the infant—different because their functional significance is quite different, although we objectively say they are the same thing—are gradually fused in the infantile perception as the same or similar things. But that can happen only when there is a refinement of differentiation so that the infant is able to separate out the very important functional differences of the different nipples, for example, from his experience with the common carrier of the nipple.

I am here attempting to set before you a course of development based on what *must* be, to account for the useful and necessary things that are done by the infant. Even though many of us as adults spend most of our time doing things that seem, at least to our friends, utterly useless, nevertheless it is an extreme and, I believe, completely unjustifiable use of inference to reach a conclusion that the infant does a great many useless and troublesome things.

---

are undoubtedly changes in an accustomed voice. To the infant, in all likelihood, it is not a question of changes in a voice, but of two different accustomed voices. But from then on, there are few things more effective at changing the immediate integration of interpersonal situations than certain tonal tricks which come to us very, very naturally because they are, in a very real sense, the second oldest thing that has been very important in our experience with producing, hearing, and interpreting the voice."]

CHAPTER 6

Infancy: The Concept of Dynamism—Part 2

The Integration, Resolution, and Disintegration of Situations

WE SHALL now consider the infant's success or misfortune in bringing about the appearance, approach, and cooperation of the good mother in connection with the satisfaction of a need. To start again with the conception of euphoria disturbed by tension, it is evident that the recurrent tension of a physicochemical need—felt, say, as the need for food—may be considered as a tendency to bring about juncture of the good and satisfactory nipple and the infant's lips, which juncture is in turn a situation necessary for nursing behavior and the satisfaction of hunger. Since the nipple is a thing that is only there now and then, I shall turn that statement around, and say that the nipple-in-lips situation, originally evoked by crying-when-hungry, is the concatenation of events which is required for beginning and continuing nursing behavior until hunger and thirst shall have been satisfied.

Work—in physical terminology, not in the popular or personal sense—is done in effecting the nipple-in-lips situation, in maintaining it, and in remedying more-or-less accidental interruption of it until hunger is satisfied, whereupon the transformations of energy which make up this work cease. Now work, or transformations of energy, is actually functional activity, which is one of the three fundamentally important aspects of all living. We may say that the tension felt as hunger tends to *integrate* the nipple-in-lips situation and to maintain this integration of the nipple and the infant's mouth as long as the tension itself continues. Considering the infant's hunger and certain other needs as the generic need for tenderness to the extent that their satisfaction requires the cooperation of an older person, we may say that the sundry tensions underlying this need for tenderness generically tend to integrate, and to maintain the integration of, sundry interpersonal infant-mother situations which are manifestly necessary for the survival of the infant. From this standpoint, the satisfaction of a need is the ceasing of an integrating tendency to manifest itself in work.

I am now reviewing from a different standpoint all the elements, ideas, and facts which I have touched upon—needs and their satisfaction, signs and their meaning, and the whole story of the very early behavior of the infant beginning with the simplest thing, namely, the nipple-in-lips situation brought about from the infant's standpoint by crying-when-hungry—in order to shed more light on what I am presenting. Thus I say that from this standpoint of the interpersonal situation, we have to consider a tension, which includes the felt tension of a need, as a tendency to integrate a situation necessary and appropriate to the satisfaction of the need; and since the infant in the early months is practically wholly incapable of getting along without a mothering one, his needs manifest themselves, even from his very earliest activities, as tendencies to integrate particular types of necessary situations with the mothering one. And from this standpoint the satisfaction of a need, the relaxation of the tension underlying the felt aspects of a need, can be said to represent the ceasing, the ending, the temporary abeyance of an integrating tendency manifesting itself in the work of maintaining the interpersonal situation. The situation brought into being by the integrating tendency lapses with cessation of the work done in its maintenance; and since the situation was necessary and adequate for the satisfaction of a need, we may say that the satisfaction of this underlying need has *resolved* the related interpersonal situation. Now you will come presently to see why I talk of situations being resolved when there is no longer any integrating tendency to maintain them.

I have been discussing the tensions of needs from the standpoint of their being integrating tendencies, tendencies to integrate appropriate and necessary situations which happen to be interpersonal. Consider now the case in which the mother is or becomes anxious, thus inducing anxiety 'in' the infant. It is evident that anxiety generically tends to interfere with the integration of the interpersonal situation necessary for the satisfaction of a need, and that if anxiety appears at any time in the course of a situation toward resolution, it will tend to disintegrate any such situation. Now I make a careful distinction in using the term *resolution* of an interpersonal situation. It is something very different indeed from the *disintegrating* of that situation. When a situation resolves itself, it ceases to exist for the time being—and actually ceases to exist at all, because it will be a new situation when the same need integrates something very like it again. This resolution or ending of an interpersonal situation comes about by the relaxing of the tension of need, by the achieving of satisfaction of the need, whereas the situation may be prevented from being integrated, or may be disintegrated—torn apart—by the occurrence of anxiety. If anxiety comes, instead of a suitable object for integration, it makes 'impossible' the integrating of a suitable situation.

Let us assume, for example, that the infant is nursing away right merrily when something makes the mother notably anxious. That anxiety, as I have long since mentioned, immediately induces, in some fashion, anxiety in the infant. Then all sorts of difficulties occur, such as letting go of the nipple, cessation of search for the lost nipple, actually repelling the nipple if it is brought near the infant's lips, and even regurgitation instead of the swallowing of milk. Now there is an important fringe of behavior connected with nursing to which I have not previously referred; I shall hint at it by saying that in certain circumstances the infant may even, on the eventuality of anxiety, act as though he were being restrained when he is held in the necessary proximity to the breast so that the nipple can be invested. This may lead to the kind of miscellaneous activity, which can in a vague way be regarded as phylogenetically evolved, by which the infant escapes situations imperiling the oxygen supply.

Now, if we consider all that can follow on the occurrence of anxiety in the mother while the infant is nursing, we will have a better impression of the difference between the resolution of an interpersonal situation when, as it were, there is no earthly reason for its continuing, and the disintegration of that situation while there is still plenty of reason for its continuing. The fact is that the nipple of an anxious mother will still give milk, and that even though anxiety appears in the midst of nursing there is still a need for food; in other words, there is plenty of tension to keep up the nursing behavior, but the interpersonal situation is destroyed—it breaks up. Here is the difference between the disintegration of an interpersonal situation and its resolution by ceasing to have any rationale, any reason for existence, for the time being.

I have already discussed needs as integrating tendencies. I now invite attention to the fact that anxiety is a disjunctive or disintegrative tendency in interpersonal relations, which opposes the manifestation of any integrative tendency in the work of creating and maintaining an interpersonal situation; anxiety so modifies the transformations of energy making up the functional activity of the infant that work is now done to escape from, or to avoid, the interpersonal situation which corresponds to the significant need. Anxiety opposes the type of work which reflects the activity of an integrating tendency; anxiety opposes those transformations of energy which manifest themselves in the investing and holding of the nipple, in the sucking activity, in the transporting and swallowing, and in sundry accessory activities which I will deal with presently. All these things are, as I say, opposed by a disjunctive tendency, of which anxiety is the present outstanding instance before us. We shall see later that, so far as interpersonal relations are concerned, anxiety is almost always, but not quite always, an outstanding ingredient in breaking up interpersonal situations which otherwise would be useful in the satisfaction of the needs of the person concerned. It is evident that the eventuality of anxiety in no way relaxes the tension of need, but only opposes it.

If we think of a particular need as a tendency to integrate a situation in which activity is directed toward the goal of satisfactory resolution of the situation, we are considering a *vector* quality in the conception of integrating tendency. We can then picture anxiety as exactly opposed to the directional component of any need with the satisfaction of which it collides. I would like to remind you of the conception of vector, which might be defined as magnitude plus direction. Now the element of direction is the very significant thing in the conception of vector. My justification for talking about vectors at this time is that an interpersonal situation is not to be considered as something static, like, for example, the situation of objects on the table before me. Statics hasn't very much to do with living.

The interpersonal situation integrated by the infant's hunger plus the mother's need to express tenderness is characterized by a direction toward the goal of satisfying the infant's hunger, and the situation manifests this direction toward the goal by the fact that activity goes on which clearly achieves that goal. Now this directional element applies to the type of consideration of need which is implied by describing the need as an integrating tendency —that is, a tendency to bring about and maintain a situation, which in turn implies change toward the resolution of that situation, which happens, from another viewpoint, to coincide with the satisfaction of the need which started the whole business.

If you think of this direction of activity toward a goal, which is implied by the tension of need, then you can think of anxiety as exactly, that is; at 180 degrees, opposed to the vector quality of the need. If you think in terms of vector addition, as it is used in physical theory, you will remember that in the parallelogram of force, one vector goes off in one direction, and another goes in another direction, and the resultant vector is accurately depicted as the diagonal of the completed parallelogram. If you think in these terms, you will realize that anxiety—which complicates, by exact opposition, the manifestation of an integrating tendency in some particular direction—can mean only a *reduction* of, or a *reversal* of, the transformations of energy concerned in the action in the situation; that is, anxiety results in *less* activity toward the goal of satisfaction, or it results in activity *away* from the achievement of that goal. Anxiety added to, let us say, hunger during the nursing situation means therefore not that something new, a diagonal, comes out of these two things. Instead, the net result is either that, although nursing goes on, there is much *less* activity; or that something which is diametrically *opposed* to nursing, to the satisfaction of the need for hunger, occurs.

Now we will come later to many situations in life where two opposing vectors *do* add up to produce a third—where there is opposition to a certain type of activity, and, somewhat in accord with the physical pattern of the parallelogram of force, a new direction of the activity results. This new vector represents, from the physical standpoint, the discharge of both integrating tendencies, which occurs, however, by the integration of a *different* situation, in which action toward resolution, the achievement of a goal, is again evident. But in the very early situation where the infant is, at least for our purpose of discussion, activated by a single need—the need for food—the appearance of anxiety results, not in a new direction of activity, but in either a reduction of nursing activity, or in the complete disintegration and avoidance of a situation suitable for nursing. And this, as I have said, can be represented in physics by drawing two vector qualities 180 degrees apart, the resultant being either a reversal of motion that was previously present, or a very marked reduction in its acceleration. While this collision of a need, which may be thought of as an integrating tendency, with anxiety has but two possible outcomes from this standpoint—very much reduced velocity, you might say, or a reversal of direction—at the same time there is more tension now involved than was concerned in the need alone. In other words, vector considerations are perfectly all right to account for activity; but a much more intricate field, namely, tensor considerations, applies to the disturbances of euphoria which are, needless to say, much greater when two opposing tensions collide than when only one of them exists.

I have now begun to talk in terms familiar to the physicist—a course which I shall pursue somewhat further in discussing the terms, work and energy. You may recall that energy is sometimes defined as the capacity for doing work; or, more carefully, as that which diminishes when work is done, by an amount equal to the work done. You may be wondering whether I shall presently be considering something like a special "mental" energy. The answer to that question is this: Energy, when I mention it, is energy as conceived in physics, and as such has two basic forms—potential and kinetic. And work, as I use the term, is conceived in its physical meaning, not something you detest but have to do for a living.

I think that it might be useful to mention at this point one of the simplest illustrations of the discrimination of potential from kinetic energy in the realm of physics, since my use of the term, potential, in any of these discussions is pretty close to the physical meaning of the term. Imagine a simple pendulum, such as you can make by attaching a plumb bob or a watch or something or other to a string and tying the other end of the string to a nail so that the watch, plumb bob, or what not, is in free space, as it is called. If you then set it to swinging, you will find that at the end of its lateral motion it stops; for an instant it stands still. It swings in one direction, pauses instantaneously, and starts swinging back. All of the energy of the pendulum is potential at the moment of its fullest swing, when it is still; but if you should ever let such a pendulum hit you on the head, you would realize that there must have been quite a good deal of potential energy in it at that moment. So potential does not mean imaginary, or something of that kind, any more than electrical potential—which is another use of the same term—is imaginary, as putting your finger on a 33,000-volt circuit would clearly suggest to you by its consequences.

The Concept Itself: Background and Implications for Psychiatry

REVIEW OF TRIBUTARY CONCEPTS

By blend of the various considerations which I have now discussed I have arrived at the point of being able to set up—I hope with some clarity—an exceedingly important conception in this theory of psychiatry. This conception is the conception of dynamism, which is, I think, a vast improvement over the ancient idea of mental mechanisms and the like.

First I would like to review some of the conceptions we have discussed which play their parts in my conception of dynamism. We have held that any living organism may be considered in terms of three ultimate factors: its communal existence with a necessary environing medium; its organization; and its functional activity. We have said that man, the person, may be considered as an organism requiring in its necessary environing medium other persons, with whom functional activity occurs, and some part of the world of culture which is implicit in personality, and which becomes organized in the person himself.

We have introduced as fundamental terms in the analysis thus far the concepts of experience, of euphoria, and of recurrent tensions of two kinds, tensions of need and tensions of anxiety, with some mention of a third kind of tension which we will discuss *in extenso* later—tensions of sleep. We have discussed these recurrent tensions as manifest in awareness as felt components, and, in relation to the environing medium, as integrating or disjunctive tendencies with respect to situations in which activity—that is, behavior—addressed to the satisfaction of needs can occur. We have indicated that the relaxation of tensions, with the relief—that is, satisfaction—of their felt components requires, in the early phases of postnatal life, tender cooperation, additional to the behavior of the infant in crying-when-hungry, crying-when-cold, and the like. We have generalized the infant's needs as those for oxygen; for water; for foodstuffs; for body temperature; and, more vaguely, for bodily integrity and freedom, and adequate physiological process, these latter perhaps being susceptible to statement as the need to be free of pain and the need to be free of restraint of bodily movement. We digressed at this point to consider the fact that delayed relaxation of naturally increasing tension, which endangers life, is attended by the appearance of the felt tension of fear, which has its particular type of crying, crying-when-afraid; and that this tension of fear could reach a maximum with the felt component called terror and activity of the sort which later in life would appropriately be called rage behavior.

We have indicated that, since the satisfaction of all the infant's needs requires tender cooperation of another, all of them may be considered as implying, at the interpersonal level, a need for tenderness. But the satisfaction of this need for tenderness, and the concurrent satisfaction of the particular tension primarily concerned, is definitely interfered with by anxiety. We have considered in some detail the relation of the infant's crying to the occurrence of tender cooperation necessary for the satisfaction of the infant's needs, and subsequently, the breathing and nursing activities, which, as it were, begin in and around the mouth. This introduced us to the conception of the zone of interaction in the communal existence of the infant with environments physicochemical and interpersonal, with particular emphasis on the oral zone, including the hearing of the infant's audible productions. The meaning of the infant's perhaps 'objectively' identical crying-when-hungry, crying-when-cold, and the like, was mentioned; all of the infant's crying communicates to the mother the infant's need for tenderness, but has no such initial general meaning to the infant, as these various forms of crying are experienced by him. That is, in the infant's experience, his various types of crying initially have no general meaning of a need for tenderness, although they all mean that to the mother.

I have said that we have considerable reason for believing that experience in its simplest, least elaborate form—that is, prototaxic experience of some momentary state of the organism—carries, as an inevitable feature of the experience itself, indication of the zone of interaction where whatever was experienced has impinged; thus, experience from the lips is definitely marked with its origin in that area and is inherently different from experience from the fingertip. Prototaxic experience is, in a way, an enduring record of the total state of the organism, including the impinging events, or rather their effects on the zone of interaction impinged with.

We then considered a number of practically inevitable eventualities in the infant's early nursing behavior, and inferred from a number of these something of their meaning in the development of the infant's experience of living. From this came a consideration of the very important conception of signs in their two basic types: the signal and the symbol, the latter being a sign of other signs, or of whole categories of signs. In addition to the previously suggested signal character of crying-when-hungry, crying-when-cold, and the like, as heard and otherwise experienced by the infant, we inferred the occurrence of four different signals which must evolve from experience of the nipple in conjunction with the lips—or, in the case of the fourth signal, in forceful disjunction with the lips; these four signals are the good and satisfactory nipple-in-lips, the good but unsatisfactory nipple-in-lips, the wrong nipple-in-lips, and the evil nipple-in-lips. The differentiation of signs of other signs or categories of signs—that is, symbols—was illustrated by reference to the early prehension of the good mother and her anxiety-evoking counterpart, the bad mother, with subsequent differentiation of the forbidding gestures which significantly characterize her.

We stressed at this point the basic relationship of a sign and the possessor or interpreter of the sign, warning against the error of objectifying the observable characteristics of anything as identical with, or necessarily related to, its signatory reality as a particular pattern in the infant's, or other organism's, experience of events. In this connection you may recall my comment about road signs, which objectively are pieces of tin on stakes, presenting patterns of reflection, but which are seen by the eye as patterns to which meaning is attached, particularly if your previous experience has included learning to drive a car and to avoid the police in so doing. The piece of tin on a stake which is stuck along the road is a sign in the police sense, but that piece of tin on a stake, and the letters on it, is a sign in our sense only insofar as it evokes its appropriate meaning in the person who perceives it. The *person* has the sign.

This point of the relationship of sign and the interpreter of the sign was developed by reviewing the communication to the mother of the infant's need for tenderness by the audible components of several different actions of the infant, which are experienced by him as behavior in the satisfaction of several needs, and for the relief of anxiety—and which are only presently to be generalized by him as evoking the good mother, or exorcising the bad mother when she unfortunately is 'produced' by crying or other activities. The nipple-in-lips was then considered from the standpoint of its constituting a situation necessary for the occurrence of nursing behavior and the satisfaction of hunger and thirst, the tension of which underlying needs could be conceptualized as recurrent forces which integrate these necessary, actually interpersonal, situations, and which perform work in maintaining them for the duration of their recurrent utility. We then reviewed anxiety from this dynamic standpoint and saw that it is not an integrating tendency, but a disjunctive one which, when coincident, exactly opposes, in the vector sense, the force of any integrative need.

Having thus come to a useful statement in the realm of the transformation of physical energy, which is the only kind of energy

I know, and the vector characteristics of two of the three genera of basic tensions (sleep not yet concerning us), I shall proceed now to a statement of the concept of dynamism.

STATEMENT OF THE CONCEPT OF DYNAMISM

Let me begin by saying that the present view of the universe, as held by a great majority of mathematicians, physicists, and other scientists, makes the discoverable world a dynamism. This is implied in the fundamental postulate that the ultimate reality in the universe is energy, that all material objects are manifestations of energy, and that all activity represents the dynamic or kinetic aspect of energy. A doctrine in which force and the conception of energy—which underlies the conception of force—is the ultimate conception or postulate would naturally be a conception of dynamism, a dynamism of the universe. Whitehead, among the philosophers, has conceived the universe as an organism,[1] and certainly there is no difficulty in seeing living organisms as particular dynamisms. Living organisms are often multicellular organizations, and the sundry kinds of living cells which in a sense compose the organism are themselves usefully conceived as dynamisms, or as subdynamisms, one might call them, which are dynamically regulated in their living in accordance with the living of the organism as a whole. Malignancies, the sarcomatous and the carcinomatous evils which befall some organisms, may be regarded as instances of the escape from such dynamic regulation of some cells of the organism which, because they have escaped this regulation, become capable of destructively independent living. They become, as it were, destructively independent dynamisms, which invade the regulated cellular structure and organization of the host organism, or the host dynamism. The unnumbered subdynamisms, the individual cells, are organized into numerous systems of dynamisms such as the kidneys, the excretory-secretory structures of the intestines, the lungs, the heart, the blood, and what not; these systems of cellular dynamisms are in turn integrated into the total dyna-

[1] [*Editors' note:* See Alfred North Whitehead, *Process and Reality;* New York: The Macmillan Company, 1929. Whitehead states, "This doctrine of organism is the attempt to describe the world as a process of generation of individual actual entities, each with its own absolute self-attainment" (p. 94), and earlier, "An actual entity is a process, and is not describable in terms of the morphology of a 'stuff'" (p. 65).]

mism of the organism so that the whole thing makes up a vast unitary system, as it may be called from the standpoint of unregenerated biology. This total dynamism of the organism cannot, however, be separated from its necessary environmental milieu without ceasing to be a living organism.

This consideration of the organism as a dynamism and made up of subdynamisms is, to some extent, illustrated by the fact that the cornea of the eye, and even the heart and other organs, can in many cases go on manifesting living, and can be perfectly capable of transplantation elsewhere without dying, even though the carrying organism has died. Thus, the major, the total dynamism, may come to an end, but some of the subsidiary dynamisms making up, in a very dynamic sense, this totality do not necessarily expire immediately.

In general, we can say that the ultimate entities usefully abstracted in the study of the morphology, or organization, of living organisms is this living dynamism, the cell. Similarly, the ultimate entity, the smallest useful abstraction, which can be employed in the study of the functional activity of the living organism is the *dynamism* itself, *the relatively enduring pattern of energy transformations which recurrently characterize the organism in its duration as a living organism.* That is perhaps the most general statement that I can make about the conception of dynamism; it reaches far beyond the realm of psychiatry, certainly throughout the realm of biology, perhaps in the thinking of some people much further. The sundry dynamisms of interest to the biologist are all concerned with energy transformations making up functional activity in the communal existence of the organism with its necessary environment, through factors of its organization. The dynamisms of interest to the psychiatrist are the relatively enduring patterns of energy transformation which recurrently characterize the interpersonal relations—the functional interplay of persons and personifications, personal signs, personal abstractions, and personal attributions—which make up the distinctively human sort of being.

THE DEFINITION OF PATTERN

I spoke, just now, of *relatively enduring patterns,* and since this term will be repeated time and again in this presentation, it may be well at this point to say a few words about the word *pattern* itself. I shall give you a definition of pattern for which I believe I am the sole authority, a situation which always awakens very great suspicion on my part. *A pattern is the envelope of insignificant particular differences.* Taxonomy, the science of classification, which is particularly important in the biological field, deals chiefly with patterns. A particular fruit may properly be called an orange if the differences in characteristics of the specimen under consideration do not, when compared with the defined ideal orange, differ in a significant degree from the defined characteristics: size, shape, verrucosity or wartiness of the skin, surface reflectance of light waves, and even such morphological details as septation—that is, how many parts it is divided into by septa in the pulp—thickness of the rind, and number and viability of contained seeds. Yet all these may vary within fairly wide limits and still their variation, or any combination of variations, does not significantly extend beyond the defined pattern, orange. Physicochemical characteristics which underlie the taste of the fruit and the smell of the fruit have a place in the pattern of its characteristics; these too may vary considerably, and you still have an orange. But *significant* variation in some of these characteristics—that is, variation which goes beyond the pattern, orange—makes the specimen under consideration some other member of the botanical world, such as a lemon or a kumquat.

Another example of insignificant particular differences may be found in the realm of hearing, which is exceedingly rich in patterns. For instance, Mozart's Quartet in F Major is experienced as that particular pattern of music despite many errors which may be made in a particular performance of it, and despite the fact that the instruments may not be very well tuned, or may, in fact, be rather strikingly out of tune. The Quartet in F Major is a pattern of musical experience, and as such can exist in spite of a good many insignificant variations in a particular performance. But the experience of these variations may become more pronounced as the result of that peculiar misuse of human ingenuity called "swinging" the classical compositions; even here one can sometimes recognize the musical pattern of a beloved masterpiece, although the current atrocity may have varied from the pattern to a point where it is not, in any musically significant sense, the masterpiece, but is a vulgarism somewhat related to it. Now here is an instance where, in my opinion, the changes deliberately introduced by the re-composer have in a very significant way destroyed that which existed before, so altered its pattern that it is ridiculous to call it what an earlier composer did. But even under these circumstances, subpatterns in the masterpiece will often stand out so vividly that they evoke a recollection of the pattern as a whole, and it suddenly dawns on us, if we have not been warned in advance, that the dubious aesthetic pleasure that we are undergoing is someone's tortured revision of some particular composition.

Heard language is entirely a matter of sound patterns. The phonemes out of which spoken words are composed or compounded are patterns of sound which do not differ too much from a culturally defined mean. The sounds out of which we build up our English words, for example, are a certain set of culturally defined areas in the continuum of possible sound variation, which can be conceived to have a certain mean which could be determined by research as, I suppose, the statistically most common area of sound that speakers of that particular phoneme in English used. But in the continuum of sound one can get a considerable distance away from this mean without causing the average hearer any difficulty whatever in spotting exactly what phoneme you were using. Culture establishes what areas of this continuum of audible sound shall be a phoneme of a particular language, and if I knew all about the phonemes of all the languages, now used or unearthed from the past, I wouldn't be vastly surprised to discover that an indefinitely large number of articulated sounds have been utilized in the establishment of the patterns which make up the phonemes of one language or another.

Not only are phonemes sound patterns approximating a culturally established norm, but words themselves are patterns of phonemes which adequately approximate a culturally established pattern. For example, I suppose many of you have a certain amount of appreciation, if not respect, for the word psychiatry, but I wonder how many of you are equal to "ps-heeatrea."[2] My venerated colleague, Adolf Meyer, during a visit with a European colleague, caught on to the fact that when this man, who spoke

[2] [*Editors' note:* This is a phonetic approximation of the Greek ψυχιατρεια.]

excellent English, spoke of "ps-heeatrea" he was referring to their common preoccupation. The joy that the old man had in this correct pronunciation of a word derived from the Greek fixed this example of a variation in word pattern in my mind.

I am harping on this to invite your attention to the great significance of the pattern of phonemal succession, and the stressing of some part of this pattern, which together make up the word. And incidentally, words, contrary to naive impressions, do not exist in dictionaries, any more than road signs exist by the side of the road. A word—that is, a word per se rather than a symbol of a word—exists, like a sign, in them that have it. Since these words are acquired by hearing them, in finding that one can imitate them, and so on, they prove to be fantastically useful in producing the illusion, at least, of communication; and in some cases —and particularly, I hope, in the present case—communication by words is not too bad. But it is patterns of sound, stress, and so on that make up the words.

It is quite probable that an acoustical recording would show your pronunciation of any word relatively commonly used in your speech to be quite different in the morning, once you have fully wakened from sleep and are feeling very fresh and energetic, from your pronunciation of that same word late in the evening, when you are much in need of sleep and are feeling fairly fatigued, if not somewhat alcoholic. These acoustically recordable sounds that you emit in saying commonplace words would be astonishingly different in the details which can be recorded by the use of physical apparatus. Yet, unless fatigue was quite extreme, or the alcoholism was marked enough to interfere with the fine movements of your throat and mouth, these pronunciations, different as they were, would sound no different whatever to you, and would be equally and precisely of the same intelligibility to the hearer. Of course, it is possible for fatigue to be sufficient to seriously impair the production of words, so that their articulation would be considered defective, and their intelligibility impaired; this happens when the words, or the syllables, or even the phonemes, especially in the case of a person who originally learned some other language, cease to fall within the limits of insignificant variation.

From this very long discussion of taxonomy, music, and words, I trust that you see that there is something, at least, in my defining a pattern as the envelope—the limit in a tridimensional or multidimensional sense—of insignificant particular differences. As long as the congeries of particular differences is insignificant, then whatever is being discussed fits the pattern, which pattern, you might say, gives it its meaning, its authenticity, or its identity.

DYNAMISMS IN PSYCHIATRY

Organisms begin by reproduction; grow; mature; resist, or repair the damage caused by, some of the noxious influences which they encounter; reproduce themselves; and, in the higher manifestations of life at least, degenerate and come to an end in death. The patterns of energy transformation which characterize their life span are only *relatively* enduring. These patterns appear, in the higher forms of life at least, by maturation; they are changed variously by growth and by favorable or unfavorable influences; and perhaps in no two recurrent manifestations are they identical in all discoverable particulars. The dynamisms which interest us are relatively enduring patterns which manifest, in some cases at least, postnatal origin by maturation, and in all cases change by experience in the occurrence of which they are a significant factor. To put this very crudely, we might say that dynamisms grow or degenerate as a result of their recurrent manifestations, but that is really a pretty mystical idea. We can be more sure of what we are talking about when we say that dynamisms are modified by experience, which has in a significant sense been brought about by their manifestation.

The thing I particularly want to emphasize about dynamisms at this point is that their manifestation in the living of the organism is, in the sense that we originally used the term, *experience* of the organism. And in a sense which will later become a little clearer, this experience of the organism is particularly related to the manifestation of the particular dynamism at work and is striking, although the change in the dynamism is insignificant from the standpoint of a pattern. It will presently appear that while these changes are insignificant so far as the pattern is concerned, they can be very significant so far as living is concerned. I reiterate this notion of a pattern to emphasize the idea that a conception such as pattern can remain valid, even though, in a long stretch of duration, the objectively observable manifestations may be quite different.

We have commented somewhat on the growth of the infant's experience by the differentiation, from the general flux of his prototaxic experience, of particular useful patterns of sentience, which is the crude stuff of perception. These patterns, which I call signs, soon come in most instances to generalize various items of experience, marked or colored by various zones of interaction. To explain further: While a given experience in the early infant is not ordinarily marked by more than one zone of interaction—although sometimes it may be—the signs come quite frequently to generalize various experiences marked, respectively, by various zones. This generalizing of experiences marked by various zones, often including vision and hearing, becomes experience in the parataxic mode. For example, when sentience arising from vision and hearing is, in a certain sense, combined with experience arising, let us say, in the tactile or thermal perceptive or kinesthetic organs of sentience around the lips, then we have an elaboration of experience which extends beyond what is meant by prototaxic experience—the earliest type of experience—and is, in fact, experience in the parataxic mode. The "usefulness" of the earliest signs resides in their facilitating the satisfaction of needs, which they accomplish by functioning in recall and foresight. These signs modify the integrating tendency responsible for their occurrence in the subsequent integrating and maintenance of particular interpersonal situations; and these situations include the activity toward satisfaction which is implied in the conception of a situation integrated by an integrating tendency.

The dynamisms of particular interest to psychiatry are of two genera: those conceptualized with primary reference to the sundry recurring tensions which manifest themselves as integrating, disjunctive, and isolating tendencies; and, on the other hand, those conceptualized with primary reference to the energy transformations characteristic of particular zones of interaction. Dynamisms of the first kind will be exemplified in our subsequent consideration, for example, of *fear;* of the anti-anxiety system which is called the *self-system*—the system involved in the maintenance of felt interpersonal security; and of *lust*, which is my particular term for certain tensions of or pertaining to the genitals, and which has an excellent historical background. Dynamisms of the second kind will be exemplified in the discussion of, for example, the *oral dynamism.* Any observable behavior may be said to manifest concomitant activity of dynamisms of both sorts, as does the phasic change in awareness concerned in sleep.

I have already stressed the pattern element of dynamism, and the fact that a dynamism is a relatively enduring pattern of energy transformation. I have attempted to hint that even though such a pattern is relatively enduring, there is nothing static about it, but that change, however insignificant, is brought about by each recurrent manifestation in living of this recurrent pattern. I have tried to get at how this change in a dynamism—its growth or degeneration, if you please—can be conceptualized. I have talked about the very early signs educed by the infant in connection with the infant's living, and have shown that these signs are "useful" in that their function in recall and foresight facilitates, makes easier, hastens (depending on what the significant criterion is) the integration of situations in which an underlying need can be satisfied. Thus I have hinted that dynamisms can and do 'include' (I am dubious about this use of a geographical word) signs and symbols, and I have attempted to give you some notion of how the accumulation of signs, the elaboration of experience into signs, facilitates life and also affects the dynamisms concerned.

I have brought forward for your consideration two grand divisions, two genera, of dynamisms that are useful conceptions. One conceives the dynamism with primary reference to the tensions which recurrently disturb the euphoria of the living creature and manifest themselves in interpersonal relations as integrating, disjunctive, or isolative tendencies of a particular sort. The second concept of the dynamism, which is equally important, is on the basis of primary reference to the energy-transformation characteristics of particular zones of interaction. We shall consider these dynamisms further as we go along.

CHAPTER 7

Infancy: Interpersonal Situations

The Concept of Personality

We shall now extend somewhat our consideration of the communal existence of the human being with the necessary environments—the physicochemical environment, the environment of infrahuman living, and the environment of other people. The concept of zones of interaction as end stations in this interaction or interpenetration has already been indicated at the start of our consideration of the concept of dynamism, and we may now say further of these zones of interaction that they may be conceived, in part, as molar physiological structures, in which there occur transformations of energy specifically concerned with the functional activity of the organism in maintaining its necessary communal existence. But these structures are structures in the activity of which there arises specific experience of the organism, always in the prototaxic mode, although it is sometimes elaborated, as, for instance, in the occurrence of signs. This experience in turn influences the subsequent manifestations of the integrating tendencies concerned in the particular functional activity, and thus introduces factors of recall and foresight, of functional history and adaptation to a foreseen goal, which is commonly meant by anticipation. These factors of recall and foresight, of functional history and adaptation to a foreseen goal, can scarcely be called details of physiological structure; but they are, nonetheless, certainly important details of the actual organism as it goes on living, and, when the organism concerned is a human being, we call them details of personality. In the present particularist sense, when we are talking as if the infant were a complete discrete entity, *personality is the relatively enduring pattern of recurrent interpersonal situations which characterize a human life.*

The concept of *interpersonal situation* necessary for the occurrence of activity in the satisfaction of a need is of fundamental importance in psychiatric theory. The nipple-in-lips, our first example of such an interpersonal situation, is integrated and maintained by the infant's need for water and food and the mother's need to give tenderness in this connection. The infant's oral zone of interaction and, generally, the mother's mammary zone of interaction are the details of the two personalities which are principally concerned in the integration of this nipple-in-lips situation. The infant's experience of the relevant oral behavior, and the mother's experience of nursing the infant are just as significantly a part of any particular nursing situation as are the physiological structures which are involved. In the ever-expanding world of the infant, it comes to be the nipple, which is a discernible characteristic of the good mother, with which he is orally integrated. In the world of the mother, it is the lips of the more-or-less personified particular infant with which her nipple is invested. The infant's personification of the good mother is the prehended pattern of her participation in recurrent nursing situations and integrations of other needful sorts which have been resolved by satisfaction. She—the infant's personification of the good mother—symbolizes forthcoming satisfaction of the sundry needs—that is, she symbolizes in turn the integration, maintenance, and resolution of situations that include her, through appropriate and adequate activity on the infant's part.

The Organization of Personifications

In what I have just said, I have introduced the idea of *personification*, which derives its importance from the fundamental importance of the interpersonal situation in understanding the phenomena with which psychiatry deals. Here, in discussing the personification of the good mother, which is formed early in infancy, we start out on the long course of attempting to understand personifications and their dynamic role. As I have said, the infant's personification of the good mother is the pattern that he in a primitive way perceives as the pattern of her participation in recurrent nursing situations and other sorts of integrations called into being by his needs, which situations have been resolved with satisfaction. Foresight, as I have said before, pertains to that which has happened, and foresight about the good mother pertains to things that have gone well. Thus the infant's personification of the good mother symbolizes the forthcoming satisfaction of the sundry needs, or, to say the same thing in a different way, symbolizes the integration, maintenance, and resolution of the situations that are necessary for the infant's appropriate and adequate action in satisfaction of his needs.

Now this personification is not the 'real' mother—a particular living being considered as an entity. It is an elaborate organization of the infant's experience. The mother's personification of the infant is not the infant, but a growing organization of experience 'in' the mother, which includes many factors only remotely pertaining to dealing with this particular 'real' infant. It is important to understand that the infant's personification of the mother is composed of, or made up from, or organized from, or elaborated out of, what has occurred in the infant's relation to what you might call the 'real' mother in satisfaction-giving integrations with her. And the mother's personification of the infant—which was sometimes rather rudimentary in the days when it was thought that the soul joined the infant at the age of seven months or so, before which I presume the infant could be called *it* instead of *he* or *she*—is not the infant and is not merely an abstract of the events that the mother has encountered when integrated with the infant; it includes also much that is only remotely related to dealing with this particular baby. The mother's personification of "her" infant, may, if he be her seventh offspring, have much less to do with experience with this infant than with the first and second of her babies. Her previous experience, in any case, would influence her experience arising in sundry dealings with this particular baby. The mother's personification of the infant includes experience when the infant is anxious as well as when he is not. It includes experience when the infant is sleeping as well as when he is awake. It includes the observation of growth changes in the infant, and a perhaps richly formulated expectation of changes yet to come. That which the personified infant signifies to or symbolizes 'in' the mother is clearly more than forthcoming satisfaction of the need to give tenderness, or to participate in the integration, maintenance, and resolution of situations integrated by the infant's immediate needs.

The mother is, as we say, a carrier of social responsibilities with respect to her child. Part of what he symbolizes to her is her recognition of these responsibilities. What these responsibilities are varies somewhat from one family group to another in any particular community, or in any particular culture area. The degree to which these social responsibilities are effectively discharged may vary greatly in the same mother with respect to different children and with respect to the same child at different times. That these responsibilities will have no effect on the rearing of the child is, if not inconceivable, at least extremely improbable. Thus when I speak of the factors which are only remotely related to dealing with the particular 'real' infant, but which nonetheless enter into and are a part of the mother's personification of the infant, I include the very extensive, very important element of the mother's responsibility to the social order of which she is a member or in which she has a part. The recognized social responsibilities which the personified infant symbolizes for the mother have something—often a great deal—to do with the situations in which the infant prehends the bad mother, and out of his experience in such situations he organizes his personification of the bad mother.

Anxiety, as a phenomenon of relatively adult life, can often be explained plausibly as anticipated unfavorable appraisal of one's current activity by someone whose opinion is significant. When it is apparent that someone is anxious in talking with us, we might ask, "What would I think were you to speak freely what is in your mind?" And very often the other person might say, "You would think less of me," or "You would be shocked at me," or something of the sort. Now that is a typical rationalization of anxiety. By rationalization we mean giving a plausible and often exceedingly inconsequential explanation. And so I say that anxiety in relatively adult people can often be explained plausibly as anticipated unfavorable appraisal of one's current activity. A mother loaded with these social responsibilities which inhere in her from her membership in a social group may come to expect criticism of her mothering activities by her husband, his mother or sister, her mother or sister, the nurse, or anyone else who observes her handling of the baby. In many instances this known or presumed disapproval, this real or fancied faultfinding with respect to her care for her offspring makes her anxious. Unless, for instance, I have very considerable and well-founded esteem for something that I do, another person's criticism of what I do, or even the suspicion that the other person feels critical toward me for what I do, is tantamount to my being anxious. Therefore, unless the mother is very clear on the social responsibilities she is undertaking to discharge, certain that she is doing at least an averagely good job at it, and clear on the reasons why other people might differ about it and criticize her for it, any criticism of her handling of the baby, any suspected critical attitude toward her handling of the baby, is apt to make her anxious. And when you remember that anxiety in the mother induces anxiety in the infant, you will understand that the induced anxiety of the infant makes him more difficult and worrisome to care for, so that his behavior may seem to justify disparagement of the mother's work with him.

The implications of this sort of vicious circle underlie the psychiatrist's interest in the dynamic composition of the family group in which a patient's infancy was spent. When I was a young psychiatrist attending conferences of very capable staff members, I would hear accounts of mental patients which sometimes went back to the great-grandparents of the patient. These accounts included details about which ones of the ascendants had gone to mental hospitals, and which ones had gone to jails, and which ones had gone to posts on university staffs, and so on. And it all ended rather nicely in a woman who married a man and bore this patient, and had a difficult or an easy labor. And the infant had or had not had a feeding difficulty (that preoccupation didn't show up when I was such a young psychiatrist, but shortly afterward), and then after a while the infant learned to walk and talk and cease to wet himself. And presently all this wonderful array of rumor and data evolved into his being before us as a mental patient. In subsequent years we got more and more interested in doing something for this mental patient so that he might cease to be a mental patient and become a member of society, to his chagrin or delight as the case might be. And then we found that we could omit the study of a good deal of this inscrutably complex heredity—about which, at best, the patient would probably have very few useful views—because out of all the rumor and data there was very little which would help us to find out why he had curiously distorted views on a good many people in his environment. Eventually we got to the point of guessing that anxiety had a lot to do with the patient's problems. But then the question was how to explain the peculiarities of anxiety. And it is from experience with the difficulties in this work of cure or treatment—a much more satisfactory concern than the mere chronicling of the patient's family history—that we finally got back to studying the development of the anti-anxiety system in human personality. Now in this presentation I am attempting to suggest how anxiety begins—what factors are influential in the beginning of anxiety in the natural history of a given person. It reaches back very, very far, and this is the reason why it is important to know the composition of the family group in which the infant spent his first months.

Consideration of the composition of the family group may indicate that persons other than the mother have exerted great influence on the earliest phase of developmental history, long before these other persons enter into significant, direct, interpersonal relations with the infant. Moreover, in a good many instances some person other than the mother does have recurring, significant, direct, interpersonal relations with even the young infant. Occasionally there is a so-called wet nurse, and not infrequently there is a nurse or an older sister who does part of the work of caring for the infant's needs in situations integrated by the nurse or sister. Any such surrogates in the mothering function also personify the infant to some extent, and these personifications of the infant include as important factors the surrogate's experience and expectations with regard to infants as a class and this infant in particular.

It may be that one of these surrogates in the mothering function will have come to manifest the peculiar expectations with respect to others to which I shall presently refer as *malevolence*. This malevolent person may behave toward the infant in ways quite other than giving tender cooperation in satisfying the infant's manifest needs; she may instead hurt and otherwise provoke fear in the infant. Since the malevolent behavior is also apt to be accompanied by anxiety and to induce anxiety in the infant, the infant's prehensions of such a surrogate come to be organized as experience of the bad mother. Let us take, for example, the situation of our mother with seven children of which the seventh is the baby now under discussion. Let us suppose that the first-born and the second-born were girls and that the first-born girl, after a fashion not uncommon in eldest children, is very difficult and is out of the house a good deal. The second-born girl is mother's helper, has had plenty to do, has felt very much rebuffed and neglected for years, and has come to be mischievous, as her aunt might call it. And now with the arrival of the seventh baby, mother's helper takes over a good part of the absolutely necessary relatively adult cooperation in looking after the baby. Now that will not include giving the baby pap, but it may certainly include keeping the baby covered, and changing the diapers, and so on. Insofar as mother's helper is malevolent—something that we will come to understand presently—the tenderness theorem will not apply in simple fashion to her dealings with the baby. And frequently or occasionally, in looking after the infant's needs, mother's helper will be rough, sound unpleasant, hurt the baby, and generally discompose him. But she will not do these things with a feeling of complete sweetness and light, because mother's helper will know quite clearly that if any of these minor atrocities to the infant were observed by mother or by someone else who told mother about them, mother's helper would get her ears boxed, or something of that kind. Now the anticipation by mother's helper of possible retribution for these little mischievous acts toward the baby is, in a sense that will presently become clear, tantamount to her being anxious as well as malicious. Under those circumstances, what the baby gets in the way of experience includes anxiety as well as fear, and that experience is, very early in infancy, the same experience that the infant has in his relation to his mother when she is anxious; therefore all such experience is organized in the rudimentary infantile personification of the bad mother. When compelling circumstances necessitate the delegation of an important part of the mothering to a malevolent surrogate, some considerable number of the infant's contacts with the mother are also apt to involve anxiety, for she can scarcely "be at peace with herself" about the mothering which her baby is receiving. There thus come to be two or more persons who recurrently induce anxiety in the infant, his prehensions of whom are organized in a single early personification of the bad mother.

It is also evident that a surrogate in part of the mothering function may be both tender and relatively free from anxiety, as may be the mother herself. In this case the infant organizes prehensions of two or more people in his earliest personification of the good mother. And in such cases, where the mother has a very good mother's helper—good in the sense of having no serious interference with the manifestation of tenderness toward the baby—then the mother will be reasonably comfortable about the mothering which her baby is receiving, and both the mother and her helper will be relatively free from anxiety. Therefore, when one or the other of these people is with the infant, the infant will have considerable experience of tender cooperation in the satisfaction of his needs and relatively little experience of anxiety. Under those circumstances, at the very start of the personifying process in early infancy there is a personification of the good mother in which the experience (from our point of view) comes from experiences with two people, but is not so differentiated by the infant.

These two of several not too uncommon instances should suffice to indicate the possible complexity of the infant's beginnings of personification, out of which beginnings will evolve his sequential personifications of the significant people who are visually and audibly differentiable within the flux of his experience. I have hinted several times thus far that as the data from the visual and the hearing receptors grow in utility in foreseeing and integrating satisfaction-giving situations, and in foreseeing and avoiding anxiety-provoking situations, differences in the persons concerned tend to appear. I have not yet said so, but I presume that differences in 'actual' persons associated with anxiety are noted by the infant before he notes differences in people involved in his getting satisfactions; the reason for this is the extremely undesirable character of anxiety and the importance of getting away from it. Perhaps in middle infancy or toward the latter part of infancy, as the infant progresses to the point where this distance data—data obtained by sight and by hearing—begins to be differentiated, its differentiation with respect to people who make the infant anxious (the mother, or the mother and a malevolent mother's helper) is on the basis of characteristics which are identical in kind, in functional significance, with those which we later call *forbidding gestures.* These forbidding gestures consist of tonal and other modifications of speech, and differences in facial posture and so on, of the mothering one.

Now I have emphasized in my two examples, first, of an anxious mother and a malevolent mother's helper, and, second, of a calm and tender mother and mother's helper, that since experience objectively related to two people may be combined in the infant's beginning personification of the bad mother, or of the good mother, this personification might be called *complex.* From our standpoint, it is complex in that it has one personification for characteristics that we would attribute objectively to two people. The meaning of this complexity deserves more than passing consideration. There is no reason for supposing that "useless" signs are organized within the infant's experience. The organization into one sign of experience with two people who regard themselves as distinct is an early instance of an exceedingly important ability which is by no means restricted to man alone in the biological series. And this organization into one sign of experience with two (to themselves) different people is *anything but* an instance of an unfortunate something which one might call "confusion." To think that the infant "confuses," in one rudimentary personification, details of his experience with two people, the mother and the surrogate, is literally to foreclose any possibility of understanding personality development. On the contrary, the infant differentiates experience arising in his encounters with one (from our point of view) identical person in organizing two rudimentary personifications, those of the good and the bad mother.

Some of you may wonder how I know this—in other words, what higher source of information I have as to what the infant of, let us say, less than the age of six months experiences. I only hope that you have been patient in your anticipation, strong in the belief that perhaps I would eventually give you a clue, which I will now attempt to do.

The probable correctness of this particular inference—that the infant differentiates his experience with a 'real' mother into two personifications, that of the good mother and that of the bad mother—is suggested by the course of developmental events in which we can participate with increasing sureness from late in infancy onward. In other words, from later data—the implication of which is quite certain—I make inferences regarding what can be observed in the young infant that seems closely and logically related to these later data, even though the actual events at this early stage are beyond participant observation, and therefore beyond a type of knowledge which is very convenient to have. It may seem that such use of inference is dangerous or even bad, but it would be exceedingly difficult to explore any new field if one did not use inference which extended from what is reasonably certain, both as to datum and implication, into the unexplored periphery of the new field. And so, in setting up this doctrine of the very earliest events in personification, I have to extend inference from what can be participated in later, backward to where it, to my way of thinking, can reasonably be inferred to begin.

The infant's differentiating and organizing of what is primarily prototaxic experience into the more complex elements of experience that I name signs, arises from a combination of two sets of factors. One of these factors is the *possibility* of thus organizing experience. It is always well to be that rudimentary in your thinking; there has to be a demonstrable possibility of something before it is reasonable to do very much with it. That there is a possibility that an infant under six months can organize signs can be, I believe, validated from careful observation of almost any six-month-old infant. So I believe that the possibility of thus organizing experience is demonstrable. I may say that it is not confined to the human, but extends, to my knowledge, as far as colts and puppies. Besides the possibility, which must be present, there has to be the factor of *functional utility* of such signs in the integration of situations necessary for the securing of satisfaction and, very soon after the beginning of life, the avoiding or minimizing of anxiety. This is the implication of my reference to "useful" and "useless"—terms which can easily be misleading. But keep in mind that when I say that a sign is "useful," and that "useless" signs are not organized in the early phase of life, what I am referring to is *functionally* useful, in the sense of facilitating some functional activity which is vital in the business of satisfying needs or avoiding anxiety. It is solely in this connection that these two dubious words—useful and useless—get into our thinking here, and I trust that the great number of other possible meanings will not creep into your thought. The point is that what the infant differentiates and organizes out of his primarily prototaxic experience is *useful* additions to his integrating tendencies, and as I have said before, these useful additions function in recall and foresight.

To repeat, there is no reason for supposing that useless signs are organized within the infant's experience. Thus there is no differentiation of a tender real mother from a tender mother's helper in the situations in which the infant satisfies his needs, for the very reason that such differentiation would in no way facilitate the satisfaction of needs in the very early months of life. And in the same way, in these earlier months of life no facilitation of the avoiding or minimizing of anxiety (mainly avoiding at this stage) would be accomplished by differentiating between an anxious mother and an anxious and malevolent mother's helper. What happens to the infant is, to all intents and purposes, identical, whether the mother or the mother's helper is involved; the only 'objective' which makes any sense is to avoid anxiety, and since anxiety is induced, it makes very little difference what the person who induces it looks like or thinks herself to be.[1]

1 [*Editors' note:* In Sullivan's 1948 lecture series he worded this somewhat differently:

"What the infant can, with reasonable probability, be believed to do rests primarily on his biological capabilities for doing it, but rests practically on the usefulness of doing it. And all that is particularly useful in the extremely dependent phase of life—early infancy—is the improvement of differentiation of those interpersonal situations that work, and those interpersonal situations that miscarry dreadfully by producing anxiety.

"In the beginning, all relations, with whatever people, which are a part of the satisfying of the infant's needs blend into a single personification which I call the good mother, to name it something; and all experience, with however many persons, which results in severe anxiety blends into a single personification which I call, to call it something, the bad mother. And the growth of differentiation, as the distance receptors begin to be more efficient and better related to one another and to the rest of the organism, is, I believe, primarily for the purpose, one might say, of becoming alert to those mis-

The young infant does not differentiate insignificant details of experience, but only the pattern, beyond whose limiting envelope events are significantly different. Forthcoming satisfaction is most significantly different from anxiety, and in the earliest months the identity of the particular person who signalizes the forthcoming satisfaction is of no moment whatever in the integration by the infant of the necessary interpersonal situation and the infant's activity in its resolution.

And here I would like to remind you of the start of this discussion by noting that even our initial example of an interpersonal situation, namely, the nipple-in-lips, is integrated and maintained doubly, in a duplex fashion, by the infant's need for water and food, and by the mother's need to give tenderness in this connection. And here I am saying that, in the earliest months of life, the infant's part in forthcoming satisfaction—his part of the integration of the nipple-in-lips, and his activity in maintaining this integration and in resolving it by having secured enough water and foodstuff for the satisfaction of his needs—has no use for, is in no way facilitated by, the inclusion of data which might seem quite significant to you or me in looking at the situation. If the carrier of the nipple gets it in the right place, within the prehensile ability of the infant's mouth, this, *provided* that the situation is free from anxiety, is tantamount to the complete integration of the satisfaction-giving situation. And that is the case in the earliest months with all the interpersonal cooperation which is necessary

carriages of things which will bring anxiety—that is, among the various things which can be perceived and organized as experience, the infant becomes alert to those that can be classed as forbidding gestures. Anything he can pick up, from the vague entities moving around him, which can be learned to be a precursor of anxiety is so incorporated. The infant learns to make this differentiation, not because he has any great skill at warding off anxiety, but because anxiety is extremely unpleasant and represents a major miscarriage of living, whereas in the rest of the infant's living the worst that can happen is that a lot of time may elapse between the appearance of need and its satisfaction. But there the device of apathy comes in to give one a rest, so that one can start over with renewed vigor at the end of the repose. However, with anxiety there is no possibility of resting or doing anything else except suffering. Thus I believe that the growth of differentiation—in the sense of refined learning, however unrefined it may be in its beginning—probably is in this area of how to get the first clues to the probability of anxiety, just as if that would be very helpful to the infant, because anxiety is such an extremely unpleasant experience."]

for the survival of the human young. There are no significant differences at the beginning, unless the carrier of whatever is needed —the relatively adult person—is anxious, in which case, as I have already stated, action and satisfaction are impaired or reversed and the infant suffers the misery of anxiety. And it is for this reason that I infer with considerable security the initial organization of two complex signs in the infant's experience, the good and the bad or anxiety-carrying mother.

Thus I have now set up for our consideration the idea that the infant is bound to have two personifications of any mothering person, barring the most incredible good fortune, and that the infant in the earliest stages of life need have only two personifications for any number of people who have something to do with looking after him. So far as the more adult persons in the infant's unknown world are concerned, each one of them is bound to have a different personification of the infant. By this time, I trust it is completely clear that personifications are not, in some metaphysical sense, the organism or the person that is personified.

Nursing as an Interpersonal Experience

The experience involved in becoming a person may be said to begin as a function of the first nursing. Prototaxic experience connected with the institution of breathing and the maintenance of body temperature probably precedes this, but it is in connection with frequently recurring activity of the oral zone that sentience, presently to be elaborated into primitive personifications, has its origin. The extraphysiological factors in the nursing situation are a growing personification of the good mother by the infant, and one or more personifications of the infant by the mother. The good mother begins as a discrimination or differentiation of the good and satisfactory nipple. That is, it is differentiated as a pattern of experience, very significantly different from the nipple of anxiety. The personification grows by the discrimination of the sundry classes of nipples that I have talked about, other than the anxiety-invested nipple, and sentience originating in distance receptor apparatus is added to the initial, more purely oral data. And by this I refer to the oral dynamism, which more or less pertains to the mouth but at this very early stage also includes the auditory channel, because all that is heard is the infant's production. Very early in life the auditory zone begins to split off as a zone of interaction in its own right. In the course of events, the sundry classes of nipples become an important part of the pattern of experience which is the personification, good mother; but even this part of the personification has expanded to include sentience from extraoral zones as remote as the prehensile hands, the buttocks, and the feet. The nursing situation still includes as its central detail the nipple-in-lips, its oldest core, as elaborated by additional data with discrimination of various classes of nipples and so on; but it now shows patterning of activity by the hands and so forth.

There may be evident discrimination between what we might call nursing-when-recumbent and nursing-when-erect. Observable accessory movements show relatively durable differences in the two cases. I am now talking of the development of personality in the infant, let us say, under six months of chronologic age. By this time there have already appeared ways of using the arms and hands, the legs and feet, and so on, in connection with the mother's body, clothing, and so forth, when nursing, which we call accessory movements. In the human, these do not, so far as I can guess, have very much to do with the getting of milk out of the nipple, but they do tend to fall into pattern, that is, they get to be, as we can very recklessly say, habitual accompaniments of nursing. And even at this early age the accessory movements—which presumably supply sentience that is organized into the personification of the good mother and makes up part of the infant's experience of the nursing behavior—show certain differences when the mother happens to be nursing while lying down in comparison with when she is nursing sitting up. And these accessory movements, particularly those of the arms and hands, are not merely something that coincides with nursing, but actually are details of behavior which may persist as patterns of activity years after a person has ceased to nurse at the breast. Some of these movements show up in states of fatigue, preoccupation, and so on, as curious manneristic movements.

More than the infant's oral zone and the mother's mammary zone is now significantly concerned in the integration of the nursing situation. And more than milk, the warmth of the mother's body, some olfactory sentience, and so forth—which were concerned in the earlier nursing—enter now into the recurring nursing experience. There are now several other important factors of sentience. For example, there is that of the infant's hands; the good mother as integrated by the infant in the nursing situation now includes elements to be grasped, pushed, pulled, rubbed, and otherwise encountered by the sensitive palmar and plantar surfaces—that is, the palms of the hands and the soles of the feet—as well as the elements of what is seen and heard in connection with the nursing situation. Insofar as all of these are sentience recurrently associated, for the infant, with the nursing situation, they can be presumed to be items in that which is personified as the good mother—which, you will remember, is anything but an appreciation of the mother as an adult human being as another adult might see her.

In some of the mammals with accessory nursing behavior, this behavior has very striking relationship to the breast, but where human beings are concerned, I think it is quite as common for a nursing infant to be toying with some of the mother's hair as to be toying with the mammary zone of her body. The fact that the accessory movements of the human infant may have very little to do with the actual mechanics, you might say, of getting milk into the mouth does not, however, lessen the real contribution of these movements to the growing personification of the source of milk, the good mother.

Zonal Needs and General Needs

Factors of biological organization which provide energy for transformation in the several zones of interaction now manifest themselves in these zones as dynamisms, and there are manifest needs to suck, to feel, to manipulate orally and with the hands, and so forth. We have already spoken of two genera of dynamisms which are of peculiar interest to psychiatry: the second of these consisted of dynamisms conceptualized with primary reference to the energy transformations characteristic of particular zones of interaction. Up to now—that is, through, let us say, the second or third month of the extrauterine life of the infant—we have considered the need for water and food which is satisfied in the nursing situation as a dynamism, an integrating tendency, which, so far as the infant is concerned, is manifested in the appropriate and adequate action. But now we have progressed to the point where we are speaking of the oral zone itself as a dynamism, and as a dynamism it manifests needs to suck, just as the hands manifest needs to feel, and to manipulate, and so on; and incidentally the oral zone also does considerable manipulation. We can speak of the oral zone and the manual zone as being in the service of another class of dynamisms—namely, the needs; but these zones, themselves considered as dynamisms, show zonal needs, of which the need to suck is a particular instance.

Now it is true of these zonal needs that they must suffice quantitatively for the resolution of situations which are integrated by general needs—that is, needs for oxygen, for water, for food, and so on; but it is equally true that the zonal needs often, if not always, exceed this necessary quantitative aspect. And the quantity concerned here is the quantity of energy which is provided in the zone of interaction for transformation in the shape of doing the work of interchange which is centered in this zone. In other words, quite early in development, the partition of energy to be transformed in the oral zone, for example, may be greater than the energy needed for the satisfaction of the needs for water and food; and this excess manifests itself in the maintenance of activity which is not needed for the satisfaction of the great general need for food and water, but begins to be the need for exercise, we might call it, of the particular zone of interaction concerned. Thus, quite early in life, the energy provided for transformation in the act of sucking may be in excess of that which is transformed in sucking for milk, and the surplus manifests itself as a need to suck which is in no sense necessarily associated with a nipple, much less with getting milk from the nipple.

Years ago a very important contribution to the probability of this whole approach to psychiatric theory was provided by the work of Dr. David M. Levy dealing with this very point, which appeared first in his study of the relation of thumbsucking to the ease with which milk was obtained from the nourishing nipple.[2] If

[2] [David M. Levy, "Fingersucking and Accessory Movements in Early Infancy: An Etiologic Study," *Amer. J. Psychiatry* (1928) 7:881–918.]

it was very easy to satisfy the need for food by sucking, then there was a great deal of sucking of other things; and the upper extremities particularly and the lower extremities to some extent provide the infant with things that can be invested by the lips and sucked. Further development of Dr. Levy's basic research in this connection was extended as far as the pecking behavior of chickens. There again it was found, under an experimental setup, that if it was extremely easy for these little birds to get a sufficiency of food, then they pecked themselves and each other, and, in fact, in some cases practically denuded each other of feathers in order to discharge the zonal need—that is, to transform the energy, provided for the securing of food by activity of the oral zone, which was in excess of the needs for food.[3]

Thus quite early in life the zones of interaction begin to be conspicuous as dynamisms in their own right, with more-or-less fixed partitions of the total vital energy for transformation in each zone; and energy is transformed only in doing work. Therefore, there is a zonal need to suck, and so on, which is quite supplementary, you might say, to the general need for food, even if necessarily related to it. If the zonal need is not adequate to the provision of food, that is a very serious business. But if the zonal need is in excess of what is required for the securing of food and water, then there is behavior for the discharge of the tension of the oral zone which is in excess of that required for the securing of food and water. The oral zone, parenthetically, is very well provided with energy for transformation, and the oral needs, in contrast to general needs, have very considerable importance in understanding personality development. So much for this consideration.

The Anal and Urethral Zones in Interpersonal Experience

Now let us look at two other important zones of interaction in the communal existence of the infant, namely, the *anal zone* and the *urethral zone*. These end stations pertain to the expulsion of food residues and excess water. The general need concerned may

[3] [David M. Levy, "A Note on Pecking in Chickens," *Psychoanalytic Quart.* (1935) 4:612–613. "On Instinct-Satiation: An Experiment on the Pecking Behavior of Chickens," *J. General Psychol.* (1937) 18:327–348.]

be called the need to be rid of more-or-less solid and of liquid waste products concerned with the communal existence and functional activity of the organism. The tensions underlying these needs are felt as the recurrent need to empty the rectum and the urinary bladder; and in the experiencing of these felt needs, tensions in two systems of neuromuscular organs are of central importance. Now, you will note that there is somewhat of a distinction here in the method of development of thought. When I spoke of the need for food and water, I did not specify any organ as of central importance in the felt need; but perhaps because the anal and urethral zones are eliminatory zones, where waste is 'thrown out,' and because of various other considerations that will be discussed, these zones and their felt needs can actually be broken down into meaningful reference to neuromuscular apparatus. Perhaps chiefly by virtue of improved survival value, the mammalian bodily organization has come to provide for the intermittent discharge of these waste products, and, especially in the case of the less fluid and much more viscous feces, for their spatial separation from the body integument.

At this point I am introducing into this discussion a group of inferences derived from my own observations, not, so far as I know, supported by observations, investigations, or experiments by anyone else, and certainly not supported by an adequate body of observation and experiment by me. I wish particularly to stress the element of provisions for the spatial separation, the separation in space, of the organism and the expelled feces. As in the case of the food and water needs of the infant, so also in the ridding of himself of the urine and feces, there is requisite the cooperation of a relatively mature mothering agency, to convey the infant away from coverings wetted by the extruded urine, and to remove the feces from the infant's body surface and from his proximity. The removal of feces entails the cleaning of soiled areas, particularly the mucocutaneous junction at the anus.

The character of the covering tissue on what we often think of as the inside of our body is, in general, very different from the covering of what we ordinarily think of as the outside of our body. Now when I speak of what is "thought of" as the inside, I am not talking about the actual, beyond-any-perchance inside.

The nasal spaces, the mouth, and the gastrointestinal tract are in a very practical sense outside the body; but they are so circumscribed by and contained in the body, for such very special purposes of the body, that the covering or membrane which separates them from what is not of the body is quite different in character from the skin and nails and hair and so on, which appear on the unquestionable outside. The particularly significant details that I wish to mention as characterizing these quasi-inside coverings are that they secrete mucus and that they have ciliary apparatus for moving things, and so on. The mucous membranes join the skin, and the place of joining is always a zone of interaction in the communal existence of the organism, although there are zones such as the ear where no such mucocutaneous junction is presented to the outer world. Where there are mucocutaneous junctions, there are really extraordinary risks to the integrity of the organism—owing to peculiarities of joining blood supplies, and one thing and another—and almost invariably there is a rich supply of receptor organs, as if to aid in protecting these comparatively delicate carpentries of two different kinds of covering membranes. The mucous membrane lining the alimentary tract ends in the anus—that is, its distal part is the anal orifice, the anus; and there, as at the lips, is a junction of mucous membrane and skin. And it is in connection with this anal end of the alimentary tract that there occurs a peculiar segregation of receptors which, while they are not in a strictly technical sense distance receptors, might be called anticontact receptors.

As I have said, the removal of feces through cooperation of the mothering agency entails the cleaning of soiled areas, particularly this mucocutaneous junction in the anus. End organs of afferent (that is, receptor) nerve channels carrying intelligence, or the basis of intelligence, inward in this anal region provide a peculiarly important part of the sentience which is marked or colored by origin in the anal zone of interaction. And this particular component of the anal sentience has this aspect, which I have just mentioned, of a quasi-distance quality, in that it determines the separation of the organism and the actual fecal mass—and by determines I do not mean that it brings it about, but that it shows whether this separation is or is not the case. In the intervals between their elimination, the feces are accumulated in a section of the alimentary canal, the tension of the muscular walls of which exert pressure against the innermost of three anal sphincters, and this pressure gives rise to the felt need to defecate. Sphincters are more or less ring-shaped muscular organs which appear where it is necessary to close a canal, and the sphincters of interest here are this set of three anal sphincters and two urinary sphincters. Incidentally, the upper end of the alimentary canal has an organization of muscle that is quite like a sphincter, which is called the *orbicularis oris*. This again is a sort of ring-shaped assembly of muscular tissue, although its precise shape is concealed by the refinements of the mouth form; its functional activity is very much more refined than that of the other sphincters and is combined with that of other muscular structures, because there is seldom occasion for any sphincter action at the oral end, except possibly when you are blowing brass wind instruments.

As I have said, the pressure of the muscular walls of the rectal part of the alimentary canal against this inner of three sphincters gives rise to the felt need to defecate. Now we must distinguish between the rectum, which is a storing space primarily, and the anal canal, which runs from the innermost sphincter through the middle sphincter, past the outer sphincter to the anus. This canal is so organized that it has to be emptied of any feces admitted into it, and gives rise to vivid sentience as long as this emptying has not been accomplished. This vivid sentience, arising from the end organs with which this canal is provided, is a particular type of discomfort, occurring when that canal is no longer being merely traversed by fecal matter, but has some in it that has to be expelled.

In later life, the expulsion of feces other than those actually in the anal canal tends to cease unless the extruded mass actually leaves contact with these quasi-distance receptors in the anus, and the detachment of each fecal mass from contact with these receptors favors the admission of another mass into the anal canal until the act of defecation has been completed. Now this is the area of data which may be proven by investigation to be erroneous, but about which I believe I have adequate basis for this presentation. It is literally true that the separation of a fecal mass from contact with the anus is necessary for ordinary completion of the act of defecation. This may seem to you a very trivial matter, but it is actually vastly more significant for theory than is a great deal that has been taught quite solemnly.

Appropriate and adequate activity of the infant in satisfying the need to defecate consists in the relaxing of the anal sphincter apparatus and the coordinate increasing in the tension of the muscular walls of the rectal canal as the anal canal empties itself. Indefinitely early in life, perhaps from the very beginning, the factor of separation from the feces begins to be important and contributes something to the experience of tenderness which is organized by the infant in his personification of the good mother.

The urine is handled by a somewhat similar combination of a cavity with muscular walls, the pressure from tension in which is exerted against the innermost of two sphincters. The canal from this first to the second sphincter must, like the anal canal, be emptied, and gives rise to vivid sentience until this has been accomplished, excepting during the actual flow of urine. Now this sentience is suspended during the actual transfer of masses which have passed the first sphincter en route to the last, and becomes significant only when that normal, functionally perfectly useful process is interrupted or is about to end. At those times, these intersphincter parts of the eliminatory canals cause vivid sentience which has the pattern of arising from their nonempty state, and disappearing when they are empty. They have ample muscular provisions for bringing about the emptying, which automatically happens unless something materially interferes. The most striking difference in the apparatus for being rid of the urine and the apparatus for being rid of the feces is that in the former there is one less sphincter.

With respect to the urinary excretory apparatus, there are important differences in the morphological organization of the male and the female, arising from the fusion of some parts of the more external reproductive apparatus with a part of the urine channels. These differences are of no special moment in the earlier stages of developmental history, and may be ignored in the stage of infancy. The urethra, the canal for the urine from the bladder to the outside, ends in an unusual mucocutaneous junction, respectively at the end of the erectile penis in the male, or in the vulva in the neighborhood of the erectile clitoris in the woman. The lining of the urethra joins with a specialized epithelium which is supplied with peculiarly characterized receptor end organs, the great import of which will appear only later in life when the development of the lust dynamism has begun through appropriate maturation.

The more significant components of sentience pertaining to the intermittent discharge of the urine arise from, first, the deeper, intersphincter part of the urethra; secondly, the distal part of the urethra; and thirdly, the surfaces closely associated with the urethral orifice. You will notice that I have not mentioned any component of pressure against the inner sphincter, which is another area of significant difference from the anal apparatus. It is the increasing pressure of the fecal mass forced by the walls of the rectum against the inner sphincter of the anal canal which is ordinarily recognized as the need to defecate. So far as the need to urinate is concerned, however, this is, so far as I know, quite unexceptionally related to the permitting of a small amount of urine to pass the inner sphincter, whereupon it strikes this peculiarly sensitive intersphincter region and gives rise to an urgent desire to urinate. To what extent pressure against the urinary sphincter may be a component of experience in this particular, I do not know, but it is very much less striking than in the anal situation.

There are significant differences in the earliest manifestation of these two excretory functions, such that the need for cooperation with respect to the urine—that is, for tenderness in connection with the satisfaction of the need to urinate—may be chiefly an aspect of body temperature protection, quite different from that assumed to be the case with regard to the feces. The urine is an aqueous saline solution, rich in dissolved nitrogenous waste products, of which urea is very conspicuous. It is usually sterile so far as bacteria and other lower organisms are concerned; in other words, it is not, as you might put it, infected with bacteria, yeasts, molds, and so on. It is entirely an excretory secretion, its quantity and contents being determined by such vital factors as the electrolyte balance of the body fluids and the nitrogen metabolism. The feces, on the other hand, consist of excretory secretion and unassimilable material taken in as, or with, food. Its composition, even its consistency, varies between wide limits. It is an excellent pabulum for the growth of a great variety of lower organisms—bacteria, fungi, and yeast—the metabolic products of which may be thoroughly noxious, not only to the infant, but to adults. This becomes increasingly true with the introduction of food substances other than the mother's milk and the corresponding dilution of the previous excretory secretions. In other words, when alimentation is proceeding perfectly in the infant, that which comes out does not include cellulose, and so on, but is only mucus and the secretion of the excretory elements of the alimentary canal; but as soon as alimentation goes wrong, incompletely digested milk and so on is added to this; and later on, when eating consists of more than milk, and indigestible substances are mixed in with the digestible, these in turn are mixed with the excretory secretions in making up the feces.

The alimentary canal is a digestive, absorbing, and excretory channel. Enzymes secreted into it at several points bring about chemical transformations productive of substances which can be usefully absorbed in aqueous solution and otherwise. Chemical changes of the kind that are here significant are a joint function of time and temperature, as is the absorptive function itself. The rate at which the food mass is transferred from the oral to the anal zones is of very real importance for survival, and the extent to which this permits adequate absorption of the useful products of digestion is a complex function of motility, water content, and osmotic tensions. In general, the intestinal contents, after the first weeks of extrauterine life, tend to be formed masses by the time they are ready for expulsion, but fluid stools may be produced under certain circumstances throughout the whole span of life.

The mothering functions necessary for the survival of the infant are, with respect to the urine, relatively simple. Besides attention to the continued excretion of this waste matter, there is chiefly the requirement that the infant shall not remain in contact with the urine long enough to interfere with the control of his internal temperature, or the damage of his integument, his neighboring skin, by maceration or soaking. Mothering with regard to the feces is quite another matter. Its prompt removal is indicated. The anal orifice needs to be cleaned, and the feces need to be inspected for the indices which they provide as to the adequacy of the alimentary function, necessary indeed to life and growth. This discrimination between the mothering function regarding the urine and the mothering function regarding the feces is important. Suppression of the urinary excretion would be a very grave problem, but beyond making sure that this does not occur, the mothering function is only to see that the infant is not wet—which would interfere with the maintenance of body temperature, the radiation of heat and one thing and another, and, if prolonged, would lead to unfortunate change in the skin. But with the feces, which are extraordinarily apt to undergo bacterial putrefaction, fungus growth, and so on, it is quite another matter. I have already mentioned that there are some facts which suggest that for completion of fecal expulsion, ideally the removal of the extruded feces from contact with the anal orifice is indicated. And because the very swiftly growing body of the infant is chiefly made up of what comes to him through successful working of the alimentary function, any hints of disturbance of that function are timely warnings of what may be very serious trouble; among the hints which anybody can discover is the character of the feces.

The anal zone of interaction thus necessarily comes to involve factors of an interpersonal character from very early in life. The functional activity centering in the anal zone often becomes involved in the manifestations of infantile anxiety, especially when the mothering one is made anxious by these details of her mothering function. By this I refer to those who find it extremely difficult to deal with the infant's soiled diapers, and so on. Here, as in the case of other needs which we have considered, anxiety manifests itself in direct vector opposition to the satisfaction of the need to defecate. Its occurrence tends to bring about retention of the feces, with increased tension of need to be rid of them. Now it is quite true that the vicissitudes of evolution have protected us from the possibility of complete suppression of the expulsion of feces because of anxiety. But the presence of anxiety tends to prolong the retention; at the same time, the more there is in the rectum, the more the pressure that is normally expressed against the internal sphincter, and the greater the need to be rid of the rectal contents. How anxiety interferes with the whole field of sentience in these two activities in the elimination of waste will become more evident presently. But we should note at this particular time that the water content of the feces is in large measure a function of the time which the food mass is retained in the alimentary canal, and the water content is the principal factor in determining the consistency of the feces. In other words, the longer the feces are retained, other factors being equal, the firmer is the consistency of the feces, and there is a point at which the feces may become so firm, and there may be such a quantity of them coalesced into a mass, that the expulsion is actually an occasion of pain—so that there may be very real suffering in connection with their transit through the anal canal. Therefore, insofar as anxiety tends to bring about retention of the feces, anxiety connected with recurrent needs to defecate may come to be—in, let us say, the fourth, fifth, or sixth month of infantile life—associated with pain in the procedure which would normally be the satisfaction of the need to defecate. Now this pain does not remove the satisfaction of defecating, but pain is never attractive, crazy ideas about sadism-masochism notwithstanding. And so one of the striking influences of anxiety, in connection with this particular zone of interaction with the environment, is that it can lead to actual physical suffering in connection with the satisfaction of the need to empty the bowels.

CHAPTER

8

The Infant as a Person

The Infant's Differentiation of His Own Body

THE ORAL zone, as I have already suggested, is an independent dynamism in the sense that while it is the principal zone of interaction in satisfying the infant's need for water and food, it also manifests an excess over needs of the energy partitioned to it; this excess appears as a need to suck, to manipulate with the lips, and so forth, quite irrespective of the need or satisfaction of hunger and thirst. In this case, there occurs what is somewhat uncertainly called 'pleasure' in the various activities which characterize the zone.

By the age of six months the infant is manifesting a variety of zonal needs and some related sign processes. Maturation has been proceeding at a great rate. The eyes, for example, converge in the way that is necessary for binocular vision and the visual appreciation of distance. That does not mean that by the age of six months the infant is particularly good at judging distance. But by the age of six months, that particular coordinate activity of the two eyeballs has matured so that the *fovea centralis*—the center of most acute vision in each retina—is pointed at the particular object being looked at. In addition, coordinate activity of two or more zones of interaction is now frequent. For some time the eyes have been turned toward sources of sound, and by the age of six months the whole head is turned in that direction quite frequently. Hand and arm movement is well developed and serves to convey to the mouth anything that is grasped. This coordination of hands and mouth is a very outstanding aspect of early coordination of two zones of interaction. The infant in these early months literally moves in such fashion as to carry anything that he can retain in his hand to his mouth, where it is tinkered with, sucked, and manipulated generally. Thus thumbs, fingers, toes, and all manner of portable objects have been explored and exploited by the mouth.

As a consequence of this manual-oral coordination, the discrimination of an exceedingly important pattern of experience begins—the differentiation of the infant's body from everything else in the universe. Perhaps this will become clearer if we compare this experience to the infant's differentiation of nipples into good and satisfactory, good and unsatisfactory, and wrong nipples; this differentiation of the nipples is primarily an *intrazonal discrimination*—that is, an organization of sentience which arises primarily within the oral zone; the eyes gradually contribute, although in the beginning they are not yet differentiated as an important zone of interaction. But in manual-oral coordination we are talking about *differentiation that is based on sentience from more than one zone.* Since the baby gets no milk when he sucks his thumb, one might think that the thumb would thus tend to fall into the class of wrong nipples—however suitable for satisfying the zonal need to suck; but the thumb is uniquely different from any nipple by reason of its being *in itself* a source of zonal sentience. *The thumb feels sucked.*

The recurrent multizonal sentience here concerned is in many ways significantly different from the recurrent multizonal sentience in which distance receptors participate with the contact receptors of the oral zone, of the fingers, or of the anus. The latter group of multizonal sentience provides experience for the growing personification of the good mother, as I have explained at some length, and for certain uncomfortable variants which contribute to the personification of the bad mother. The infant's appropriate activity—although it is often adequate for the evocation of the good mother, the good and satisfactory nipple, the good mother's satisfaction-insuring cooperation—is not uniformly effective. Sometimes it is, at least for a time, wholly ineffectual. Sometimes it miscarries badly, and the bad mother appears, approaches, and results in anxiety and, in some cases, in actual pain.

But the infant's appropriate activity to secure the thumb-in-lips situation, once it has been patterned, is always adequate, unless it is opposed by anxiety. Of course, a certain amount of what we shall later discuss as trial-and-error learning is necessary for the infant to be reasonably sure of getting the thumb into the mouth, but, as the neuromuscular apparatus matures, it comes to be pretty dependable. It fails only when the infant is anxious. But in this case it is a failure which is not organized as such, but is instead part of the growing system of experience 'with' anxiety—that is, the experience of being anxious. And when the infant is anxious, anxiety is so much more conspicuous than are the matters opposed by anxiety that failures of this kind are not organized as failures of the activity to create the thumb-in-lips situation. In this thumb-in-lips situation there are *no* failures organized as such in the infant's experience; and the uniform success of this performance is thus significantly distinguished in multizonal experience by its invarying approximation to its foreseen achievement. This is in contrast to the activity with respect to producing the mother and getting food, being cleaned, being covered, and so on, which even though adequate and appropriate may on occasion fail. Needs are differentiated, so far as the infant is concerned, by their foreseen satisfaction. Foreseen satisfaction of hunger may, at least temporarily, miscarry rather badly. But foreseen satisfaction of the zonal need to suck when the thumb-in-lips situation is that which is appropriate is *invariably* followed by the achievement of the satisfaction. So here is an important distinction between this situation and all those previous situations which were obviously relevant and significant to the infant.

By the time the infant is six months old, grasping, the kinesthetically sensed [1] transporting by the hand to the mouth, and the oral sucking and other manipulation of anything thus presented to the mouth—all these are well advanced, along with visual and other accompanying sentience in many cases. But in the infant's experi-

[1] By "kinesthetically sensed" I refer to those types of receptor processes which acquaint us with the position of our joints and so on, or, more specifically, the position of joint surfaces and tension against joint surfaces and so on, and by which, after we have had a great deal of experience, we learn where our extremities are. The movement of these surfaces gives us our acquaintance with, or sentience about, the geometry of the body. Getting the thumb into the mouth involves learning how the elbow, the wrist, and other joints feel, or having prototaxic experience which is effective in bringing about adjustments of muscular movement, and so on.

ence, of all that which is thus grasped, transported, and manipulated, only the parts of his own body which he can get into his mouth, generally his thumb, uniformly and invariably feel sucked and orally manipulated. Thus of all the things which are transported to the mouth, which in actual fact amounts to practically everything which can be moved, the thumb is the only one that feels sucked at the same time that the mouth 'feels sucking.'

Now it is true that the hand feels a variety of events connected with the oral manipulation of sundry objects transported to the mouth, but these manual experiences and their coincident oral experiences are of a relatively wide variety. The hand feels all sorts of things—a ball, a block, or the rods of the crib, let us say. The hand may feel the ball or the block, or something of that kind, at the same time that the mouth is feeling the ball or the block, but the feeling in the hand and the feeling in the mouth, so far as we have any reason to suppose at this time, are not particularly connected with an object. There is sentience from the hand, and this does add up in the course of time to a great deal of acquaintance with objects; and there is very vivid sentience from the lips and mouth, which also adds up to a great deal of acquaintance with objects. But there is no particular reason for thinking of these as being either necessarily or probably organized into any unitary conception of the particular object. This is entirely the contrary of the experience with the thumb-in-lips. All these feelings of the hand with objects other than the thumb which are presented to the mouth combine in the organization of sentience about living among portable objects, so to speak; but the invariant coincidence of the manual-tactile sentience and the sundry oral elements of sentience is not present in these cases.

There may be frequent occasions of fairly sustained coincidence of manual sentience from grasping a nursing bottle and oral sentience from manipulating its attached nipple, but the relation of felt oral and manual needs, and the foresight of satisfaction by activity to integrate the appropriate situation is by no means invariably successful. And this situation of nursing bottle and nipple—by the age of six months or shortly afterward, the infant can grasp and hold the bottle and keep the nipple in approximation to the mouth—does really depend on somebody's providing the nursing bottle, and on the bottle's remaining within reach if it is dropped, which events are by no means invariable concomitants with the infant's wanting the bottle. As a matter of fact, infants very commonly have to go to the same length to get the nursing bottle that they do to get the milk-giving nipple of the mother —that is, they have to cry—and by the age of six months they often cry plenty without anything happening. So while there is the invariant relationship of the foreseen satisfaction connected with the thumb-in-lips, there is anything but this invariant relationship connected with any situation in which there is something intermediate, as it were, between the hand and the lips. The thumb-in-lips is dependable, and is independent of evoking the good mother; the infant can bring it into being, as it were, without cooperation—in isolation from any of his personifications, whether of the good mother or the bad mother. While he cannot live by sucking his thumb, and cannot thus satisfy recurrent needs for food and water, he has matured and profited enough by the organization of his experience to be self-sufficient in respect to satisfying this particular oral zonal need which, as I have said before, generally exceeds in its available transformable energy that which is required for the necessary nursing behavior.

The relatively invariant coincidence of felt need, foresight of satisfaction by adequate and appropriate activity, and independence of cooperation by an at least dimly prehended other person in securing the anticipated satisfaction—all these will come presently to be an important part of a master pattern of experience to which reference is made by the use of the word "my," and more particularly "my body," and, by the sophisticated, "my mind" or even "my soul." Bear in mind that I am for the moment omitting experiences in which anxiety opposes—to the point of preventing—adequate and appropriate activity, which as I have said tends to bring about the organization of experience-with-being-anxious, or experience-while-being-anxious, or anxiety-colored experience, and therefore does not add to the organization of data about the need and its satisfaction. The thumb-in-lips situation is the first we have encountered in which two zonal needs are satisfied by one adequate and appropriate activity that the infant can perform without cooperation of a chronologically more mature person—in which there is no need for evoking the good mother and no danger, at this particular stage, of evoking the bad mother. It is the first situation in which there is an *invariant* coincidence of the felt need and the foresight of its satisfaction by certain activity which is always adequate and appropriate, with the satisfaction of the two zonal needs.

This is a pattern of experience, or it is a kind of experience that will be organized in a pattern. This is an extremely important pattern, for it is the pattern which will evolve, with further experience throughout years and years, into a symbol—a very complex, meaningful, and rich sign; and this sign is the organization of data to which one refers as "my body" and which may include, in a certain less exact sense, practically anything to which "my" is applied seriously. I am not, of course, suggesting that the infant's experience in sucking his thumb and feeling it sucked immediately blossoms out into a considerable formulation of his body. But it is the point of departure for this formulation; it is the type of experience, or the type of activity sequence, which is more or less paradigmatic of experience which will presently be said to include "my body." And for various reasons which will concern us later, it is this pattern, "my body," which has so much to do with the very firmly entrenched feelings of independence, of autonomous entity, if you please, which have been a great handicap to the development of a grasp on interpersonal relations, and which are behind what I have for many years called the delusion of unique individuality.[2] The importance of trying to see how this extraordinary pattern of experience characterized by "my" comes into being, why it has to be as it is, and how it appears as early as perhaps the sixth month of extrauterine life, is that it gives us some idea of how extremely troublesome it is to strip off, from this grand division of experience, the later elaborations which are vicious and misleading in complicating human interpersonal relations. Any important central development of experience that begins so early has roots which are extremely difficult to get at rationally or to formulate.

[2] [*Editors' note:* See Sullivan's paper, first given as a lecture in 1944 and published posthumously with minor revisions, "The Illusion of Personal Individuality," *Psychiatry* (1950) 13:317–332.]

To sum up briefly the beginnings of this experience, by mid-infancy the hands are exploring all reachable parts of the infant's life space and are encountering a variety of objects which fall into two grand divisions, the self-sentient and the non-self-sentient. The thumb is the classical example of what I mean by the self-sentient. It is discovered not by the hand but by the mouth, or rather by hand-mouth cooperation. The mouth feels the thumb, and the thumb feels the mouth; that is self-sentience. This, as I have said, is the point of departure for an enormous development. But the hands, not in connection with the mouth, proceed to contribute a great deal of sentience which is elaborated in this same general field, and the basis of elaboration is that some of the things which the hands encounter are not only felt by the hands but feel the hands, although many of the things that the hands encounter are felt by the hands but do not feel the hands. Prehension about the former (the self-sentient) becomes additional pre-information or information which will presently be organized as the conception of the body; and prehension about the latter (the non-self-sentient) will presently, but distinctly later, be part of the elaborate group of conceptions and misconceptions which is external reality—that which is outside the body.

One might glibly say that the infant is now 'learning about' his own body. But this objective language, by which one might describe in general terms what the infant is doing as something observed, is extremely misleading, so far as contributing to the study of development of personality is concerned. A great deal of what might be read into the infant's behavior cannot, for the best reasons on earth, be the case from the infant's standpoint.

The Influence of Anxiety on the Infant's Acquaintance with His Body

The infant's acquaintance with that which is infant—that which is self-sentient, which feels as well as is felt—does not proceed very far in most directions before it encounters very powerful influences brought to bear by the more mature persons making up the infant's objectively verifiable world. The reason for the infant's not even being free to get acquainted with his own body is a blend of two things, one of which we have touched on at some length before: first, the social responsibility carried by the mothering one to take her infant and turn out a decent, acceptable human being; and, second, a variety of beliefs entertained by the mothering one, some of which may be valid—that is, pretty good approximations to something inhering in the universe and, in particular, in the raising of infants.

One of these bodies of social responsibility and belief soon begins to interfere with the thumb-in-mouth situation. The tendency of the manual zone is not only to grasp and transport to the mouth, but also to pull, and tinker, and so on. Because of this effect of the manual zone on things that it contacts, and because of the present eruption of teeth, it is believed—and, I have no doubt, correctly in some instances at least—that too much of this thumb-in-mouth or hand-in-mouth will result in an aesthetically unfortunate, and perhaps even digestively unfortunate, distortion of the teeth, such that if it is not interfered with, the baby will presently have what is called buckteeth. And this would necessitate expensive, tedious, and, to the child, very unwelcome orthodontic intervention for the sake of beauty. So it becomes to many mothering ones important to do something about the infant's initial venture in self-sufficiency—thumb-sucking. And as time passes, a varying degree of anxiety, identifiable to the infant as the undergoing of forbidding gestures and so on, is brought to bear to interfere with the infant's very important discovery that his body is, in a curious sense, invariably dependable. Thus the infant's activity in satisfying, by sucking his thumb, excess zonal needs pertaining to the mouth is apt to be brought under stern prohibition by the mothering one. So far as I know, this stern prohibition does not ever appear immediately, and even if it did, the infant would suck his thumb when the mother was not around. Thus the thumb-in-lips experience invariably takes places; we do not expect to find an infant who has not sucked his thumb. Nothing less than restraint apparatus to keep the hand away from the mouth would prevent an infant from doing so, and it is quite possible that the result of such very early restraint would be anything but a human being as we like to think of one. Thus there always occurs this discovery by the infant of what might presently be called by a variety of names such as self-sufficiency or (and this name is much more distressing to me) autoerotic perfection. But, as I have said, it is only a matter of time in most cases before this discovery by the infant becomes subject to strong pressure from the carrier of culture who is looking after the infant, lest there be evil effects from it.

By the exploration of the hands, as I have said, many things besides the mouth are discovered—among them, the feet, the umbilicus, the anus, and the external genitals. So far as I have yet detected in my very casual contact with infant-rearing, most mothering ones see nothing the matter with the infant's feeling of the umbilicus; by the time the infant has sufficient dexterity of the upper extremities to do so, the umbilicus will presumably be very nicely healed, and, therefore, there is no great risk of fatal infection. And since one of the deeply ingrained motor patterns seems to be a general motion of curling up, it is quite early that, for instance, a foot and a hand are brought into contact with each other; and that is all right from the mother's point of view.

But an equally convenient kind of exploration, from a geometrical standpoint—namely, feeling of the perineal region, the anus and the external genitals—is, in the estimation of the mothering one, a very different matter indeed. As I suggested before, there is a certain reason, probably ingrained in the organization of the human being, for keeping a certain distance from at least stale feces. Particularly in the northwestern European culture, if a culture area may be so described, the idea of the noxious character of the feces and even the noxious character of the anal region is very strikingly implanted. The hand manipulating the anus, as any mother knows, will shortly be the hand that is in the mouth; thanks to the great development of the doctrine of germs and to the doubts about physical and sexual purity and cleanliness—which are written into the so-called Christian underpinnings of Western culture, built in turn on the Jewish foundations—many mothers feel that a finger conveying anything from the perineal region to the mouth would be disastrous. Thus any exploration of the fecal mass by the hands of the baby, or any tinkering around the area that is touched by the fecal mass, frequently is extremely repellent to the mothering one. And even if these things are not so regarded by the mothering one, she will know that they are so regarded by a large number of other people. Thus the sooner she can get her young to leave that part of the body alone, the better for their standing as potential members of the community in which they live. And, therefore, while in a good many cases there is some pretty strong forbidding of much sucking of the thumb, there is almost invariably pretty strong forbidding of any tampering with the expelled feces or the anal orifice itself.

The social responsibilities and beliefs pertaining to the place of lust in life are somewhat different from those which apply to the expelled feces and the anal orifice itself, although they are all too frequently confused—that is, literally welded together. These beliefs and social responsibilities—the dangers to public decorum and personal standing in the community which presently will relate to what one does with and about one's genitals and other people's genitals—lead to the necessity for strong forbidding on the part of the mothering one of the infant's explorations of the external genitals by the hand.

Thus anxiety, and all sorts of blended feelings in which anxiety is an element, can be evoked in the mothering one with regard to the culturally strong taboos about feces—and even dirt, insofar as it comes to have a more or less fecal connotation—and about handling, or even looking at, the external genitals. The extent to which anxiety in the mothering one, and blended emotions in which anxiety composes an important part, can attach to these two fields of activity is very widely variable. On the one hand, the mothering one's attitude can be what I would say is simply necessary for the infant's becoming a person suitable for life in his particular community—that is, a gradual discouragement of interest in the extruded fecal mass and in the sentient anus, which feels as well as is felt, and in the genitals, which similarly feel as well as are felt. The mother may discourage this from very clear consideration of the customs and beliefs and interests which are acceptable in the community and in the community as she presumes it will develop by the time her young participate actively in it. On the other hand, the mothering one's attitude may be a state of practically sustained, very severe anxiety because baby handles his penis, let us say, or a state of sustained and severe anxiety over his getting his hands soiled with feces. This sometimes amounts to what a psychiatrist without previous acquaintance with the behavior would call frank, severe mental disorder—that is, major psychosis on the part of the mothering one. And this attitude can very successfully obliterate, by inducing intolerable anxiety in the infant, any possible chance of his catching on to what is happening. Thus the social responsibilities and beliefs of the mothering one are apt to interfere to a startling extent with the infant's very dependable, independent, appropriate and adequate action for the satisfaction of purely zonal needs. This may lead to all sorts of efforts by the mothering one—forbidding gestures which get more and more unpleasant, if not actually the inculcating of pain or the use of incredible orthopedic interferences—which are apt to be enforced to segregate out these zones of "ownness" as belonging to that queer thing which we shall shortly discuss as the area of personality called *not-me*.

Thus the development of the pattern of experience which will presently be manifest as the very extensive symbol organization called "my body" gets a good many additions and limitations from the mothering one who may be the embodiment of culture, prejudice, mental disorder, or what not; and so I believe it perfectly safe to say that no one can become a person with just a mature attitude toward his body—in other words, simply with that degree of information which can be acquired by the use of human abilities as they mature.

The Learning of Facial Expressions

Lest we lose track of a great deal that is going on by mid-infancy —that is, by the age of six to eight months—I want to call attention to another very important type of interpersonal process which has been at work. And the interpersonal process involved in the learning of facial expressions is closely related to the experience of "my body" and might be called one of the vicissitudes of ownness.

We are provided with muscular apparatus, fixed to the bones and cartilages of the head, which is capable of doing a great many useful and necessary things for the survival of the underlying animal and therefore of the person. Many of these muscular structures are immediately under a comparatively thin layer of covering—skin and some fatty tissue, and so on. The effector aspect of these muscles—the nerve centers and the muscular tissue itself—

is capable of a very striking manifestation of postural tonicity. A great many of the skeletal muscles are also capable of this postural tonicity but in a much less refined fashion. This postural tonicity has no immediate reference to, shall I say, the simplest function. For instance, the simplest function of these muscles in my arm is to pull up my arm, and they are ordinarily, except when I am asleep or under general anesthetic, maintaining a posture so they can immediately pull, if properly innervated; that is, when I am resting my hand on my thigh, these muscles do not just go flabby and hang down, so to speak. Instead, they come to rest in a posture which permits me immediately to move my forearm when I tighten these muscles. We speak of that as a postural tension, and, in the case of the arm muscles and many others, this postural tension is essentially a sort of active resting condition, so that immediate results can be brought about if there are to be changes in geometry.

With a good many of these effector structures around the face, the postural tensions are much more differentiated than in the case of the arm. And, while it is true that a person who is so mad that he could bite a tenpenny nail, as the expression has it, will be maintaining very high postural tension in his masseter or biting muscles, still these extreme examples of what we call emotional expression, or expressive postures, are not anywhere near easily equated with preparation, or resting preparedness for action, of these muscles. There is actually an enormous amount of change in the appearance of the surface of the face that can be brought about by shifting the pattern of postural tensions in a great many muscles in the face.

By mid-infancy, solely because of contact with the mothering one and any other significant people, the infant has learned certain patterns of postural tension of the face that are right and wrong. Among the most important of all these learnings is the coordination of posture and change of posture—that is, the expressive movement—of the face which is ordinarily called smiling. It might be thought, and in fact I am sure that for many years it has been taught, that we are born with instincts, or something of that general class, for smiling, and, I suppose, for expressing all sorts of things from respectful admiration to frank disgust. But that charmingly simple idea undergoes a little damage when we lift our eyes from our own community and bring them down on the very young in a strikingly alien culture area, such as, for example, Bali or one of the Micronesian Islands in the period before the war and the diffusion of Western culture. In these places, oddly enough, some human beings seem not to have the instinct to smile in the sense that we know it, but instead an instinct to smile in a very different way, so different that you wouldn't recognize it as a smile until you noticed what the others did in a similar situation. The point is that man has an unending, a numerically enormous, number of possible resting states of the face, and a still more enormous number of transitions in resting states of these so-called expressive muscles. Thus a truly astounding number of so-called expressions is possible, and it is by the organization of initially prototaxic experience, later elaborated further into combinations of sentience from various zones, that the infant gradually picks out from this numerical multitude rough approximations to what the culture-carriers esteem as expressions. That is literally the way that a great deal of our facial expression comes into being.

Facial expressions are always a blend of both postural tensions and motion. That is to say, a fixed frown, for example, rapidly loses its capacity to communicate to anyone, and becomes recognized as a feature. But prescribed changes from certain momentarily fixed postural tones to certain other momentarily fixed postural tones has immense and dependable communicative capacity for those who know each other—that is, for denizens of the same or approximately the same culture. These expressions are learned —and this learning is by trial and error under the influence of anxiety or the absence of anxiety. Insofar as there is success, there is nothing forbidding, no discouraging disturbance of euphoria. Insofar as things fail there is a disturbance of euphoria, again because of the social responsibility, and the expectation of the development of intelligence, and all sorts of things which the mothering one has about the infant. Thus people literally learn to express their emotions by trial-and-error approximations under the influence of anxiety. Now I am not talking here of how the infant looks very early in life when he is crying, but I am talking about how the infant looks when he is crying by the time he is twelve months old, by which time his crying shows a good deal of influence by the expectations, the use of minor forbidding gestures, the anxiety, and so on of the mothering one.

The Learning of Phonemes

I am now going to touch briefly on another type of learning which manifests itself in mid-infancy, and which I shall presently discuss in more detail. Provided the underlying human animal has not had any genetic or pathological misfortunes, by the sixth to eighth month a form of learning appears which is a manifestation of human potentialities of simply overwhelming importance in subsequent life: this is not trial-and-error learning under the influence of anxiety, but it is trial-and-error learning by human example or by human model. Here it is not the anxiety-tinted or euphoria-protecting attitude of the mothering one which determines success, but it is the infant's already developed coordination of two zones of interaction. We have touched upon one development of coordination which does not have human example—namely, the getting of the thumb into the lips. That appears to be arranged by a rather astounding connection in the central nervous system in the human and certain closely related species, the mouth being an enormous source of data in the early acquaintance with reality. But the coordination of two zones that I am now referring to is a coordination in which, when we first mentioned it, we did not separate the zones—this was when we spoke of the infant's hearing his own crying. I am now talking about hearing as an independent zone of interaction. The delicate coordination of sound production with activities of the hearing zone is now proceeding by maturation, and the infant is now 'experimenting'[a] in approximating sounds heard, needless to say, from others. There is no need for the infant to approximate sounds heard from himself—they are there, they always have been there. One of the first things we mentioned was the birth cry, which I suggested that the infant heard, but that was probably heard by bone conduction or anyway by solid conduction. But now I am talking about the long process of learning by trial and error from example, by

[a] When I use such words as "experimenting" in talking about the infant, you must understand that this is all illusory language and that I don't mean quite what you might find in the dictionary.

which the infant begins to approximate sounds *made by him* to sounds *heard by him.* And this development, which originally appears in rather curious noises commonly called gurgling and cooing, proceeds in the next few months through babbling to the actual close approximation of those particular stations in the continuum of sound which are the phonemes out of which the speech of the people significant to the infant is constructed. Now this cannot occur if the infant cannot hear, and it could not occur if the infant were living in an utterly mute and silent environment. But, barring these circumstances, as early as the eighth month after birth the coordination of the ear-receptor and the voice-producing apparatus is already beginning to manifest itself in what are literally the preliminaries to acquiring the capacity to make the right phonemal sounds, out of which all the stupendous structure of language will presently have its being.

CHAPTER 9

Learning: The Organization of Experience

I NOW want to take up an area of very great importance which I have never gotten very well under control. It is undoubtedly a field which requires multidisciplined thinking, and some of the people who could perhaps add most valuably to such a multiple approach are, unhappily, people who feel that psychiatrists have no business in this neighborhood—a form of craft-union antagonism which, I trust, will gradually fade into history. The topic I now wish to discuss is learning—that is, the organization of experience.

So far, the processes of maturation of the underlying animal have not yet included any of the more or less epoch-marking developments which will later concern us—such as the acquisition of language, in contrast to the very few sounds that are identified by others as words; the need for compeers with whom to interact; and the other maturations that mark off the eras of personality development. But still there has been a truly astounding series of maturations of the underlying capabilities, and by the end of the ninth month the infant is manifesting pretty unmistakable evidence of processes which are of the pattern of, or are rudimentary instances of, a very great deal of that which is peculiarly the human way of life. Maturation has progressed, thereby bringing into being capabilities of the underlying human animal for becoming a human being, and experience has been organized in the opportunities which are provided both by the cooperation with the mothering one, and by the rather incidental physical environment of objects and the like.

Thus by the end of the ninth month of infancy there are organizations of experience which are manifested in recall and foresight in many of the categories of behavior that make up the fully human type of living. Needless to say, these organizations are imperfectly developed. But the point is that they are manifested in patterns which make it highly probable that the rudiments of a large area of human living are already organized by the end of the ninth month. These organizations appear as growth of the dynamisms concerned, both with respect to the integration and maintenance of suitable situations, and with respect to the vector quality (the appropriateness and adequacy) of behavior in the resolution of the various situations—that is, with respect to the achievement of satisfaction as a goal. To say this a little differently, the close observation of situations, as early as the end of the ninth month, shows that there is considerable organization of experience which can be called the development of the appropriate dynamisms for integrating and maintaining situations, and for the choice—and I am using that word very broadly—of the appropriate and adequate energy transformations or activities for the achievement of the resolution of the situation—that is, for the satisfaction of the need which is involved.

This growth may be considered to result from sundry learning processes which rest on the necessary basis of serial maturation of capacities of the underlying animal, coupled with the opportunity for manifesting the ability concerned; in most cases the opportunity still involves an element of cooperation with the mothering one—that is, it is interpersonal. First, one always has to have the maturation of the capability; and secondly, one must have appropriate and useful experience, so that the ability, the actually demonstrable transformations of energy in activity addressed to the goal, appears; and experience of the type that we can call learning processes has a very great deal to do with the latter.

Learning by Anxiety

I am now going to set up a heuristic classification of the processes of learning. The first of all learning is, I think, beyond doubt in immediate connection with *anxiety*. I have already tried to suggest, and will again and again suggest, that severe anxiety probably contributes no information. The effect of severe anxiety reminds one in some ways of a blow on the head, in that it simply wipes out what is immediately proximal to its occurrence. If you have a severe blow on the head, you are quite apt later to have an incurable, absolute amnesia covering the few moments before your head was struck. Anxiety has a similar effect of producing useless confusion, and a useless disturbance of the factors of sentience which immediately preceded its onset, a phenomenon which is so striking that in later life the great problem of psychotherapy is very often centered on this very matter of getting the patient to see just when anxiety intervened, because that area is disturbed in such a way that it is almost as if it had not been.

Less severe anxiety does permit gradual realization of the situation in which it occurs, and there is unquestionably, even from very early in life, some learning of an inhibitory nature; that is, the transfer of attributes of "my body" to the "not-me" aspect of the universe. But regardless of all these refinements, the first greatly educative influence in living is doubtless anxiety, unqualified.

Vastly more important, in fact perhaps astoundingly important in its relation to our coming to be human beings acceptable to the particular society which we inhabit, is the next process of learning, which is learning on the basis of the *anxiety gradient*—that is, learning to discriminate increasing from diminishing anxiety and to alter activity in the direction of the latter. As I have said before, this notion of gradients can perhaps be illustrated by the distribution of amoebae in the water near, let us say, a hot spring. The conduction of heat in the water will result in a temperature gradient from extremely high, utterly beyond the temperature limits of life, down to a temperature lower than that in which the amoebae live most successfully. There is a certain optimum temperature for the growth of the amoebae, and at that point the concentration of amoebae will be very high. But because of peculiarities in the amoebae, or peculiarities in physical space which can hold only a certain number of amoebae, the concentration of amoebae will grade off both ways. There will be some amoebae in a rapidly declining triangle, we might say, toward the hotter water, and there will be some, perhaps the more underprivileged amoebae, trailing off as a tail into the colder water. What attenuates the concentration of amoebae, particularly in the direction of the hot water, is their avoidance of temperatures which are intolerable to their processes, which is no more mysterious than anything else that goes on in any of the living. Since these amoebae are influenced by that particular manifestation of energy called heat, they rise to a maximum very rapidly at a certain distance from the hot water, and decline to a minimum rather more slowly in the direction of the cold water.

Very early in human life there begins to be discrimination as to when euphoria is diminishing—that is, when one is getting more anxious; and this is really the discrimination of a gradient. The all-or-nothing character of anxiety and euphoria has disappeared very early in life—in fact, I doubt that it ever existed—and an immense amount of what is human behavior in any society is learned simply on the basis of this gradient from anxiety to euphoria. For example, the satisfaction of rubbing the anal region with the finger, let us say, might carry such rapidly increasing anxiety under certain circumstances—namely, in the presence of the mothering one, the social censor—that really quite early in life there might be learning about this. The infant might learn, first, that this is not to occur when the mothering one is around, which is, more or less, learning by pure anxiety; and secondly, that the peculiar circumstance of fiddling with this area through a blanket—even though the infant does not recognize the blanket as such—seems much less strikingly characterized by very rapidly mounting anxiety. And so, presently, direct manipulation of the anus may be restricted to periods of somnolence; or, if the impulse is quite strong, some mediate performance may be engaged in.

Now, if I make myself at all clear, you will realize that I am indicating here the formulation for a type of process of really staggering importance; I have never found a satisfactory name for this process, and therefore still use the good old term of the most traditional psychoanalytic standing—*sublimation*, the long-circuiting of the resolution of situations, chiefly those pertaining to zonal needs—a long-circuiting which proves to be socially acceptable. However, in considering this stage of infancy, one should not think in terms of impulses, social acceptability, and so on, but should realize that the actually describable and intelligible factor is the anxiety gradient, and that learning by the anxiety gradient often includes irrational tricks that permit satisfaction without encouraging notable anxiety. Needless to say, this begins at a time when anything like consensually valid formulation is simply inconceivable.

> [Thus the infant] learns to chart a course by the anxiety gradient. Simple performances which would relax the tension of some needs have to be made more complicated in order that one may avoid becoming more anxious. Before he is very many months of age, the child will be showing full-fledged *sublimation*, in the sense of quite unwittingly having adopted some pattern of activity in the partial, and somewhat incomplete, satisfaction of a need which, however, avoids anxiety that stands in the way of the simplest completely satisfactory activity. . . . Whether it recurs in the second or the fifty-second year of chronological age, sublimation is, unwittingly, not a matter of conscious thought of a communicable sort, but rather the outcome of referential processes in the parataxic mode, in the service of avoiding or minimizing anxiety. . . .[1]

This unwitting development, which is the pattern of sublimation, becomes an important element in learning to be human—that is, in learning to behave as one should behave in a given society.

Other Learning Processes

The next important learning process is learning by *trial and success* of techniques for the relief of the tensions of needs. For example, in order to satisfy the zonal need to suck, the infant learns how to get the thumb into the proper position in the mouth. That is literally done by trial movements of the extremities, aided by a certain amount of visual sentience and a good deal of kinesthetic sentience. There are quite a number of misses and some hits, the hits being successes in getting the thumb into the mouth; and it is these successes that become stamped in as 'habits'—although 'habit' has many unfortunate connotations. In other words,

1 [*Editors' note:* All the quotations in this chapter, including this one, are from Sullivan's "Tensions Interpersonal and International: A Psychiatrist's View," in *Tensions That Cause Wars*, edited by Hadley Cantril; Urbana, Ill.: Univ. of Ill. Press, 1950, pp. 95–98.]

the successes are the patterns of sentience and effector impulse which work.

Thus while unnumbered of the manipulative attempts of the infant's hands, for example, fail—which is, perhaps, in infancy not too astounding—some of them succeed. And again, diligent study of the infant shows that a success has a really remarkable fixing power. In other words, that which works, however wrongly designed, is very apt to become part of the activity resources of the person, which is true even in adult life. And so, second only to learning by the anxiety gradient is the learning of how to do things by trial and success.

In late infancy and from then on through life, an important process of learning is by *rewards and punishments.* Probably this kind of learning exists earlier in infancy, but this is more difficult to be sure of, since there it would have to depend on empathic factors.

The rewards which encourage learning in the very young probably begin with *fondling,* pleasure-giving manipulation of the child. They take in general the pattern of a change from relative indifference to the child to more or less active interest in and approval of whatever he seems to be doing. The need for "audience response" becomes conspicuous remarkably early in human life.

The punishments are commonly the inflicting of *pain,* the refusal of contact or of attention, and of course, the inducing of anxiety—a very special punishment. I know of no reason why punishment should be undesirable as an educative influence excepting it be anxiety-ladened. Pain has a very useful function in life and loneliness and the foresight of enforced isolation, the "fear of ostracism," is bound to be an important influence from early in the third stage of development.

The next very important learning process is *trial-and-error learning by human example,* or from human example. I have already mentioned this in discussing facial postures; smiling, as I have said, appears pretty early, while a number of other instances of this kind of learning can invariably be observed in late infancy—that is, very definitely under the age of eighteen months, and probably by the age of twelve months. In this kind of learning, unlike the manipulative learning, the error is important. The success is, you might say, just too good to be important. When success is achieved, the problem is finished. Success in manipulation, on the other hand, has the effect of immediately stamping in a pattern of behavior. But the error in this particular way of learning—learning from human example—is to be kept clearly in mind. It is what one observes as part of the content of consciousness, in those who are mature enough to communicate clearly their experience.

[Not only is this kind of learning probably exemplified in the patterning of facial expressions, but] it is certainly the chief agency in the acquisition of *language*. The phonemes of any system of speech have simply nothing to do with any but cultural necessity. The child learns to approximate from among an indeterminately great variety of vocal sounds that he utters, the particular sound-areas that are used by the significant people around him. In the same way, he picks up the patterns of tonal melody in their speech; often being able to reproduce the tonal, melodic, progressions of speaking well in advance of his "use" of any word.

The only other very important process in learning that I know of is the very refined process which Spearman called the *eduction*[2]—more or less the pulling out—of relations. This comes to be a highly complex capacity, rather strikingly, but by no means exclusively, restricted to the human. It is a capacity—of the most infinite complexity—of our nervous systems which enables us to get more and more to see relations which endure in nature and therefore are to a truly remarkable degree dependable. Spearman built up tests for superior intelligence which depended practically entirely on the capacity to educe, or to grasp, an increasingly complex series of relations which characterize the world as known.

The first instances of this sort of learning to live are purely matters of inference, but it is entirely reasonable to believe that some of the elementary mechanical-geometric relations pertaining to "parts" of a very important preconceptual "object," presently to be named *my body*, are prehended quite soon after birth.

And this process of educing relations can be observed in the infant in certain rudimentary aspects of his interpersonal relation with the mothering one before the use of words.

Every important process in learning which I have been able to formulate is illustrated, at least in rudiment, before speech. I would like to emphasize again the fact that beyond any perchance,

[2] [*Editors' note:* See Chapter 5, footnote 1.]

as early as or before the end of the tenth month in many instances, so much learning of sounds by trial and error, or from human example, appears that the baby sounds to a person at a little distance as if he were talking to himself. This is a truly amazing instance of human ability. I would like to remind you that in your dealings with friend and foe, stranger and intimate acquaintance, modifications and stresses in the tonal patterns of your remarks can do things which no words qua words could do. When you see how very early and how extremely important this form of learning is, and how basically important are the things which are learned, oh, so long before communicable thought can take place, you may perhaps feel a little more impressed with the importance of the phase of infancy.

CHAPTER 10

Beginnings of the Self-System

Three Aspects of Interpersonal Cooperation

WE HAVE got our human animal as far, in the process of becoming a person, as the latter part of infancy, and we find him being subjected more and more to the social responsibilities of the parent. As the infant comes to be recognized as educable, capable of learning, the mothering one modifies more and more the exhibition of tenderness, or the giving of tenderness, to the infant. The earlier feeling that the infant must have unqualified cooperation is now modified to the feeling that the infant should be learning certain things, and this implies a restriction, on the part of the mothering one, of her tender cooperation under certain circumstances.

Successful training of the functional activity of the anal zone of interaction accentuates a new aspect of tenderness—namely, the additive role of tenderness as a sequel to what the mothering one regards as good behavior. Now this is, in effect—however it may be prehended by the infant—a *reward,* which, once the approved social ritual connected with defecating has worked out well, is added to the satisfaction of the anal zone. Here is tenderness taking on the attribute of a reward for having learned something, or for behaving right.

Thus the mother, or the parent responsible for acculturation or socialization, now adds tenderness to her increasingly neutral behavior in a way that can be called rewarding. I think that very, very often the parent does this with no thought of rewarding the infant. Very often the rewarding tenderness merely arises from the pleasure of the mothering one in the skill which the infant has learned—the success which has attended a venture on the toilet chair, or something of that kind. But since tenderness in general is becoming more restricted by the parental necessity to train, these incidents of straightforward tenderness, following the satisfaction of a need like that to defecate, are really an addition—a case of getting something extra for good behavior—and this is, in its generic pattern, a reward. This type of learning can take place when the training procedure has been well adjusted to the learning capacity of the infant. The friendly response, the pleasure which the mother takes in something having worked out well, comes more and more to be something special in the very last months of infancy, whereas earlier, tenderness was universal when the mothering one was around, if she was a comfortable mothering one. Thus, to a certain extent, this type of learning can be called learning under the influence of reward—the reward being nothing more or less than tender behavior on the part of the acculturating or socializing mothering one.

Training in the functional activity of the oral-manual behavior—that is, conveying things by the hand to the mouth and so on—begins to accentuate the differentiation of anxiety-colored situations in contrast to approved situations. The training in this particular field is probably, in almost all cases, the area in which *grades of anxiety* first become of great importance in learning; as I have already stressed, behavior of a certain unsatisfactory type provokes increasing anxiety, and the infant learns to keep a distance from, or to veer away from, activities which are attended by increasing anxiety, just as the amoebae avoid high temperatures.

This is the great way of learning in infancy, and later in childhood—by the grading of anxiety, so that the infant learns to chart his course by mild forbidding gestures, or by mild states of worry, concern, or disapproval mixed with some degree of anxiety on the part of the mothering one. The infant plays, one might say, the old game of getting hotter or colder, in charting a selection of behavioral units which are not attended by an increase in anxiety. Anxiety in its most severe form is a rare experience after infancy, in the more fortunate courses of personality development, and anxiety as it is a function in chronologically adult life, in a highly civilized community confronted by no particular crisis, is never very severe for most people. And yet it is necessary to appreciate that it is anxiety which is responsible for a great part of the inadequate, inefficient, unduly rigid, or otherwise unfortunate performances of people; that anxiety is responsible in a basic sense for a great deal of what comes to a psychiatrist for attention. Only when this is understood, can one realize that this business of whether one is getting more or less anxious is in a large sense the basic influence which determines interpersonal relations—that is, it is not the motor, it does not call interpersonal relations into being, but it more or less directs the course of their development. And even in late infancy there is a good deal of learning by the anxiety gradient, particularly where there is a mothering one who is untroubled, but still intensely interested in producing the right kind of child; and this learning is apt to first manifest itself when the baby is discouraged from putting the wrong things in the mouth, and the like. This kind of learning applies over a vast area of behavior. But in this discussion I am looking for where things are apt to start.

Training of the manual-exploratory function—which I have discussed in connection with the infant's getting his hands near the anus, or into the feces, or, perhaps, in contact with the external genitals—almost always begins the discrimination of situations which are marked by what we shall later discuss as *uncanny emotion*. This uncanny feeling can be described as the abrupt supervention of *severe anxiety*, with the arrest of anything like the learning process, and with only gradual informative recall of the noted circumstances which preceded the extremely unpleasant incident.

Early in infancy, when situations approach the 'all-or-nothing' character, the induction of anxiety is apt to be the sudden translation from a condition of moderate euphoria to one of very severe anxiety. And this severe anxiety, as I have said before, has a little bit the effect of a blow on the head, in that later one is not clear at all as to just what was going on at the time anxiety became intense. The educative effect is not by any means as simple and useful as is the educative effect in the other two situations which we have discussed, because the sudden occurrence of severe anxiety practically prohibits any clear prehension, or understanding, of the immediate situation. It does not, however, preclude recall, and as recall develops sufficiently so that one recalls what was about to occur when severe anxiety intervened—in other words, when one has a sense of what one's action was addressed to at the time when everything was disorganized by severe anxiety—then there come to be in all of us certain areas of 'uncanny taboo,' which I think is a perfectly good way of characterizing those things which one stops doing, once one has caught himself doing them. This type of training is much less immediately useful, and, shall I say, is productive of much less healthy acquaintance with reality, than are the other two.

Good-Me, Bad-Me, and Not-Me

Now here I have set up three aspects of interpersonal cooperation which are necessary for the infant's survival, and which dictate learning. That is, these aspects of interpersonal cooperation require acculturation or socialization of the infant. Infants are customarily exposed to all of these before the era of infancy is finished. From experience of these three sorts—with rewards, with the anxiety gradient, and with practically obliterative sudden severe anxiety—there comes an initial personification of three phases of what presently will be *me*, that which is invariably connected with the sentience of *my body*—and you will remember that *my body* as an organization of experience has come to be distinguished from everything else by its self-sentient character. These beginning personifications of three different kinds, which have in common elements of the prehended body, are organized in about mid-infancy—I can't say exactly when. I have already spoken of the infant's very early double personification of the actual mothering one as the good mother and the bad mother. Now, at this time, the beginning personifications of *me* are *good-me*, *bad-me*, and *not-me*. So far as I can see, in practically every instance of being trained for life, in this or another culture, it is rather inevitable that there shall be this tripartite cleavage in personifications, which have as their central tie—the thing that binds them ultimately into one, that always keeps them in very close relation—their relatedness to the growing conception of "my body."

Good-me is the beginning personification which organizes experience in which satisfactions have been enhanced by rewarding increments of tenderness, which come to the infant because the mothering one is pleased with the way things are going; therefore, and to that extent, she is free, and moves toward expressing tender appreciation of the infant. Good-me, as it ultimately develops, is the ordinary topic of discussion about "I."

Bad-me, on the other hand, is the beginning personification which organizes experience in which increasing degrees of anxiety are associated with behavior involving the mothering one in its more-or-less clearly prehended interpersonal setting. That is to say, bad-me is based on this increasing gradient of anxiety and that, in turn, is dependent, at this stage of life, on the observation, if misinterpretation, of the infant's behavior by someone who can induce anxiety.[1] The frequent coincidence of certain behavior on the part of the infant with increasing tenseness and increasingly evident forbidding on the part of the mother is the source of the type of experience which is organized as a rudimentary personification to which we may apply the term bad-me.

So far, the two personifications I have mentioned may sound like a sort of laboring of reality. However, these personifications are a part of the communicated thinking of the child, a year or so later, and therefore it is not an unwarranted use of inference to presume that they exist at this earlier stage. When we come to the third of these beginning personifications, *not-me,* we are in a different field—one which we know about only through certain very special circumstances. And these special circumstances are not outside the experience of any of us. The personification of not-me is most conspicuously encountered by most of us in an occasional dream while we are asleep; but it is very emphatically encountered by people who are having a severe schizophrenic episode, in aspects that are to them most spectacularly real. As a matter of fact, it is always manifest—not every minute, but every day, in every life—in certain peculiar absences of phenomena where

[1] Incidentally, for all I know, anybody can induce anxiety in an infant, but there is no use cluttering up our thought by considering that, because frequency of events is of very considerable significance in all learning processes; and at this stage of life, when the infant is perhaps nine or ten months old, it is likely to be the mother who is frequently involved in interpersonal situations with the infant.

there should be phenomena; and in a good many people—I know not what proportion—it is very striking in its indirect manifestations (dissociated behavior), in which people do and say things of which they do not and could not have knowledge, things which may be quite meaningful to other people but are unknown to them. The special circumstances which we encounter in grave mental disorders may be, so far as you know, outside your experience; but they were not once upon a time. It is from the evidence of these special circumstances—including both those encountered in everybody and those encountered in grave disturbances of personality, all of which we shall presently touch upon—that I choose to set up this third beginning personification which is tangled up with the growing acquaintance of "my body," the personification of *not-me*. This is a very gradually evolving personification of an always relatively primitive character—that is, organized in unusually simple signs in the parataxic mode of experience, and made up of poorly grasped aspects of living which will presently be regarded as 'dreadful,' and which still later will be differentiated into incidents which are attended by awe, horror, loathing, or dread.

This rudimentary personification of not-me evolves very gradually, since it comes from the experience of intense anxiety—a very poor method of education. Such a complex and relatively inefficient method of getting acquainted with reality would naturally lead to relatively slow evolution of an organization of experiences; furthermore, these experiences are largely truncated, so that what they are really about is not clearly known. Thus organizations of these experiences marked by uncanny emotion—which means experiences which, when observed, have led to intense forbidding gestures on the part of the mother, and induced intense anxiety in the infant—are not nearly as clear and useful guides to anything as the other two types of organizations have been. Because experiences marked by uncanny emotion, which are organized in the personification of not-me, cannot be clearly connected with cause and effect—cannot be dealt with in all the impressive ways by which we explain our referential processes later—they persist throughout life as relatively primitive, unelaborated, parataxic symbols. Now that does not mean that the not-me component in adults is infantile; but it does mean that the not-me component is, in all essential respects, practically beyond discussion in communicative terms. Not-me is part of the very 'private mode' of living. But, as I have said, it manifests itself at various times in the life of everyone after childhood—or of nearly everyone, I can't swear to the statistics—by the eruption of certain exceedingly unpleasant emotions in what are called nightmares.

These three rudimentary personifications of *me* are, I believe, just as distinct as the two personifications of the objectively same mother were earlier. But while the personifications of me are getting under way, there is some change going on with respect to the personification of mother. In the latter part of infancy, there is some evidence that the rudimentary personality, as it were, is already fusing the previously disparate personifications of the good and the bad mother; and within a year and a half after the end of infancy we find evidence of this duplex personification of the mothering one as the good mother and the bad mother clearly manifested only in relatively obscure mental processes, such as these dreamings while asleep. But, as I have suggested, when we come to consider the question of the peculiarly inefficient and inappropriate interpersonal relations which constitute problems of mental disorder, there again we discover that the trend in organizing experience which began with this duplex affair has not in any sense utterly disappeared.

The Dynamism of the Self-System

From the essential desirability of being good-me, and from the increasing ability to be warned by slight increases of anxiety—that is, slight diminutions in euphoria—in situations involving the increasingly significant other person, there comes into being the start of an exceedingly important, as it were, secondary dynamism, which is purely the product of interpersonal experience arising from anxiety encountered in the pursuit of the satisfaction of general and zonal needs. This secondary dynamism I call the *self-system.* As a dynamism it is secondary in that it does not have any particular zones of interaction, any particular physiological apparatus, behind it; but it literally uses all zones of interaction and all physiological apparatus which is integrative and meaningful from the interpersonal standpoint. And we ordinarily find its ramifications spreading throughout interpersonal relations in every area where there is any chance that anxiety may be encountered.

The essential desirability of being good-me is just another way of commenting on the essential undesirability of being anxious. Since the beginning personification of good-me is based on experience in which satisfactions are enhanced by tenderness, then naturally there is an essential desirability of living good-me. And since sensory and other abilities of the infant are well matured by now—perhaps even space perception, one of the slowest to come along, is a little in evidence—it is only natural that along with this essential desirability there goes increasing ability to be warned by slight forbidding—in other words, by slight anxiety. Both these situations, for the purpose now under discussion, are situations involving another person—the mothering one, or the congeries of mothering ones—and she is becoming increasingly significant because, as I have already said, the manifestation of tender cooperation by her is now complicated by her attempting to teach, to socialize the infant; and this makes the relationship more complex, so that it requires better, more effective differentiation by the infant of forbidding gestures, and so on. For all these reasons, there comes into being in late infancy an organization of experience which will ultimately be of nothing less than stupendous importance in personality, and which comes entirely from the interpersonal relations in which the infant is now involved—and these interpersonal relations have their motives (or their motors, to use a less troublesome word) in the infant's general and zonal needs for satisfaction. But out of the social responsibility of the mothering one, which gets involved in the satisfaction of the infant's needs, there comes the organization in the infant of what might be said to be a dynamism directed at how to live with this significant other person. The self-system thus is an organization of educative experience called into being by the necessity to avoid or to minimize incidents of anxiety.[2] The functional activity of the

[2] Since *minimize* in this sense can be ambiguous, I should make it clear that I refer, by minimizing, to moving, in behavior, in the direction which is marked by diminishing anxiety. I do not mean, by minimize, to "make little of," because so far as I know, human ingenuity cannot make little of anxiety.

self-system—I am now speaking of it from the general standpoint of a dynamism—is primarily directed to avoiding and minimizing this disjunctive tension of anxiety, and thus indirectly to protecting the infant from this evil eventuality in connection with the pursuit of satisfactions—the relief of general or of zonal tensions.

Thus we may expect, at least until well along in life, that the components of the self-system will exist and manifest functional activity in relation to every general need that a person has, and to every zonal need that the excess supply of energy to the various zones of interaction gives rise to. How conspicuous the 'sector' of the self-system connected with any particular general need or zonal need will be, or how frequent its manifestations, is purely a function of the past experience of the person concerned.

I have said that the self-system begins in the organizing of experience with the mothering one's forbidding gestures, and that these forbidding gestures are refinements in the personification of the bad mother; this might seem to suggest that the self-system comes into being by the *incorporation* or *introjection* of the bad mother, or simply by the introjection of the mother. These terms, incorporation or introjection, have been used in this way, not in speaking of the self-system, but in speaking of the psychoanalytic superego, which is quite different from my conception of the self-system. But, if I have been at all adequate in discussing even what I have presented thus far, it will be clear that the use of such terms in connection with the development of the self-system is a rather reckless oversimplification, if not also a great magic verbal gesture the meaning of which cannot be made explicit. I have said that the self-system comes into being because the pursuit of general and zonal needs for satisfaction is increasingly interfered with by the good offices of the mothering one in attempting to train the young. And so the self-system, far from being anything like a function of or an identity with the mothering one, is an organization of experience for avoiding increasing degrees of anxiety which are connected with the educative process. But these degrees of anxiety cannot conceivably, in late infancy (and the situation is similar in most instances at any time in life), mean to the infant what the mothering one, the socializing person, believes she means, or what she actually represents, from the standpoint of the culture being inculcated in the infant. This idea that one can, in some way, take in another person to become a part of one's personality is one of the evils that comes from overlooking the fact that between a doubtless real 'external object' and a doubtless real 'my mind' there is a group of processes—the act of perceiving, understanding, and what not—which is intercalated, which is highly subject to past experience and increasingly subject to foresight of the neighboring future. Therefore, it would in fact be one of the great miracles of all time if our perception of another person were, in any greatly significant number of respects, accurate or exact. Thus I take some pains at this point to urge you to keep your mind free from the notion that I am dealing with something like the taking over of standards of value and the like from another person. Instead, I am talking about the organization of experience connected with relatively successful education in becoming a human being, which begins to be manifest late in infancy.

When I talk about the self-system, I want it clearly understood that I am talking about a *dynamism* which comes to be enormously important in understanding interpersonal relations. This dynamism is an explanatory conception; it is not a thing, a region, or what not, such as superegos, egos, ids, and so on.[3] Among the things this conception explains is something that can be described as a quasi-entity, the personification of the self. The personification of the self is what you are talking about when you talk about yourself as "I," and what you are often, if not invariably, referring to when you talk about "me" and "my." But I would like to make it forever clear that *the relation of personifications to that which is personified is always complex and sometimes multiple;* and that *personifications are not adequate descriptions of that which is personified.* In my effort to make that clear, I have gradually been compelled,

[3] Please do not bog down unnecessarily on the problem of whether my self-system ought to be called the superego or the ego. I surmise that there is some noticeable relationship, perhaps in the realm of cousins or closer, between what I describe as the personification of the self and what is often considered to be the psychoanalytic ego. But if you are wise, you will dismiss that as facetious, because I am not at all sure of it; it has been so many years since I found anything but headaches in trying to discover parallels between various theoretical systems that I have left that for the diligent and scholarly, neither of which includes me.

in my teaching, to push the beginnings of things further and further back in the history of the development of the person, to try to reach the point where the critical deviations from convenient ideas become more apparent. Thus I am now discussing the beginning of the terrifically important self-dynamism as the time when —far from there being a personification of the self—there are only rudimentary personifications of good-me and bad-me, and the much more rudimentary personification of not-me. These rudimentary personifications constitute anything but a personification of the self such as you all believe you manifest, and which you believe serves its purpose, when you talk about yourselves one to another in adult life.

The Necessary and Unfortunate Aspects of the Self-System

The origin of the self-system can be said to rest on the irrational character of culture or, more specifically, society. Were it not for the fact that a great many prescribed ways of doing things have to be lived up to, in order that one shall maintain workable, profitable, satisfactory relations with his fellows; or, were the prescriptions for the types of behavior in carrying on relations with one's fellows perfectly rational—then, for all I know, there would not be evolved, in the course of becoming a person, anything like the sort of self-system that we always encounter. If the cultural prescriptions which characterize any particular society were better adapted to human life, the notions that have grown up about incorporating or introjecting a punitive, critical person would not have arisen.

But even at that, I believe that a human being without a self-system is beyond imagination. It is highly probable that the type of education which we have discussed, even probably the inclusion of certain uncanny experience that tends to organize in the personification of not-me, would be inevitable in the process of the human animal's becoming a human being. I say this because the enormous capacity of the human animal which underlies human personality is bound to lead to exceedingly intricate specializations—differentiations of living, function, and one thing and another; to maintain a workable, profitable, appropriate, and adequate type of relationship among the great numbers of people that can become involved in a growing society, the young have to be taught a vast amount before they begin to be significantly involved in society outside the home group. Therefore, the special secondary elaboration of the sundry types of learning—which I call the self-system—would, I believe, be a ubiquitous aspect of all really human beings in any case. But in an ideal culture, which has never been approximated and at the present moment looks as if it never will be, the proper function of the self-system would be conspicuously different from its actual function in the denizens of our civilization. In our civilization, no parental group actually reflects the essence of the social organization for which the young are being trained in living; and after childhood, when the family influence in acculturation and socialization begins to be attenuated and augmented by other influences, the discrete excerpts, you might say, of the culture which each family has produced as its children come into collision with other discrete excerpts of the culture—all of them more or less belonging to the same cultural system, but having very different accents and importances mixed up in them. As a result of this, the self-system in its actual functioning in life in civilized societies, as they now exist, is often very unfortunate. But do not overlook the fact that the self-system comes into being because of, and can be said to have as its goal, the securing of necessary satisfaction without incurring much anxiety. And however unfortunate the manifestations of the self-system in many contexts may seem, always keep in mind that, if one had no protection against very severe anxiety, one would do practically nothing—or, if one still had to do something, it would take an intolerably long time to get it done.

So you see, however truly the self-system is the principal stumbling block to favorable changes in personality—a point which I shall develop later on—that does not alter the fact that it is also the principal influence that stands in the way of unfavorable changes in personality. And while the psychiatrist is skillful, in large measure, in his ability to formulate the self-system of another person with whom he is integrated, and to, shall I say, "intuit" the self-system aspects of his patient which tend to perpetuate the type of morbid living that the patient is showing, that still, in no sense, makes the self-system something merely to be regretted. In any event, it is always before us, whether we regret or praise it. This idea of the self-system is simply tremendously important in understanding the vicissitudes of interpersonal relations from here on. If we understand how the self-system begins, then perhaps we will be able to follow even the most difficult idea connected with its function.

The self-system is a product of educative experience, part of which is of the character of reward, and a very important part of which has the graded anxiety element that we have spoken of. But quite early in life, anxiety is also a very conspicuous aspect of the self-dynamism *function.* This is another way of saying that experience functions in both recall and foresight. Since troublesome experience, organized in the self-system, has been experience connected with increasing grades of anxiety, it is not astounding that this element of recall, functioning on a broad scale, makes the intervention of the self-dynamism in living tantamount to the warning, or foresight, of anxiety. And warning of anxiety means noticeable anxiety, really a warning that anxiety will get worse.

There are two things which I would like to mention briefly at this point. One is the infant's discovery of the unobtainable, his discovery of situations in which he is powerless, regardless of all the cooperation of the mothering one. The infant's crying for the full moon is an illustration of this. Now even before the end of infancy, it is observable that these unattainable objects gradually come to be treated *as if* they did not exist; that is, they do not call out the expression of zonal needs. This is possibly the simplest example of a very important process manifested in living which I call *selective inattention.*

The other thing I would like to mention is this: Where the parental influence is peculiarly incongruous to the actual possibilities and needs of the infant—before speech has become anything except a source of marvel in the family, before it has any communicative function whatever, before alleged words have any meaning—there can be inculcated in this growing personification of bad-me and not-me disastrous distortions which will manifest themselves, barring very fortunate experience, in the whole subsequent development of personality. I shall soon discuss some typical distortions, one of the most vicious of which occurs in late infancy as the outcome of the mothering one's conviction that infants have *wills* which have to be guided, governed, broken, or shaped. And when, finally, we come to discuss concepts of mental disorders we will have to pick up the manifestations of a few particularly typical distortions, in each subsequent stage from the time that they first occur.

CHAPTER 11

The Transition from Infancy to Childhood: The Acquisition of Speech as Learning

The Consistency and Sanity of the Parental Efforts at Education

IN LATE infancy, there are increasing efforts by the parents, principally the mothering one, to perfect the socialization, or the beginning socialization, of the infant. In this socialization process, I wish to emphasize the element of *frequency* in the infant's experience, which is important in any relatively inadequate creature's learning of complex entities, or acquiring of complex patterns of behavior—and this is more and more the situation which the infant is really in. And along with the element of frequency, the element of *consistency* must be grasped as very important; consistency may be considered a function of frequency, insofar as consistency means repetition of a particular pattern of events, just as inconsistency means a reduced frequency of a pattern of events or a greater variety of patterns of events. Many of the difficulties which show up from the end of the first year of life onward may prove to be the accumulating results of inconsistencies in the efforts of the acculturating parent to teach the infant what is what. The extent to which the parent fails to provide anything like an invariant pattern of events takes on very great significance at the time when the child is using speech as his outstanding acquisition, say, in the third year of life; but it is improbable that the parental influence which is strikingly inconsistent at that time was anything like wholly consistent at, say, the end of the first year of life. Therefore, it is rather difficult to say just when deviations in the consistency and frequency of interpersonal events begin to bear on the development of personality.

Now besides the elements of consistency or inconsistency, frequency or infrequency, in the interpersonal events to which the infant is subjected, there is also to be considered another element, which I call, in the absence of a better word, the *sanity* of the educational efforts. By sanity I mean the parental modification of these efforts in accordance with the infant's capacity for observation, analysis, and elaboration of experience at a given time. Let me mention a few negative examples which possibly will illustrate what I am driving at.

One instance might be described as the doctrine of the will, which is a result of parental misinformation—all too easy to acquire and to retain in this civilization. Now I cannot at this time discuss *in extenso* the roots from which arises the illusion that we have a more-or-less all-powerful, or at least magically potent, will. But I do wish to invite your attention to the disastrous effects of treating a year-old baby as if he were being willfully troublesome. No matter what any of us may believe about the will, I think that most of us would not push the idea of the powerful will so far as to include the twelfth month of life after birth. But some parents do, and become involved in all sorts of curious, if not subpsychotic, attempts to guide, direct, break, manage, and so on, the self-willed infant.

My second example of, shall I say, insanity in the socializing influences brought to bear from the twelfth month onward is one which is much less conspicuously based on unutterable misconceptions of personality development. This is the subjection of the infant to a person, to a mothering one, who regrets the fact that the infant must grow up, and in a good many ways encourages him to stay put. Thus she provides experience, rewards, and anxiety in a fashion that works against the process of maturation in her offspring, and will presently, unless something changes radically in their relationship, literally be trying to keep the child young.

Another example of what I would consider a lack of sanity of educative effort is the idea that the infant must be clean and dry by, let us say, the age of fifteen months, an achievement of which the mother is insufferably proud. I have encountered pretty dependable evidences of a history of early training of this kind in quite a number of gravely—in fact, quite hopelessly—disordered people. I believe that I am correct in saying that the only way one could get an infant of fifteen months to be clean and dry would be by setting up terrific anxiety barriers to the development of anything like practical, useful, helpful feelings about the perineal area in the evolution of the concept "my body" and all its relationships to the concept "me."

In a very much more considerable number of disturbed, disordered personalities, I have uncovered another vicissitude of early training which can be regarded as not sane, and which I have already discussed; this is what I used to call the primitive genital phobia, where the parent is fearsomely upset by the infant's tinkering with the external genitals. Before the end of infancy, well before there is any speech behavior, all sorts of incredible orthopedic devices—marbles in the pajama back, bandages, and this and that—are sometimes used to prevent this supposedly dreadful component of the infant's manual exploratory performances. Insofar as such training occurs before the genital sentience is well integrated into experience, it can only be incredibly unrelated to anything that is any good to us in later life. Even insofar as it comes after the special sentience of the genitals—which you must remember is quite limited until the lust dynamism has matured—there too it represents, as it were, a hole punched in the totality of "my body," and is responsible for certain peculiarities encountered in later life, such as desiring to be masturbated by somebody else but having a dreadful time if one masturbates oneself, and so forth. Such easily misunderstood intricacies of the later so-called sex life are the outcome of quite seriously deviated personality development beginning before childhood.

Now these instances of "insanity" that I am laying before you may be generalized under a topic I have previously touched on—namely, the parental expectations about the infant, which are a part of the personification of the infant existing in the mothering one. Even in this realm of pure expectation on the part of the parents, a peculiar viciousness may appear as the infant approaches the end of infancy, by which time the infant has acquired, to a certain extent, expressive posturings of the face, the so-called expressions of pleasure and displeasure, and so on, and has lost much of the peculiar lineaments which are the rule at birth and a few months afterward. So it is that, in certain families and with certain mothering ones, the expectations about the infant now begin to take on color on the basis of whom the infant is alleged to look like, and whom the infant is now detected to be showing signs of "taking after." And the person whom the infant is supposed to look like, or take after, may be either a real parent or relative or even a mythological ancestor. In certain situations, these fancied resemblances in looks or in behavioral rudiments are very much more important, in the formulation of behavior by the mothering one, than are the infant's looks or behavior as they might be observed by someone with scientific detachment. Where parental expectations bring about this kind of situation, certain accidental events actually begin to take precedence over, and thereby interfere with, certain learning processes that were already started, which I shall touch on presently.

Overt and Covert Processes

I want now to develop further some points that I have not developed adequately as I went along. As I have discussed recall and foresight previously, the discussion has centered around the influence of past experience on living, if that past experience has recurred frequently enough—or has been otherwise sufficiently marked by importance—for it to be organized into signs. The function of organized experience in present behavior can be called, in part, the manifestation of sign processes in recall and foresight. Up to the ninth or tenth month the observer has nothing to work on other than inference, in convincing himself of the importance of this organized experience. It is not subject to clear, objective demonstration, but has to be inferred from what can be observed.

Now at this point I wish to make a perduring distinction—a distinction that will be important from infancy to the end of living—between what can be observed by a participant observer, and what can never be so observed but must always be the result of inference from that which is observed. And this is the distinction between *overt processes* in interpersonal relations and *covert processes*.[1]

A great deal that I have described thus far has concerned covert processes, and has been arrived at as a result of inference. As soon as speech behavior appears, it begins to be what it forever after will be, a wonderfully good index to the probability of the correctness of the inference. Moreover, in the latter months of infancy, there are better grounds for making certain inferences about the covert processes because of the beginning manifestation of the phenomenon of *delayed behavior*. I have spoken earlier of how the tension of anxiety acts in direct vector opposition to needs. It is now possible to observe in the young that needs themselves rather unmistakably manifest a certain hierarchical organization. Sometimes hunger takes precedence over something else that is going on, and behavior calculated to satisfy hunger—or behavior in the pursuit of the satisfaction of hunger—interrupts, as it were, something else that was going on; but, when the hunger is satisfied, instead of sleep supervening, the interrupted activity is resumed again, and has apparently been waiting in a sort of quiescent state until the more potent motivation worked itself out or was satisfied. Occasionally one will see, when the interrupted activity is resumed, that there has actually been some change in its situational pattern. It is to be inferred from this observation that something has certainly been going on in connection with the delayed or interrupted motivation, at the same time that the more potent motivation was moving on to satisfaction. Such inferred activity I call covert activity, in contradistinction to that which is clearly manifest.[2]

[1] I did not always use these terms; at one time I talked about implicit processes instead of covert ones. I have now abandoned the word implicit, because it has picked up so many shades of meaning which are troublesome or irrelevant to what I am attempting to communicate that some other word in common use has seemed more desirable. The discrimination of covert, as against overt, serves just as nicely.

[2] As a matter of fact, I have picked up a good deal of data which suggest that it may be possible to infer covert processes from delayed behavior manifested by the infant even before the age of six weeks. If these data are correct, they mean that covert symbol operations in connection with zonal

Thus by the end of infancy and on the threshold of childhood, one does see what can only, I think, be explained as the continuation of symbol operations behind a screen, one might say—the screen being the presenting activity, the energy transformation connected with the satisfaction of a stronger need. It is as if some sign processes had been going on during the period that behavior in the satisfaction of an intercurrent need was in progress, and the whole thing had progressed covertly. This sort of thing one can see in oneself very well, the most distinguished example being perhaps the phenomenon of how greatly puzzled one may be about some problem in the afternoon or evening, and how perfectly lucid one may be about the same problem early next morning after one has slept on it.

Now these covert processes might be taken to be extremely private, and also not at all directly susceptible to the type of social patterning, of educative change, which most certainly applies to quite a substantial part of the overt behavior of the year-old infant. In origin, however, these covert processes have been derived from the organization of experiences which were essentially interpersonal, however little the personification of the other person may have developed in the infant. Perhaps the only time when it is not possible to recognize covert processes as interpersonal phenomena is when a kind of synthesis of interpersonal events has taken place —as might often happen in these processes—by which one has arrived at new conclusions by combining old experiences in a new fashion; when that has happened there may seem to be no direct connection with specific interpersonal events.

As I further develop the topic of the self-system and its function, it will become clear, I believe, that many covert processes which were all right at the age of, let us say, twelve months, have been rigidly excluded from the repertory of the older person, chiefly by dint of learning under the guidance of anxiety; and that any possibility of the appearance of these covert processes promptly brings out a degree of anxiety that is ordinarily sufficient to interfere with their appearance.

---

and general needs show up in a rudimentary form amazingly early in the postnatal life of the human young.

The Learning of Gesture and Language

Of the learning that goes on from the end of the first year, the immediately and vastly important congeries is the acquisition of overt behavior which belongs to what might well be called two grand divisions of interpersonal communicative behavior, namely, those of gesture [8] and of language. In order to suggest the great importance of the gestural performance of speech, I might point out that it is only in quite restricted fields of living—for example, when a scientist is being a good scientist—that language behavior is stripped of gestural components. Most people would find such rigidly defined language behavior rather more soporific than communicative.

The learning of gestures, by which I include the learning of facial expressions, is manifested by the infant, certainly well before the twelfth month, in the learning of the rudiments, one might say, of verbal pantomime. And this learning is, in good measure, learning by trial-and-error approximation to human example. Quite recently I observed the most amazing instance of this, in my exceedingly limited experience. My most recent full-time nurse was delivered, now about eleven months ago, of a robust infant whom I saw for the first time, after my fashion of interest in infants, within the last month. During this visit I was utterly amazed to notice that under our conversation the infant was carrying on a very interesting conversation of his own. I discovered that what had caught my attention was the beautiful tonal pattern. Only perhaps fifty percent of the sounds were, I would say, good phonemal stations in the English language, but the melody, the pattern of tone, was speech; it was what our speech would be like if speech were not articulate. In other words, before this infant was twelve months old, he had, by trial-and-error learning from what he heard—he was being raised in a very vocal home—

[8] [*Editors' note:* Sullivan used "gesture" in a somewhat broader sense than is usual; in other lectures, and in other parts of this lecture, it becomes clear that by gesture he included, not only facial expressions and pantomime with other parts of the body, but also the melody, rhythm, and emphasis of speech. In other words, by gesture he referred to the "expressive," as opposed to the "denotative" aspects of speech—terms which he used in the 1948 lecture series.]

gotten the melodic progression of speech very nicely within his competence, so that there was nothing obviously infantile in it. It was so startlingly like speech that I could distinguish it only by careful listening, and only after I listened for a while could I tell that it included many things that would never be English words. Here was an example of the very early acquisition of a very large part of the gestural aspects of speech.

I might suggest that the acquisition of mannerisms through trial-and-error learning by human example is by no means confined to early life. The number of chronologic adults who are big chunks of mimicry, particularly regarding the gestural aspects of speech, is amazing. Psychiatrists often find that patients begin to sound like them; even though the phonemes they use, if analyzed, would prove to be quite different, the tonal gesture, melody, and so on, come to resemble theirs. In one instance, I could no longer tell which of two people was speaking to me on the telephone, although they once were quite easily identified by what came over the telephone. As a particular instance, I have one old friend who, for some reason that I have never felt free to investigate, fairly early in his professional career acquired the habit of turning on his smile for a moment as if a switch were operating it, and then suddenly switching it off. I have watched among some of his colleagues the acquisition, well along in professional life, of certain degrees of skill at this flashlight smile. Thus I suggest to you that what begins here in the very last stage of infancy doesn't stop then.

Even before the era of childhood, learning of the gestural aspects of speech, and so on, is already manifest; and this business of picking up more and more of the nonverbal, but nonetheless communicative, aspects of speech behavior is well established by that time and continues to be one of our manifest abilities, even if unnoted, for a very long period thereafter. In other words, before speech itself is actually possible—that is, literally during what I consider infancy—a great deal of learning can not only be incorporated into speech behavior, but is actually quite clearly manifest in those infants who are not especially handicapped by anxiety. The first thing which the infant unquestionably picks out from the verbal performances of the mother is the progression of tones and silences—and remember that silence is as much a part of speech as sound is; this progression is more or less the rhythmic tonal pattern to which all domestic animals are apt to show quite specific sensitivity. I trust that I have given some little notion of how early the various components appear that finally add themselves up to language behavior—the remarkably early abilities to catch on to vocal melodies and grosser sound patterns, and to perfect—by trial-and-error learning from the human examples around one—the refined little patterns or subpatterns of sound which make up the phonemal stations used by the language of the home.

The Roles of Reward and Indifference in the Learning of Language

Now I want to invite your attention to effects that the responses of the mother and other significant persons have on these abilities. Quite early, I suppose by the eighth or ninth month, the infant is spacing things like "da" so that it comes out "da-da-da" and presently "da-*da*-da." This means that the element of melodic repetition, the rhythmic tonal business, is already being caught on to by the infant. In this process some things like "dada" happen to be said at an appropriate time, so that an enthusiastic parent is apt to wonder if it isn't an attempt to say "mama" or "papa" or something else, and there is a certain amount of response. If by any chance "mama" is said, that is considered proof that the child has learned to call mother something (which I think is almost infinitely improbable), and there is a strong tender response. I think this is about all there is to it, although I am sure it won't endear me to parents. Thus out of the infant's mere repetitive syllabic experimentation, those experiments which happen to come somewhere near what is supposed to be appropriate baby talk get themselves stamped in, and so meet with much response, reiteration, and attention from the mothering one. When the learning has progressed to the point where different syllabic forms, different combinations of phonemes, and some vague attempts to imitate what is heard get said, there actually appears the beginning of the extremely rich development of sounds, tonal patterns, rhythms, and what not that make up the various great and small languages of the world, including the baby's private language. It is at this time, when the baby is saying things other than mere dada's and caca's and mama's, that the element of learning by reward enters in, so that the child's satisfaction in making vocal noises and hitting, by trial and error, on things that he has heard is now augmented by the tenderness of the mothering one. In addition, there comes in another great teaching influence, which I have not previously stressed—teaching by, of all things, *indifference*. Although it has been there all the time, it takes on particular significance only when the element of teaching by the reward of additional tenderness becomes a conspicuous part of the infant's life. This teaching by indifference is the paradigm of one of the most powerful influences to which man is subjected in later life, which I will, at the cost of getting entirely off the beam, mention as the fear of ostracism.

The very important element in the development of the baby's language is that while a lot of his vocal inventions receive reward, a great many of them do not provoke any response in the mother —and, needless to say, the busier she is and the less imagination she has, the greater will be the proportion of vocal inventions which receive no response. These latter are good only for what little zonal satisfaction there may have been in the hearing of them, and so they tend to drop out, for they don't accomplish anything—they get no special returns. Therefore, perhaps to an extraordinary extent, from the twelfth to the eighteenth month, the vocal efforts which in the presence of the mothering one do not happen to hit the right area fail of frequent repetition. As interpersonal relations grow, this element of socialization under the influence of indifference—which is a case neither of reward by tenderness nor of anxiety, but just a case where nothing happens —becomes pretty powerful.

Autistic Language

In the stage where this learning is well under way the baby develops a language, not the mother's language, not English (I am assuming that it is an English-speaking home), but the baby's own language. It is pertinent to note Edward Sapir's statement that ". . . the elements of language, the symbols that ticket off experience, must . . . be associated with whole groups, delimited classes, of experience rather than with the single experiences themselves." [4] And it is under this interpretation of language—which incidentally is the only interpretation that I have ever heard that made any sense—that we find the baby developing a language in which there is a certain amount of consensus that a particular sound refers to a particular class of events—that is, to a particular class of experience. For example, let us suppose that when the mother brings the nursing bottle or the bowl of food or whatever year-olds use, the baby, by sheer accident, were to say "ha." Now, under certain circumstances, which I cannot possibly discuss, a situation might be set up so that the next time this happens he again would say "ha," whereupon the mother would become much impressed by the probability that "ha" refers to food. And very quickly "ha"—a perfectly good word—does refer to food. It doesn't happen to be very useful in talking to Aunt Mary, who is a rare visitor in the house, but she can be told about it. The point is that it is in a sense a perfectly good language—and such language grows rather rapidly—but it has exceedingly little widespread communicative power. It is what we will later come to name *autistic;* [5] it is rather dangerous to describe it as the baby's private language, for its evolution is not private at all. Certain sound combinations have come, through the influence of the mother, to mean certain types of events. Needless to say, if there are nurses and the like running around the place, this baby language will not have even approximate communicative power to any one of them. In any case, the communicative power of this language is limited because it is all a language of nouns; incidentally, when it comes

[4] [Edward Sapir, *Language: An Introduction to the Study of Speech;* New York: Harcourt, Brace and Co., 1921; p. 11.]

[5] [*Editors' note:* Sullivan says that autistic is ". . . an adjective by which we indicate a primary, unsocialized, unacculturated state of symbol activity, and later states pertaining more to this primary condition than to the conspicuously effective consensually validated symbol activities of more mature personality" (*Conceptions of Modern Psychiatry;* New York: W. W. Norton & Company, 1953, second edition; p. 17).

Patrick Mullahy has described Sullivan's "autistic" as a "subspecies of the parataxic . . . . a verbal manifestation of the parataxic" ("A Theory of Interpersonal Relations and the Evolution of Personality," the same reference, p. 126).]

to verbs, the learning is much more deliberate, in the sense that the mothering one tries to teach their use.

I have discussed the baby's inventing words by establishing connections between a particular enunciated tonal pattern and a particular event or object, and the baby's learning to approximate particular words taught it by the mothering one. Now here are two classes of words that are being built into the baby's vocabulary, so to speak, both of which are autistic, in that only rarely is there a clear relation between a word and the really significant denotation of that same word in language used for communicative purposes among adults. Furthermore, in many, many instances the mother has satisfied some need that I do not understand very well by exposing the infant for a long time, even before the appearance of an autistic language, to sundry distortions of the communicative speech of the society in which she lives, which are called "baby talk." Some of this baby talk has taught the infant the significant approving and forbidding melody patterns of speech. Some of it is imagined to be of educative value because it is supposed to be the sort of speech that the baby can himself manage. However, I am afraid that there is very seldom any correlation between the amount of baby talk the baby hears and his abilities for learning words.

Language as Syntaxic Experience

Insofar as there happens to be a coincidence between the dictionary meanings of words and the infant's prehension and organization of experiences and activities by nouns and verbs—to that extent the language of the very young is beginning to manifest what I shall henceforth discuss as *experience in the syntaxic mode.* In fact, the first unquestionable organization of experience in the syntaxic mode is in the realm of the two great genera of communicative behavior, gesture and speech. And since the syntaxic, as we will later show it, is closely related to such things as the illusion of volition, I should stress that syntaxic symbols are best illustrated by words that have been consensually validated. A consensus has been reached when the infant or child has learned the precisely right word for a situation, a word which means not only what it is thought to mean by the mothering one, but also means that to the infant. Incidentally, an enormous amount of difficulty all through life arises from the fact that communicative behavior miscarries because words do not carry meaning, but evoke meaning. And if a word evokes in the hearer something quite different from that which it was expected to evoke, communication is not a success.

As I have indicated, the first instances of experience in the syntaxic mode appear between, let us say, the twelfth and the eighteenth month of extrauterine life, when verbal signs—words, symbols—are organized which are actually communicative. Of course, a vast deal of what goes on during this period of life is not in the syntaxic mode: there is uncommunicative action by the mother—and wholly uncommunicative behavior as far as the infant's zonal satisfactions are concerned; and there is even the beginning of his avoidance of forbidding gestures, which is the initial manifestation of the infant's self-system.

Reverie: Nonverbal Referential Processes

As the baby's true autistic language develops—which I endeavored to illustrate with my example of "ha" meaning food—we begin to observe evidences of something generically identical with the great body of processes later called *reverie.* And reverie shows at this early stage somewhat of the relationship of the covert and overt, in that the baby carries on, with or without an audience, a certain amount of exercise in his language, first audibly, that is, overtly. Gradually, the language becomes more and more covert, by which I do not mean that he tends to be more and more silent. But his behavior begins to show the process of delay, even with respect to vocalization, so that we are able to presume that there is a change, as it were, from audible to perhaps silent speech. I hope, however, that you will be more-or-less magically protected from translating my remarks into Watsonian psychology and from assuming that I mean a gradual transition from overt to implicit laryngeal behavior. As a matter of fact, I think that speech is very much more a function of the ears that it is of the larynx, and I imply absolutely nothing about moving muscular tensions, and so on, when I talk about the internalization, if you please, or the becoming-covert of processes which have been overt. Certainly we all know that the reverse can be true and that quite often processes which for a long time have been covert can manifest themselves overtly.

As I have said, even in the first half of the second year of life, there is some evidence of what can properly be called the reverie process, which will continue throughout life. The infant is now provided with a baby language—an autistic language, since it has arisen out of coincidences, and so on, in the actual experience of the infant, and has only to a very limited extent been subjected to precise language teaching. In the second year of life such reverie processes as go on must be presumed to be in this purely autistic language. So far as language process is concerned, reverie continues all through life to be only infrequently and in special circumstances of a type that, if it were expressed, would be clearly meaningful and communicative to a hearer. Only those reverie processes which are in preparation for the expression of something, for the communication of something, take on the attributes which we at least hope our spoken and written thoughts will show. Reverie continues to be relatively untroubled by grammatical rules, the necessity for making complete sentences, and so on.

Incidentally there are people who seem completely staggered when one talks about nonverbal referential processes—that is, wordless thinking; these people simply seem to have no ability to grasp the idea that a great deal of covert living—living that is not objectively observable but only inferable—can go on without the use of words. The brute fact is, as I see it, that most of living goes on that way. That does not in any sense reduce the enormous importance of the communicative tools—words and gestures. It is probable that, up to the age of—let us say—three or four, words, mostly still of the child's special language, are used very much as pictures might be used in a book; they decorate, concentrate, or illuminate, referential processes which are not verbal but which are the manifestation of experience in the parataxic mode organized at various times earlier, such as the identification of good and useless nipples, and so on, that I have already talked about.

The Symbolic and the Nonsymbolic

I would like at this point to take up a type of abstract separation of things, supposed to be helpful in thought, which has developed considerable hold in the field of social-psychological theory: namely, the separation of all activity, overt or covert, into the symbolic and the nonsymbolic. I once thought it could be usefully added to this presentation of psychiatric theory, but now I think that it is not relevant. The distinction between the covert and the overt is self-evident when once made; and as long as one is dealing only with the first eighteen or twenty months of life, it is quite easy to make this second abstraction of symbolic and nonsymbolic, which can then be projected into later life. The idea is roughly this: the infant behaves nonsymbolically when he is taking nourishment from the breast; and the child behaves symbolically when he calls an inanimate toy "kitty." Now, I have no inclination whatever to argue the fact that there are activities provided for by the organization of central nervous and muscular tissue, and so on, at birth, such as the elaborate apparatus which actually makes sucking a fact and swallowing a fact. Perhaps the first time that anything happens it is nonsymbolic. But from the very beginning the cooperation of older people is necessary for infantile survival; and from the very beginning the potent influence of anxiety permits the organization of experience, prevents the organization of experience, or gradually shoos the direction of experience into approved channels. Thus it is quite obvious that a great deal of what goes on by the time one is a year old, even if it is inborn, is very highly symbolic. I have emphasized from the beginning that recall and foresight are conspicuous even, according to Jennings, at the level of the amoeba. Wherever the phenomenon of recall and foresight is clearly manifested in the human being so that something can be extracted in the way of communication about it, one finds this very definite anticipation of some achievement connected with it. I am afraid that, for practical purposes, all human behavior so purely and unquestionably manifests the organization of experience into what are in effect signs—whether signals or symbols—that an attempt to discriminate intelligibly in human behavior between what is symbolic and what is nonsymbolic is far more misleading than it is helpful. Therefore, without denying that there may be purely nonsymbolic performances in human beings, I would say that for the purposes of psychiatric theory I am concerned exclusively with covert and overt symbolic activity—that is, with activity influenced by the organization into signs of previous experience in terms of satisfaction, or in terms of avoiding or minimizing anxiety.

CHAPTER 12

Childhood

The Role of Language in the Fusion of Personifications

We shall now more or less depart from our prolonged stay in infancy. In my discussion of language behavior, I hope it was made clear that the infant's success in the field of language behavior carries a very, very high premium so far as favorable, tender response of the significant elder figures is concerned. The extraordinary value that comes to invest verbal behavior, especially as it manifests itself in the school years, is one of the important factors which make it difficult for us to be aware of reverie processes that are in a relatively simple parataxic mode of experience, or even of some reverie processes that are in highly developed forms of the parataxic mode. Verbal behavior takes to itself, in the case of all those who are not born deaf-mutes, qualities bordering on the really magical; for instance, a good many of us, even though we are properly invested with the degree of doctor of this or that, show quite often and quite clearly that we depend on really magical potencies in certain of our verbal behaviors. And in psychiatric practice, we encounter chronological adults whose unearthly dependence on the potency of verbal behavior is, quite clearly, the outstanding characteristic of their difficulty with others.

Now among the things brought about in the very early phases of childhood largely by the peculiar power of language behavior is a fusion of personifications. So far as awareness is concerned, this fusion is final and absolute; but, so far as personality is concerned, it need not be anything like so complete. I am speaking now of what has, up to this stage, been the double personification of the mothering one, or the collection of mothering ones—the personifications of the good mother and of the bad or evil mother. Thanks in no small part to the incredible power which verbal behavior seems to exercise in interpersonal situations, and to the great energy devoted by the more mature people around the very young child to equip him with this most important of all human tools, language, it becomes quite impossible for the child to carry forward any striking surviving evidence of his earliest impression of two mothers—one who gives tenderness and cooperation in the satisfaction of needs, and one who carries anxiety and interferes with the satisfaction of needs. Although this dichotomy pertaining to one real person can go on at the lower strata, you might say, of personality, it can scarcely survive very long the high-pressure acculturation which makes one person "mama," and possibly another person "sister," or something like that. Thus no matter how thoroughly organized the two separate personifications of the good mother and the bad mother were, their individuality is lost or fused into a later personification, in the process of learning language. But this fusion is not to be taken to be comprehensive. In other words, all the attributes organized in infancy in the personification of the bad mother are not necessarily or probably present in the personification of mother as it begins to be conspicuous in childhood; and it is scarcely possible under any circumstances that all the attributes of the good mother of infancy can be fused into the childhood personification of mother. Under certain circumstances, we see evidence which makes this last statement practically beyond doubt; that is, in later life the person seeks, and can quite clearly be proven to be seeking, someone who will fit fairly closely the personification of the good mother, in aspects which are not shown in the personification of the 'real' mother. The peculiarly complex way in which personifications of one stage of personality enter into personifications at a later stage of personality —although very seldom totally—is, to a considerable extent, due to the unique power of vocal verbal behavior, and to the very high premium that is put on the acquisition of verbal behavior in childhood and the succeeding developmental eras, as long as one is in organized educational situations.

The Theorem of Escape

I want now to carry further the development of the self-system, which I began to outline a while back, and to present what I have formulated as the *theorem of escape.* The self-system, unlike any of the other dynamisms posited to organize knowledge about interpersonal relations, is extraordinarily resistant to change by experience. This can be expressed in the theorem that *the self-system from its nature—its communal environmental factors, organization, and functional activity—tends to escape influence by experience which is incongruous with its current organization and functional activity*. This peculiarity of the self-system must be grasped if one is either to comprehend personality in terms of this system of psychiatry, or to engage in the types of therapeutic intervention which this system implies. When last I touched on the self-system, I spoke of its being of purely experiential origin, and I said that, unlike the dynamisms of needs, it did not rest on peculiarities of the physicochemical communal existence of the underlying human animal. The self-system is derived wholly from the interpersonal aspects of the necessary environment of the human being; it is organized because of the extremely unpalatable, extremely uncomfortable experience of anxiety; and it is organized in such a way as to avoid or minimize existent or foreseen anxiety.

But I want to repeat that the character of situations which provoke anxiety is never completely to be grasped. It is quite clear that since anxiety in the mother makes the infant anxious, we cannot expect the infant to understand very much about what caused anxiety; what is perhaps a little harder to see is that, in chronological adults, there is this same fringe of the simply undiscoverable about circumstances which cause anxiety. As we get older we like to feel that we can name or explain things and this conceals from us, in part, this never-completely-to-be-graspable character of situations which provoke anxiety. There is an old story about how sick the patient feels when he has a bad pain and how much more comfortable he feels when the doctor says, "Oh, it is only appendicitis." That is a small instance of how much better we feel when we have a verbal tag by which, it seems, a novel set of facts is made familiar—if only to somebody else. So it is with a great many of the things that we recurrently do inefficiently and inappropriately—we feel much better, more worthy, if we can rattle off a string of words, which is often about as effective as the traditional woman's explanation of the mysterious: "I did it *because*." Actually, in a very long psychiatric career I would say that I have come to have more and more affection for the rationalization which ends with "just *because*"; the more words that follow, the harder it is to figure out how much is personal verbalism—rationalization, as it is called—and how much is an important clue to something that one ought to see.

Thus, however much we as adults may be able to talk about situations which provoke anxiety, we almost never grasp the character of such situations—certainly the child never grasps them. Hence all additions to the self-dynamism are either *imperfect observations* of the circumstances that have caused anxiety, and of the successful interventions of the self-system to minimize or avoid repetition of these circumstances; or certain *definite inventions* by which more complex operations are built out of simpler ones, new things are made by recombining the old—a concept which I shall discuss shortly. Furthermore, the culture itself is based on no single great general principle that can be grasped even by a genius, but is based instead on many contradictory principles. And it is in education for life in the culture that we have all experienced a great deal of our anxiety.

Whereas any recurrent experience will quite soon be added to, and will modify, the manifestations of any dynamism in the satisfaction of needs, the particular structure and functional activity of the self-system is such that a person can go through a whole series of consistent failures of what we call security operations—which is the typical performance when the self-dynamism is the central motor of activity—without learning much of anything. In fact, the chances are that self-system activity will come in *more* readily at the faint hint of anxiety-provoking situations, but still without showing the type of profit from failures that would appear in connection with the satisfaction of more biologically conditioned needs. We can see, when we study this curious insensitivity to experience, that the patterns of experience which are not profitable are all characterized by not being understandable or analyzable in terms of the tendencies already incorporated in the self-system.

Needless to say, the lifelong tendency of the self-system to escape profit from experience is not absolute. But I want to emphasize this general tendency of the self-system. I have gone to the trouble of formulating a theorem about it in order to emphasize that we are being perfectly irrational and simply unpleasant if we expect another person to profit quickly from his experience, as long as his self-system is involved—although this is a very reasonable anticipation in all fields in which the self-system is not involved. This does not make the self-system rigidly incapable of change in central characteristics from infancy onward; quite the contrary. Because of the general effect on personality which accompanies every newly matured need or capacity in the early stages of each developmental phase, the functional activity of the self-system invariably does change somewhat in direction and characteristics; and it is at those times that the self-system is peculiarly open to fortunate change. The self-system, so far as I know, can, in any personality system, be changed by experience; but the experience, or rather the set-up in which such change can be expected, often has to be very elaborate and very considerably prolonged. The resistance of the self-system to change as a result of experience is in large part the reason why, in therapy, we find it profitable to think in terms of complexly organized, rather prolonged, therapeutic operations by which we gradually build up a series of situations which requires the self-system to expand—that is, to take in experience which had previously, because of selective inattention or otherwise, had no material effect on the patient's susceptibility to anxiety, in particular interpersonal situations.

Sublimation

To return to our discussion of very early childhood, I now invite attention to what happens with regard to the young child's activity concerned with the pursuit of the satisfaction of *needs*—activity which by now is both covert and overt. These needs are by now not only those clearly concerned with the necessary communality with the physicochemical world—needs for food, water, oxygen, and the elimination of waste products—but also include an ever-increasing complement of zonal needs. This latter category includes the need to manifest every capability that matures—what we see as the child's pleasure in manifesting any ability that he has achieved. The refinements of behavior patterns and of covert processes—which were earlier a matter of inference but which now become objectively verifiable—arise from the maturation of new capacities and from past experience; and these refinements can in some cases now be categorized as improved information about 'reality,' as it is commonly shorthanded. All this leads to the invention of new patterns from old, and to the learning of data from interpersonal situations with the acculturating adults, in the fashions I have described already.

Among these inventions there is one pattern of behavior change—a refinement of behavior patterns and covert processes—which is, according to my definition, of very broad significance. As usual, I have been too lazy or inefficient to find a term for this pattern of behavior change, or referential process change; and so I will again, with the same discontent that I have experienced for at least ten years, say that I am talking about my variant on *sublimation.* As I have already indicated, when I talk about sublimation I am not discussing exactly what Freud had in mind when he set up the terms; my thinking about sublimation makes it a very much more inclusive process than a study of classical psychoanalysis might suggest. The manifestations of what I shall continue to call sublimation, for want of a better term, appear in late infancy, become conspicuous in childhood, and become very conspicuous indeed in the succeeding period. Since this is the label of a very important manifestation of changes in behavior and referential pattern, let me make a somewhat precise statement about it:

Sublimation is the unwitting substitution, for a behavior pattern which encounters anxiety or collides with the self-system, of a socially more acceptable activity pattern which satisfies part of the motivational system that caused trouble. In more fortunate circumstances, symbol processes occurring in sleep take care of the rest of the unsatisfied need.

Now this is the first time that I have laid particular stress on the *unwitting.* I hope that I have prepared the way for it by my discussion of covert living in all of us. In the infant, these covert processes which can be inferred to go on certainly cannot be conceived to be within the infant's awareness, his clear recognition or grasp. As I have already suggested, I believe that in both the more distinguished and the more commonplace performances of each of us in our living, all but the last step—or all but the last few steps—usually goes on quite exterior to anything properly called the content of consciousness, or awareness. Thus by unwitting, or unnoted, I refer to the great congeries of covert referential processes which must have occurred, but whose occurrence is completely unknown to the person concerned, and is only to be inferred from the evidence of what the person does know and does notice—in other words, from what occurs within his so-called field of consciousness. To use the term sublimation in the sense that I use it, one must keep track of the fact that it occurs exterior to the field of conscious content; the reason for that is intricate but nonetheless important, and will perhaps be made clear when we come to discuss particular patterns of so-called mental disorder. What happens in the kind of sublimation that I am now trying to describe is that a need collides with anxiety at the behest of the social censor or acculturating person; a notable example of this—although, of course, no example is perfect—is the very young child who wants to put his thumb in his mouth but his thumb is soiled with, say, feces. If we find that this very young child, when his fingers are soiled in this particular way, always or very frequently picks out a particular toy and sucks it, then we may actually feel with reasonable certainty that there has been a 'substitution' of the experience of sucking this toy, in place of the experience of putting this particular type of soiled thumb in the mouth. When something like this happens in late infancy, we can scarcely presume that it is the result of much thinking on the part of the infant, and for this reason it seems to be a peculiarly good instance by which to call attention to the way sublimation occurs all through life. The person never figures it out. It occurs and is continued, but it is unwitting. And what occurs, and what is continued, is a partial satisfaction of the needs; and this partial satisfaction has been substituted for the satisfaction of the need which has collided with anxiety, which is being prohibited by forbidding gestures of the significant people around. What has been substituted, what appears in lieu of this particular need-satisfying behavior, will be something which is not disapproved, or not so much disapproved—something which is not a target of self-system activity, however primitive this activity may be.

This sublimation, or peculiar substitution of goal may be, and in fact is, in a notable proportion of all instances, almost completely satisfying, so that there is very little leftover, unsatisfied need. In my illustration, in which the finger soiled with feces is not to be gotten anywhere near the mouth, the substitution of a toy cannot satisfy the need concerned, because that need includes the combination of sucking satisfaction and being-sucked satisfaction, whereas the toy is insensate. Now what becomes of the excess need which is not satisfied by these long-circuited, socially approved techniques? In many instances the excess need can be discharged by covert operations. In the adult who leads a fairly busy life, the great time for covert operations of that kind is during sleep; although it doesn't have to be, it very commonly is. In childhood this covert satisfaction does not have to be pushed into sleep, and in later childhood the unsatisfied components of some forbidden activity in the satisfaction of needs can be found to be faithfully reflected in expressed fantasy performances. The point is that the excess of need which is not satisfied by the sublimation is discharged by covert or overt symbolic performances which do not collide particularly with social censure—that is, which are not particularly associated with anxiety. Needless to say, there are some patterns of behavior and covert process in the pursuit of satisfactions that can scarcely be subjected to this process. When we discuss adolescence, we will discover that this is true of lust, at least in my view. Certain zonal needs which form part of the lust pattern may be sublimated, but if one depends on such processes for handling the whole thing, trouble is right around the corner, if not already present.

A great deal of what is called learning is made up of the refinement of behavior, and the change of covert referential processes, which are accomplished by this relatively simple process of sublimation—by combining activity in partial satisfaction of a need with other patterns of action—perhaps purely in the pursuit of security, perhaps partly in the pursuit of other satisfactions—so that anxiety is successfully avoided. But, while this sort of thing makes up an important part of learning, one cannot expect that the person who learned it will know all about how it was learned. When the so-called substitution is undertaken clearly within awareness, the educative process very rarely works effectively, if it works at all. I hear every now and then that the young child should be given every opportunity to understand just why certain things are required. If this were necessary, we might possibly reach maturity anywhere from sixty to a hundred and forty years of age, and I doubt that many people would put up with the tedium. So it is that a very important part of education for living in an essentially irrational culture is found in this type of refinement of behavior and covert process which occurs exterior to awareness, but which has the pattern of giving up immediate, direct, and complete satisfaction of a need, and of utilizing instead some partially satisfying, socially approved pattern, discharging any excess need in sleep or in some other way.

The Disintegration of Behavior Patterns

In less successful child-training projects—that is, in family groups that are not estimable in the skill, ingenuity, and understanding with which they try to discharge their social responsibilities—the first instances of the *disintegration* of behavior patterns and patterns of covert process under the force of anxiety occur quite early in childhood. This, which is somewhat different from sublimation, gets somewhere near the area of the not-me personification which I spoke of earlier. I am now considering a situation in which a pattern of behavior in the pursuit of satisfaction, and the exercise of recall and foresight in connection with this satisfaction, are *stopped* by the mothering one; then, depending on the character of the need—which in turn depends somewhat on the evolutionary stage of the personality concerned—either there is a great deal of trouble, in the sense that the behavior is, in fact, not abandoned by the child, and more and more anxiety piles up in the personality, so that one might say the *whole of living* is rather disorganized; or this *particular pattern* of behavior and covert process is disintegrated. But what is disintegrated does not, in that process, cease to be; it does not, like a coin in the magician's palm, vanish without a trace. And what becomes of patterns of behavior and covert process which have been disintegrated by frontal application of anxiety—which come into complete collision with the self-system so far as it is developed? Since the recombining of activities in this very simple pattern of sublimation presumably has not come off this time, there may be a recombining of activities in more complex patterns of activity—a number of which are best revealed in the mental disorders which we shall presently consider—or there may be *regression,* so-called, to earlier patterns.

Now the conception of regression is often utilized as a pure verbalism; that is, psychiatrists often use the term to brush aside mysteries which they do not grasp at all. I do not want anyone to think, when I use the term regression, that it is some great abstruse whatnot that can be used to sound intelligent about the mysterious. And the notion that regression is something rare, something highly morbid, and so on, can be dismissed on the strength of one very easy observation: that in the course of the life of any child, you can observe, practically at twenty-four hour intervals, the collapse, when the child gets thoroughly tired, of patterns of behavior which are not very well stamped in. Quite commonly before sleep, the child resumes earlier patterns of behavior that are no longer shown in the more alert periods of his life. When the patterns of motivational systems are, however, well established, then such diurnal disintegration is either very much less conspicuous or not in evidence at all. For example, a child who has otherwise entirely desisted from sucking his thumb quite commonly resumes sucking his thumb just before falling asleep. The zonal needs which were concerned in sucking the thumb have in various ways been refined, expanded, and so on; but with the supervention of the state called fatigue, the more complex, more recently evolved patterns of satisfaction-giving behavior, and incidentally security-protecting behavior, fall apart, as it were, and an earlier stage of direct satisfaction of the particular zonal need concerned reappears. Now that is genuinely an example of regression of behavior pattern, and from it, I believe, you can deduce the limits to which this particular conception can rationally be pushed.

The Theorem of Reciprocal Emotion

I want next to take up the vicissitudes in early childhood of the group of personifications which are presently to be fused in the personification of the self—namely, the personifications called good-me and bad-me, and the vestigial, vague personification of not-me. Since at this time there is a steady increase of the socializing influence by the more adult environment, the experiences which can be incorporated into the personification of bad-me grow through these earlier stages of development, and the 'naturalness' of good-me becomes much more open to exception.

In connection with the vicissitudes of the personifications which presently will culminate in the personified self, I would like to refer to a formulation which carries forward, and greatly modifies, the initial theorem of tenderness. My initial theorem stated, approximately, that the evidence of needs, as manifested by the infant, calls out tender cooperative behavior on the part of the mothering one. This is true of the period of the infant's complete dependence, but in childhood the social responsibility of the mothering one begins to interfere with it. Thus *from early childhood onward another general statement might be applied to interpersonal relations*, which, for want of a better name, I once called *the theorem of reciprocal emotion*, or reciprocal motivational patterns: *Integration in an interpersonal situation is a reciprocal process in which (1) complementary needs are resolved, or aggravated; (2) reciprocal patterns of activity are developed, or disintegrated; and (3) foresight of satisfaction, or rebuff, of similar needs is facilitated.*

When I state here that complementary needs are resolved or aggravated, you will observe that this is a change from the theorem of tenderness, in which the complementary needs were definitely resolved. But for the more general purpose—that is, in interpersonal situations from early childhood onward—we find that while there are complementary needs, the fact that a person needs tenderness may bring tenderness, or it may bring a denial of tenderness, or frank anxiety which aggravates the need for tenderness. The second part of my theorem is that reciprocal patterns of activity are developed or disintegrated. We saw, when we discussed the infant, that there was a steady growth on the part of the infant of nursing behavior, and so on, and on the mothering one's part there was certain cooperation with this extending pattern of nursing behavior. But from the more general standpoint, just the reverse may be true; previous patterns of cooperative activity in an interpersonal situation may now be disintegrated, because the mother supposes that the growth of the infant permits of his being educated away from things that she tolerated earlier. And the third part of my theorem is that the foresight of satisfaction, or rebuff, of similar needs is facilitated. The facilitation of the foresight of satisfaction is a particular instance of the continued improvement of behavior in the pursuit of satisfactions, which takes place when the interpersonal situations encourage such improvement. And the facilitation of foresight of rebuff is an instance where self-system processes are called out to interfere; what is foreseen is not the satisfaction of needs, but the forbidding gestures and the anxiety which will attend the direct manifestation of the needs.

So far as the positive aspect of this theorem manifests itself, complementary needs are resolved in the interpersonal relations one lives through; reciprocal patterns of activity are developed, refined, made more perfect; and there is foresight of how satisfaction can be gained more quickly, or continued longer, by improved performance. Now all of that gives rise to experience which is naturally entirely congruous with the personification of good-me, and is manifested, as we can sometimes observe from the vocal and other expressions of young children, as their happiness and pride —to miscall it in traditional terms—in the use of their abilities. But with the increase of pressure toward socialization of the young, naturally the negative side of this reciprocal process appears; needs are aggravated because they are thwarted, and patterns of activity have to be sublimated or disintegrated, and in certain cases rebuff —the probability of unfavorable outcome of behavior—is clearly foreseen as a part of the process of getting rid of those patterns.

Further Developments in the Self-System

Now all the experiences which arise from these situations tend naturally to fit into the personification of bad-me. And in addition, thanks to the general pattern of childhood training in this culture at least, certain peculiar additions to the self-system are cultivated. You recall that all that is the self-system arises in interpersonal relations, and from the elaboration of experience in interpersonal relations. And the peculiar additions I refer to are the development of a presumably biological reaction which we call *disgust*—which represents an elaboration of something that is always present, the capacity to empty the stomach in a reverse direction—and a still further elaboration of part of the experience of being disgusted in what is called the emotion of *shame*.

To go on with the growth of the still tripartite personifications of what will later be the personified self—good-me, bad-me, and not-me—I should like to discuss how a variety of elements in the teaching of language interfere with the more satisfactory development of the personified self. This interference occurs when the behavior of the acculturating older people teaches the young child that certain vocal processes can have a propitiatory effect with respect to items of bad behavior which otherwise are strongly associated with anxiety—that is, which are generally so forbidden that they would be as much as possible sublimated, or they would be disintegrated.

To some extent, I suppose, every one of us in our very early formative years—perhaps all through childhood, and certainly later in the juvenile period—had opportunities to learn that certain combinations of words and gestures would minimize, if not remove, the danger of anxiety which we could clearly foresee in connection with certain behavior, since we had already learned that this behavior endangered our feeling of interpersonal security—that is, was definitely disapproved. Now insofar as a verbal statement by a child is taken by the acculturating adults to have a superior quality of reality to other of his behavioral acts, the child is being trained to be incapable of dealing with life. That is just all there is to it. Yet in a good many homes, the following kind of statement is a conspicuous ingredient in the alleged education of the young: "Willie, I told you not to do that. Now say you are sorry." This is a classical instance of what I mean by propitiatory gesture. If Willie dutifully says he is sorry, that is supposed to markedly mitigate the situation, although it is something that Willie is almost absolutely incapable of understanding—if, in fact, anyone can understand it. The effect of this sort of thing is that it interferes with and delays the fusion of good, bad, indifferent, and unknown aspects into the personified self, and it continues, beyond a reasonable term, the maintenance of the tripartite personification with respect to *my body*. And so you will hear these same children telling you later on, "Oh, I didn't do that, it was my hand," or "Oh, mama, I've been bad," and so on, which are not particularly fortunate evidences of education.

During childhood something striking comes to happen to one of the components of the generic need for tenderness, which characterizes the infant from very early. This component I have referred to, in theoretic explanation of certain later idiosyncrasies, as the need for physical contact. In childhood an elaboration of this need is manifested, first, as a need for participants and, later, as a need for an audience. Late infants and young children like most emphatically to play with mother, to engage in certain exercises with mother which satisfy certain zonal muscular needs, and so on; and at a later stage they have a definite preference for putting on their performances in the presence of the tenderness-giving, approval-giving elder person. But if there are too many demands of other kinds on the mother, or if she has too many other children or is too ignorant of what it is all about, or if there are a variety of other circumstances, including mental disorder on her part, or crazy ideas about the child's will or spirit or what not—then, quite frequently, the child encounters such consistent rebuff of his expressed needs for tenderness that his behavior and covert processes concerned with the expression of the need for tenderness have to be subjected to change. Quite a bit of this can fit into the conception of sublimation, because the more fortunate of these children discover that when sublimations occur, tenderness is again forthcoming, and everything is fine. But a good many of them do not have that experience, and are literally compelled to disintegrate the behavior patterns and covert operations which would manifest themselves as the need for tenderness, because they foresee—on the best grounds possible, namely, frequency of occurrence—the rebuff of any need for tenderness that they manifest. In that case, after a certain time, a pattern of behavior develops which is as if bad-me had become the central part of the picture; there is literally the substitution of malevolent—"mischievous" is usually the word mother uses to tell Aunt Agatha about it—behavior when there is a need for tenderness. I shall discuss this development further, because it is very important in understanding many of the difficulties we have with our patients and others in later life.

CHAPTER 13

Malevolence, Hatred, and Isolating Techniques

Required Behavior and the Necessity to Conceal and Deceive

I NOW want to discuss further the very interesting phenomenon of one's becoming malevolent, and we will see if we can approach a consensus. The gross pattern of a great many things that happen in childhood, as compared with the infantile phase of personality, includes two conspicuous elements. One, as has been emphasized, is the acquisition of not only private but communicative language, with the great returns which the learning of this vitally important human tool always carries with it. But the second element, so far as actual development of interpersonal relations goes, is the more significant difference between the two epochs; it can be stated in terms of required behavior. At birth the infant can do practically nothing to assure his own survival. During infancy, he learns only the grossest culture patterns about zonal and general needs. But throughout the era of childhood there is an increasing demand for his cooperation. The child is expected to do things which are brought to his attention or impressed on him as requirements for action by the authority-carrying environment —the mother, increasingly the father, and perhaps miscellaneous siblings, servants, and what not.

In childhood—in contradistinction to at least the first two-thirds of the infantile period, and, one rather hopes, the whole infantile period—a new educative influence, *fear,* is brought to bear; we touched on this earlier, but we have not given it very much attention, since it has not so far had remarkable significance with respect to personality development. The discrimination between fear and anxiety is a vital one. Very severe fear and very severe anxiety, so far as I know, feel the same—that is, the felt component is identical—but the discrimination between these two powerful disjunctive processes in life is at times vital. Anxiety is something which I believe is acquired by an empathic linkage with the significant older persons, whereas fear is that which appears when the satisfaction of general needs is deferred to the point where these needs become very powerful. And of these general needs, the need which we particularly want to deal with here is the need to be free from painful sensations. Pain is here defined, not figuratively, but in its most obvious central meaning, hurt—that which occurs, for instance, as a result of sufficient pressure on, or incision into, the actual physical organization, or from misadventures in the internal function of some of the vital organs.

In childhood, perhaps not universally nowadays, but still with great frequency in almost all cultures I think, the child, in contradistinction to the infant, is presumed, at certain times, to deserve or require punishment; and the punishment I am talking about is the infliction of pain. Such punishment can be practically free from anxiety, or it can be strongly blended with anxiety. A parent who very methodically feels that a certain breach of the rules calls for a certain more or less specified form and amount of pain can administer it with no particular anxiety, although possibly with some regret, or possibly with singularly neutral feelings as one might have in training a pet. Many parents, however, for a variety of reasons subject the child to anxiety as well as pain. But insofar as punishment, the causing of pain, is used in its own right as an educative influence, this means a new type of learning—namely, learning enforced by a growing discrimination of the connection between certain violations of imposed authority and pain.

Frequently the child is subjected to punishment—pain with or without anxiety, but almost always with anxiety in this case—where he could have foreseen it except that the pressure of a need, zonal or otherwise, made the foresight ineffective in preventing the behavior. In a much more significant, although necessarily quite infrequent, group of circumstances, there comes punishment—pain with, almost invariably in this case, plenty of anxiety—under circumstances which are such that the child could not possibly have foreseen such an outcome from the behavior. This is particularly likely to happen with irritable, ill-tempered parents who are afflicted by many anxiety-producing circumstances in their own lives, and who tend rather strikingly to take it out on the dog or the child or what not.

Thus we see in childhood a new educative influence which shows up very definitely as actual fear of the capacity of the authority-carrying figure to impose pain. It is a peculiarity of the difference between anxiety and fear that, under fortunate circumstances, the factors in the situation in which one was hurt can be observed, analyzed, identified, and incorporated in foresight for the future, while in the case of anxiety that is only relatively true, at best; and if anxiety is very severe, it has, as I have said before, almost the effect of a blow on the head. Thus one has very little data on which to work in the future—we might almost say there is nothing in particular to be elaborated into information and foresight.

In childhood, the increased effort of the parents to teach, to discharge their social responsibility, and—I regret to say—to discharge a good many of the more unfortunate peculiarities of their personality produces, in many cases, a child who is "obedient" or a child who is "rebellious," and this outcome may appear fairly early. Of course the pattern may alternate in the same child, and have a very definite relationship to the existent personifications of good-me and bad-me; in reasonably healthy circumstances, good-me tends fairly definitely to be associated with obedience—but still with a considerable measure of freedom to play and so on—and rebelliousness tends to be part of the personification of bad-me.

In this stage of development—when the parents are making increasing efforts to teach the child, when his abilities are maturing, and when he is organizing past experiences and exercising his fantasy, his covert processes in play and make-believe—there is invariably, from very early, a beginning discrimination by the child among the authority-carrying figures, and later, but still quite early, a beginning discrimination of authority situations. In other words, almost all children learn certain indices that stand them in reasonably good stead as to when it is extremely unsafe to violate authority and when there is some chance of 'getting away with it.' This is, I think, a healthy discrimination which provides useful data, although under certain circumstances, of course, when the parental figures are overloaded with inappropriate and inadequate ways of life, it can be very unfortunate in the way of experience for later life. As the presumed relationship of more-or-less complete dependence of the infant on the mothering one is suspended and the father gets more and more significant, this discrimination by the child of different authority figures and authority situations, insofar as it succeeds—that is, gives information that proves reasonably dependable in foreseeing the course of events—contributes definitely to the growth of and importance of foresight in interpersonal relations. But insofar as the authority figures are confusing to the child and insofar as the authority situations are incongruous from time to time so that, according to the measure of the child's maturing abilities and experience, there is no making sense of them—then, even before the end of the thirtieth month, let us say, we see instances in which the child is already beginning to suffer a deterioration of development of high-grade foresight. In such cases it is quite probable that, in later stages of development, conscious exercise of foresight, witting study of how to get to a more-or-less recognized goal, will not be very highly developed.

Among the things that almost always attend the training of the child to take part in living, to 'cooperate' with the parent, to carry out instructions, to do chores and so on, is very frequently the imposition on the child of the concepts of duties and responsibilities. That is certainly good preparation for life in a social order; but again in cases where the parents are uninformed or suffering from unfortunate peculiarities of personality, this training in concepts and responsibilities includes as a very important adjunct (adulterant perhaps) a great deal of training—that is, experience which is presumed, erroneously I think in a great many cases, to be educational—in which the idea of *ought* is very conspicuous.

When it comes to putting into words an adequate statement of the cultural prescriptions which are generally required in the socialization of the young, one really is confronted by a task which requires most remarkable genius. Had culture grown as the work of a single person or a small group of greatly gifted people, almost crushed under their responsibility for their fellow man, then it is quite possible that one could build up a great structure of statements of what principles govern under all sorts of situations, and the result would be a coherent and rationally understandable social system. But that has been nowhere on earth, that I know of, very strikingly the case; possibly the nearest approach to such a social order is to be found in the regimented groups which have characterized various people at various times. For example, there is at least an attempt to embody often subtly contradictory requirements in such things as army regulations; but people who are really diligent students of army regulations frequently discover that it requires only a minor effort to discover a little conflict in authority, and such a conflict provides room for interpreting a situation according to which of the conflicting authoritative statements apply. But, as I was saying, such regulations do provide a rough approximation to this ideal of a rational culture, in that pretty ingenious people, many of them actively interested in maintaining the peculiar social organization of the military, have done their damndest to put plain statements of *ought* and *must* into words which could be understood by the comparatively uninitiated.

But when it comes to imposing the prescriptions of the culture on the child, these prescriptions are often most glaringly contradictory on different occasions, so that they require complex discrimination of authority situations. Moreover the child is incapable for a good many years of comprehending the prescriptions in terms of their possible reasonableness. And more important than anything else, out of the irrational and impulse-driven type of education by anxiety, and by reward and punishment—that is, tenderness and fear—a great many children quite early begin to develop the ability to conceal what is going on in them, what actually they have been doing behind someone's back, and thus to deceive the authoritative figures. Some of this ability to conceal and to deceive is literally taught by the authority-carrying figures, and some of it represents trial-and-error learning from human example—that is, by observing and analyzing the performances, the successes and failures, of siblings, servants, and the like.

Verbalisms and 'As If' Performances

Now these growing abilities to conceal and to deceive tend very early to fall into two of the important patterns of inadequate and inappropriate behavior—considered from the broad point of view—which become troublesome in later life and get themselves called mental disorders or processes in mental disorder. I hope that I have communicated by this time a very firm conviction that no pattern of mental disorder which is purely functional, as it is called—that is, which is an inadequate and inappropriate way of living with other people and with one's personifications—includes anything which is at all novel as to human equipment. Everything that we see in the symptomatology of these nonorganic—that is, nondefect—situations has its reflection in kind, if not in degree, in the developmental history of every one of us. And so, when we get to, let us say, mid-childhood, it is not uncommon to discover that the child has become fairly skillful at concealing what might otherwise bring anxiety or punishment—at deceiving the authority-carrying figures as to the degree or nature of his compliance with their more-or-less recognized demands.

The first of these two patterns we touched on previously—namely, verbalisms which are often called rationalizations, in which a plausible series of words is offered, regardless of its actual, remarkable irrelevancy, which has power to spare one anxiety or punishment. The degree to which verbalisms constitute elements in inadequate and inappropriate living which we call mental disorder, whether mild or severe, is truly remarkable. If you think that this is not a very powerful tool, you overlook its amazing significance in the service of the self-system, in the very striking characteristic of the self-system which makes favorable change so difficult—namely, the self-system's tendency to escape from experience not congruent to its current directions.

But the second pattern is even more impressive than verbalisms: it is the unfortunate—in the sense of being concealing and deceptive—learning of the value of *as if* performances. There are two grand divisions of these. One of them, far from being necessarily troublesome in personality development, is an absolutely inevitable part of everybody's maturing through childhood; and this is the group which perhaps may be called *dramatizations.* A great deal of the learning which the child achieves is on the basis of human examples, and these examples are at this phase authority-invested. The child will inevitably learn in this fashion a good deal about the mother, and, as the father personification becomes more conspicuous, about the father; and this trial-and-error learning by human example can be observed in the child's playing at *acting-like* and *sounding-like* the seniors concerned, and, in fact, playing at *being* them. Probably the progression literally is that one tries first to *act like* and one tries then to act *as if one were.*

In the earlier half of childhood, this inevitable part of one's learning to be a human being becomes a rather serious concern—in terms of what may show up later—only when these dramatizations become particularly significant in concealing violations of cooperation and in deceiving the authority-invested figures. In these latter cases, for a variety of reasons, some of which we will touch on briefly, these dramatizations tend to become what I could perhaps safely call sub-personifications. The roles which are acted in this way that succeed in avoiding anxiety and punishment, or that perhaps bring tenderness when there was no performance based on previous experience to get tenderness, are organized to the degree that I think we can properly call them *personae;* they are often multiple, and each one later on will be found equally entitled to be called *I.* To describe this type of deviation from the ideal personality development, I long since set up the conception of me-you patterns, by which I mean often grossly incongruent ways of behaving, or roles that one plays, in interpersonal relations with someone else. And all of them, or most of them, seem just as near the real thing—the personification of the self—as can be, although there is no more making sense of them from the standpoint of their representing different aspects of durable traits than there is of translating Sanskrit before you understand language. While these dramatizations are very closely related to learning to be human, they can even in these early days begin to introduce a very strikingly irrational element in the personification of the self.

The other group of these *as if* performances to which I wish to refer is perhaps best considered under the rubric of *preoccupations*. I would like to say a few words about one of my cocker spaniels, because it perhaps makes the point better than anything else I can think of now. This particular dog has always been the most diminutive in a litter of six; she has been kept with two others in this litter to the present time. The two others are a rather large male and a very shrewd and, shall I say, domineering female. The little bitch whom I am attempting to discuss was quite often the butt of the unquestionably painful vigor of the male and the unquestionably clever domineering of the female. Probably as a result of this, this little dog very conspicuously indeed took to remaining apart from her brother and sister, and could be observed very diligently digging great holes and trenches in the environment. This was literally quite a complex performance, in that each scoop of dirt that was flung out between her hind legs had to be examined carefully lest it contain something edible or otherwise interesting; the little dog would dig furiously in one of these mammoth excavations, rush around, examine the dirt thrown out, go down and get another shovel full—a tremendous activity for literally hours at a time. Somehow there seemed to be a stipulation that as long as she was so hard at work, the other two would leave her alone most of the time. But time has passed; she has been rescued from her unhappy submersion in the bigger siblings; and nowadays she treats them very roughly when she meets them. Now the trash man is outstanding around our place as a stimulus for provoking fear in the dogs—they are all quite upset when he shows up and to some extent are afraid of the mammoth truck and the din and so on that goes on about it. But when he is around, this little dog, alone out of the whole family, goes out and barks furiously at him. But she stops, after almost every third bark, to dig frantically, and to rush around and examine the dirt again, and then she goes back and roars furiously at him again. It is not, I think, too much to infer that this dog is really very timid, having had excellent reasons for being afraid in the past, but that she became so accustomed to being saved in the past by being preoccupied with her digging that the excess of fear in this situation leads to the reappearance of her preoccupation with digging.

In the human being, preoccupation as a way of dealing with fear-provoking situations or the threat of punishment, and of avoiding or minimizing anxiety appears quite early in life. And quite often the irrational and, shall I say, emotional way in which parental authority is imposed on the child, teaches the child that preoccupation with some particular onetime interesting and probably, as it turns out, profitable activity is very valuable to continue, not because it is any longer needed for the maturation of abilities or for satisfaction in new abilities, but as a preoccupation to ward off punishment and anxiety. Now if these performances are not only successful in avoiding unpleasantness, but also get positive reward by the child's being treated tenderly and approved, that naturally sets him on what will later be a strikingly complex way of life—that to which we refer as the *obsessional*.

Anger and Resentment

I have touched previously on learning by doing certain things in play *like* mother or *like* father, and by playing at *being* mother and father. There is one particular phase of this type of learning which is very evident in our ordinary contact with our fellow being, as well as in the psychiatrist's contact with the patient or vice versa. This is learning, from authority figures, a peculiar way of avoiding or neutralizing a fear-provoking situation. You may remember that earlier we spoke of how behavior that could be called, generically, rage behavior arose even in the extremely young when certain types of physical restraint were imposed which produced terror, particularly restraint that might interfere with the breathing movements. Now in punishment situations where pain is to be inflicted, there is invariably an element of restraint of freedom of movement—a particularly deliberate attempt on the part of the punishing person to interfere with the child's escaping the actual physically enforced pain. This, I believe, would, in any very young child who had missed disastrous experience up to then, lead to a movement in the general direction of such fear that rage behavior would be called out. But rage behavior doesn't have any particular value in this situation. And so, since the possibility of analysis and discrimination, and the exercise of foresight are already fairly well under way by now, instead of rage itself occurring as a frequent eventuality, what might be described as a version of its felt component—namely, anger—comes to be quite important. Especially in circumstances in which children are punished by an angry parent—but in all cases sooner or later, if only from improving discrimination of the progression of forbidding gestures in the authority-invested adults—everyone learns the peculiar utility of anger; I think that this statement is probably precisely true, although some people also learn that anger itself can bring a great deal of punitive treatment. But children invariably—or so nearly invariably that we don't need to pay a vast deal of attention to the exceptions—in their play are angry with their toys; and later they are angry with their imaginary companions. And the patterns of the child's being angry, the circumstances when it is suitable, and so on, are pretty much profits from his experience with the authority-carrying adults among whom he lives; what the child tends to show, in general, is that his toy, or whatever, has violated his authority in connection with the business of his *being* mother or *being* father. From this beginning, almost everyone—at least almost all the more fortunate of the denizens of our world—come to use anger very facilely, very frequently; and they use it when they would otherwise be anxious. In other words, it comes to be the process called out by mild degrees of anxiety in a truly remarkable number of people. But when one is around the age of thirty months, it may or may not be that one is well trained in the use of anger with the authority-carrying adults; in the more unhappy parental situations, one does not get very much encouragement that way, in partial result of which it comes about that in certain unhappy homes, children well into the school years have tantrums, which are in essence unmodified rage behavior.

In a great many other unfortunate homes children develop a complex modification of this rather simple use of anger. This more complex modification is the classical outcome of a situation in which the child is going on his way perfectly all right, so far as he can see, whereupon punishment, almost always with anxiety, is discharged upon the child for activity the forbidden aspect of which could not have been foreseen by the child—where there is no possibility of his understanding what the punishment is for. Or the punishment may be for activity so attractive that the possibility of punishment, even though foreseen, was ignored. In those circumstances, a great many children learn that anger will aggravate the situation, and they develop what we properly call *resentment*. Thus resentment is the name of the felt aspect of rather complex processes which, if expressed more directly, would have led to the repressive use of authority; in this way resentment tends to have very important covert aspects. In the most awkward type of home situation, these covert processes are complicated by efforts to conceal even the resentment, lest one be further punished; and concealing resentment is, for reasons I can't touch on now, one of our first very remarkable processes of the group underlying the rather barbarously named 'psychosomatic' field. In other words, in the concealing of resentment, and in the gradual development of self-system processes which preclude one's knowing one's resentment, one actually has to make use of distribution of tension in a fashion quite different from anything that we have touched on thus far. And these processes, which have nothing to do with activity such as a tantrum or something of that kind, are utilized for getting rid of tension so as to avoid activity which would otherwise be revealing, be noticed, and bring punishment.

The Malevolent Transformation

All these generalities about childhood acculturation are background for the circumstances under which the child develops in the direction, not of being obedient or being rebellious, but of being malevolent. Now the ways that malevolence shows in childhood may be numerous. Thus there are so-called timid children whose malevolence shows by their being so afraid to do anything that they just always fail to do the things that are most urgently desired. The great group is the frankly mischievous, and from there we may progress to the potential bully, who takes it out on some younger member of the family, and on the pets, and so on.

But under what circumstances does so remarkable and, may I say, so ubiquitous a thing as malevolence appear as a major pattern of interpersonal relations in childhood? A great many years of preoccupation with this problem has eventuated in a theory which is calculated to get around the idea that man is essentially evil. One of the great social theories is, you know, that society is the only thing that prevents everybody from tearing everybody to bits; or that man is possessed of something wonderful called sadism. I have not found much support for these theories—that man is essentially a devil, that he has an actual need for being cruel and hurtful to his fellows, and so on—in the study of some of the obscure schizophrenic phenomena. And so as the years passed, my interest in understanding why there is so much deviltry in human living culminated in the observation that if the child had certain kinds of very early experience, this malevolent attitude toward his fellows seemed to be conspicuous. And when the child did not have these particular types of experience, then this malevolent attitude was not a major component.

And the pattern that appeared was approximately this: For a variety of reasons, many children have the experience that when they need tenderness, when they do that which once brought tender cooperation, they are not only denied tenderness, but they are treated in a fashion to provoke anxiety or even, in some cases, pain. A child may discover that manifesting the need for tenderness toward the potent figures around him leads frequently to his being disadvantaged, being made anxious, being made fun of, and so on, so that, according to the locution used, he is hurt, or in some cases he may be literally hurt. Under those circumstances, the developmental course changes to the point that the perceived need for tenderness brings a foresight of anxiety or pain. The child learns, you see, that it is highly disadvantageous to show any need for tender cooperation from the authoritative figures around him, in which case he shows something else; and that something else is the basic malevolent attitude, the attitude that one really lives among enemies—that is about what it amounts to. And on that basis, there come about the remarkable developments which are seen later in life, when the juvenile makes it practically impossible for anyone to feel tenderly toward him or to treat him kindly; he beats them to it, so to speak, by the display of his attitude. And this is the development of the earlier discovery that the manifestation of any need for tenderness, and so on, would bring anxiety or pain. The other elaborations—the malevolence that shows as a basic attitude toward life, you might say, as a profound problem in one's interpersonal relations—are also just an elaboration of this earlier warp.

A start in the direction of malevolent development creates a vicious circle. It is obviously a failure of the parents to discharge their social responsibility to produce a well-behaved, well-socialized person. Therefore, the thing tends to grow more or less geometrically. Quite often the way in which the parents minimize or excuse their failure to socialize the child contributes further to his development of a malevolent attitude toward life—and this is likely to be on the part of the mother, since it is difficult to picture a malevolent transformation's occurring at all if the mother did not play a major part in it. A particularly ugly phase of this is found in cases in which the mother is very hostile toward the father, and has exceedingly little sympathy or satisfaction with him; so from very early in the child's life, she explains the increasingly troublesome character of his behavior, his manifestation of as much malevolence as is safe, by saying that he is just like his father in this particular, or just like his father's younger brother, or something of that kind. While the initial references of this kind communicate very little information, their continuation for long enough does tend to warp the child's personification of himself in the direction of something detestable, to be avoided and so on, thereby making very important contributions to his conviction that he will always be treated thoroughly badly.

And in the long course of development, even more subtly destructive are the instances where malevolence has come about because the mother is malevolent toward the child, in which case quite frequently, from very early, there is a good deal of verbal reference which takes the curious form of saying to aunts, uncles, neighbors, and others, "Yes, he has a bad temper just like me," or, "Yes, he is rebellious just like me." One should keep in mind that the mothering one is bound to be significant in all personality evolutions—she can't be otherwise; now when the child gets so that he doesn't think it safe to live among people because he is just like the person that he has to live with, and he gets punished a lot for it, the situation becomes a bit difficult, to say the least. The question arises: If it is all right for mother, why not for me?

Let me conclude by saying that the general conception of malevolence is of very considerable importance. It is perhaps the greatest disaster that happens in the childhood phase of personality development, because the kind of 'ugly'—as it is often called—attitude which it produces is a great handicap to the most profitable experience one could have in subsequent stages of development. It is from the second stage of personality development that a good deal of the foundations of one's attitude toward authoritative figures, superiors, and so on, is laid. So one often learns costly ways of getting around anxiety-provoking and fear-provoking situations—costly in the sense that one never feels exceedingly good or worthy; and these ways of avoiding such situations are not greatly contributory to one's useful information and foresight about living. Thus there can occur this very serious distortion of what might be called the fundamental interpersonal attitude; and this distortion, this malevolence, as it is encountered in life, runs something like this: Once upon a time everything was lovely, but that was before I had to deal with people.

CHAPTER 14

From Childhood into the Juvenile Era

The Meaning of the Arrest of Development

SO FAR we have only touched on much that is often discussed as an arrest of development, a term which is much bandied about in discussions of psychiatry, but which needs more than the mere utterance of the words for some of its implications to become clear. I refer to our discussions of the *as if* performances and the transformation of attitudes and interpersonal relations in the direction of malevolence. These may not be immediately evident as an arrest of development. But, as I said before, the transformation toward malevolence might very easily prevent a great deal of profit from subsequent developmental experience. And the use of dramatizations, obsessional preoccupations, and so on, to avoid anxiety and punishment does actually very seriously interfere with the undergoing of subsequent experience, with analysis and synthesis; if the child is encouraged by various influences to make use of a good deal of obsessional substitution and dramatization, there is literally a slowing down of healthy socialization in lieu of the customary useful unfolding of the repertory of interpersonal motivation and behavior patterns. Arrest of development does *not* imply that things have become static, and that from thenceforth the person will be just the same as he was at the time that development was arrested. The conspicuous evidence of arrest and deviation of personality development is, at first, delay in the showing of change which characterizes the statistically usual course, and later, the appearance of eccentricities of interpersonal relations, which are often anything but self-evident signs of the developmental experience which has been missed or sadly distorted. Thus there is nothing static about arrest of development; but the freedom and the velocity of the constructive change are very markedly reduced. Sometimes, from quite early, the persistence of certain characteristics of the self-system strongly suggests a static condition. But that is not as real as it may seem; even if the self-system seems to be quite unchanged from year to year—or very slightly changed from year to year—nonetheless, experience does occur and is elaborated in personality. Thus, the so-called arrest of personality really means that the returns from opportunity are very markedly reduced. As we go on, it will become more and more impressive to notice the consequences, in subsequent stages of development, that attend unfortunate interferences in particular stages.

Gender as a Factor in the Personification of the Self

Certain influences in childhood make for the growth of the personified self, the personifications "me" and "we," along what I choose to call *gender* lines—and I use this term to avoid too easy a confusion between what I am about to discuss and the notion of sexuality, which becomes highly meaningful only much later in life. At this point I want to call attention to an ancient observation of mine which I think has been rather widely accepted in some related fields: that the child is influenced by the fact that the parent who is of the same sex as the child has a feeling of familiarity with the child, of understanding him; while the parent of the other sex has a surviving, justifiable feeling of difference and of uncertainty toward him. Thus, with boys the father feels more comfortable than with girls; and so he is convinced that he is right in his expectations of his sons, and he is less inclined to think twice, perhaps, in reaching a judgment of disapproval or the like. And the contrary is the case with the mother. The result is that each authority figure treats the child of the other sex in a way which is somewhat favorable to the, shall I say, more rational, more insightful education of the child. This is one of the ubiquitous factors that can be misconstrued as having something to do with a conception such as that of the Oedipus complex, which has enjoyed very great vogue in the fairly recent past of psychoanalytic theory.

The additions to the personified self on the specific basis of whether one is a boy or a girl are advanced notably by two influences: One is the child's play at being the authority figure of his own sex. And the other is the influence of so-called rewards and punishments—particularly interest and approval, in contrast with indifference and disapproval—and sometimes the influence of shame and guilt, which in many ways is the obverse of the *ought* business that we talked about previously, with respect to the roles that the child is playing, is observed to be playing, or later, says that he is playing. These influences tend to educate the child with peculiar facility in the social expectations of his particular sex, in the sense of gender, and to inculcate many of the cultural prescriptions. Thus when the girl catches on in play to something that seems very feminine, this play gets a certain amount of applause, interest, and support from the mother—at least it does if the mother happens to still endorse the feminine. In this way, as the result of the authority figure's attitude toward particular items of play, many of the cultural prescriptions of how one behaves when one grows up are transmitted to the child. The play is, in truth, to a considerable extent trial-and-error learning by human example. But this influence of approval, disapproval, praise, blame, appeal to shame, and the inculcation of guilt are worth mentioning.

The Learning of Cultural Prescriptions for Overt Behavior

There is another strong influence in transmitting certain of the cultural prescriptions to the child, which brings about more rapid transition in the personifications of the child than would occur simply from play and maturation, and so on. This is the very widespread practice of telling or reading stories to the child. These are in general of two types: They may be socially approved moral tales which have become ingrained in the culture because they set forth complex ethical ideals in a fashion that can be grasped by a child. Or they are inventions of the authority figure which may be actually pretty far from the socially approved moral stories and a very special function of the parental personality; the child is apt to be particularly impressed by long-continued stories in which a parent takes the trouble to carry the imaginary protagonists night after night through new adventures. A study of the influence of both kinds of stories has, so far as I know, never been made very rigorously. But certainly their influence on the young, early in childhood, or perhaps all through childhood, often appears in personality studies which are made many, many years later.

In this way, children get the impression that they should be governed by certain influences which we call social values, or judgments, or the ethical worth of certain types of behavior. These notions, since they are primarily in the parataxic mode, do not necessarily have much of anything to do with the observed behavior of the parents, or the child's opinions of the parents. Often these values continue to exist in notable magic detachment from the actual living experience of the child himself. They are apt to be particularly rich soil for the production of verbalism; and these verbalisms, for the very reason that they are derived from moral stories or the like which are part of the cultural heritage, have an effect in impressing the other person which is quite magical.

This is a special aspect of a very important discrimination which grows in the child between what can be expressed, demonstrated, shown, or said, in contrast to what goes on but must be treated as if it did not—which amounts in the last analysis to that which can be overt behavior and that which must remain covert in the presence of authority figures. A special instance of this process is the pointless question, which is the bane of many parents at times and is the kind of process that is commonly encountered in the history of those people who do not come to have adequate ways of living. This occurs when the child has caught on to the fact that certain things about which he needs some information are taboo for any demonstration or discussion; whereupon the child begins to ask questions which do not express what is being sought in the way of information. Of course, at the stage I'm discussing, speech itself is not particularly communicative, so that it is never too wise to assume that what a child says means what those words would ordinarily be taken to mean. But what I'm driving at is the situation in which the child *could* indicate the need for information much more clearly, but is prevented by anxiety and the threat of punishment. Therefore, he begins another kind of indirect behavior, which is not to be confused with obsessional preoccupations or dramatizations: he asks the question, but he adds an autistic element to take the place of that which cannot quite be inquired about. The older the child gets, the nearer these autistic elements are to word combinations that actually refer to something, so that the child may make perfectly rational, diligent inquiries about why mother and father are always doing this and that in the morning when he really wants to know why mother and father do not say a word to each other when they wake to join the day. In other words he really wants to know why they're both morose and have nothing to do with each other except possibly in putting the food on the table and getting it eaten, and that sort of thing. This is a field which is actually quite mysterious to the child, first, because the child is scarcely capable of being morose, and therefore has no particular aptitude for understanding the demonstrations of moroseness; and secondly, because he is under such a necessity for participant play—of play with parental audience and so on—that it would scarcely be possible for him even to imitate morose behavior most of the time. So here is something puzzling and disturbing to the child; but any poking around in this field brings anxiety or the actual threat of punishment by a strong forbidding attitude. And so in an attempt to catch on to something which is ununderstandable, the child begins to ask questions that are beside the point. Now they aren't beside the point to the child, but the anxiety element requires that the child shall use words to *conceal* what is being inquired about, if you want to put it that way. Thus in the child's apparently pointless and sometimes tediously repetitive questions, the question is actually an autistic combination of words which refers to what the child wants to know, and not to what the parent supposes the question pertains to. Toward the end of childhood, as the development proceeds, this process becomes more complicated. The element of questioning for questioning's sake, which may be a form of malicious mischief, may actually become quite rational—that is, the child may ask an immense number of questions about things about which he is really questioning, but he may still do it because there is some very puzzling and disturbing element in the interpersonal relations around him which he is, or feels, prohibited from investigating.

Throughout childhood, as I've already hinted, there is what is often called very active imagination—that is, all sorts of toys are used for temporary investiture with traits of personality, traits of humanness. There is gradually a capacity to do this entirely by referential process—in other words, the child doesn't need anything concrete, but can have a perfectly 'imaginary' plaything. As I have indicated, a good deal of learning is attendant upon the parents' interest in these imaginary plays, imaginary conversations, and so on.

In this connection, an element is introduced to the child which often crops up over the years as an exceedingly disturbing sort of experience. At this stage, while the distinction between overt and necessarily covert processes may be fairly clear at times, it sometimes happens that what is supposed to be covert—that is, what the child knows ought not to be revealed—quite simply gets itself revealed, because of the child's very limited grasp on many things. For example, without intending to communicate anything to the authority figures, the child may speak aloud, just because this is exercise of his vocal abilities and part of his imaginary play; the child's ideas, or rudimentary ideas, are picked up by the parent who hears this, and rewards or punishments, particularly the latter, are poured out on the child, to his quite profound mystification. This is likely to give the child the idea that there is something violable about his covert processes, so that the authority figures know things that he is attempting to conceal, that he does not wish to exhibit, that he knows are dangerous to show. Under some circumstances, this kind of experience begins a group of processes in recall and foresight which literally amounts, in later life, to a feeling at times that one's mind can be read, or can at least be wonderfully accurately suspected. And along with this feeling—I think purely because of cultural artifacts—the child is very apt to get the notion that somehow or other this ability is connected with the eyes, a conception which later appears in the hackneyed and, so far as I am concerned, profoundly erroneous notion that one's eyes are in some curious fashion the windows of one's soul, through which people can observe evil within one, and all that sort of thing. If this sounds a little odd to you, you are rather fortunate, because it is one of the survivals of childhood experience which is regarded as a very remarkable delusion when it appears in the content of a psychosis in later life. And incidentally, it's quite essential, if I am to achieve what I am gunning for in this discussion, that you realize that anything that seems to you to be very remarkable indeed in the content of a psychosis is just something that you haven't placed in your own developmental history.

The Growing Necessity for Distinguishing between Reality and Fantasy

There is, as I have said before, a very considerable need for participation of the parents in the child's play, at least as an attentive audience and if possible as people who perform a role, unless there are siblings who serve this purpose. In a good many instances, circumstances do not permit very much of this audience behavior of the authority figures, and the child is actually lonely; and loneliness at this stage is a foreshadowing of the loneliness which we will be discussing later. The 'lonely' child, the child who cannot obtain the presence and participation, however passive, of elder folk, inevitably has a very rich fantasy life—that is, he makes up for the real deficiencies by multiplying the so-called imaginary personifications which fill his mind and influence his behavior.

Of course, it is necessary to remember that the young child probably does not recognize fantasy as such. The young child knows a lot about the "reality" of a cup, a spoon, or of certain toys which are actually experienced. But with the exception of objects which he has actually experienced, he has only very limited ability to distinguish between fantastic objects and objects which have aspects of what we ordinarily call reality. Thus, a good many things which have no 'reality' but which are built up in the child's mind from the example of the authority figures, or from the maturing needs of the child himself, are of approximately the same reality as the perfectly real things—at least as long as they continue to be effective in covert process and play. As a matter of fact, the perfectly real things—that is, 'real' to the adult—are very heavily invested by the child with [autistic] [1] referential process, so that this kind of 'reality' and his fantasy are indistinguishable to him. And in turn the things which we as adults come to take so very seriously—like policemen, and traffic signals, and all that sort of thing—of course have none of the significance to the child that they have to us. Toys are useful to the very young child for the purpose of discharging newly matured abilities: they do not have any of these relationships which cause us to carry collision damage insurance on automobiles. In other words, the distinction between what anyone would agree was real and what is unutterably the child's own is of no particular moment in this very early stage. The only exception to this is in the field of anxiety-provoking phenomena. But, in general, I believe that if the child under thirty months, for example, considers that performances of the mothering one which did not occur are valid, this is no particular evidence of oncoming difficulty in later life. If the needs and the security operations of the child of this age happen to result in remarkable 'falsifications' of what really happened, I see no reason why this should imply anything more than that the child is alive.

By the end of childhood, the pressure toward socialization has almost invariably fixed a big premium on carefully sorting out that which is capable of being agreed to by the authority figure. This is the first very vivid manifestation in life of the role of consensual validation, by which I mean that a consensus can be established with someone else. Consensually validated symbols underlie almost all operations in the syntaxic mode; what distinguishes syntaxic operations from everything else that goes on in the mind is that they can under appropriate circumstances work quite precisely with other people. And the only reason that they come to work quite precisely with other people is that in actual contact with

1 [*Editors' note:* Autistic has been inserted, since Sullivan seems to be contrasting here the autistic referential processes of the child with the referential processes of the adult—processes which are in the adult more syntaxic in regard to "reality."]

other people there has been some degree of exploration, analysis, and the obtaining of information. The business of socializing the child so that what the parents call purely imaginary events are not reported as true, as actually having happened, is so important as an introduction to the next phase of socialization that, as I say, it is enforced by the end of childhood on practically everyone. The lonelier the child has been, the more striking may be the child's need of effort—need of continuous recall and foresight—to fix these distinctions between what, as we say, actually happened and what was part of fantasy process.

In the next phase of development one can make shocking mistakes and get oneself laughed at, punished, and so on, for reporting what we call lively fantasy as real phenomena. If only because that in itself can be so disconcerting, a 'lonely' child has a natural bent toward social isolation, which is one of the relatively unfortunate outcomes of the next era of development. Here is another of these rather circular processes, approximating a vicious circle: already the child has had to develop a very rich fantasy life to make up for the lack of audience and of participation by the authority figures, and from this lack the child is apt to be relatively undeveloped in the very quick discrimination of what is his private fantasy and what may be consensually validated; that in turn exposes the juvenile to ridicule, punishment, and what not, and so tends to give the feeling of risk in life. This feeling of risk is quite distinct from what I discussed before in talking about the transformation of personality toward malevolence. Risk suggests danger of injury and of anxiety; and malevolence is a peculiar transformation which comes from a convinced foresight of these things. The risk that I am now talking about is not so much a transformation of personality as a partial arrest in the socializing process. It is this which makes people around you not so much enemies as unpredictable sources of humiliation, anxiety, and punishment with respect to what you communicate; and that naturally tends to reduce the freedom and enthusiasm of your communication.

The Change in the Role of Playmates in the Juvenile Era

Perhaps I can illustrate the egocentric nature of much of childhood by an example which may for the moment seem tangential but which really supports much of what I have been saying. Nowadays children are not infrequently put in a formal educative situation before they are quite through with this era of childhood. I believe nursery schools often have members who, according to my schematization, would be children. In these nursery-school situations there is a commonly observed phenomenon—so-called egocentric speech. You see, by late childhood, speech has become a great field for play and a very considerable aid in one's fantasy life. A child in a nursery-school setting will talk a blue streak, apparently to another child; but his talk is not at all influenced by, for instance, the other child's starting to talk, or the other child's going away.

As childhood progresses, a time is reached when there is very rapid acceleration of change in the character of fantasy; and this change is in the direction of burying, losing interest in, forgetting, or modifying what may in very early childhood have been truly incredibly fantastic imaginary playmates, and toward a direction of attempting to personify playmates very like oneself. Where circumstances do not contradict the possibility, there is a beginning of truly cooperative action with other people of about the same age. But even in the case of children who have grown up with no possibility of playing with other children, who are born on remote farms, or in other isolated places, this change in play or change in imagination appears. The child now begins to have rather realistic imaginary playmates, while before a great deal of his imaginary accouterments, his imaginary toys, and so on were strikingly fantastic. Now they begin to be as like him as can be, rather than to be things like the pictures in the *Wizard of Oz* or something of that sort. I refer to all this as the maturation of the need for compeers, which ushers in what it seems best to call the *juvenile era,* which is particularly the period of formal education, as required by law, in this nation at least.

CHAPTER
15

The Juvenile Era

I NOW want to give a hurried sketch of the exceedingly important juvenile era. Much of what I will be talking about is actually accessible to all of us—namely, a good many of the factors which contributed to the growth and direction of personality in the years between entrance in school and the time when one actually finds a chum—the last landmark which ends the juvenile era, if it ever does end. In the succeeding phase of preadolescence, in the company of one's chum, one finds oneself more and more able to talk about things which one had learned, during the juvenile era, not to talk about. This relatively brief phase of preadolescence, if it is experienced, is probably rather fantastically valuable in salvaging one from the effects of unfortunate accidents up to then.

But the importance of the juvenile era can scarcely be exaggerated, since it is the actual time for becoming social. People who bog down in the juvenile era have very conspicuous disqualifications for a comfortable life among their fellows. A vast number of important things happen in the juvenile era. This is the first developmental stage in which the limitations and peculiarities of the home as a socializing influence begin to be open to remedy. The juvenile era has to remedy a good many of the cultural idiosyncrasies, eccentricities of value, and so on, that have been picked up in the childhood socialization; if it does not, they are apt to survive and color, or warp, the course of development through subsequent periods.

It is in general true that, as one passes over one of these more-or-less determinable thresholds of a developmental era, everything that has gone before becomes reasonably open to influence; this is true even in the organization of the self-system, which, as I suppose I cannot stress too much, is remarkably inclined to maintain its direction. The changes which take place at the thresholds of the developmental eras, as outlined here, are far-reaching; they touch upon much of what has already been acquired as personality, often making it somewhat acutely inadequate, or at any rate not fully relevant for the sudden new expanding of the personal horizon. Thus the beginning phase of a developmental era may considerably affect those inappropriate aspects of personality which emerge from what the person has undergone up to then. People going into the juvenile era are all too frequently very badly handicapped for acquiring social skill. Take, for example, the child who has been taught to expect everything, who has been taught that his least wish will be of importance to the parents, and that any obscurities in expressing what he is after will keep them awake nights trying to anticipate and satisfy his alleged needs. Now picture what happens to that child when he goes to school. Or take the petty tyrant who rules his parents with complete neglect of their feelings. Take the child, on the other hand, who has been taught to be completely self-effacing and docilely obedient. These are just a few of the many greatly handicapping patterns of dealing with authority which the home permits or imposes on the child. All these children, if they did not undergo very striking change in the juvenile era, would be almost intolerable ingredients, as they grew up, in a group of any particular magnitude.

In this culture, where education is compulsory, it is the school society that rectifies or modifies in the juvenile era a great deal of the unfortunate direction of personality evolution conferred upon the young by their parents and others constituting the family group. There are two contributions to growth in the juvenile era, the experience of social subordination, and the experience of social accommodation.

In considering *social subordination*, it should be noted that in the juvenile era there is a great change in the type of authority, and in the kind of subordination to authority. The social order, by requiring formal education, provides a succession of new authority figures who are often fortunate in their impersonality. Thus the child is exposed to such variegated authority-carrying figures as the schoolteachers, the recreational directors, the crossing policemen, and so on. Some of these new authority figures have pretty highly stereotyped limitations on the authority they may exercise; in every case, they are almost certainly quite different from the figures in the home, in their exercise of authority and their regard for and interest in the young juvenile. In his relations with his teacher and the various other adult authority figures who now appear, the juvenile is expected—as the child had begun to be by his parents—to do things on demand; and he is given rewards, punishments, and so on, with respect to compliance, noncompliance, rebellion, and what not. But there are more-or-less formally enforced limits to each of these new authorities. At the same time, there is the possibility for the juvenile to see the interrelation of the behavior of his compeers to success or failure with the new authority figures. And in addition to the adult authorities, there are in almost every school situation malevolent juveniles—bullies. Part of the incredible gain in ability to live comes from one's finding a way of getting by under the episodic and destructive exercises of authority by such compeers.

Occasionally some figure in the home is of such great social importance that the new authority figures are intimidated and treat the child as exceptional. For example, the psychiatrist may see an adult in treatment who is the son of an important politician, and may discover that the potency of this politician-father had so altered the freedom with which corrective authority could be imposed on his son that to an extraordinary extent the person as an adult continues to suffer from warp acquired at home as a child. But even under extraordinary circumstances of birth and rank, there occurs some correcting of the more eccentric aspects of adjustment to authority as soon as the child leaves the home.

In almost all cases, however, the more emphatically effective contribution of the juvenile era is that of *social accommodation*—that is, a simply astounding broadening of the grasp of how many slight differences in living there are; how many of these differences seem to be all right, even if pretty new; and how many of them don't seem to be right, but nonetheless how unwise one is to attempt to correct them. This arises from the contact with, and necessity for a certain amount of accommodation to, people of about the same age with a great variety of personal peculiarities. Some of these juveniles are treated with the utmost crudeness by other juveniles. At this stage—if only because the juvenile has just come from the home situation and his previous experience has been with older and younger siblings, or with really imaginary playmates—there is a truly rather shocking insensitivity to feelings of personal worth in others. Thus the school years are a time when a degree of crudeness in interpersonal relations, very rarely paralleled in later life, is the rule. But, in spite of this, the opportunity which is laid before the young juvenile for catching on to how other people are looked upon by authority figures and by each other is an exceedingly important part of the educative process, even though it is one to which no particular attention is conventionally given. A great deal of this educative experience, which tends to correct idiosyncrasies of past socialization, is never discussed as such. Ten, fifteen, or twenty years after one has left the juvenile era, the experience is extraordinarily inaccessible to ready recall, if, for instance, one is undergoing an intensive study of personality.

The rate of growth of personality through all these earlier phases is truly amazing. We realize this more and more as we begin to analyze the enormous number of rather exquisite judgments which one uses in directing one's life in an incoherent culture among people with many specific limitations and individual abilities and liabilities. And the amount of education for life that comes from the juvenile era is immensely important. The juvenile can see what other juveniles are doing—either getting away with, or being reproved for—and can notice differences between people which he had never conceived of, because previously he had had nothing whatever on which to base an idea of something different from his own experience.

Authority Figures as People

Perhaps the most startling aspect of the juvenile acculturation, and the last of the enormous accessions to personality in the juvenile era, is the beginning differentiation of the childhood authority figures—parents and their homologues—as simply people. Failure in this very discrimination of parents as people is often strikingly reflected much later in life. This discrimination is, to a considerable extent, first gained by discovering merits in particular teachers and then discovering demerits in certain other teachers, with or without communication of these experiences to the authority figures at home. But if there has been anything like a healthy development up to this time, these observations *are* discussed in the home. As a result of all this, if it works right, the juvenile gradually has an opportunity to pare the parents down from godlike figures to people. Another great tributary to this type of learning, which appears in most juveniles probably when they are well on in the second grade, is that they learn from other juveniles about their parents. The story most often heard of these earlier school years is, "My father can lick your father"; but it is more important to note that there is simply an amazing amount of checking on the relative virtues and weaknesses of one's parents, especially if there has been no major disaster to development this far. There is no reason in the world why a juvenile should not come out of this period convinced that few people have parents as good as his—that can happen. But if he comes out of the juvenile era with no freedom to compare his parents with other parents, with teachers, and so on—if they still have to be sacrosanct, the most perfect people on earth—then one of the most striking and important of the juvenile contributions to socialization has sadly miscarried.

Competition and Compromise

Now, it is traditional to say—and the tradition is well justified by our observations on inadequate and inappropriate living in chronological adults—that there are two genera of learning which are practically the special province of the early school situation —competition and compromise. They are sufficiently important that certain provisions for them are made in the primary education of all cultures that value these things at all. Unfortunately, competition is the one that gets far more encouragement, although it is perhaps the one that is beginning to sink in importance. The juvenile society itself encourages competitive efforts of all kinds, and in the juvenile himself, I should say, such competition is natural. In addition, the authority figures encourage competition—that is, they do in any culture that values competition. There are some cultures that do not value competition; in those cultures, the tendencies of juveniles to compete appear, but are subjected to inhibitory influence by the authority figures. In our culture, these tendencies are rather vigorously encouraged, so much so, in fact, that if one is physically handicapped or, for some other reason, very bad at competitive performances that are *de rigueur*, then one is practically taught that one is not really fit to be around—that there is something rather profoundly wrong with one.

The other of this pair of elements, compromise, is also invariably enforced by the juvenile society itself, and to a certain extent is encouraged by the school authorities or the juvenile authority figures. Both competition and compromise, while very necessary additions to one's equipment for living with one's fellows, are capable of being developed into outstandingly troublesome traits of the personality. In what I call chronically juvenile people one sees a competitive way of life in which nearly everything that has real importance is part of a process of getting ahead of the other fellow. And if there is also a malevolent transformation of personality, getting the other fellow down becomes the outstanding pattern in the integration of interpersonal relations. This is another of these instances of arrest of development, which is not to say that a chronic juvenile continues in a great many ways to be strikingly like a person, let us say, in the fifth grade of grammar school; it merely means that there are warps in the freedom for interpersonal relations which relate back to the juvenile developmental phase and to particularly unfortunate experiences there. Now under some circumstances compromise also becomes a vice, so that we find people going on from the juvenile era who are perfectly willing to yield almost anything, as long as they have peace and quiet, as they are apt to put it. And that is another unfortunate outcome of juvenile socialization.

Control of Focal Awareness

Thus the juvenile era is the time when the world begins to be really complicated by the presence of other people. The full educational effort, insofar as that effort is formalized by the school curriculum, by the teaching, and so on, is addressed to the extinction of the autistic from the expressed thought and other behavior of the juvenile. And this learning of successful ways of expression and successful types of performance covers so much ground and receives so much encouragement from all sorts of educative influences—all the way from anxiety to carefully awarded prestige with one's fellows—that by the end of the sixth, seventh, or eighth grade, a person of normal endowment has given up a great many of the ideas and operations which, in childhood, and in the home, were all right. This, I believe, is the principal factor entering into the so-called latency period, which was one of the important early psychoanalytic concepts. The effect of the juvenile era is, literally, to make it hard to recall what went on in childhood unless it turns out to be perfectly appropriate and easily modified to meet the strenuous attempt by the society to teach the young to talk, to read, and to "act right."

This giving up of the ideas and operations of childhood comes about through the increasing power of the self-system to control focal awareness. And this in turn comes about because of the very direct, crude, critical reaction of other juveniles, and because of the relatively formulable and predictable manifestations of adult authority. In other words, the juvenile has extraordinary opportunity to learn a great deal about security operations, to learn ways of being free from anxiety, in terms of comparatively understandable sanctions and their violations. This is quite different from anything we have discussed up to now. And insofar as the sanctions and the operations which will avoid anxiety make sense, can be consensually validated, the self-system effectively controls focal awareness so that what does not make sense tends to get no particular attention. That is, effective manifestations of awareness are sternly shepherded by anxiety to be more or less in the syntaxic mode—the mode of experience which offers some possibility of predicting the novel, and some possibility of real interpersonal communication.

This control of focal awareness results in a combination of the fortunate and the unfortunate uses of selective inattention. The sensible use is that there is no need of bothering about things that don't matter, things that will go all right anyway. But, in many cases, there is an unfortunate use of selective inattention, in which one ignores things that do matter; since one has found no way of being secure about them, one excludes them from awareness as long as possible. In any case, the self-system controls, from well on in the juvenile era, the content of consciousness, as we ordinarily call it—that is, what we know we're thinking about—to a very striking extent.

Sublimatory Reformulations

A part of the educational effort, of course, pertains to the acquiring of rote data and information which is not in any particular sense personal; thus juveniles are taught a great many things that seem to have nothing to do with them, but which they have to know in order to get by the teachers. But I am concerned here with the juvenile educative process which is tributary to success in living. Insofar as it is tributary, it is very largely a manifestation, not of rational analysis and valid formulation, but of the sublimatory reformulation of patterns of behavior and covert process. As I have said before, this reformulation occurs when a way of behavior that is socially approved is unwittingly substituted for a part of the motivational pattern that is not acceptable to the authority figures and is not tolerated or regarded with esteem by one's fellows; and when this happens there is some remainder of unsatisfied need which is worked off in private reverie process, especially during sleep.

A very great deal of one's education for living, unfortunately, has to be this sort of sublimatory, strikingly unwitting 'catching-on to' how to get a good deal of satisfaction, although not complete satisfaction. Since it is unwitting, it is not particularly represented in useful understanding of one's behavior. But insofar as it is not overloaded, this process gives one great surety in what one is doing; and one's certainty is not even disturbed by the fact that somebody else may reason better to a different end. Thus when a juvenile acquires a pattern of relating himself to someone else which works and is approved, he simply *knows* that what he is doing is right. And this certainty comes about because there is, in the juvenile era, an increasing power of the self-system to control the contents of awareness, and because the acquisition of the pattern is itself unwitting. Since there is no particular reason for anyone to try to bring into the juvenile's awareness how he arrived at these reformulations of behavior, most of us come into adult life with a great many firmly entrenched ways of dealing with our fellow man which we cannot explain adequately. Even in adult therapy, it is fairly difficult for the psychiatrist to attract enough of the patient's attention to one of these sublimatory reformulations to get him to realize that there's something about it quite beyond explaining. People are not even particularly vulnerable to inquiry in this area, because, by the time anybody is apt to be investigating it, they have a whole variety of devices for heading off awkwardness.

Of the learning which goes on in the juvenile era, a very great amount of it, as I have said before, pertains to competitive and compromising operations to preserve some measure of self-esteem, a feeling of personal worth. As the juvenile era progresses—as one gets into fifth, sixth, seventh, and eighth grades—one has to notice, from this standpoint of the competitive and the compromising operations in which the self-system is involved, the other person concerned. And the other person will be in one of the three groups of significant people that make up the world of the juvenile—the family, the nonfamily authorities, and the other juveniles. The nature of our social system is such that the juvenile alternates between immediate contact with the family group—no juvenile is apt to be able to throw off the influence of the family group—and immediate contact with the school, in its double aspect of authority carriers and other juveniles.

Ostracism

But as the juvenile era goes on, one of its enormously forceful social implements is generally manifest in a segregation into groups within the juvenile society itself—that is, the other pupils in the school—which is a reflection of a good deal of the sickness of the larger society in which juvenility is set. An inevitable outcome of differences in background, differences in abilities, differences in speed of maturations, differences in health, and so on, is the establishment of more-or-less in-groups and out-groups. There are often in-groups with respect to one group of things and in-groups with respect to another; and there are often corresponding out-groups in these various areas. But in most juvenile societies there are a certain number of juveniles who definitely are excluded from very much association with those other juveniles who certainly seem to stand high in the esteem of the school authorities, or in the esteem of the juvenile society in general. The segregating influence which makes some people get along fine together, and apparently rate high with the teachers and with the crossing policemen, or which makes them very important to other juveniles even if they rate very low with the authorities—this segregating influence is sharp, and, to the unfortunate juvenile, quite mysterious. One's experience with these people who are in the right place, who have prestige as a group of juveniles—a very loose group, but still a numerical group at least—is apt to make one feel what can now be perfectly correctly called *ostracism.* Thus juveniles, unless fortunate, can feel ostracized; and if they're quite unfortunate, they get a liberal education in how they are kept ostracized.

In any large group of school children habitually in contact with each other, some of the juveniles will definitely suffer from ostracism by a considerable number of others; but these relatively ostracized out-group youngsters have interpersonal relations one with another. Although these relations to some extent take the curse off the ostracism, they usually do not show enough ingenuity or magical potency to make this unlucky group an in-group. And insofar as these associations with other unfortunate juveniles fail, this experience is not tributary to good self-esteem. In other words, members of out-groups, even if they are fairly successful in maintaining internal competition and compromises, usually show pretty durable evidences of their having been in an inferior position with respect to other compeers whom they were compelled to respect, however painfully and unwillingly, because of their social preferment.

Stereotypes

In the juvenile era, one of the additions to acquaintance with social reality which is almost always encountered is the growth of patterns of others' alleged personalities, which, in a great many cases, amount to actual stereotypes. It is apparent that a great many of us make practical use of stereotypes when we say, "He acts like a farmer." This does not usually mean that we have made a great many observations of farmers and have segregated from all these observations a nuclear group of durable and important traits which are found only in farmers; more probably we are really referring to a stereotype, which may be completely empty of any validifiable meaning. In the juvenile era, the growth of stereotypes which will later disfigure one's ability, or interfere with one's ability, to make careful discriminations about others goes to really lamentable lengths in some instances. These are the stereotypes of persons never encountered in reality, or—perhaps next most troublesome—stereotypes of large groups of humanity on the basis of a solitary instance or a very few instances. Thus, for example, in my own early years, by a series of irrelevant accidents, I heard things said about Jews, but I didn't know any Jews. Because of an extremely fortunate accident of what seemed to be otherwise a very unpleasant developmental history, I did not have very much interest in these vague rumors that I'd never seen exemplified, and so I did not adopt this stereotype. Therefore I emerged into the adult world with some curiosity about these people, whom I thought of as extraordinary, since my own acquaintance with them resulted almost entirely from perusing Holy Writ. I am glad that I did not fix in my mind some of the alleged attributes of Jews which I might have found lying around in certain juveniles, which in turn they, having no actual experience with them, had taken over from parents and other authority figures. Otherwise, I am quite certain that I would have been richly supplied with stereotypes. And these would have been much harder to correct later than was my curiosity as to what the devil the people who wrote the Old Testament must have been like.

Stereotyping can be a source of very real trouble in later life, especially if one is going into a field of work like psychiatry, where the extremely important thing to do is to observe participantly what goes on with another person. If you have a number of implicit assumptions that have not been questioned by you for twenty or twenty-five years about the alleged resemblance of the person before you to some stereotype that you have in your mind, you may find yourself greatly handicapped, for these stereotypes are often viciously incomplete and meaninglessly erroneous.

A great deal of this stereotyping is stamped in, in the juvenile era. Since there is so much to be done in this era and so much pressure on the juvenile to take over any successful patterns for doing it, in our type of school society at least, one of the conspicuous outcomes is that a great many juveniles arrive at preadolescence with quite rigid stereotypes about all sorts of classes and conditions of mankind. One of these stereotypes is about people of the opposite sex. Unless something fortunate intervenes, juveniles pretty nearly have to adopt gross stereotypes of juveniles of the other sex. If you think back to your experience in, say, the first grade, with a particularly attractive playmate who happened to be of the other sex, you may remember how that relationship changed as you went on in juvenile society. And you may realize that, in spite of all experience which was contrary to the stereotype, you almost had to adopt, by the time you were on the verge of preadolescence, what might be described as the juvenile stereotype of the "girls" or the "boys"—whichever the other sex was—and govern yourself accordingly—publicly at least.

Sometimes there are stereotypes about teachers which are all too easy to accept because of previous unpleasantness with authority figures. Quite often there are stereotypes of juveniles' relations to teachers; and if one is actually teacher's pet, or simply for some reason the teacher is especially interested in one, one has to act under the aegis of the juvenile stereotype of the teacher's pet, and cannot therefore derive any simple profit from what would otherwise be a fortunate accident. I suppose, if only because of the speed with which the awesome varieties of people and behavior are impressed on the juvenile, it's hard indeed to avoid organizing—accessible to awareness—crude classifications of people, performance, and so on, which really are irrational and which later become troublesome stereotypes.

Supervisory Patterns

Stereotyping, to a striking extent, also characterizes the evolution of the juvenile's own self-system, insofar as the personifications of the self are concerned. An almost inevitable outcome of the most fortunate kind of juvenile experience is the appearance of what I call *supervisory patterns* in the already very complex system of processes and personifications that make up the self-system. These supervisory patterns amount in certain instances to subpersonalities—that is, they are "really" imaginary people who are always with one.

Perhaps I can make my point by mentioning three of these supervisory patterns that everyone knows most intimately from very prolonged personal experience. When you have to teach, lecture in public, as I am doing, or do any talking in which it's quite important that the other fellow learns something from you, or thinks that you're wonderful, even if obscure, you have as a supervisory pattern a personality whom I might call your *hearer*. Your hearer is strikingly competent in judging the relevancy of what you are saying. This hearer patiently listens to all your harangues in public and sees that the grammar is stuck together and that things that are too opaque are discussed further. In other words, it is really as if a supplementary, or a subordinate, personality worked like thunder to put your thoughts together into some semblance of the English language. My hearer—my particular supervisory pattern—has a certain rather broad composition, which is built out of a great deal of experience in being an essentially solitary, overprivileged juvenile, surrounded by numerous people who were not free from envy. Thus my supervisory pattern is such that I often adjust my remarks fairly well to the needs of, let us say, fifty percent of my audience. Some people's hearers seem to have been even more singularly uninformed about other people than mine, and these hearers let pass, as adequate and proper, expressions which communicate to very few indeed of those that hear them. But in any event, it is as if there were two people—one who actually utters statements, and another who attempts to see that what is uttered is fairly well adjusted to its alleged purpose.

All of you, whether or not you have a diligent hearer, have now long had, as a supervisory pattern, the *spectator*. The spectator diligently pays attention to what you show to others, and do with others; he warns you when it isn't quite cricket, or it's too revealing, or one thing and another; and he hurriedly adds fog or camouflage to make up for any careless breach. And if any of you write seriously, or even write detective stories, you have another supervisory pattern of this kind—your *reader*. I have been very much interested in the character of my reader, never quite interested enough to conduct an extended investigation to discover his actual origin; but enough to know that he's a charming pill, practically entirely responsible for the fact that I almost never publish anything. He is bitterly paranoid, a very brilliant thinker, and at the same time an extraordinarily wrongheaded imbecile. Thus when I attempt to use the written language to communicate serious thought, I am unhappily under constant harassment to so hedge the words around that the most bitterly critical person will be unable to grossly misunderstand them, and, at the same time, to make them so clear that this wrongheaded idiot will grasp what I'm driving at. The result is, as I say, that I write almost nothing. I usually give it up in the process of revising it.

These supervisory patterns ordinarily come into being in the juvenile era and persist, with some refinements, from then on. Their presence in the self-system may well be stressed from another standpoint: They are only a small part of this very elaborate organization, which we all come to have, for maintaining our feeling of personal worth, our self-respect, for obtaining the respect of others, and for insuring the protection which positions of prestige and preferment confer in our particular society.

Social Judgments and Social Handicaps

In the course of the juvenile era, particularly toward the close of it, one is invariably exposed to judgments and suspected judgments which can be called one's reputation as a juvenile. And in a good many cases, there are very great discrepancies—often quite worthy of inspection in the course of later study of personality—between one's reputation with nonfamily authorities, with other juveniles, and with the family society. With other juveniles, one's reputation is particularly determined by the in-groups and by those juveniles who are manifesting what is called leadership in its more rudimentary form—another of the phenomena of juvenile society as it gets on.

Now, the sorts of things that make up one's reputation in these three areas of the social world may be suggested if I run over only a few of the contrasts that are, I suppose, with one through life. A person is popular, is average, or is unpopular. In juvenile society, being average has special qualities; for instance, people who can't be popular are much happier being average than being unpopular. Another one of these contrasts is being a good or a bad sport, particularly for males in this culture. Or again, a person is unquestionably bright, or average, or dull. One is assured, or average, or socially diffident. One is superior, or average, or unfortunately inferior with respect to the progress of one's development in interpersonal relations—that is, as we ordinarily say it, in personality development. One is, in other words, outstanding in one's capacity for understanding and invention of new interpersonal patterns, and so on; or one is below average—that is, literally backward in the evolution of interpersonal relations. There can be very real foundations for a juvenile's being backward in this area, if, for example, ill health comes at critical periods and cuts him out of school recurrently, or if something prevents his participation in games which enjoy great prestige in that particular school group. It can come about because of social handicap; this social handicap may be the reputation of one's father as the neighborhood drunkard—things of that kind, which one was not fortunate enough to discover a way to get around. In the good old days, it might be nothing more fatal than the fact that your mother had divorced and remarried. All these things may literally provide such a handicap that one is pretty slow in developing social accommodation. And some of these social handicaps are very real indeed. One of the things which time and time again has shown itself to have been quite disastrous in the history of patients was the social mobility of the parents, which took the juvenile from one school to another at frequent intervals, so that he was always being introduced as a stranger to another group of juveniles. Other things being equal, if one is getting on at all fortunately in juvenile society, it's a very good thing to stay in that group of juveniles throughout the period, or certainly until near the end of the juvenile era. Otherwise one will actually show considerable inferiority in acquiring the complement of interpersonal aptitudes which the juvenile era, at its best, confers. Of course, if one is in a very unfortunate position in a group of juveniles, it is perhaps fortunate if one can get out of it. But continuous upheaval in schooling—and this is strikingly true with service personnel—is apt to leave a very considerable handicap in this and subsequent phases of development.

The Learning of Disparagement

In addition to all this, there are certain more obscure factors which may make one backward, as it were, in growing up. With respect to one's reputation, and particularly with respect to one's superior profit or inferior profit from the juvenile era, there are rather important influences which may be exerted by the parental group. The particular one that I shall use as an instance is only one of many unfortunate influences which the parents may exercise, which tend to reduce profit from the juvenile era. This is a parental morbidity of security operations, such that the juvenile is taught to disparage others—a common phenomenon on the American scene. It may be the way, for instance, that the significant figure in the home handles a juvenile "misfortune," such as being average instead of superior. It may occur because the parental figure has always disparaged all people who made her or him uncomfortable. It may occur because one or both parents feel threatened by the revealing nature of juvenile communication and so disparage teachers and other people with whom they feel compared. This disparaging business is really like the dust of the streets—it settles everywhere. It is perhaps not so disastrous in the juvenile era as it is from then on; but it is very disastrous at any time. If you have to maintain self-esteem by pulling down the standing of others, you are extraordinarily unfortunate in a variety of ways. Since you have to protect your feeling of personal worth by noting how unworthy everybody around you is, you are not provided with any data that are convincing evidence of your having personal worth; so it gradually evolves into "I am not as bad as the other swine." To be the best of swine, when it would be nice to be a person, is not a particularly good way of furthering anything except security operations. When security is achieved that way, it strikes at the very roots of that which is essentially human—the utterly vital role of interpersonal relations.

In the juvenile era this kind of security operation, literally and very significantly, interferes with adequate analysis of personal worth. In other words, if another boy does well and little Willie reports it to mother, and mother promptly knocks the spots off the other boy and his family, that tends to indicate that little Willie's impression of how the other fellow was behaving was groundless, or that the rewards which the other fellow's behavior got from teachers, and so on, were undeserved. In other words, one is encouraged to feel incapable of knowing what is good. Learning from human examples is extremely important, as I have stressed; but if every example that seems to be worth emulating, learning something from, is reduced to no importance or worth, then who are the models going to be? I think that this is probably the most vicious of the inadequate, inappropriate, and ineffectual performances of parents with juveniles—this interference with a sound development of appreciation of personal worth, by universal derogatory and disparaging attitudes toward anybody who seems to stand out at all. It is in this way that parents are apt to very markedly handicap the 'sane' development of standards of personal worth in their young. To that extent—barring great good fortune in subsequent eras of personality development—they literally guarantee that their children will be barely better than the other swine.

The Conception of Orientation in Living

By the end of the juvenile era, with any good fortune, one has gotten to the point at which it is quite proper to apply the conception of *orientation in living,* as I use the term. *One is oriented in living to the extent to which one has formulated, or can easily be led to formulate (or has insight into), data of the following types: the integrating tendencies (needs) which customarily characterize one's interpersonal relations; the circumstances appropriate to their satisfaction and relatively anxiety-free discharge; and the more or less remote goals for the approximation of which one will forego intercurrent opportunities for satisfaction or the enhancement of one's prestige.* The degree to which one is *adequately oriented* in living is, I believe, a very much better way of indicating what we often have in mind when we speak about how "well integrated" a person is, or what his "character" is in the sense of good, bad, or indifferent.

The juvenile actually has an opportunity to undergo a great deal of social experience, in contrast to the child, who cannot have any orientation in living in the larger world. To the extent that the juvenile knows, or could easily be led to know, what needs motivate his relations with others, and under what circumstances these needs—whether they be for prestige or for anything else—are appropriate and relatively apt to get by without damage to self-respect, to this extent the person has gotten a great deal out of his first big plunge into socialization. If this comes off successfully, he inevitably has established some things which we can really call his values, from the pursuit of which he will not be deflected by other things that come along and might be obtained; in other words, a striking aspect of good orientation in living is the extent to which foresight governs the handling of intercurrent opportunities.

To the extent that a juvenile has been denied an opportunity for a good orientation in living, he will from henceforth show a trait which is a lamentable nuisance: he will be so anxious for the approval and unthinking immediate regard of others that one might well think he lived merely to be liked, or to amuse. And in some cases, that, I fear, is about true.

So, if one has been fortunate in the juvenile era, his orientation in living among other people is fairly well organized. And if his orientation in living is not well organized, his future contributions to the human race will probably be relatively unimportant or will be troublesome, unless he has very good fortune in the next succeeding phases of personality development.

CHAPTER 16

Preadolescence

Need for Interpersonal Intimacy

JUST AS the juvenile era was marked by a significant change—the development of the need for compeers, for playmates rather like oneself—the beginning of preadolescence is equally spectacularly marked, in my scheme of development, by the appearance of a new type of interest in another person. These changes are the result of maturation and development, or experience. This new interest in the preadolescent era is not as general as the use of language toward others was in childhood, or the need of similar people as playmates was in the juvenile era. Instead, it is a specific new type of interest in a *particular* member of the same sex who becomes a chum or a close friend. This change represents the beginning of something very like full-blown, psychiatrically defined *love*. In other words, the other fellow takes on a perfectly novel relationship with the person concerned: he becomes of practically equal importance in all fields of value. Nothing remotely like that has ever appeared before. All of you who have children are sure that your children love you; when you say that, you are expressing a pleasant illusion. But if you will look very closely at one of your children when he finally finds a chum—somewhere between eight-and-a-half and ten—you will discover something very different in the relationship—namely, that your child begins to develop a real sensitivity to what matters to another person. And this is not in the sense of "what should I do to get what I want," but instead "what should I do to contribute to the happiness or to support the prestige and feeling of worth-whileness of my chum." So far as I have ever been able to discover, nothing remotely like this appears before the age of, say, eight-and-a-half, and sometimes it appears decidedly later.

Thus the developmental epoch of preadolescence is marked by the coming of the integrating tendencies which, when they are completely developed, we call love, or, to say it another way, by the manifestation of the need for interpersonal intimacy. Now even at this late stage in my formulation of these ideas, I still find that some people imagine that intimacy is only a matter of approximating genitals one to another. And so I trust that you will finally and forever grasp that interpersonal intimacy can really consist of a great many things without genital contact; that intimacy in this sense means, just as it always has meant, closeness, without specifying that which is close other than the persons. Intimacy is that type of situation involving two people which permits validation of all components of personal worth. Validation of personal worth requires a type of relationship which I call collaboration, by which I mean clearly formulated adjustments of one's behavior to the expressed needs of the other person in the pursuit of increasingly identical—that is, more and more nearly mutual—satisfactions, and in the maintenance of increasingly similar security operations.[1] Now this preadolescent collaboration is distinctly different from the acquisition, in the juvenile era, of habits of competition, cooperation, and compromise. In preadolescence not only do people occupy themselves in moving toward a common, more-or-less impersonal objective, such as the success of "our team," or the discomfiture of "our teacher," as they might have done in the juvenile era, but they also, specifically and increasingly, move toward supplying each other with satisfactions and taking on each other's successes in the maintenance of prestige, status, and all the things which represent freedom from anxiety, or the diminution of anxiety.[2]

1 [*Editors' note:* Sullivan's use of the terms "collaboration" and "cooperation" should be kept in mind throughout this section. By cooperation, he means the usual give-and-take of the juvenile era; by collaboration, he means the feeling of sensitivity to another person which appears in preadolescence. "Collaboration . . . is a great step forward from cooperation—*I* play according to the rules of the game, to preserve *my* prestige and feeling of superiority and merit. When we collaborate, it is a matter of *we*." (*Conceptions of Modern Psychiatry*, p. 55.)]

2 [*Editors' note:* Up to this point, this chapter is taken from 1944–1945

Psychotherapeutic Possibilities in Preadolescence

Because of the rapidly developing capacity to revise one's personifications of another person on the basis of great interest in observation and analysis of one's experience with him, it comes about that the preadolescent phase of personality development can have and often does have very great inherent psychotherapeutic possibilities. I believe I have said earlier that it is at the developmental thresholds that the chance for notable favorable change tends to segregate itself. Although the structure of the self-system is such that its development in general is rather powerfully directed along the lines it has already taken, it is much more subject to influence through new experience, either fortunate or unfortunate, at each of the developmental thresholds. The fact that the self-system can undergo distinct change early in each of the developmental stages is of very real significance. For it is the self-system—the vast organization of experience which is concerned with protecting our self-esteem—which is involved in all inadequate and inappropriate living and is quite central to the whole problem of personality disorder and its remedy. And it is this capacity for distinct change in the self-system which begins to be almost fantastically important in preadolescence.

During the juvenile era a number of influences of vicious family life may be attenuated or corrected. But in the Western world a great deal of the activity of juveniles is along the lines of our ideals of intensely competitive, invidious society; only recently—and, I fear, still quite insularly—has there been any marked social pressure toward developing the other aspects of the same thing, the capacity to compromise and cooperate. Because of the competitive element, and also because of the juvenile's relative insensitivity to the importance of other people, it is possible that one can maintain throughout the juvenile era remarkably fantastic ideas about oneself, that one can have a very significantly distorted personification of the self, and keep it under cover. To have a very

---

lectures, rather than from the series on which this book is primarily based, since this portion is missing in the latter series because of failures of recording equipment. The material corresponds, however, to the outline in Sullivan's Notebook.]

fantastic personification of oneself is, actually, to be very definitely handicapped. In other words, it is a misfortune in development.

Because one draws so close to another, because one is newly capable of seeing oneself through the other's eyes, the preadolescent phase of personality development is especially significant in correcting autistic, fantastic ideas about oneself or others. I would like to stress—at the risk of using superlatives which sometimes get very tedious—that development of this phase of personality is of incredible importance in saving a good many rather seriously handicapped people from otherwise inevitable serious mental disorder.

I may perhaps digress to the extent of saying that for some years I have had no negative instance to the following generalization: As a psychiatrist and a supervising psychiatrist, I have had occasion to hear about many male patients who find all relationships with other men occasions for considerable tenseness and vigilance, and who are uncomfortable in all their business, social, or other dealings with other men; of this group, I have found without exception that each one has lacked anything like good opportunities for preadolescent socialization. (I am confining my remarks to male patients here because the female picture is more complicated and I have less material on it.) These male patients may have what they call very close friends of the same sex, may even be overt and promiscuous homosexuals; but they are not at ease with strange men, they have much more trouble doing business with other men than seems to be justified by the factual aspects of the difficulty, and they are particularly uncertain as to what members of their own sex think of them. In other words, I am practically convinced that capacity for ease, for maximum profit from experience, in carrying on the conventional businesses of life with members of one's own sex requires that one should have been fortunate in entering into and profiting from relations with a chum in the preadolescent phase of personality development.

It is self-evident, I suppose, that I am conspicuously taking exception to the all-too-prevalent idea that things are pretty well fixed in the Jesuitical first seven years. This idea has constituted one of the greatest problems for some anthropologists who have tried to translate psychiatric thought into anthropologically useful ideas. The anthropologists have noised at them from all sides the enormous importance of infantile experience—meaning experience certainly under the age of eight. Yet one of the most conspicuous observations of an anthropologist working anywhere is that children of the privileged, who are raised by servants, do not grow up to be like the servants. That is a little bit difficult for an anthropologist to reconcile with the tremendous emphasis on very early experience. My work has shown me very clearly that, while early experience does a great many things—as I have been trying to suggest thus far—the development of capacity for interpersonal relations is by no means a matter which is completed at some point, say, in the juvenile era. Very far from it. And even preadolescence, which is a very, very important phase of personality development, is not the last phase.

Preadolescent Society

Except in certain rural communities, there occurs in preadolescence the development of at least an approach to what has long been called by sociologists "the gang." I am again speaking rather exclusively of male preadolescents, because by this time the deviations prescribed by the culture make it pretty hard to make a long series of statements which are equally obviously valid for the two sexes. The preadolescent interpersonal relation is primarily, and vastly importantly, a two-group; but these two-groups tend to interlock. In other words, let us say that persons *A* and *B* are chums. Person *A* also finds much that is admirable about person *C*, and person *B* finds much that is admirable about person *D*. And persons *C* and *D* each has his chum, so that there is a certain linkage of interest among all of these two-groups. Quite often there will be one particular preadolescent who is, thanks to his having been fortunate in earlier phases, the sort of person that many of these preadolescent people find useful as a model; and he will be the third member, you might say, of many three-groups, composed of any one of a number of two-groups and himself. At the same time, he may have a particular chum just as everybody in this society may have. Thus these close two-groups, which are extremely useful in correcting earlier deviations, tend at the same time to interlock through one person or a few people who are, in a very significant sense, leaders. And incidentally, let me say that many of us are apt to think of leadership in political terms, in terms of "influence" and the "influential." We overlook the fact that influence is exerted by the influential in certain conspicuous areas other than that of getting people to do what the leader wants done. The fact is that a very important field of leadership phenomena—and one that begins to be outstandingly important in preadolescence—is opinion leadership; and understanding this and developing techniques for integrating it might be one of the few great hopes for the future.

Thus some few people tend to come out in leadership positions in preadolescent society. Some of them are the people who can get the others to collaborate, to work with understanding and appreciation of one another toward common objectives or aims, which sometimes may be crimes, or what not. And others are the leaders whose views gradually come to be the views of a large number in the group, which is opinion leadership. This kind of leadership has certain fairly measurable and perhaps some imponderable aspects. One of its reasonably measurable aspects is that people whose development, combined with their intellectual abilities, has given them the ability to separate facts and opinions, tend to be considered by the others as well informed, right in their thinking about things of interest at that particular stage, and thus tend to do the thinking for a good many of the others because of the latter's unfortunate personality warp. And the time when these leaders in opinion do the thinking almost exclusively is when there are serious problems confronting the members of the group. The level of general insecurity about the human future is high at this stage of development, and in any case probably increases when serious problems arise, whether they occur in the preadolescent gang or in society as a whole. It is at those times that perhaps far more than half of the statistical population—handicapped by lack of information, by lack of training, and by various difficulties in personal life which call out a good deal of anxiety, which in turn interferes with practically everything useful—has to look to opinion leadership for anything like reassuring views or capable foresight. Thus an important part of the preadolescent phase of personality development is the developing patterning of leadership-led relationships, which are so vital in any social organization and which are, theoretically at least, of very great importance in relatively democratic organizations of society.

I have suggested that an important aspect of the preadolescent phase is that, practically for the first time, there is consensual validation of personal worth. Now it is true that some children are fortunate, indeed; through the influences to which they have been subjected in the home and school, they are about as sure as they can be that they are worth while in certain respects. But very many people arrive in preadolescence in the sad state which an adult would describe as "getting away with murder." In other words, they have had to develop such remarkable capacities for deceiving and misleading others that they never had a chance to discover what they were really good for. But in this intimate interchange in preadolescence—some preadolescents even have mutual daydreams, spend hours and hours carrying on a sort of spontaneous mythology in which both participate—in this new necessity for thinking of the other fellow as right and for being thought of as right by the other fellow, much of this uncertainty as to the real worth of the personality, and many self-deceptive skills at deceiving others which exist in the juvenile era, may be rectified by the improving communication of the chums and, to a much lesser extent but nonetheless valuably, by confirmatory relations in the collaboration developed in the gang.

Types of Warp and Their Remedy

We might next look at a few of the warped juveniles who can receive very marked beneficial effect from the maturation of this need for intimacy and from preadolescent socialization, who can at this stage literally be put on the right road to a fairly adequate personality development. For example, there are egocentric people, who go from childhood through the juvenile era and still retain literally unlimited expectations of attention and services to themselves. Some of these people you know as those who sulk when something doesn't suit them; some of them are people who have tantrums under certain circumstances. If the families of these juveniles are so influential that the more adult members of the school community hesitate to "break" the juveniles of these undesirable "habits," then about the last chance they have of favorable change is based on their need for getting along with a chum in preadolescence. As juveniles, they have been classified quite uniformly by other juveniles as thoroughly bad sports; there is a distinct tendency for other juveniles to avoid them, to ostracize them, in spite of some necessity for accommodating to them which is imposed by the influence of the family. It is quite possible that in preadolescence such a person will establish his chumship with some other ex-juvenile who is more or less on the fringe of ostracism, and who had been in the out-group of the juvenile society. That looks as if it wouldn't be too good; and in some instances it is not so good, as I will note later. But it is very much better than what was going on before. Not infrequently people of this kind go through the comparatively brief period of preadolescence and come out very much less inclined to expect unlimited services from others, very much nearer the ideal of a good sport who can "take it," and who doesn't require very special treatment. In other words, two unfortunate juveniles thrown together by their unfortunate social status as juveniles may, under the influence of this growing need for intimacy, actually do each other a great deal of good. And as they show some improvement they will become less objectionable to the prevailing preadolescent society and may actually get to be quite well esteemed in the gang. But the risk is that these bad sports, these self-centered or egocentric juveniles, now formed into two-groups, may carry their resentment and misery from the ostracism they have suffered to the length of seeking out and identifying themselves with the most antisocial leadership which can be found.

However, the notion that preadolescence readily consolidates a criminal, antisocial career is the most shocking kind of nonsense, which overlooks almost all instances which happen to be negative. It happens that there is more literature on antisocial gangs than there is on the vastly favorable aspect of preadolescent society. I believe that a study of preadolescent society in the very worst neighborhoods would reveal tendencies other than those leading toward becoming minor criminals. And in some very bad neighborhoods, while there are gangs which are antisocial, there are also gangs which are very much less antisocial, if not actually constituting a constructive element in the neighborhood. In any event, the socialization is bound to happen; and if the setting is bad enough, it's quite possible that the organization will be against the world and will tend to implant that attitude as a reasonable purpose for social action.

Some juveniles arrive in preadolescence strikingly marked with the malevolent transformation of personality which I have discussed previously at some length. All too many of them, because of this malevolent transformation, take their time in establishing a chumship, or may actually fail to do so. But the drive connected with this need for intimate association with someone else is so powerful that quite frequently chumships are formed even by malevolent people. And the entrance into one of these two-groups, which in turn is integrated into the preadolescent gang, provides experience which definitely opens the mind anew to the possibility that one can be treated tenderly, whereupon the malevolent transformation is sometimes reversed, literally cured. More commonly, it is only ameliorated, because the malevolent transformation is apt to have quite a cramping effect on the very easy amalgamation of malevolent two-groups into larger organizations.

There is a variety of other peculiarities that more or less survive the juvenile period. For example, there is the person who feels that something is wrong with others if they don't like him—in other words he really feels perfectly entitled to being universally liked. This kind of person never learns, in the juvenile era, that that is not a reasonable attitude toward life. In the school society, such a person ordinarily has to handle his disappointments by derogatory rationalizations and disparagement of others, for which he generally is set an excellent example in his home. These folk, getting into the preadolescent socialization, quite often gain enough in security from the intimacy with their chums to enable them to really open their minds and discuss these other unpleasant people who don't seem to like them, in a fashion that is illuminating, both as to the real worth of the others and as to some of their own traits which may not be very endearing. Thus preadolescence tends actually to correct to a notable extent one of our most vicious forms of morbidity—the tendency to pull people down because one isn't quite big enough to be comfortable with them. Needless to say, preadolescence does not always cure this, but it tends to mitigate it.

Isolated juveniles, people whom one would expect to go on indefinitely in a rather 'schizoid' way of life, sometimes, by very fortunate preadolescent experience, come out remarkably well able to handle themselves, to develop the social accommodation which did not really reach them in the juvenile period; and this is because of the peculiarly intimate consensual exchange which goes on in preadolescence. On the other hand, social isolation may make it very difficult to establish the type of intimacy which preadolescence calls for; and it may often delay preadolescence so that there is only a brief time, before the puberty change, in which to consolidate the benefits of the preadolescent period.

One of the more warped kinds of juveniles is the one who will not grow up. He is sometimes popular, but often he is unpopular. In any event, he is apt to become increasingly unpopular as the juvenile era wears itself out. This kind of person can properly be called irresponsible. He doesn't want to take on anything that he can avoid; he wants to remain, if you please, juvenile. He wants to be as young as possible, in that he has a real unwillingness to bend the knee to our society's necessities with respect to others. Here again maturation of the need for intimacy sometimes has very marked beneficial effect; on the other hand, it may not work out that way, and he may get into an irresponsible gang. But I do not want you to think that antisocial gangs are in any notable proportion of instances made up of people who were irresponsible juveniles. Whether the gang activity is constructive or destructive in its relationship to the larger society which houses it has nothing in particular to do with the types of warp in the personalities involved in it, but is more a function of what is acceptable as leadership.

In summing up these various warps, one might say that, as long as the warp is not so great as to preclude any undergoing of the preadolescent era, the formation of these new intimacies will provide some consensual validation for all of the warps—that is, one gets a look at oneself through the chum's eyes. To the extent that that is accomplished the self-system concerned is definitely expanded, and its more troublesome, inadequate, and inappropriate functions are reduced to the point that they become unnecessary.

I should like to mention a few more things that are not quite warps but which might come to be the basis for inadequate and ineffectual living, were it not for the preadolescent influence. Some people go through the juvenile phase with a very favorable record; they are wonderful in sportsmanship, they are very skillful in compromise, or they are just so bright that everybody in the juvenile society profits. Now comes the preadolescent need for intimacy. Any one of these people is apt to be integrated in a two-group with a more average person. And in this interchange in the preadolescent society, some of these very successful juveniles get the first great clue to the fact that they are not going to be carried through life on a silk cushion, and they learn to accept this fact. They discover that if they are lucky enough to have gifts, these gifts carry responsibilities; and that insofar as gifts are used for the discharge of social responsibilities, one is to a certain extent spared the great evil of envy and all the destructive practices which envy carries in its wake.

A somewhat similar group of juveniles are those who have very high intelligence and rate well with teachers, but who are unpopular and unsuccessful with other juveniles—a fact which teachers seldom notice, since they are mainly preoccupied with their pupils' learning. In preadolescence, the drive of the need for intimacy may turn this high intelligence to good use, and literally provide the ex-juvenile with an opportunity for using his intelligence to learn how to be one with others.

Finally, perhaps, I should touch on those who, because of illness or social handicaps or what not, have hung behind all through the juvenile era. Here too the preadolescent intimacy may literally give them, as it were, so much of a helping hand that they come near to catching up with what they have missed in the juvenile era in the way of competition, compromise, and socialization.

The factors that count in the two-groups of preadolescence are: the personal suitability of the people thrown together and then tied together by their need for intimacy; the intensity of the relationship which is achieved; and the durability of the relationship, or the progressive direction of change in those instances in which the relationships have not proved durable throughout preadolescence. This last might result from change of residence of the parents; or there might be factors in the two-group itself that make for disintegration, each of the components then becoming integrated with someone else.

I want particularly to touch on the intensity of the relationship, because it is easy to think that if the preadolescent chumship is very intense, it may tend to fixate the chums in the preadolescent phase, or it may culminate in some such peculiarity of personality as is ordinarily meant by homosexuality—although, incidentally, it is often difficult to say what is meant by this term. Actual facts that have come to my attention lend no support whatever to either of these surmises. In fact, as a psychiatrist, I would hope that preadolescent relationships were intense enough for each of the two chums literally to get to know practically everything about the other one that could possibly be exposed in an intimate relationship, because that remedies a good deal of the often illusory, usually morbid, feeling of being different, which is such a striking part of rationalizations of insecurity in later life.

Perhaps I can illustrate this point by telling you how, by an extraordinary concatenation of events, I was once able to find out something about the adult lives of a onetime preadolescent group who had attended school together in a small Kansas community. I first had access to this information through a man who had been one of the preadolescents in the school, and I was later able to follow this up and get rather complete information on the group. This particular man was an overt homosexual. During his preadolescence, he had been distinctly in the out-group, if only with respect to so-called mutual masturbation and other presumably homosexual activity which went on in this group of boys as preadolescent pals; that is, he had not participated in any of the mutual sexuality which went on in the terminal phase of preadolescence in this group. There was one other preadolescent who had not participated in it, and I was able to track him down. I found that he also had become an overt homosexual. Those who had participated in mutual sexuality were married, with children, divorces, and what not, in the best tradition of American society. In other words, relationships of what might be described as 'illegitimate' intimacy toward the close of the preadolescent period had not conduced to a disturbed type of development in adolescence and later; the facts showed something quite different.

The great remedial effect of preadolescence occurs not only by direct virtue of the intimacy in the two-group, but also because of the real society which emerges among the preadolescents, so that the world is reflected in the preadolescent microcosm. The preadolescent begins to have useful experience in social assessment and social organization. This begins with the relationship which the two-groups come to have to the larger social organization, the gang. The chums are identified as such, and are literally assessed by all other two-groups—and this is not in terms of who they are, but of how they act, and what you can expect from them in the social organization. This is an educative, provocative, and useful experience in social assessment. The fact that one looks out for oneself and is regarded as incredibly individual and what not begins very strikingly to fade from the center of things; and that is an exceedingly fortunate experience to have had. And the gang as a whole finds that it has a relationship to the larger social organization, the community, and that it is assessed by the community. Community acceptance of the gang is likely to depend on whether or not the gang is antisocial, and it may also depend on how widely representative the gang is.

Within the gang, experience in social organization is reflected in how closely integrated the gang is, how stable its leadership is, and how many leaders for different things there are. Sometimes there are preadolescent gangs in which you would find, if you made a careful study, that the members maintain subordination to a number of different leaders, each for different circumstances, which is really pretty refined social organization in miniature.

Disasters in Timing of Developmental Stages

As the preadolescent goes on toward the puberty change, the effect of previous experience on rate of maturation becomes peculiarly conspicuous. The time of the puberty change may vary considerably from person to person—in contrast to the time for the convergence of the eyes in infancy, for instance, which can be predicted almost exactly. This difference in time of puberty maturation may occur partly because of certain biological and hereditary factors; but I know, from considerable data, that factors of experience are also involved. Certain peculiarities of earlier training are so extraordinarily frequent in cases of so-called delayed puberty that one suspects that this training has literally delayed the maturation of the lust dynamism.

One of the lamentable things which can happen to personality in the preadolescent society is that a particular person may not become preadolescent at all promptly—in other words, he literally does not have the need for intimacy when most of the people of about the same age have it, and therefore he does not have an opportunity of being part of the parade as it goes by. But then this person, when preadolescence is passing for most of his contemporaries, develops a need for intimacy with someone of his own sex and may be driven to establishing relationships with a chronologically younger person. This is not necessarily a great disaster. What is more of a disaster is that he may form a preadolescent relationship with an actually adolescent person, which is perhaps more frequently the case in this situation. This does entail some very serious risk to personality and can, I think, in quite a number of instances, be suspected of having considerable to do with the establishment of a homosexual way of life, or at least a 'bisexual' way. And, as I have already hinted, there is definitely a possibility of going no further than preadolescence. The fact that one can be preadolescent for perhaps two years longer than others in one's particular group of young people is nowadays frequent enough to be a study in itself. The number of instances of schizophrenic disorder which are precipitated by one of the chums' getting well into adolescence while the other remains preadolescent is, in my experience, notable.

If adolescence is delayed, it would not have any particular importance, and might actually be somewhat advantageous, as long as one were sure of having a reasonable number of equally delayed people with whom to maintain the type of intimacy which characterizes preadolescence. It is only when chumships are broken up, and the preadolescent society is disorganized by the further maturation of nearly all the members, that great stress may be applied to the personalities which are not able to move on the same time schedule. Sometimes these people who are delayed in puberty have a progression of chums from people of their own age to younger ones, which is somewhat hard on the status of both in the preadolescent organization, tending to exclude both from what would normally be the society of the younger. I suppose the best thing that can happen—next to having a number of confreres who are also slow in maturing—is to be able to take the early stage of adolescence before one has really gotten to it, which is sometimes possible; that is, the adolescent change means a moving of an interest toward members of the other sex, but one can often find an eccentric member of the other sex who also has not undergone the puberty change, but is glad to go through the motions. That reduces the stress on one's feeling of personal worth and security which delayed adolescence may otherwise bring. The delayed completion of the preadolescent phase of personality, together with a shift from the group with which the preadolescent has been developing to marginal groups of adolescents, is, I think, apt to be pretty hard on this younger person; that is, he is, in a sense, the victim of marginal groups of adolescent people, who are actually having plenty of trouble themselves and who are apt to develop a very lively interest in sexual operations with this preadolescent whose adolescence has been delayed. In certain instances, at least, these operations are very costly to the personality when finally the puberty change and the phases of adolescence begin.

In a given person, the beginning of adolescence, as far as personality development is concerned, takes place at an indefinite time; that is, although it does not take place overnight, it is observable at the end of a matter of months, instead of years. Early adolescence, in my scheme of development, is ushered in by the beginning of the array of things called the puberty change, by the frank appearance of the lust dynamism. And the frank appearance of the lust dynamism is, in a great many instances, manifested by the intrusion, into fantasy or the sleep-life, of experience of a piece with the sexual orgasm; in other instances, where there has been preliminary genital play, and so on, it is manifested by the occurrence of orgasm in certain play. Lust is the last to mature of the important integrating tendencies, or needs for satisfaction, which characterize the underlying human animal now well advanced to being a person.

In our society, the age when early adolescence appears varies within three or four years, I think. This remarkable developmental discrepancy which is possible among different people of the same chronological age—a vastly greater discrepancy than occurs in the maturing of any of the previously discussed needs—is one of the important factors which makes adolescence such a time of stress. And incidentally, only by studying a different social organization from ours could one see how much less a time of stress the period of adolescence might be. In certain other societies, where the culture provides a great deal more real preparation for adolescence than ours does, the extraordinarily stressful aspect of adolescence is not nearly so conspicuous. There are, however, certain elements of the puberty change and its associated adolescent phase of personality organization that are not to be overlooked in any social order; those are the ones associated with the remarkable speeding up of certain growth factors which, for example, makes people clumsy and awkward who were previously quite skillful and dexterous. Thus there are always, or almost always, some stresses concerned with this very rapid maturation of the somatic organization which is ushered in by the puberty change. But so far as the psychological stresses are concerned, they are more apt to result from disasters in timing than from anything else.

The Experience of Loneliness [3]

Before going on, I would like to discuss the developmental history of that motivational system which underlies the experience of loneliness.

Now loneliness is possibly most distinguished, among the experiences of human beings, by the toneless quality of the things which are said about it. While I have tried to impress upon you the extreme undesirability of the experience of anxiety, I, in common apparently with all denizens of the English-speaking world, feel inadequate to communicate a really clear impression of the

[3] [*Editors' note:* Several times, in the series of lectures which has been used as the basis for this book, Sullivan has made reference to a later discussion of loneliness. Yet this discussion does not appear in this particular series, probably through an oversight. We have therefore included here a discussion of loneliness from a 1945 lecture.]

experience of loneliness in its quintessential force. But I think I can give you some idea of why it is a terribly important component of personality, by tracing the various motivational systems by developmental epochs that enter into the experience of loneliness. Of the components which culminate in the experience of real loneliness, the first, so far as I know, appears in infancy as the need for contact. This is unquestionably composed of the elaborate group of dependencies which characterize infancy, and which can be collected under the need for tenderness. This kind of need extends into childhood. And in childhood we see components of what will ultimately be experienced as loneliness appearing in the need for adult participation in activities. These activities start out perhaps in the form of expressive play in which the very young child has to learn how to express emotions by successes and failures in escaping anxiety or in increasing euphoria; in various kinds of manual play in which one learns coordination, and so on; and finally in verbal play—the pleasure-giving use of the components of verbal speech which gradually move over into the consensual validation of speech. In the juvenile era we see components of what will eventually be loneliness in the need for compeers; and in the later phases of the juvenile era, we see it in what I have not previously mentioned by this name, but what you can all recognize from your remembered past, as the need for acceptance. To put it another way, most of you have had, in the juvenile era, an exceedingly bitter experience with your compeers to which the term "fear of ostracism" might be justifiably applied—the fear of being accepted by no one of those whom one must have as models for learning how to be human.

And in preadolescence we come to the final component of the really intimidating experience of loneliness—the need for intimate exchange with a fellow being, whom we may describe or identify as a chum, a friend, or a loved one—that is, the need for the most intimate type of exchange with respect to satisfactions and security.

Loneliness, as an experience which has been so terrible that it practically baffles clear recall, is a phenomenon ordinarily encountered only in preadolescence and afterward. But by giving this very crude outline of the components that enter into this driving impulsion, I hope I have made it clear why, under continued privation, the driving force of this system may integrate interpersonal situations despite really severe anxiety. Although we have not previously, in the course of this outline of the theory of personality, touched on anything which can brush aside the activity of the self-system, we have now come to it: Under loneliness, people seek companionship even though intensely anxious in the performance. When, because of deprivations of companionship, one does integrate a situation in spite of more or less intense anxiety, one often shows, in the situation, evidences of a serious defect of personal orientation. And remember that I am speaking of orientation in living, not orientation in time and space, as the traditional psychiatrists discuss it. I have already given my conception of orientation in living in discussing the juvenile era. Now this defective orientation may be due, for instance, to a primary lack of experience which is needed for the correct appraisal of the situation with respect to its significance, aside from its significance as a relief of loneliness. There are a good many situations in which lonely people literally lack any experience with things which they encounter. . . .

Loneliness reaches its full significance in the preadolescent era, and goes on relatively unchanged from thenceforth throughout life. Anyone who has experienced loneliness is glad to discuss some vague abstract of this previous experience of loneliness. But it is a very difficult therapeutic performance to get anyone to remember clearly how he felt and what he did when he was horribly lonely. In other words, the fact that loneliness will lead to integrations in the face of severe anxiety automatically means that loneliness in itself is more terrible than anxiety. While we show from the very beginning a curiously clear capacity for fearing that which might be fatally injurious, and from very early in life an incredible sensitivity to significant people, only as we reach the preadolescent stage of development does our profound need for dealings with others reach such proportion that fear and anxiety actually do not have the power to stop the stumbling out of restlessness into situations which constitute, in some measure, a relief from loneliness. This is not manifest in anything like driving force until we arrive at the preadolescent era.

CHAPTER 17

Early Adolescence

THE EARLIER phase of adolescence as a period of personality development is defined as extending from the eruption of true genital interest, felt as lust, to the patterning of sexual behavior which is the beginning of the last phase of adolescence. There are very significant differences, in the physiological substrate connected with the beginning of adolescence, between men and women; but in either case there is a rather abrupt change, relatively unparalleled in development, by which a zone of interaction with the environment which had been concerned with excreting waste becomes newly and rapidly significant as a zone of interaction in physical interpersonal intimacy. In other words, what had been, from the somatic viewpoint, the more external tissues of the urinary-excretory zone now become the more external part of the genital zone as well. The change, from the psychological standpoint, pertains to new needs which have their culmination in the experience of sexual orgasm; the felt tensions associated with this need are traditionally and quite properly identified as *lust*. In other words, lust is the felt component of integrating tendencies pertaining to the genital zone of interaction, seeking the satisfaction of cumulatively augmented sentience culminating in orgasm.

There is, so far as I know, no necessarily close relationship between lust, as an integrating tendency, and the need for intimacy, which we have previously discussed, except that they both characterize people at a certain stage in development. The two are strikingly distinct. In fact, making very much sense of the complexities and difficulties which are experienced in adolescence and subsequent phases of life, depends, in considerable measure, on the clarity with which one distinguishes three needs, which are often very intricately combined and at the same time contradictory. These are the need for personal security—that is, for freedom from anxiety; the need for intimacy—that is, for collaboration with at least one other person; and the need for lustful satisfaction, which is connected with genital activity in pursuit of the orgasm.

The Shift in the Intimacy Need

As adolescence is ushered in, there is, in people who are not too much warped for such a development, a change in the so-called object of the need for intimacy. And the change is from what I shall presently be discussing as an isophilic choice to what may be called a heterophilic choice—that is, it is a change from the seeking of someone quite like oneself to the seeking of someone who is in a very significant sense very different from oneself. This change in choice is naturally influenced by the concomitant appearance of the genital drive. Thus, other things being equal and no very serious warp or privation intervening, the change from preadolescence to adolescence appears as a growing interest in the possibilities of achieving some measure of intimacy with a member of the other sex, rather after the pattern of the intimacy that one has in preadolescence enjoyed with a member of one's own sex.

The degree to which the need for intimacy is satisfied in this heterophilic sense in the present-day American scene leaves very much to be desired. The reason is not that the shift of interest toward the other sex in itself makes intimacy difficult, but that the cultural influences which are borne in upon each person include very little which prepares members of different sexes for a fully human, simple, personal relationship together. A great many of the barriers to heterophilic intimacy go back to the very beginnings of the Western world. Just to give a hint of what I am talking about, I might mention the so-called double standard of morality and the legal status which surrounds illegitimate birth. One can get an idea of the important influence of cultural organization and cultural institutions on the possibilities of relationships in adolescence which are easy and, in terms of personality development, successful, by studying a culture very significantly different from our own in this respect. For some years I have recommended in this connection Hortense Powdermaker's *Life in Lesu.*[1] There, the institutions bearing on the distinction between the sexes are very significantly different from ours, and the contrast between our institutions and theirs perhaps sheds some light in itself on unfortunate aspects of the Western world.

But to return to our culture: The change in the need for intimacy—the new awakening of curiosity in the boy as to how he could get to be on as friendly terms with a girl as he has been on with his chum—is usually ushered in by a change of covert process. Fantasy undergoes a rather striking modification—a modification almost as abrupt and striking as the sudden acceleration of somatic growth which begins with the puberty change and leads, for instance, to the awkwardness which I have mentioned. And there may also be a change of content in overt communicative processes, both in the two-group and in the gang. That is, if the preadolescents are successfully progressing toward maturation and uniformly free from personality warp, this interest in members of the other sex also spreads into the area of communication between the chums, even though the one chum may not be quite up to the other and may be somewhat opposed to this new preoccupation with girls. In the more fortunate circumstances, this is presently a gang-wise change, and those who are approximately ready for it profit considerably from this last great topic of preadolescent collaboration—the topic of who's who and what's what in the so-called heterosexual world. If the group includes some members whose development is delayed, the social pressure in the group, in the gang, is extremely hard on their self-esteem and may lead to very serious disturbances of personality indeed. As I have previously hinted, it is not uncommon for the preadolescent phase to fade imperceptibly into the early adolescent phase, and for gang-wise genital activity to become part of the pattern of the very last stage of preadolescence or the verge of adolescence. Thus one not uncommonly finds at this point that the lust dynamism is actually functioning and governing a good part of group activity, but this

[1] [Hortense Powdermaker, *Life in Lesu: The Study of a Melanesian Society in New Ireland;* New York: W. W. Norton & Co., Inc., 1933.]

is very definitely oriented to that which is to follow with members of the other sex.

In this change from preadolescence to adolescence, there has to be a great deal of trial-and-error learning by human example. A considerable number of those at the very beginning of adolescence have some advantage in this learning by virtue of having already acquired data from their observation of and experience with a sibling of the other sex not very far removed from them in developmental age; these data which had been previously unimportant are now rapidly activated.

I believe that according to conventional, statistical experience, women undergo the puberty change somewhat in advance of men; in a great many instances, this leads to a peculiar sort of stutter in developmental progress between the boys and the girls in an age community so that by the time most of the boys have gotten really around to interest in girls, most of the girls are already fairly well wound up in their problems about boys. From the standpoint of personality development, it would be convenient if these things were timed slightly better; but I suppose that in the beginning when everything was arranged—I've never had any private information on the subject, by the way—procreation was fully as important as a feeling of self-esteem is now in a highly developed civilization. And so women get ready for procreation quite early; in fact one of the important problems of adolescence is how to avoid the accident of procreation.

Various Collisions of Lust, Security, and the Intimacy Need

After lust gets under way, it is extremely powerful. In fact, if one overlooks his experience with loneliness, he may well think that lust is the most powerful dynamism in interpersonal relations. Since our culture provides us with singular handicaps for lustful activity rather than with facilitation, lust promptly collides with a whole variety of powerful dynamisms in personality. The most ubiquitous collision is naturally *the collision between one's lust and one's security;* and by security I mean one's feeling of self-esteem and personal worth. Thus a great many people in early adolescence suffer a lot of anxiety in connection with their new-found motivation to sexual or genital activity—and I use those words interchangeably. Besides the puzzlement, embarrassment, and so on, which the culture practically makes certain, there are lamentably too many instances of people who already have a rather profound warp with respect to the general area of the body which is concerned. I have called this the primary genital phobia, which is not entirely to be interpreted on the basis of the usual ideas about phobia. By primary genital phobia I refer to an enduring warp of personality which is often inculcated in late infancy and early childhood and practically converts that area of the body into something not quite of the body. In discussing the excretory function and the exploratory power of the hand, I have commented on the incredible efforts made by certain parents to keep the young child from handling the genitals, from exploring and getting sensations from them. In cases in which this is successful, that area of the body becomes distinctly related to that area of personality to which I long since referred as the not-me. It is almost impossible for the adolescent who has this type of warp to arrive at any simple and, shall I say, conventional type of learning of what to do with lust. Therefore, as that person becomes lustful, he has the energy of the genital dynamism added to loneliness and other causes for restlessness; thus his activity with others becomes comparatively pointless, which almost certainly is humiliating and is not a contribution to his self-esteem. Or he may actually have some fairly serious disturbance of personality because of the outstanding power of the lust dynamism and the comparative hopelessness of learning how he, in particular, can do anything about it. Thus a person in this era may know a good deal about what other people do, but if he finds he can't do it himself, he doesn't feel quite up to the average.

Not only does lust collide with the need for security, but *the shift in the intimacy need may also collide with the need for security*. In early adolescence, the need for intimacy, for collaboration with some very special other person, reaches out toward, and tends to settle on, a member of the other sex. Now the ways in which this may collide with self-esteem are numerous, but there are a few particular instances that I want to bring to your attention. Quite often we discover that the young reach adolescence very much to the discontent of their elders in the home. In those situations it is not uncommon to find that there has been no serious taboo by the family group against the development of a chum relationship or even against membership in a gang; but now as the interest begins to move toward members of the other sex, there does begin to be strong repressive influence brought to bear on the adolescent by the family group.

One of the most potent instruments used in this particular is ridicule; many an adolescent has been ridiculed practically into very severe anxiety by parents who just do not want him to become, as they think of it, an adult interested in such things as sex, which may get him diseased or what not, or may result in marriage and his leaving home. Ridicule from parents and other elders is among the worst tools that are used on early adolescents. Sometimes a modification of ridicule is used by parents who are either too decent to use ridicule or are unaware of its remarkable power; and this modification takes the form of interfering with, objecting to, criticizing, and otherwise getting in the way of any detectable movement of their child toward a member of the other sex. This can go to the point of being a pathological performance which we call jealousy, in which the parent literally gets incredibly wrapped up in the rudimentary two-group that the adolescent is trying to establish with some member of the opposite sex. We will touch on jealousy again when we get around to discussing the particular group of difficulties in living which are called paranoid states. It should merely be noted at this point that jealousy is invariably a matter of more than two people, and that very often everyone concerned in jealousy is pretty fantastic—that is, there are a great many parataxic processes mixed up in it. Sometimes the third person concerned is purely a parataxic delusion on the part of the jealous person. So much for merely a few high spots on the type of collisions between the feeling of personal worth and the change in the direction of the need for intimacy.

There are also *collisions between the intimacy need and lust.* In establishing collaborative intimacy with someone, four varieties of awkwardnesses are common, of which the first three—embarrassment, diffidences, and excessive precautions—make up one group. The fourth represents one of our magic tricks of swinging to the other extreme to get away from something that doesn't work, which I call the *not* technique. In other words, you know what an apple is, and if you were under pressure enough you could produce an imaginary truth, *not apple*, made up entirely of the absence-of-apple characteristics. Thus, one of the ways of attempting to solve this collision between the intimacy need and lust is by something which is about the opposite of diffidence—namely, the development of a very bold approach in the pursuit of the genital objective. But the approach is so poorly addressed to the sensitivities and insecurities of the object that the object is in turn embarrassed and made diffident; and so it overreaches and has the effect of making the integration of real intimacy quite improbable.

A much more common evidence of the collision of these two powerful motivational systems is seen among adolescents in this culture as the segregation of object persons, which is in itself an extremely unfortunate way of growing up. By this I refer to the creating of distinctions between people toward whom lustful motivations can apply, and people who will be sought for the relief of loneliness—that is, for collaborative intimacy, for friendship. The classical instance is the old one of the prostitute and the good girl. The prostitute is the only woman who is to be thought of for genital contact; the good girl is never to be thought of in that connection, but only for friendship and for a somewhat nebulous future state referred to as marriage. When this segregation has been quite striking, this nebulous state takes on a purely fantastic character. Nowadays, the far more prevalent distinction is between sexy girls and good girls, rather than this gross division into bad and good women. But no matter how it comes about that the other sex is cut into two groups—one of which can satisfy a person's loneliness and spare him anxiety, while the other satisfies his lust—the trouble with this is that lust is a part of personality, and no one can get very far at completing his personality development in this way. Thus satisfying one's lust must be at considerable expense to one's self-esteem, since the bad girls are unworthy and not really people in the sense that good girls are. So wherever you find a person who makes this sharp separation of members of the other sex into those who are, you might say, lustful and those who are nonlustful, you may assume that this person has quite a cleavage with respect to his genital behavior, so that he is not really capable of integrating it into his life, simply and with self-respect.

These sundry collisions that come along at this stage may be the principal motives for preadolescents or very early adolescents getting into 'homosexual' play, with some remarkable variations. But a much more common outcome of these various collisions—these difficulties in developing activity to suit one's needs—is the breaking out of a great deal of autosexual behavior, in which one satisfies one's own lust as best one can; this behavior appears because of the way in which preadolescent society breaks up, and because of the various inhibitions which have been inculcated on the subject of freedom regarding the genitals. Now this activity, commonly called masturbation, has in general been rather severely condemned in every culture that generally imposes marked restrictions on freedom of sexual development. That's very neat, you see; it means that adolescence is going to be hell whatever you do, unless you have wonderful preparation for being different from everyone else—in which case you may get into trouble for being different.

Incidentally, problems of masturbation are sufficiently common, even among the wise, so that a word might be said here regarding what seems to be a sound psychiatric view of the matter. The question sometimes arises as to whether masturbation is good or bad. Now whenever a psychiatrist is confronted by such a question, he may well take it under advisement to see whether he can reformulate it into a question that he can, as a psychiatrist, deal with; psychiatrists don't dispense these absolute qualifications of good or bad. The nearest we can approach such values is to decide whether a thing is better or worse in terms of the interpersonal present and near future. From this approach, one can note that in this culture the developmental progress in connection with the adolescent change is handicapped by both lack of preparation and absolute taboos on certain freedoms; but lust *combined with* the need for intimacy frequently does drive the victim toward correcting certain warps in personality and toward developing certain facilities, certain abilities, in interpersonal relations. There is no way that I know of by which one can, all by oneself, satisfy the need for intimacy, cut off the full driving power of loneliness, although loneliness can be manipulated or reduced to a certain extent. But through autosexual performance one can prevent lust from reaching tension sufficient to break down one's barriers. For that reason, the entirely exclusive use of autoerotic procedures can contribute to the prolongation of warp, which in turn contributes to the continued handicap for life of the person concerned. It is from this viewpoint alone that I would consider that masturbation, as the *only* solution for the sundry collisions that lust enters into, is worse than almost anything else that is not definitely malevolent. Needless to say, such an argument becomes meaningless if, as is so often the case in genital behavior, the autoerotic performance is not fixed and exclusive but is incidental or occasional. Arguments against masturbation based on anything other than this particular reason seem to me to smack more of unanalyzed prejudice on the part of the arguer than of good sense.

Fortune and Misfortune in Heterosexual Experimentation

My next topic is the rather important one of the fortune and misfortune which the early adolescent has in his experimentation toward reaching a heterosexual type of experience. In the olden days when I was distinctly more reckless than now, I thought that a good many of the people I saw as mental patients would have been luckier in their adolescence had they carried on their preliminary heterosexual experimentation with a good-natured prostitute —that is, this would have been fortunate in comparison to what actually had happened to them. Not that I regard prostitutes as highly developed personalities of the other sex; but if they happen to be in the business of living off their participation in genital sport and are friendly, they at least will know a good deal about the problems in this field that earlier adolescents encounter, and will treat them with sympathy, understanding, and encouragement; but unfortunately, a great many of these experiments are conducted with people who are themselves badly, though differently, warped. The number of wretched experiences connected with adolescents' first heterosexual attempts is legion, and the experiences are sometimes very expensive to further maturation of personality. If there has been a lively lustful fantasy and little or no overt behavior with respect to the genitals—which incidentally will tend very strongly to characterize everyone who has this primary genital phobia I have spoken of—then it is almost certain that on the verge of an actual genital contact, precocious orgasm will occur in the man; and this precocious orgasm suddenly wipes out the integration and just leaves two people in a practically meaningless situation although they had previously made immense sense to each other. Such an occurrence reflects very severely on the self-esteem of the man concerned and thereby initiates a still more unfortunate process which is apt to appear as impotence. The recollection of so disastrous an occurrence, which has been in terms of anxiety pretty costly, is quite apt to result in either of two outcomes: there may be an overweening conviction that that's the way it's going to go, that one just hasn't any 'virility,' that one's manhood is deficient; or there may be frantic attempts to prove otherwise, which, if they were kept up long enough, would work. Unless there has been some genital activity, or unless the woman is quite expert in reducing the anxiety of the male, or even his sexual excitement, this precocious orgasm is very apt to be a man's introduction to heterosexual life. Needless to say, it has about as much true significance as drinking a glass of water—that is, if one could accept it in perfectly calm and rational fashion, it would prove absolutely nothing except that it had occurred once, and one could subsequently see whether it was going to be typical behavior or whether it was an accident. It usually isn't typical unless its effects are disastrous, in which case it can be stamped in as a sort of morbid way of handling one's incapacity to integrate true lustful situations, or as a channel for various other things which I shall discuss presently.

In other instances in which there is a lack of experience and considerable warp in the personalities concerned, lust may carry things through to orgasm, usually of only one partner; but immediately upon the satisfaction of the lust dynamism and the disintegration of the situation as a lustful situation, the persons concerned may become the prey of guilt, shame, aversion, or revulsion for each other, or at least this may be true for one of the people concerned. And this experience is not a particularly fortunate addition to one's learning how to live in the world as it is. A much less usual, but also unfortunate, event in this initial experimentation in genital activity is that if it has gone pretty well it may become a high-grade preoccupation. This is usually to be understood on the general theory of preoccupation and is just as morbid as any other preoccupation. Since lust has a peculiarly strong biological basis, and, in some people, may be an ever recurrent and very driving force in early adolescence, this preoccupation with lust can lead to serious deterioration of self-respect because of the unpleasant situations one is driven into, because of the disapproval one encounters, and because this type of preoccupation literally interferes with almost any commonplace way of protecting one's self-esteem. A great many people whose self-esteem has been somewhat uncertain, depending on scholarship only, find their standing as students rapidly declining as they become completely preoccupied with the pursuit of lust objects. Thus they become the prey of severe anxiety, since their only distinction is now being knocked in half.

With truly distressing frequency, these sundry problems connected with early adolescence cause the persons concerned to turn to alcohol, one of the great mental-hygiene props in the culture, with unfortunate results. I sometimes think alcohol is, more than any other human invention, the basis for the duration and growth of the Western world. I am quite certain that no such complex, wonderful, and troublesome organization of society could have lasted long enough to become conspicuous if a great number of its unhappy denizens did not have this remarkable chemical compound with which to get relief from intolerable problems of anxiety. But its capacity for dealing with those problems naturally makes it a menace under certain circumstances, as I scarcely think I need argue. Like a good many other props which temporarily remedy but do not in any sense favorably alter cultural impossibilities, it is costly, not to all, but to too many. A peculiarity of alcohol is that it interferes very promptly with complex, refined referential operations, particularly those that are recent—that have not been deeply and extensively involved in the whole business of living—while it does not particularly disturb the older and more essential dynamisms of personality. It definitely poisons the self-system progressively, beginning with the most recent and most complex of the self-system's functions. So personality under alcohol is less competent at protecting itself from anxiety, but practically all the anxiety is experienced later, retrospectively. Since the self-function, which is, of course, very intimately connected with the occurrence of anxiety, is inhibited and disturbed by alcohol, but one's later recall is not, one experiences the anxiety in retrospect, you see. And the problems that get one all too dependent on alcohol are, I think, the problems of sexual adjustment, which hit hardest in early adolescence.

The Separation of Lust from Intimacy

I want next to discuss misfortunes of development in early adolescence in which there is, as the outstanding characteristic, a separation of those interpersonal relations motivated by lust from those based on the need for intimacy—that is, motivated by loneliness. This sharp division is merely a very much more extensive and enduring deviation of personality than the kind of classification of heterophilic objects—for example, into good women and bad women—which I previously mentioned. The need for intimacy has been gradually developing along its own lines from very ancient roots, while lust has only recently and vividly appeared. The complex outcomes of these developmental interpersonal relations which are scarcely parallel and are actually divergent are a very rich source for problems which concern the psychiatrist. Some people are unfortunate enough to sublimate, as we still have to call it, their lust—that is, to partially satisfy it while connecting it with socially acceptable goals. This is, as I would again like to remind you, an extremely dangerous overloading of possibilities, which is very apt to collapse in a lamentable way. I am postponing a discussion of what happens to lust under these circumstances. But the intimacy need sometimes shows itself as follows: A member of the other sex who is in a good many ways like the parent of that sex may become invested with full-fledged "love" and devotion. Another, not so striking instance, is the pseudo-sibling relation. There are, of course, many jokes in the culture about the girl who is willing to be a sister to you. But I wonder if you realize how many unfortunate early adolescents get by with the appearance of personality development by striking up one of these pseudo-sibling relationships, which can be mistaken by others for a satisfactory move toward developing a solution for the problems of lust and loneliness. Another change of this kind is, we might say, a prolongation and refinement of the separation of good and bad girls: All women are good—too good; they are noble, and one cannot approach them for anything so something-or-other as genital satisfaction. And there is the alternative of that, in which all women are regarded as extremely unattractive, unsuited to anything but a particular kind of hateful entanglement which becomes practically official business.

In the process of trying to separate one's need for intimacy from one's need for genital integration, certain peculiarities of personality appear which we will later discuss as *dissociation.* Among the people with these peculiarities of personality pertaining to the need for intimacy, there is the one who feels pursued by the other sex and actually spends a lot of time in trying to avoid being hounded by the other sex. There is also the true woman-hater—that is, the man who literally feels the most strenuous antipathy to any but the most superficial relation with members of the other sex. When lust is dissociated—and components in lust are quite frequently dissociated—such things occur, even from early adolescence, as the celibate way of life, in some cases with accessible lustful fantasies, and in other cases with no representation of lustful needs in awareness. This latter can go so far that actually there are no recollections of any content connected with what must have been the satisfaction of lust in sleep; in other words, there are nocturnal orgasms, but there is never any recollectable content at all. When one encounters that sort of thing, one thinks immediately that something has gone very radically wrong with the personality. Another manifestation in this field is what I call, in terms of a man's viewpoint, horror of the female genitals; even though the man considers that women are all right, and in fact, in many instances, may make a very good approach to them, the actual attempt at a physical intergenital situation causes the man to be overcome with a feeling which is literally uncanny, which is quite paralyzing. As I have already hinted, all these uncanny feelings refer to the not-me, and are, by this stage of personality, practically always signs that there is serious dissociation somewhere in personality. Another solution of this kind is to fall into a homosexual way of getting rid of lust; this is accompanied either by liking, by indifference, or by aversion toward the partner, or by revulsion or by fascination for the whole type of situation.

In this special group of disturbances of development, there are also the instances in which the genital drive is discharged with infrahuman or nearly infrahuman participation—that is, some of the lower animals are used as genital partners, or people are used whom the person has so much prejudice against that he scarcely considers them to be human. Very occasionally human ingenuity leads people who suffer from primitive genital phobia to invent what are called masturbating machines. This is a phenomenon that gets a good deal of attention, more than it deserves, and is, supposedly, very interestingly connected with paranoid states. As a matter of fact, it does coincide more than occasionally with later paranoid states, but this relation has been vastly overaccentuated.

The Isolated Adolescent

Finally, I want to mention here the misfortune of isolation in early adolescence, which is quite different from the developmental disturbances I have just discussed. This misfortune of isolation in adolescence has affected quite a number of the people whom you meet in ordinary life, or whom the psychiatrist encounters in his practice. Perhaps because the community is very small, or perhaps because of peculiar home circumstances or something of the sort, the isolated adolescent does not have other adolescents with whom to fraternize, is not thrown into contact with members of the other sex of approximately the same developmental phase. Such people are, from a theoretical standpoint, rather interesting because of the progression of their reverie processes; as they go from preadolescence into adolescence, the chief characters in their long-continued fantasies shift toward the other sex. The extent to which lustful covert processes are added to their fantasies depends, to an extraordinary degree, on the extent to which mediate educational influences have provided some basis for covert processes. Sometimes one finds people who, simply because of their isolation, have not reached the point of having particularly lustful reverie processes, so that when the lust dynamism comes along, it discharges itself largely in sleep; and this in itself may not represent a grave disturbance of personality. If we could study some of these isolated people—or rather if they were, in spite of entire lack of experience, clever at communication, which is almost unheard of—it would be interesting to see what the nocturnal development of covert processes connected with the satisfaction of lust is like. Some of these isolated early adolescents suffer a particular handicap from this reverie substitution for interpersonal experience, in that they develop quite strongly personified imaginary companions; and the singularly personal source of the idealized characteristics may be a severe barrier later on to finding anybody who strikes them as really suitable for durable interpersonal relations.

Failure to Change the Preadolescent Direction of the Need for Intimacy

I have said that, along with the maturation of the lust dynamism, but by no means in absolute temporal coincidence with it, there is, in the fortunate, a shift in the intimacy need toward seeking friendship with a person who is different, a member of the other sex. But I now want to consider the accidental development in which the *lust dynamism matures but there is no change in the preadolescent direction of the need for intimacy*. In this case there is added to the impulse which makes for the cultivation and cherishing of a friend of the same sex, all the force of the lust dynamism with its drive for genital interaction with someone or something. And in these instances transient or persisting homosexual organization of the interpersonal relations is usual, with the genital drive handled in a variety of ways. The first of these ways is by known homosexual reverie processes that are surrounded by precautions which protect the self-esteem, at least partially, of the person who entertains them. This is generally accompanied by autogenital discharge of lust, coupled with an avoidance of, or an indifference to, members of the other sex, and social distance toward members of the same sex. Thus, while there is a movement toward satisfying lust in the isophilic or monosexual two-group, there is either no encouragement for mutual genital satisfaction or no capacity to recognize such encouragement—or in some cases there is even such great fear of the perineal area that mutual genital satisfaction would be impossible. Thus the coincidence of lust with the continuing preadolescent direction of the intimacy need leads to fantasies of what we can call a homosexual character, coupled with various guarding operations, security operations, to prevent their being discovered or suspected. But in order that this may succeed, there must be some satisfaction of lust; and the way that almost all people find for that is self-manipulation. Along with this there is, in boys, usually either an active avoidance or a definite indifference toward girls, although one of the best precautions invented by these delayed people is finding an accepted woman who gives the social appearance of normal development, but who has no expectations of the man. And almost invariably, in these solutions, we see an increase in the social distance between the person concerned and certain boys other than the chum who is the object of the reverie processes. And incidentally, while I have been discussing this largely from the viewpoint of boys, the parallel is perfectly possible in women.

Another of the ways by which the genital drive is handled in this situation is by known—that is, conscious—homosexual reveries which are associated with inadequate precautions to conceal them and with severe anxiety as a result of rebuffs, fancied or real. This often leads to hateful behavior, or to "masturbation-shame," and to a variety of other miseries which are hard for the person to express; but he knows, or can very readily come to know, that these miseries are associated with his homosexual reverie practices.

A third of the difficulties to which man is heir at this juncture and under these circumstances is a situation in which there are covert processes not accessible to awareness—in other words, unconscious processes, to use the old-fashioned term—which are attended by pseudo-heterosexual practices with or without an attenuation of the contact with members of the same sex. This sort of thing is often a precursor of a lifelong course of searching for the 'ideal' woman—or the 'ideal' man, if the person concerned is a woman—with the recurrent discovery of serious imperfections in each candidate for this ideal role. And this type of situation is the classical field for the appearance of the extremely unpleasant tension of jealousy. Jealousy is, I think, in some ways even less welcome than anxiety; and when I say that, I am almost engaging in hyperbole, because anxiety, if at all severe, is *utterly* unwelcome. But jealousy, in my experience with people who really suffer it, seems to come very close to providing an adequate picture of the now old-fashioned Christian hell.

Yet another solution of this failure of the intimacy urge to change its objective to the other sex is the turning to homosexual ways of life which are either so anxiety-ridden as to be scarcely distinguishable as achieving lustful satisfaction, or are definitely admixed with hateful, malevolent motivation, so that while lust may be satisfied more-or-less incidentally, what is most vividly remembered is the malicious mischief connected with the thing. And finally, as an outcome of this continuation of the isophilic intimacy need, a satisfying and relatively secure homosexual way of life may be established, sometimes by trial-and-error learning, quite often from example.

Any of these five typical outcomes which I have mentioned may come presently to include unsatisfactory, but security-giving, heterosexual performances. The outcome which is least apt to culminate in this sort of elaborate masking operation is the anxiety-ridden and hateful homosexual practice. But there are plenty of instances in which these people also finally either set up housekeeping with a common-law wife, or go through the motions of marrying, and even have children, but mostly for security reasons.

Maturation of the Lust Dynamism in the Chronic Juvenile

In addition to these situations in which there has been no change in the preadolescent need for intimacy as the lust dynamism has matured, the situation arises in which there is *maturation of the lust dynamism in those not yet preadolescent.* In other words, a person who is chronically juvenile reaches the time when the lust dynamism matures and goes into action. Arrest in the juvenile era is not by any means an extraordinarily unusual developmental disorder among people in this culture and in these times. The striking instance of this, as seen later in life, is what I call the juvenile ladies' man. You probably are familiar with the story of Don Juan and know how much the conception of Don Juanism has appeared in some of the psychiatric literature; to the extent that I have studied such people, they have proven to be these lustful juveniles. I might describe another outstanding manifestation of this kind by the use of slang terms—women who are customarily called "teasers" and men whom I call "hymen hunters." These people in general engage in more or less refined boasting, frequently have an insatiable interest in pornography, and have simply an overweening necessity for being envied for their women or their men. In fact, I have known some of them who really kept something very like a stable, for different occasions using different people, some of whom were supposed to be appropriate for public appearance. This is the sort of thing which happens when lust matures in a person whose preadolescent expansion of personality has simply been foredoomed and thus has failed to occur. In the sort of outcomes I have described, the person has done something with lust other than falling rather gravely ill—which, incidentally, is not an uncommon outcome of adolescent maturation in those who have serious warp of personality.

The Lust Dynamism as a Psychobiological Integrating Apparatus

I have already discussed some of the more or less typical outcomes that occur in people whose difficulties in development become very seriously complicated, in early adolescence, by the addition of the lust dynamism, although they have not passed into grave disturbances of personality. Now at this point, because we shall presently be moving into the area of difficulties of living rather than of difficulties in development, I should like to review lust as a dynamism, hoping that you remember something of our now fairly distant discussion of the concept of dynamism. Lust is in many ways a peculiarly illuminating example of a dynamism, partly because it comes along when so much of one's referential apparatus, so much of one's capacity to think and to communicate, is pretty well established and pretty well perfected. You may recall that in discussing the concept of dynamism we said that human dynamisms are relatively enduring patterns which manifest, in some cases at least, postnatal origin by maturation and, in all cases, change by experience in the occurrence of which they are significant factors. We then said that these dynamisms can be conceptualized from two viewpoints: first, with primary reference to the sundry recurring tensions manifesting as integrating, disjunctive, and isolative tendencies; and second, with primary reference to the energy transformations characteristic of the particular zones of interaction involved.

The lust dynamism—the last and the most conspicuous and illuminating of all the dynamisms, but nonetheless probably a model of every one of them, may most simply be considered as an organization of apparatus provided by the underlying human organism. This is a purely psychobiological consideration, but nonetheless important. We find that, considered solely as the property of an organism—that is, from the standpoint of psychobiology—lust can be broken up immediately into three kinds of *integrating apparatus*. By integrating apparatus I refer to organizations of tissue and function which hold the psychobiological organism in an organic unity. These three kinds of integrating apparatus are the autacoid system—that is, the endocrine or ductless gland system; the vegetative nervous system; and the central nervous system.

The first, the autacoid system, provides a tying together of the whole, by the simple device of pouring potent chemicals into a circulating fluid. In the lust dynamism, the pouring of this potent chemical into the blood stream determines whether you can have outward manifestations of lustful excitement, or whether you will fail therein. Thus the autacoid element is such that the administering of testosterone propionate, which is a synthetic chemical closely related to some of the testicular hormones, produces the appearance of something very like lust in a man; and a corresponding native hormone can be isolated which, injected into a woman, produces something very like lust. Now a person who was not at all given to very minute study of his interpersonal impulses would report to you, if he were a male, that testosterone made him lustful. However, the autacoid mechanism is not the whole thing; these very powerful chemical agents circulated in the blood stream and lymph are not all there is to being lustful.

The next great integrating apparatus involved in the lust dynamism is the vegetative nervous system, consisting of what is often referred to as the autonomic and the sympathetic nervous systems. Thus, in men, by the time the seminal vesicles are sufficiently distended there is restlessness, and, other things being equal, lust will appear; and somewhat comparably in women, at or around the time of the menstrual change, quite frequently lust will appear. If there is any difficulty with the vegetative part of the incredible integrating apparatus concerned in lust, one might feel lust, but one cannot demonstrate to a partner the necessary preliminaries for the discharge of lust, such as moistening of the vagina or erection of the penis.

And the third great integrating apparatus concerned in the dynamism of lust is the central nervous integrating apparatus. Everyone has probably, at some time, had the experience of gazing at certain art objects and promptly feeling lustful excitement. And it is not so awfully difficult to provoke lust by an appropriate series of remarks, which again reflects the intervention of the integrating apparatus of the central nervous system and includes a vast deal of symbol operations—a pretty far cry from, say, the administration of testosterone. Without the participation of this apparatus, a person would never know that lust was appropriate, unless something seized, or penetrated, the genital apparatus. If the other two integrators were active at that time, he would, after a fashion, respond, but he would not particularly enjoy it.

The Lust Dynamism as a System of Zones of Interaction

Now I pass to a field much more appropriate to psychiatry—that of considering the *lust dynamism as a system of zones of interaction.* When we touched on zones of interaction before, we suggested that all zones of interaction with the environment, considered in the borderline area of psychobiology and psychiatry, were characterized by three significant groups of characteristics: their receptor aspects, their eductor aspects, and their effector aspects. And now let me throw out only a few hints of the aspects of the lust dynamism—the late-comer among the great dynamisms of life—that fit into this frame of reference as zones of interaction with the environment.

In the receptor aspect of the lust dynamism there are the genital-tactile, the genital-visceral, and the aspect pertaining to the "erogenous areas." The peculiar *tactile* sensitivities of the genitals are such that if something touches the delicate mucosa of the genitals—whether it be the hands of a partner, a fly, or merely microscopic organisms like Trichomonas—there is an acute central awareness of specially marked sensations very clearly associated with the genital area. Although such sensations begin at an early age, in some cases practically in late infancy, they become part of the lust dynamism itself only later, when the two other types of receptor function mature.

In addition to the genital-tactile influx, there is the *genital-visceral* influx, which is carried over entirely separate channels, but is just as apt to provoke lust as the other. That is, lust, as experienced, is as often a result of tensions in unstriped muscles as it is of the stimulation of local tactile units. For example, a man can be excited, with lust as a result, by tension suffered by either the seminal vesicles or the prostate or both; or a woman, by tension suffered by the Fallopian tubes, the uterine mucosa, and the vaginal mucosa.

Quite exterior to these two fields of influx to the central nervous system, there are, after the maturation of the lust dynamism, very important influxes from other areas—the so-called "*erogenous areas*" of the body, some of which are fixed by the structure of the organism, and some of which are fixed by the experience that one has had earlier in life. In everyone, this erogenous zone is rather diffusely spread over the region of the perineum. In women, the nipples are quite generally erogenous zones. In other words, anything moving about on the surface of the nipples is apt, just like stimulation of the genitals or tension in the viscera, to be accompanied by the activation of the lust dynamism. But in either sex, any area of the body may be involved, although 'individual' variation is wide and depends on previous experience. So much for the receptor aspect of the zones of interaction.

Next we shall discuss briefly the *eductor aspect* of this system of zones of interaction called the lust dynamism. It was Spearman [2] who formulated the eduction of relationships from the data that

[2] [See Chapter 5, footnote 1.]

flow into the mind as the basis for *knowing*—one of the most profound observations, so far as the needs of psychiatrists are concerned, of the nature and manifestations of human intelligence. When I speak here of the eductor aspect of the zones of interaction, I am referring to the *knowing*—the understanding, interpretation, recognition, and contemplation of goals—which is involved in the lust dynamism considered from the standpoint of a system of zones of interaction. There are three grand divisions of what happens in the region that we call our "mind," by which we ordinarily refer to our capacity to grasp what is the case, and what should be done about it. These are facilitory, precautionary, and inhibitory referential processes. The first of these processes facilitates the identifying of situations which might be appropriately integrated by the lust dynamism. And incidentally, most people seek diligently to cultivate their facilitory symbol operations with respect to achieving lustful integrations. Precautionary measures have been taught us by the difficulties of dealing with tenderness and other motivation which calls for the kindly intervention of others. Precautionary activities enable us to conceal the fact that we are motivated by lust, and tend to protect us from very brutally making fools of ourselves. And frankly inhibitory processes make it difficult or impossible to add up the activities of the receptor apparatus into a statement that lust is present. Any denizen of the Western world has plenty of elaborate apparatus for inhibiting integration in the interest of lust, when such integration would collide with the self-system, or with particular aspects of it. I think that everyone, carefully searching his past, may remember times when he was singularly restless and uncomfortable, which, in retrospect, he will see meant the unrecognized presence of lust; and this lust was unrecognized not because it is hard to know lust, but because there was some powerful impulse active to inhibit its recognition.

And we finally come to what one is more likely to know about from personal experience—the *effector* aspects of the zones of interaction concerned in the lust dynamism. The effector aspects of the zones of interaction connected with lust—to offer the crudest kind of an analysis, leaving out unnumbered interesting aspects—are five in number. The first is the vasomotor-erectile effector aspects of the urethro-genital zone of interaction with the environment, which is often first manifest at birth—but perhaps not consciously—and which is manifest recurrently, from birth onward. This is a complicated performance of obstructing venous return and increasing blood supply, which is illustrated not only in the genitals but also in the nose and sundry other parts of the body—the genitals and the nose being the most troublesome, in this climate at least. Besides the vasomotor-erectile—and appearing very much later, around the time of the puberty change—are the purely secretory effector aspects of the urethro-genital zone of interaction and its system of zones, consisting in the male of such things as the production of a dense but highly lubricant mucus by the Cowper's glands, the production of an anything-but-dense albuminous fluid by the prostate, and the production of a complex nutritive albuminous fluid by the epididymis and probably the seminal vesicles. In the female, there is the secretion of mucus and the hydrogen ion concentration proper for the spermatozoa.

As another very important aspect of the effectors, there are those massive patterns of skeletal behavior which we lump scientifically under the rubric "copulatory posture and movement." The copulatory posture and movements are very complicated. They are one of the few things which faintly support the notion that the concept of instinct is not utterly irrelevant to human beings, for they come without calling, almost as if a little instinct still survived in our incredibly culture-ridden life.

Among the effector apparatus there is also the orgasmic complex of integrated movements, which, again, matures in the puberty change; to some extent this existed before as parts, but these are now suddenly integrated. The orgasmic movements are built up, in men, primarily on the capacity for clonic spasm in the prostatic urethra, with which a man is born so that he is able to expel urine. But this becomes, suddenly in the puberty change, very closely and emphatically (from the sensory or receptor standpoint) coordinated with spasm of the walls of the seminal vesicle, which had not previously occurred. So here we find movements of unstriped muscle, which earlier were used only to expel the last drops of urine, suddenly integrated with the expulsive activity of the container of semen in the male—a coordination which had not been present at all before the puberty change. This is accompanied by the most vivid central representation, comprising that extremely strongly marked experience which represents the satisfaction of the lust dynamism.

But there are still further effector aspects of the zones of interaction which make up the lust dynamism. If the lust dynamism is successfully satisfied, a series of changes restores the apparatus to, shall I say, a resting condition which is called, traditionally, detumescence. There seems to be evidence that in women detumescence is a somewhat longer process, but here too the women's erogenous zones, including the breasts, also shrink and come to rest in comparative insensitivity after the orgasm. In both men and women, after the apparatus has been restored to a resting condition, the lust dynamism, under external or internal provocation, can again become a very powerful organizer of a remarkable part of our capacity for contact with external events.

The Lust Dynamism as a Pattern of Covert and Overt Symbolic Events

Now I wish to consider the lust dynamism neither as an integrating apparatus nor as a system of zones of interaction, but as *a pattern of covert and overt symbolic events*—that is, events meaning something, if you please, which are either inferable or observable. The covert and overt symbolic events which are included in manifestations of experience with respect to the lust dynamism include experience in the prototaxic, the parataxic, and less often in the syntaxic modes. Experience in the prototaxic mode, while it is particularly obvious in the instance of primary genital phobia, is present in any case. The parataxic mode is perhaps more apt to be the major element in the symbol operations connected with lust than it is with any one other dynamism, because the culture is so very hard on consensual validation and syntaxic operations with respect to lust. Experience of covert and overt symbolic events is concerned with six major rubrics. The first rubric is the *observation and identification* of the following: (*a*) the felt aspects of the integrating tendency—that is, lust per se; (*b*) the interpersonal situation as including an 'object'—presumably another person with whom a lustful situation can be integrated, if only in fantasy; (*c*) the interpersonal situation as otherwise characterized —that is, not merely as to the other person, but with respect to the suitability of the situation for probable satisfaction, the collateral factors which may make lustful excitement strangely irrelevant (for example, the unwisdom of getting intensely sexually excited about your opponent in the traffic court); and (*d*) the interpersonal situation as characterized with respect to anxiety, which is very important indeed in the lives of most of us.

Now these aspects of observation and identification are, in fortunate situations, supplemented by *foresight*, which is the second of these six rubrics. That is, after observation and identification, there comes foresight, although it is sometimes only rudimentary, and is often by no means extended. And, following the foresight, which is in a sense my way of referring to decision, there comes, third, *activity in pursuit of or in avoidance of the goal*, which is the discharge of lust. At the same time, there are in all real situations—and this is my fourth rubric of experience—sundry, often seemingly irrelevant, *covert accompaniments* of the last-mentioned —that is, processes which can be detected only by inference, which accompany action in pursuit of or in avoidance of the goal. In other words, I refer to a good deal that is going on in the 'mind.'

Regardless of whether integration by the lust dynamism has been effected or avoided, and regardless of the extent of the discharge of lust, there is, later on, *retrospective and prospective, witting and unwitting analysis* of this particular experience, which is my fifth rubric. That is, there is analysis of what has happened recently, with a view to what may happen again. And incidentally, if, in the days of the Puritans, everyone's development of acquaintance with experience regarding lust had depended on *witting* analysis, I think that lust might have disappeared, along with the human race. How much is witting and how much is unwitting depends on one's cultural background, and not on anything else. Thus whether one has pursued the goal of lustful satisfaction, or avoided it, there is always in the experience concerned with any particular episode some review and prospective analysis, with the idea of improving one's capacity for achieving contentment and success in this field of life. Finally, and this is my sixth rubric, in some instances—and, fortunately, this is not always the case—

there are *more complex processes* concerned in the experience, which may replace the retrospective and prospective analysis, or may just complicate it. And these reflect, however obscurely, the personality warp of at least one person concerned in the situation in which the lust dynamism is the principal system of integrating tendencies.

The Lust Dynamism as a System of Integrating Tendencies

And this brings me to my next and more important point. Having reviewed the lust dynamism as a system of covert and overt symbolic events, I should now like to discuss it as a system of integrating tendencies—that is, as an integration of those characteristics of people which integrate situations with other people. In other words, this is an elaborate system of motives which get us involved with others or lead us to avoid them.

The lust dynamism is a *system of integrating tendencies:*

(1) of which the unanalyzable elements have *matured in earlier stages of development* and have *been modified by experience of satisfaction* or *experience with anxiety*, or both, and in some cases with signs of *disintegrative change* or *elaboration in dissociation.*

(2) in which the *anxiety-marked components are widely varied* from person to person, because of inadequacies in the culture complex and their accentuation by resulting family-society and school-society peculiarities.

(3) of which some components are almost always, in this culture, *unrepresented in focal awareness*, whether their lack of representation be due to selective inattention, to masking processes, to misinterpretation, or to the manifestation of a dissociative process in the self.

(4) which is often related to acute or persisting *disorientation in living*, and to the disastrous disturbance of self-esteem.

(5) which, in the handicapped, may come to channel the partial satisfaction of a variety of other integrating tendencies—and thus may come to seem preternaturally important.

(6) of which the recurrent partial satisfaction leaves residual motivation to be discharged in sleep and in waking reverie processes in a way that may undermine self-esteem, or may call for precautionary processes or social distance—which in turn seriously reduce the chances of fortunate experience in life.

Statement (1) is the simplest of these possible views of the lust dynamism. In other words, the integrating tendencies which are systematized in the lust dynamism have matured over various stages of one's past, and have, since maturation, been subjected to experience and to the various characteristics of experience which we have considered thus far, such as change to avoid anxiety, disintegration to avoid anxiety, or actually development in dissociation.

Statement (2) reflects the fact that our culture is the least adequate in preparing one for meeting the eventualities of sexual maturity, which is another way of saying we are the most sex-ridden people on the face of the globe. In (4), I suggest that the lust dynamism is *the* system of integrating tendencies often related to acute or persisting disorientation in living.

When I mention the handicapped in statement (5) I refer to those people who have had disasters in the stages of development before adolescence. I might illustrate this rubric by saying that if your resentment at authority should find in lustful activities a discharge which, though only partial, was better than nothing, then, insofar as you suffered authority, lust and lustful activities would come to be unreasonably, extravagantly important in your life. Thus in those who have had serious warp in personality, the lust dynamism is a system of integrating tendencies which may provide a channel for the obscure and unrecognized satisfaction of many thwarted integrating impulses having no direct connection with lust. The persistently juvenile person who finally reaches genital maturity advertises this fact to the high heavens to those who investigate him. Psychiatrists have tended to overlook the very rich source of data on this particular point because of the seeming essential dullness of the persistently juvenile person and the social insignificance of his life with others.

Patterns of Manifestation of the Integrating Tendencies of the Intimacy Need and Lust

Now I have given you, with a feeling of deep apology for the condensation that has characterized it, something like a theoretically justifiable, if not definitive, variety of approaches to the meaning of the lust dynamism. It is important to realize that everything said of the lust dynamism applies to every dynamism; but because the lust dynamism happens to come along so late in life, it is a particularly informative example of dynamisms in general. I shall presently try to suggest the rich variety of human life with respect to every dynamism by some cold mathematical adumbrations of the possible patterns of adjustment called out in part by the lust dynamism. But first, since these things do not stand alone, I would like to go back to the idea of orientation of living and to defects therein as they are related to the two very powerful integrating tendencies that characterize adolescence—lust and the need for intimacy. In discussing disturbed or inadequate orientation in the later phases of adolescent living and thereafter, one cannot, except for purposes of clarity of thinking, separate the manifestation of these two very powerful motivating systems of human life. But though these systems are intricately interwoven, at the same time they are never identical.

I have already tried to suggest something of the broad basis, in the developmental history of everyone, for the feeling ordinarily called loneliness, which is the exceedingly unpleasant and driving experience connected with inadequate discharge of the need for human intimacy, for interpersonal intimacy. Since it seems to me that no amount of emphasis will be extravagant in this connection, let me again comment on the major integrating tendencies which gradually come to be concerned with the experience of loneliness. It begins in infancy with an integrating tendency that we know only by inference from pathological material later, but which we nonetheless accept unhesitatingly—a need for contact with the living. And its next great increment is a need for tenderness—for protective care delicately adjusted to immediate situations. This need continues into childhood. But in childhood a need for adult participation is added—that is, a need for the interest and participation of significant adults in the child's play. This activity takes the form of expressive play necessary to provide the child with equipment for showing what he feels, in manual play necessary for the coordination of the very delicate and intricate relationships of vision and the prehensile hands, and so on, and in verbal play, which is the basis of all the enormously important acquisitions to personality which are reflected by verbal behavior and abstract thought. All of these activities become more pleasure-giving to the child because of the adults' participation. By the juvenile era, there is added the need for compeers, as indispensable models for one's learning by trial and error; and this is then followed by a need for acceptance which is perhaps to most of you known by its reverse, the fear of ostracism, fear of being excluded from the accepted and significant group. And added to all these important integrating tendencies, there comes in preadolescence the need for intimate exchange, for friendship, or for —in its high refinement—the love of another person, with its enormous facilitation of consensual validation, of action patterns, of valuational judgments, and so on. This becomes, in early adolescence, the same need for intimacy, friendship, acceptance, intimate exchange, and, in its more refined form, the need for a loving relationship, with a member of the other sex. Now this is the great structure which is finally consolidated, made meaningful, as the need for intimacy as it characterizes late adolescence and the rest of life.

I have now reviewed the history of one powerful integrating tendency—the need for intimacy—and I have already given my views of lust, the other of these major integrating tendencies. At this point I shall endeavor to give some idea of the possible varieties of intricately interwoven patterns of these tendency systems.

The theoretical patterns of manifestation of the two powerful integrating tendencies, the need for intimacy and lust, may be classified:

(1) on the basis of the intimacy need and the precautions which concern it—as autophilic, isophilic, and heterophilic;

(2) on the basis of the preferred partner in lustful integrations,

or the substitute therefor—as autosexual, homosexual, heterosexual, and katasexual;

(3) on the basis of genital participation or substitution—as orthogenital, paragenital, metagenital, amphigenital, mutual masturbation, and onanism.

In creating the rubrics with respect to the need for intimacy (1), I have turned to the old Greek term *philos*, meaning "loving," since the need for intimacy in its highest manifestations is unquestionably love—and while love has been many things to many people, the common denominator pertains to interpersonal intimacy. All the manifestations, morbid and successful, of this need for intimacy, may be grossly classified under the three rubrics of *autophilic*, *isophilic*, and *heterophilic*. We will use these three rubrics to describe a 'person'—and I use person here in the sense of that which we hypothesize to account for what we see or experience. In the autophilic person, there has been no preadolescent development; or such preadolescent development as took place has been disintegrated because of profound rebuff, and he has been returned to a state before preadolescence in which the capacity to love is, if manifest at all, concentrated within his personification of himself. The autophilic is always a misfortune and a deviation of development. An isophilic person has been unable to progress past preadolescence, and continues to regard as suitable for intimacy only people who are as like himself as possible, in significant fashions—that is, members of his own gender. A heterophilic person has gone through the preadolescent period and made the early adolescent change in which he has become intensely interested in achieving intimacy with members of what, in this culture, is most essentially different—the other sex. The isophilic is, for a period of two-and-a-half to three-and-a-half years, a normal phase of every successful development; but this phase may continue through life. And the heterophilic represents the last stage of development of the need for intimacy; many achieve this phase even though they are unable to leave late adolescence.

Now I invite you to consider (2) and (3), which underlie all that I have already said of the lust dynamism. The first of these refers to the gross characteristics of integrations which seek the discharge of the lust dynamism, which are directly related to recognized lust and its satisfaction; for these I use the term *sexual* —and do not confuse this with the term "erotic." In my classification of sexual behavior on the basis of the preferred partner, the *homosexual* and the *heterosexual* are obviously related to preadolescent and early adolescent phases of development. The *autosexual* represents an earlier stage—that is, although lust has matured, the preadolescent and adolescent eras have not been reached. The *katasexual* refers to passing beyond the confines of the human species—that is, the dead or infrahuman creatures are the preferred lustful partners—and this represents a very complex substitution for things which one experiences as impossible to want.

And finally, I would like you to consider the lust dynamism in terms of (3) the participation of the *genitals* in covert and overt, witting or unwitting, lustful performances; and here I am talking about a region of the body. Situations principally integrated by lust are sexual situations; but at the same time the patterning of this behavior depends on the part played by the genitals, as well as the lustful character of the situation. On the basis of one's genital participation with another, or with a substitute, I have named six rubrics, most of which are neologisms of my own invention. *Orthogenital* situations are characterized by a preferred integration of one's genitals with their natural receptor genitals—genitals of the sexually opposite type. In *paragenital* situations, one uses the genitals as if they were seeking an appropriate opposite type of genitals, but does so in behavior which is not related to the procreation of one's kind. A common example is being masturbated by someone else, in which case the hand is the paragenital receptor of one's genitals; other examples are the passive role in fellatio or the active role in pederasty. In *metagenital* situations, one's genitals need not be involved at all, but the other person's genitals are involved. The most obvious example is masturbating someone else; other examples are taking the passive role in pederasty or the so-called active role in fellatio. In *amphigenital* situations, for which the French have adopted the term "soixante-neuf," either homosexual or heterosexual groups of two people take a singularly analogous if not identical relationship to the genitals of each and the substitutes of each. Besides these, there are the relatively primitive performance of *mutual masturbation* and the quite primitive performance of *onanism.*

Now I do not like to coin freak terms, but what these terms represent is terribly significant. And the terrible significance is this: In this culture the ultimate test of whether you can get on or not is whether you can do something satisfactory with your genitals or somebody else's genitals without undue anxiety and loss of self-esteem. Therefore the psychiatrist who has to consider the life problems presented by people who come to him has to have some way of organizing thought regarding this last phase of interpersonal adjustment. To accomplish that I have had to set up what are, so far as I know, unique inventions: the resolute separation of the need for intimacy from the lust dynamism; and the distinction between the *general interpersonal objective* of the lust dynamism, and the *particular activities* which the genitals—the center of the lust dynamism, one might say—have in preferred adjustive effort.

Since I have set up three classifications of intimacy, four classifications of the general interpersonal objective of the integration of lust, and six classifications of genital relationship, this results in seventy-two theoretical patterns of sexual behavior in situations involving two real partners. As a matter of fact, there are only forty-five patterns of sexual behavior that are reasonably probable; six are very highly improbable, and the rest just aren't possible. From this statement, I would like you to realize, if you realize nothing else, how fatuous it is to toss out the adjectives "heterosexual," "homosexual," or "narcissistic" to classify a person as to his sexual and friendly integrations with others. Such classifications are not anywhere near refined enough for intelligent thought; they are much too gross to do anything except mislead both the observer and the victim. For example, to talk about homosexuality's being a problem really means about as much as to talk about humanity's being a problem.

The reason why I attempt to set up careful classifications in this field is this: It is almost always essential for the psychiatrist, when he ventures into remedial efforts for serious developmental handicaps, to pay attention to the place of lust in the difficulties of the person. And let me make it clear that lust, in my sense, is not some great diffuse striving, 'libido' or what not. By lust I mean simply the felt aspect of the genital drive. And when I say that the psychiatrist must usually pay attention to this, I do not mean that problems in living are primarily or chiefly concerned with genital activity. But I am saying, of people in this culture who are chronologically adult, that their problems in interpersonal relations quite certainly will be either very conspicuous in, or exceedingly well illustrated by, the particular circumstances governing their handling of the emotion of lust. While this statement is, I believe, strikingly true of Northwestern European culture, I would say, although I have no evidence on the matter, that it is not true of certain other cultures.

By the time a person has plunged into early adolescence, he has either largely overcome all the crippling handicaps to personality that he has encountered, or his development in adolescence will be badly warped. And since lust cannot be eliminated from personality any more than hunger can, data on personality warp as seen in a person's sexual behavior is bound to be useful to the psychiatrist, for instance; I mean here the broad conception of sexual behavior, including reverie processes and any evidences of dissociated processes, which I shall discuss presently. But to think that one can remedy personality warp by tinkering with the sex life is a mistake, even though it is a very convenient doctrine for psychiatrists who are chronic juveniles. It may provide them with fees for enjoying their interest in pornography; but if one is a serious psychiatrist, it is apt to be the hardest possible way to tackle one's task. When difficulties in the sex life are presented by a patient as his reason for needing psychiatric help, my experience has demonstrated rather convincingly that the patient's difficulty in living is best manifested by his very choice of this as his peculiar problem. In other words, people don't go to psychiatrists to be aided in their sexual difficulties; but they do sometimes present this as their problem, and such problems show, when properly understood, what ails their living with people. It is only an exceptional person who is able to have his sex life as his major interpersonal activity; only such a person could correctly present to a psychiatrist, as his greatest difficulty in living, a sexual problem. Thus let me warn my fellow psychiatrists: If you want to do psychiatry that can well be crowded into a lifetime, see if you can't find something besides the sexual problem in the strangers that come to you for help. Quite frequently it is no trick at all to find something very much more serious than the sexual difficulty; and quite often the sexual difficulty is remedied in the process of dealing with the other problems. You may notice that there is a slight difference here between my views and some of the views that have been circulated in historic times.

CHAPTER 18

Late Adolescence

THE MARK which, to my way of thinking, separates early adolescence from late adolescence is not a biological maturation but an achievement. Such a discrimination as that between early and late adolescence would not be needed in a social organization in which the culture provided facilitation and capable direction for the achievement of adequate and satisfactory genital activity. But in our own and allied cultures, every taboo from the religious to the political is applied to this last of our developmental achievements.

Late adolescence extends from the patterning of preferred genital activity through unnumbered educative and eductive steps to the establishment of a fully human or mature repertory of interpersonal relations, as permitted by available opportunity, personal and cultural. In other words, a person begins late adolescence when he discovers what he likes in the way of genital behavior and how to fit it into the rest of life. That is an achievement of no mean magnitude for a large number of the denizens of our culture. The failure to achieve late adolescence is, in fact, the last blow to a great many warped, inadequately developed personalities. Because this kind of experience is such an all-absorbing and all-frustrating preoccupation, it often constitutes the presenting difficulty which precedes the eruption of very grave personality disorder in a large number of people; it is of course by no means the actual difficulty.

The Importance of Opportunity

The outcome of late adolescence is so much a matter of accident that whether one continues to be, dynamically, a late adolescent throughout life, or actually achieves something that might reasonably be called human maturity, is often no particular reflection on anything more than one's socioeconomic status and the like. Opportunity, as I have used it in my definition, is now a matter of other people and of the institutional or gross social facilitation and prohibition. A psychiatrist sees people who could have gone much further had they had a chance at the educational experience which others at this time of life are able to undergo.

We cannot escape the fact that many people who have had excellent developmental opportunity are caught, perhaps chiefly because of the culture, in circumstances in which there are exceedingly restricted opportunities for further growth. For example, suppose that the eldest son in a rather large family in the lower economic cadres finds himself suddenly in the position of wage earner for the family because of the death of the father. Now if this eldest son has had excellent developmental opportunity up to that point, it becomes practically certain that he will take over a large measure of the responsibility for giving the younger siblings opportunities. Along with his taking over of the responsibilities previously carried by his father, there will be a corresponding very marked reduction of his opportunities to live and learn. Thus there is no gainsaying the 'real' factors entirely outside of the developmental history of the person concerned.

Yet at the same time there are people who, with all the educational opportunities in the world, simply do not have the capacity to adequately observe and analyze the opportunities which come to them, because of inherent defect or because of various types of warp which they have not been able to correct in time. The only chance that such a person has then—except by an act of God—is through psychiatry. And how small that chance is has become more and more overwhelmingly apparent to me the longer I live.

Growth of Experience in the Syntaxic Mode

Insofar as the long stretch of late adolescence is successful, there is a great growth of experience in the syntaxic mode. Consider, for example, a person from a fairly well-knit community and a pretty good home, who has fortunately achieved a patterning of his genital behavior. If he then goes to a university, he is given several years of truly extraordinary opportunity to observe his fellows, to hear about people in various parts of the world, to discuss what has been presented and observed, to find out, on this basis, what in his past experience is inadequately grasped, and what is a natural springboard to grasping the new. In other words, for the fortunate, the educational opportunity provided by living at a university is very great.

But this is also the time when people who are not that fortunate, or who are not interested in further education, are attempting to establish some way of making a living, as wage earners, or exploiters of their fellow man, or something or other. Within limits, the kind of experience obtained is much the same as at a university, except for the probable lack of the broad, cultural interest which we trust characterizes all higher formal education. But the education in how to make a living, how to get on with people in the same line of work, is similarly a source of a great deal of observational data, and provides great possibilities for interchange of views, for expanding of one's limitations, and for the validating of one's hunches. Thus, once a person who is not very seriously warped has got the sex problem settled reasonably well, whatever he does is bound to broaden his acquaintance with other people's attitudes toward living, the degree of their interdependence in living, and the ways of handling various kinds of interpersonal problems—much of which is learned by trial and error from human example. In other words, in late adolescence one refines relatively personally-limited experience into the consensually dependable, which is much less limited. Just as in preadolescence a very remarkable, if sketchy, social organization develops on the basis of the people actually available for social organization, so in late adolescence everyone is more or less integrated into society as it is. Some of those whose opportunities are great are potentially able to integrate literally with the world society—to be at home in the world. Those who are working as apprentices in machine shops, for example, have, needless to say, vastly less opportunity in terms of geographical and cultural scope. But still they are now, from the viewpoint of society, going concerns in every way—provided with the franchise, expected to pay income tax, and the like. In general, late adolescents are adults in the eyes of the law, and have all the benefits and handicaps thereunto appertaining. Thus they have to take on a good many responsibilities which are written into the culture; they may have evaded these responsibilities thus far, but now they have to develop ways of at least giving the appearance of meeting some of them. If they are fortunate, their growth goes on and on; they observe, formulate, and validate more and more; and at the same time, their foresight continuously expands so that they can foresee their career line—not as it inevitably will be, but in terms of expectation and probability, with perhaps provisions for disappointment.

Inadequate and Inappropriate Personifications of the Self and Others

Now the fact that a great many people don't seem to get very far in this phase of personality development is to be understood primarily from the consideration of the role of anxiety in their living, which is, in turn, a way of referring to self-system functioning within the personality. Long since, I mentioned the peculiar tendency of the self-system to govern 'witting' experience, so that one tends to be strangely unchanging in spite of what might be called objective opportunities for observing and analyzing, and learning and changing. And when it comes to finding out why people do not profit from experience and why people get so short a distance toward maturity in long stretches of time, one has primarily to consider the nature and functional activity of the self-system in the person concerned. At the level where communication is fairly easy, this critical opposition of anxiety, of self-system function, is manifest as inadequate and inappropriate personification of the self. People have come to hold views of themselves which are so far from valid formulations that these views are eternally catching them in situations in which the incongruity and inappropriateness are about to become evident, whereupon the person suffers the interference of anxiety. And as I have said before, when anxiety is severe, it has almost the effect of a blow on the head; one isn't really clear on the exact situation in which the anxiety occurred. A phenomenon which is very much more important in the later phases of personality development is that people become extremely agile at responding to minor hints of anxiety. By that I don't mean that the person warns himself, "You will be anxious presently if you are not careful"—not at all. But nevertheless the appearance of just a little anxiety serves to deflect living away from the situation, just as the amoebae are deflected away from the hot water, as I have mentioned much earlier.

Thus the most accessible aspects of the self-system in many late adolescents show such superficially incomprehensible falsifications in the person's view of himself that he is not apt to learn very much in this field unless somebody goes to a great deal of trouble to put him through educative experience. And this kind of experience is fraught with relatively severe anxiety which—as I hope you will grasp by now—people put up with only when they can't help themselves. When the imperative necessity for change is recognized through psychiatric or similar experience, then most people are able to stand some anxiety, although I suppose this varies on the basis of individual past experience. To say that a person is able to stand some anxiety is another way of saying that he is able to observe previously ignored and misinterpreted experience in such fashion that his formulation of himself and of living can change in a favorable direction. One might suppose, then, that anybody who has had considerable anxiety ought to have made wonderful progress in development. But the joker to that is that the overwhelming conviction of the necessity for change is, in other than special circumstances, utterly lacking in people who suffer a great deal of anxiety. In fact, they expect to go on indefinitely as they are; they can't do anything about it; and when you attempt to show them what might be done about it, they get still more anxious and know that you are bad medicine and avoid you. What I am attempting to suggest at this point is that there is a very considerable difference between being very much in the grip of anxiety, mild or severe, and, as it were, 'coming to grips' with a source of anxiety, mild or severe.

Now I shall have to digress long enough to remove any shadows of voluntaristic meaning from my use of such expressions as "coming to grips" with anxiety and "confronting" anxiety. There seems to be very little profit in psychiatry from dependence on any such idea as the mysterious power of the will. I think I have touched on this before in discussing the evil effects of the doctrine of the will on development. In a society in which people are usually quite proud of their will and are noisy about it, I would like to warn psychiatrists that the less voluntaristic their language, and the more utterly free their thinking from convictions about the will, the further they will be able to get in understanding and perhaps favorably influencing their patients. So when I speak of the confronting of anxiety, I do not mean that a psychiatrist asks a patient to pull himself together and exert his will so that he will not so easily yield to the threat of anxiety. What the psychiatrist does, if he accomplishes anything in this particular, is to so nurture in the patient correct foresight of the near future that it becomes intolerable to be always running away from minor anxiety. The appearance of anxiety is in no sense connected with any mythological or real will; it is connected with experience which has been incorporated into and become a part of the self-system and with the foresight of increasing anxiety in connection with the self-system. The problem of the psychiatrist is more or less to spread a larger context before the patient; insofar as that succeeds, the patient realizes that, anxiety or not, the present way of life is unsatisfactory and is unprofitable in the sense that it is not changing things for the better; whereupon, in spite of anxiety, other things being equal, the self-system can be modified.

In addition to inadequate and inappropriate personifications of the self, there are, attendant upon that, and in congruity with it, inadequate and inappropriate personification of others. Such inadequacy and inappropriateness of secondary personifications—secondary because to most people they seem less important than a person's personification of himself—may apply broadly to everyone, or specifically to stereotypes of certain alleged people. A person cannot personify others with any particular refinement except in terms of his own personification of himself and in terms of more-or-less imaginary entities related by the 'not' technique to his personification of himself. If you regard yourself as generous, then you tend to assume that others will be generous; but since you have a good deal of experience not in keeping with that, you personify many people as ungenerous, *not* generous. Now that doesn't give you any particularly good formulation of what they are; they are just different and opposite from you in one of your better aspects. Thus, to a remarkable degree this limitation in the personification of others is based on inappropriate and inadequate personification of oneself. Particularly troublesome are the inadequate and inappropriate personifications by what I have referred to as stereotypes, which again reflect the limitations in the personification of the self. We often encounter the most accessible part of such things as prejudices, intolerances, fears, hatreds, aversions, and revulsions that pertain to alleged classes of people. Now these stereotypes may concern newsboys, the Jews, the Greeks, the Communists, the Chinese, or what have you. They are, needless to say, not based on adequate observation, analysis, and consensual validation of data about the people concerned.

Stereotypes reflect inadequate and inappropriate elements in one's own self-system; thus all the special stereotypes are either poor imitations of ingredients in the personified self, or—even more inadequate in terms of providing a guide in life—they are *not* elements from the personification of the self. For example, the view that the Irish are all politicians can be held with perfect impunity and peace of mind either by people who show remarkable political gifts, or by those who show remarkable political imbecility. That is, if you are a good politician you can stereotype a whole ethnic group or biethnic group with this characteristic, and if you are a rotten politician you can simply stigmatize a group with a *not* variant of yourself.

Incidentally—to continue a little further with the subject of prejudice and stereotypes—I am myself inclined to think that the Irish are pagans. Now there is no shadow of doubt in my mind that any sort of searching study of the current residents of Ireland would toss up a great many instances in which the term pagan would be irrelevant, in any meaningful sense. What I have in mind is that in many ethnic groups or ethnic communities which are vigorously Christian in their protestations, one can find, as soon as one gets into actual informative interchange with their members about their religious convictions, a truly wonderful survival of types of attitude toward transcendental power and so on which have very little indeed to do with Christian prescriptions. The Irish, who happen to be my ancestral people, are a little better known to me than are, for example, the Chinese; and so I feel—

after the best modern pattern—perfectly free to make a wisecrack about the underlying religious attitude of my people. But, thank God, I know that it may or may not make any sense; I wouldn't think of staking anything on it. It is all right for parlor conversation with good friends, preferably Irish. But if I say it often to other people, I may very unhappily present them with an opportunity to clinch an uninformed prejudice, which is usually done by nailing it onto a preceding one. Whether such remarks are amusing wisecracks which may be used for little prestige purposes, and so on, as doubtless my comment about the pagan Irish is, or whether they are a device for avoiding any growth of intelligence, information, and consensual agreement about whole huge sections of the human race, largely depends on the extent to which the prejudice expressed reflects a serious limitation in the personification of the self.

The purposes served by these stereotypes are many. But the alleged purpose which almost any unsophisticated person will immediately produce under suitable circumstances is one of the saddest commentaries on the misfortunes of personality in our world and time: namely, that they are very useful guides for dealing with strangers. Quite simply, they are not. They are, insofar as they are important, exactly the opposite of guides for dealing with strangers; they are inescapable handicaps in becoming acquainted with strangers. And to that extent they are chiefly effective in denying one any opportunity for spontaneous favorable change in the corresponding limitation in one's personification of oneself.

Parataxic Processes to Minimize Anxiety

In further commenting on the critical opposition of anxiety and the self-system to favorable growth in late adolescence, I would like to call attention to the parataxic processes concerned in avoiding and minimizing anxiety. These processes extend from selective inattention—which to a certain extent covers the world like a tent—through all the other classical dynamisms of difficulty, to the gravest dissociation of one or more of the vitally essential human dynamisms. And incidentally, while I once liked the rubric, dynamism of difficulty, it has lost its charm over my years of attempting to teach psychiatry, because the conviction grew among some of the people who encountered this usage that these dynamisms represented peculiarities shown by the morbid. On the contrary, I believe that there are no peculiarities shown by the morbid; there are only differences in degree—that is, in intensity and timing—of that which is shown by everyone.[1] Thus whenever I speak of dynamisms I am discussing universal human equipment, sometimes represented almost entirely in dreadful distortions of living, but still universal. And the distortions arise from misfortunes in development, restrictions of opportunity, and the like. Thus the interventions of the self-system which are striking in this late adolescent phase—that is, in chronologic maturity—cover the whole field of what we like to talk about as being psychiatric entities—mental disorders, if you please.

Restrictions in Freedom of Living

Another way of approaching the general topic of the self-system's prevention of favorable change in the late adolescent phase is to consider restrictions in freedom of living, with their complex processes for the discharge of the integrating tendencies that are restricted. This is a different approach to what we have already discussed and is an attempt to highlight certain things which we have not noticed before.

By restrictions in freedom of living, I refer here to the limitations that arise 'internally,' because of handicaps in one's past, and not to the restrictions which come under the broad classification of opportunity, which I have touched on before. Restrictions in freedom of living are attended by complex ways of getting at least partial satisfaction for what one's restrictions prevent and by further complex processes, in the shape of sleep disorders and the like, for discharging dangerous accumulations of tensions. These restrictions may be usefully considered from the standpoint of restricted contact with others and of restrictions of interest. Restricted contact with others may range from the early develop-

[1] I am always in these remarks eliminating the organic; in other words, if someone shoots away half of a person's skull, he will not be thereafter in the central field of my psychiatric interest—not that psychiatry might not grow from studying him.

ment of a strikingly isolated way of life, with such great social distance that one has to continue to deny oneself a great deal of useful, educative, and consensual validating experience with others, to circumscriptions of oneself on the basis of factors such as prejudice, caste, and class, if one happens to be in a very small minority.

But in a great many instances, the restrictions in freedom of living are very much more striking in the sharp circumscriptions of interest; large numbers of aspects of living are, as it were, taboo—one avoids them. Sometimes a compulsory restriction of living growing out of warp in the past is masked in the shape of pseudo-social rituals and interests which look like something quite different from a restriction. And these rituals seem to raise the person concerned above the level of the common horde and take on great distinction, at least to him and his ilk. The example I am going to give concerns *devotion to games*, and in this instance devotion to bridge. Since I got into quite serious trouble with a very distinguished and greatly respected anthropologist by this example of bridge, I judge that it has some power to fix interest, and so I will use it again. Now I have never played much of anything well; I think probably my vulgar taste is well handled by casino or hearts; certainly it isn't anywhere near up to bridge. My example concerns a very select group of women in New York who have great socioeconomic opportunities. They do little each day but get out of bed and prepare for the bridge club, to which they repair with minimum talk to their husbands or chauffeurs and there spend many hours in a very highly ritualized interchange with their fellows, whereupon they are content with life and repair to bed again. I hope that you begin to get a notion of what I mean by pseudosocial ritual; in this case, each person is busily engaged with people, but nothing particularly personal transpires. I believe that most of these people would be willing to agree that it would be rather better—aside from considerations of displaying their clothing, and so on—if they could sit in cubicles with one-way screens directed toward the cards. There would be less distraction from people coughing and sneezing and so on, and they could therefore perform their function in life more comfortably. While this is an extreme example of pseudosocial ritual, there are a remarkable number of people who have ways of being social as the devil without having anything to do with the other people concerned. They live by very sharply restricted rules.

Another of these restrictions in living is the development of ritual avoidances and ritual preoccupations. Regardless of your political leanings, you have probably all experienced with your confreres ritualized avoidance in matters of political thought. For example, this kind of avoidance might appear if you talked to your banker about the necessity for further New Deal legislation. To give a personal example, on the rare occasions that I get to a barber shop, I am duly shorn by a good fellow veteran of the First World War whom I cherish both because he is a very public-spirited citizen who does a great deal of welfare work, and because he is a good barber and keeps quiet. I so detest the business of having my hair cut that I wish to at least approach dozing, and conversation is extremely unwelcome. But one day as I was getting my hair cut, the radio had some tweet on about Henry Wallace, and the barber denounced Henry Wallace very succinctly. I remarked that, well, I knew the man and liked him very much. I feel that, like some of the rest of us, he is not always possessed of the most brilliant and far-reaching foresight, but he has occasionally had some remarkably good ideas, which is enough to give a person standing with me. It was not difficult after that to repose during the time I was in the barber chair. Five or six months later, when Henry Wallace was boosted out of the Department of Commerce, the subject came up again; in other words, it was an important matter. Now this barber has no real desire to quarrel with me about anything, but my comment about Wallace had disturbed part of his ritual avoidance machinery; and this disturbance was attached to me, since he's got good enough recall to know how I disturbed him. And so the topic was developed further. But we still patronize each other for all that.

Now all these ritual avoidances and preoccupations give one a feeling that one is making some sense in an important area of living. Actually one is not making any sense at all, because one is completely inaccessible to any data. Besides the political, there is the 'society' aspect; here again great sections of life are closed off by supposedly rational definitions which, on careful scrutiny, turn out to be simply ritualistic avoidances. The same is true in the world of art; and those who have dealt with natural and unnatural sciences may have noticed much the same thing at annual meetings and the like. And God knows the world is filled with ritual avoidances and preoccupations under the name of religion.

Of course, I can quite respect a person for being clear as to what he is interested in and what he is not particularly interested in. For instance, there is no earthly reason why I should be frantically interested in the theory of money. There is no reason on earth why I should labor to develop an aesthetic appreciation of painting, or of unnumbered other things in which I have only vestigial interest. I could not conceivably be adequately interested in anything like the whole field of internal medicine. But if no one can even *talk* to me about Dadaism, for instance, or the Baptists, or the theory of money, it is not because my life course has concentrated a great deal of my satisfaction and security in a particular field; it is because my security depends on *avoiding* a particular field or a particular subject. Life, I suppose, has never been all equally interesting to any one person or within the capacity of any one person. I am quite sure that as the primal horde came out of prehistory there was some specialization among the denizens; certainly there was specialization in the bearing of children, and such a specialization as that would surely call for further specializations. Ritual avoidances and preoccupations may superficially look the same as specializations, but they actually mean that you cannot enter a certain field; any interest moving toward that field immediately arouses anxiety which prohibits any further movement in pursuit of information.

Self-Respect and Human Maturity

From all that I have suggested you may see that it is no extraordinary use of inference to presume that self-respect is necessary for the adequate respect of others. There are many people who respect many people they don't know, but that isn't what I am talking about. It is safe to say that people who respect no one except people they don't know do not respect themselves. And people who are very high in self-respect—that is, whose life experience has permitted them to uncover and demonstrate to their own satisfaction remarkable capacity for living with and among others—are people who find no particular expense to themselves connected with respecting any meritorious performance of anyone else. One of the feeblest props for an inadequate self-system is the attitude of disparaging others, which I once boiled down into the doctrine that if you are a molehill then, by God, there shall be no mountains. In a good many ways one can read the whole state of a person's self-respect from his disparagement of others. The disparagement is built of two ingredients, that which one 'despises' about oneself, and a great many *not* operations. Thus the person who greatly respects himself for his "generosity," which is probably always of a very public character, finds an incredible number of people ungenerous, stingy, mean, and so on. I think it has been known from the beginning of recorded thought that a person who is very bitter toward others, very hard on his fellow man for certain faults, is usually very sensitive to these particular faults because they are secret vices of his own. Insofar as self-respect has been permitted to grow without restrictions, because of comparatively unwarped personal development or because warp of personal development has been remedied, there is no expense, no feeling of impoverishment, no hints of anxiety connected with discovering that somebody else is much better than you are in a particular field. It is lamentably true that in so highly specialized and intricate a social organization as almost any extant culture is, it is virtually certain that there are very few top figures in any complex operation. Most people are not as good as the very few, and many people are much worse than the average. But there is such an enormous field for living that one does not have to depend on what one is not good at, and therefore one has no particular need for keeping a bookkeeping record on how many people are worse in a field in which one is bad. But some people, because of certain warps in personal development, make this an outstanding operation, in order to reduce anxiety from invidious comparisons with others.

I should like now to say a few words about human maturity—a subject I always treat extremely casually, partly because it is not a problem of psychiatry, although it could be extrapolated from psychiatry. But the actual fact is that an understanding of maturity eludes us as psychiatrists who are students of interpersonal relations, for the people who manifest the most maturity are least accessible for study; and the progress of our patients toward maturity invariably removes them from our observation before they have reached it. Thus a psychiatrist, as a psychiatrist, doesn't have much actual data. But one can guess a few things. I would guess that each of the outstanding achievements of the developmental eras that I have discussed will be outstandingly manifest in the mature personality. The last of these great developments is the appearance and growth of the need for intimacy—for collaboration with at least one other, preferably more others; and in this collaboration there is the very striking feature of a very lively sensitivity to the needs of the other and to the interpersonal security or absence of anxiety in the other. Thus we can certainly extrapolate from what we know that the mature, insofar as nothing of great importance collides, will be quite sympathetically understanding of the limitations, interests, possibilities, anxieties, and so on of those among whom they move or with whom they deal. Another thing which can quite certainly be extrapolated is that, whether it be by eternally widening interests or by deepening interests or both, the life of the mature—far from becoming monotonous and a bore—is always increasing in, shall I say, importance. There is no reason to entertain for an instant the notion that it would be too bad to become mature, because then one might get bored to death; quite the contrary. It is certain that no person, whether mature or terribly ill, is proof against any possibility of anxiety or fear, or against any of the needs that characterize life. But the greater the degree of maturity, the less will be the interference of anxiety with living, and therefore the less nuisance value one has for oneself and for others. And when one is mature, anything which even infinitesimally approximates the complexity of living in the world as we know it today is not apt to become boring.

PART III

Patterns of Inadequate or Inappropriate Interpersonal Relations

CHAPTER

19

The Earlier Manifestations of Mental Disorder: Matters Schizoid and Schizophrenic

I AM now beginning a discussion of the patterns of inadequate or inappropriate interpersonal relations which are ordinarily referred to as mental disorders, mild or severe. By adding "mild or severe," I wish to indicate that the topic of mental disorders covers all sorts of things, from minor accidents, such as unhappily being unable to remember an important person's name when you are about to request a favor from him, to the most chronic psychosis in the mental hospital. And so—as nearly as I can discover—if the term, mental disorder, is to be meaningful, it must cover like a tent the whole field of inadequate or inappropriate performance in interpersonal relations.

To begin with, I must make it clear that I am not dealing with all those disorders of living which arise primarily because of more-or-less clearly biological defect. On these I will have nothing in particular to say, although I believe that this theory of psychiatry will make evident to the more thoughtful how primary biological defect can influence the developmental course and the necessary preparation for living as a person among persons. Primary biological defect can be either inborn and manifest from the beginning, as in the case of the very unfortunate imitations of human beings called idiots; or it may be as recondite as a particular vulnerability to life, which manifests itself, for instance, in premature old age or premature senile deterioration (Alzheimer's disease), or in the arteriosclerotic changes and the senile psychoses. All these things refer much more to the innate constitution of the living matter that makes up the human body than they do to life experience, although, as I have indicated from time to time, life experience may have some influence on the timing of the manifestation of the defect. But it is quite clear that there are people so well endowed by heredity that they can survive very, very stressful circumstances for many years without marked destructive elevation of blood pressure or serious deterioration of the walls of the blood vessels such as occurs in arteriosclerosis; such people can go on into their eighties, perhaps even past the middle of the eighties, with no material senile changes, such as we see in the senile psychoses. Thus there is a large body of phenomena ordained by heredity which probably have fundamentally important bearing on the course of life. But what I am discussing is the difficulties of living which arise far more from misfortunes in developmental history than from any innate endowment.

Developmental Events Tributary to the Not-Me

To open this discussion of 'mental disorders'—or patterns of inadequate and inappropriate action in interpersonal relations—I want to take up more fully the 'natural history' of the conception of *not-me*, which I could only hint at in connection with late infancy and early childhood. The not-me is literally the organization of experience with significant people that has been subjected to such intense anxiety, and anxiety so suddenly precipitated, that it was impossible for the then relatively rudimentary person to make any sense of, to develop any true grasp on, the particular circumstances which dictated the experience of this intense anxiety. As I have said, very intense anxiety precipitated by a sudden, intense, negative emotional reaction on the part of the significant environment has more than a little in common with a blow on the head. It tends to erase any possibility of elaborating the exact circumstances of its occurrence, and about the most the person can remember in retrospect is a somewhat fenestrated account of the event in the immediate neighborhood. If, for example, a parent has had a subpsychotic fear of the infant's becoming a lustful monster and has gone off the deep end whenever the infant was discovered to be holding the penis or fondling the vulva—then we expect that the personality of the infant as it develops will show a sort of hole in that area, in the sense that any approach to the genitals will ultimately lead to the appearance of a feeling which has scarcely evolved beyond sudden, intense, all-encompassing anxiety. All this almost undifferentiated, sudden, violent anxiety is experienced as *uncanny* emotion; that is, if a person had a good grasp on the word, he would say, in trying to describe what was happening to him, that he felt uncanny. In later life, this all-encompassing anxiety shows some slight elaborations, which are hinted at by four words in our language—awe, dread, loathing, and horror. Although these four words suggest the possibility of discriminating between various uncanny emotions, actually the experiences are pretty much indistinguishable, which is borne out by the descriptions offered by highly articulate people.

While there is an awfulness connected with all of the uncanny emotions, *awe* itself is one of them. From it, of course, we get our term "awful," although the connection has been lost in the history of English. Awe is perhaps the least oppressively sudden and the least paralyzing of these uncanny emotions; in fact, it is in many adults called out only by unexpected, stupendous manifestations of nature, or of man's works, stirring some of the more fantastically autistic reveries of the past. Thus upon entering certain buildings which have great architectural beauty, one may feel awe, which, if the building happens to be a church, may carry with it curiously early thinking about the nature and actual presence of the deity, for example. And many people, when they first climb the hill and look into the Grand Canyon, have a paralyzing emotion which is anything but really an attractive experience, but yet is not horrible. One is, as it were, lifted utterly out of the context of life and is profoundly impressed.

The other three terms connected with the uncanny emotions speak very much more of the dreadful character of the experience; they are dread itself, loathing, and horror. Loathing is that peculiar combination of physical illness and other extremely unpleasant things which some not particularly articulate people have described to me as an intense desire to vomit without the capacity to even feel nauseated—which in its way is rather impressive. And horror is the uncanny emotion that all of you have known at least once, probably in your sleep. Horror is a simply paralyzing combination of what I like to call revulsion—a feeling of almost total desire to be elsewhere and away from all this sort of thing—coupled again with a great desire to vomit, and perhaps a tendency to have diarrhea and one thing and another; and at the same time there is literally a sort of paralysis of everything, so that nothing really goes on except this awful and—if it can possibly be avoided—never-to-be-repeated experience.

All these things seem to be rather of the essence of sudden attacks of all-paralyzing anxiety; and this anxiety can be induced very early in one's life by the sudden outburst, in a significant person, of extremely unpleasant emotions. And this is the foundation, if you please, of certain experience structures in personality that can be for practical purposes, because of their later manifestations, referred to as the not-me—in contrast to good-me and bad-me. Good-me and bad-me, as I have said, are the basis of lifelong ingredients of consciousness—that is, there is no person who is not, in the privacy of his own covert operations, perfectly clear on the fact that he has a number of unsatisfactory and undesirable attributes which he is busily engaged in concealing, or excusing, or what not, and that he also has some good traits, among the others; and these are the outgrowths of the initial dichotomy of good-me and bad-me. But only under exceptional circumstances are there any reflections in consciousness—that is, in awareness—of that part of one's life experience which I have called not-me—a sort of third rudimentary personification.

Evidences of Dissociation

In addition to every other form or process elaborated into the self-system for the avoiding or minimizing of anxiety or for the concealing of anxiety, the self-system has, in practically every instance, some aspects which can be said to be—and this is highly figurative language—directed to keep one safe from any possibility of passing into that extremely unpleasant state of living which can be called the uncanny emotions; and these aspects of the self-system can only be inferred, except in case of disaster. Depending on one's distant past, this group of self-processes may be fairly extensive or may be minor indeed. The manifestations of such self-functions, as experienced by practically everyone, are actually called out by progressions of processes in sleep which become so explicit, in some allegedly impossible aspect of personality, that they suddenly call into action self-system processes which are ordinarily in abeyance at night. The result is that one suddenly awakes with a more-or-less shivery feeling of having been in the presence of something dreadful. Now the nightmare, as it is ordinarily encountered, may or may not represent matters actually touching upon the not-me component in personality. But in a good many ways the smaller the content of the nightmare and the more tremendous the emotion—the more utterly shattering the recollection of the emotional state—the more you may surmise that some process in sleep has all too emphatically connected with this particular component of personality, which is ordinarily only inferentially evident, and which is the result of the most disastrous contacts with sudden and violent anxiety in the early years.

In later childhood, the basis provided by the not-me experience of early childhood may either grow or may be more or less stationary, depending on the experience at that time. In that era, the more fortunate people develop precautionary and propitiatory processes concerned with manifestations of what was previously bad-me, and disintegrate those motivational systems that get them into very serious trouble, with either reorganization—sublimatory or otherwise—of the disintegrated motivational system, or regressive reactivation of earlier patterns of behavior for such components as are not reorganized. But in the later childhood of more fated people who, for instance, lose a parent in childhood and get instead a very bad imitation, or are sent to an inferior institution, or something like that, there may begin to be very clear evidences of this exceedingly important system of processes to which we refer as *dissociation.*[1]

In dissociation, the trick is that one shall carry on within aware-

[1] Dissociation is unfortunately made rather too important in *Conceptions* [Sullivan, *Conceptions of Modern Psychiatry; op. cit.*], in which I did not take enough time to emphasize all the other things that go on besides dissociation.

ness processes which make it practically impossible, while one is awake, to encounter uncanny emotion. You see, dissociation can easily be mistaken for a really quite magical business in which you fling something of you out into outer darkness, where it reposes for years, quite peacefully. That is a fantastic oversimplification. Dissociation works very suavely indeed as long as it works, but it isn't a matter of keeping a sleeping dog under an anesthetic. It works by a continuous alertness or vigilance of awareness, with certain supplementary processes which prevent one's ever discovering the usually quite clear evidences that part of one's living is done without any awareness. I am practically ready to say that the dissociat*ing* components of self-system processes have their most classical manifestation in obsessive substitution for difficulties in living. Certainly there seems to be no clear line between people who have, as their prevailing ineffective, inappropriate, and inadequate interpersonal process, substitutive processes of the obsessional type, and those who, under certain circumstances, suffer episodes of schizophrenic living. And so, while it would be rather unreasonable, at this point, to say that the great wealth of substitutive processes found in this culture are all clear evidences of serious dissociations, I believe that when our theoretical formulations have progressed a little further on the basis of better study of data, we will find that that may be just the case. In any event, there is such a close parallel between the difficulties of working with really important substitutive processes and the difficulties in working with schizophrenic processes that the distinction again becomes minor. And when I say really important substitutive processes, I mean the use of substitution in very important areas of living. Quite strikingly, in this day and age, substitutive processes are used to conceal extreme vulnerability to anxiety at the hands of practically anyone. One finds in a great many of the more severe obsessional people, as we call them in the vernacular, a great degree of what they call hatred, but what actually, on more close scrutiny, proves to be their shocking vulnerability to almost anybody with whom they are integrated. And the obsessional substitutions which make up such conspicuous and troublesome aspects of their lives are simply all-encompassing attenuations of contact which protect them from their abnormal vulnerability to anxiety.

Thus one should look upon obsessional substitution as perhaps an outstanding instance of what goes on in the self-system in order to keep something utterly excluded from awareness, so that there is no possibility of its eruption into awareness.

Whenever dissociated systems of motives are involved, we find a relative suspension of awareness as to any effects that these motives have. That suspension of awareness may be as minor as the relatively trifling and almost ubiquitous disturbance of awareness to which I give the term *selective inattention*, in which one simply doesn't happen to notice almost an infinite series of more-or-less meaningful details of one's living. But even selective inattention is very impressive when one observes that it could not possibly act so suavely, and so eternally at the right times, unless there was continuous vigilance lest one notice what for some obscure reasons one is not going to notice. Selective inattention is, more than any other of the inappropriate and inadequate performances of life, the classic means by which we do not profit from experience which falls within the areas of our particular handicap. We don't *have* the experience from which we might profit—that is, although it occurs, we never notice what it must mean; in fact we never notice that a good deal of it has occurred at all. That is what is really troublesome in psychotherapy, I suppose—the wonderfully bland way in which people overlook the most glaring implications of certain acts of their own, or of certain reactions of theirs to other people's acts—that is, what they are apt to report as other people's acts. Much more tragically, they may overlook the fact that these things have occurred at all; these things just aren't remembered, even though the person has had them most unpleasantly impressed on him.

I'm going to digress for a moment to give an instance of the circumvention of selective inattention, which involves one of my more gross acts of unkindness. There is a drugstore at which I frequently have to purchase this and that; and during the war years it had among its clerks at the soda fountain a person who, I am quite sure, would be shown by intelligence tests to be a low-grade moron. Not only was he quite lacking in intelligence, but also—in which I sympathize with him, as I do with everyone who deals with the public—he showed a very rare collection of hostilities to customers, so that whatever you asked for, he would dutifully, when he got around to it, bring you something else. Having suffered from this repeatedly, I was extremely unpleasant on one particular occasion and said, "What is that, huh?" And he said, "Water. Didn't you ask for it?" And I said, "*Get me what I asked for!*" Whereupon the poor bird tottered off under the unpleasantness and got me what I had asked for. But the great joker is that the next time I saw him he grinned at me and immediately got me what I asked for. Now, that humbled me, because his inattention was not as complete as I had thought. He profited from an unpleasant experience, and, by God, that's more than some of us do. If he had acted as I expected, it would have been a classical instance of selective inattention; he would never have noticed that almost always he brought people things they didn't want. And therefore, of course, any occasion such as I provoked would be utterly novel, inexplicable—just an instance of deviltry on my part. The great joker was that it didn't seem to be. This story to the contrary, I hope I have given you a notion of how suavely we simply ignore great bodies of experience, any clearly analyzed instance of which might present us with a very real necessity for change.

Among the other evidences of dissociation—in addition to selective inattention and the dissociative processes such as obsessional substitution—there are certain relatively uncommon marginal observations which go on in awareness in unusual interpersonal situations; and these observations have a touch of the uncanny about them. And the uncanny in this very mild sense is what I call revulsion. Revulsion is a certain sort of chilled turning away from things, quite different from chronic detestations, such as I have for yolk of egg—a detestation in which there is no shadow of anything except a realization that were I to taste it again it would be as unpleasant as ever. Revulsion is something else: you have a little disturbance in your belly and so on, and you aren't at all inclined to think what would happen if you had gone further. And in the course of average living, evidences of dissociation may also appear as certain disturbances at night, from which one is awakened with nothing except uncanny emotion—a feeling that one was having a damned unpleasant dream which was lost in the process of awakening. Much more occasionally one recalls fragments of dreams which were clearly associated with horror, dread, or what not. These are almost invariably uninterpretable as they are ordinarily reported. Only when psychotherapy becomes fairly well established can a person ordinarily stand the strain of having fairly clear dissociated processes revealed in his dreams.

Along with these detectable ingredients of awareness, there are, when there is dissociation of major motives, certain gross items of behavior which we call *automatisms*. And while I say that this happens when there is dissociation of major motives, I presume that this is true in any instance of dissociation, although it is very much harder to see when the motives are not major. Automatisms can be very massive performances under certain circumstances, although they are minor movements in general; and sometimes they are such extreme things as tics, convulsions of certain muscle groups, and so on, which seem about as far removed from meaningful behavior as possible. A graphic instance of these automatisms can be frequently seen in the more populated areas such as Manhattan. Those of you who are men may have discovered, as you're walking down the street, that quite a number of other men look at what is called the fly of your pants, and look away hastily. Many of them raise their eyes to yours—apparently, insofar as you can interpret, to see if they have been noticed. But the point is that some of them, if they encounter your gaze, are as numb and indifferent as if nothing had occurred. Others of them blush and are obviously very much disturbed. In the latter, it has not been an automatism; if being detected in this act is very embarrassing to the person who manifested it, then the act has had meaning to him. But when such an act is automatic—the manifestation of dissociated motivation—it is not embarrassing to be detected. Even if it were brought emphatically to the attention of the person who manifested it, his natural inclination would always be to deny that it had occurred. If, perhaps with a photograph, you could demonstrate that it had occurred, the person would still feel completely blank as to what on earth it could have arisen from, what it could mean. Thus major systems in dissociation—and I presume all dissociated experience—manifest themselves in certain disturbances of behavior, or certain gross behavioral acts, whose single distinction is the fact that their occurrence is either unknown, or at least meaningless, to the person who shows them.

In more major automatisms, one 'finds oneself,' with very considerable disturbance, in very awkward situations into which one has apparently walked with one's eyes shut, so to speak; and this discovery leads to uncanny emotion. Sometimes one realizes that one has been in a really curious state of mind during the time that one got into this awkwardness; and this state of mind might be labeled *fascination*. When fascinated, one is actually engaging in molar behavior which gets one into a situation where the manifestations of a dissociated impulse would be appropriate. That seldom happens; instead one 'finds oneself' with thoroughly disagreeable fringes of horror, dread, revulsion, or something of the kind, and extricates oneself, usually with a distinct feeling of being badly shaken by the experience.

Possibility of Reintegration of Dissociated Systems

Dissociated systems are founded in early life; their greatest chance of automatic remedy, and also their greatest contributions to danger to the personality, occur in the preadolescent and adolescent phases of development. Many people have come out of preadolescence and early adolescence in distinctly less risk, so far as their future is concerned, than when they began these eras. But at the same time, anyone familiar with mental-hospital admission rates knows that very grave disturbances of personality often occur in the instance of the delayed preadolescent or during the phases of adolescence. In general, important aspects of personality existing in dissociation are not reintegrated except under extremely fortunate circumstances. One of these fortunate circumstances is found in preadolescence, as I have already said, when the development of the need for intimacy can lead to very considerable improvement of the partition of energy between the not-me component and the other components of personality. And at the same time that this new integrating tendency is being called out by maturation, certain eventualities are likely to occur which may have favorable influence in reintegrating a dissociated tendency system. Among these fortunate eventualities of preadolescence and adolescence are the reintegration by what I call "deliberate fugue"; the reintegration "as if by misadventure while asleep"; and the reintegration by "adjustment to the uncanny."

To begin with, perhaps I should explain what I mean by fugue. A fugue, in the sense in which I use the term, is literally a relatively prolonged state of dreaming-while-awake—that is, one acts a dream with every conviction that one is awake, and one actually is awake, as far as a bystander can tell. Fugues sometimes occur in the perhaps partially organic, if not wholly organic, state of epilepsy, although fugues, in the sense I'm now discussing, are by no means restricted to the epileptic. Fugues are part of the onset of some very serious mental disorders, although sometimes the occurrence of a fugue is all that is needed to avoid the onset of very serious mental disorder. But in any case, when one is in a fugue, as I am trying to describe it, one *believes* that one is awake, one *acts as if* one were awake in many important particulars, and everyone else *presumes* one is awake. But the relationship with circumambient reality and with the meanings to which things attach from one's past is, to a certain extent, as fundamentally and as absolutely suspended as it is when one is asleep. And there are certain absolute barriers to recall, which are to be understood only on the basis of their being minor indications of a very prolonged state of sleep.

Now preadolescents and adolescents sometimes approach situations in what I call *deliberate fugues:* that is, a person braces himself with an attitude of "Well, hell, let's take a chance on anything once." He then plunges into some situation, with a sort of tightening up of everything, often keeping his eye on something irrelevant—that is, preoccupying himself with things really tangential to what he is after. This has striking resemblances to an active fugue state, although without the literal cutting-off of certain aspects of past history that a true fugue shows. In this state one has experiences which under other circumstances would precipitate a psychosis. And by a sort of attenuating process, by which the whole thing adds itself to conscious experience slowly, one survives it and is the better for it.

I have mentioned that reintegration of dissociated tendencies may be initiated, as it were, by misadventure, particularly in connection with the relative abeyance of security operations as if one were asleep. That is, one gets into situations primarily motivated by the dissociated system, as if one were asleep. This, again, is a very tricky business, and it is a mistake to accuse a person of having falsely claimed to be asleep in such situations. The longer we deal intimately with personalities in this very risky area, the more we realize that we have no absolute criterion for sleep and that there are unquestionably a number of levels of sleep. The true fugue, for example, is of the essence of sleep, but no criterion that we could ordinarily apply would show it to be anything remotely like what we think sleep is. Thus one may hear of a youngster who has found himself in some presumably very disturbing experience because he had fallen asleep, although he knows all about it; one may think this a little bit curious and be inclined to doubt it, but one should proceed cautiously. I'm not sure he isn't simply telling the truth. In other words, these misadventures, when one may or may not have been asleep, are perhaps the next step between the "deliberate fugue," where one decides to pull ahead and take the consequences, and the true fugue, where one has no more clarity on what has happened to one than if one were profoundly asleep.

The last method by which dissociated systems may be reintegrated—and one I have difficulty putting into words—is what I call the "adjustment to the uncanny." This is probably in some ways a function of the mythology that has been incorporated in one's earlier experience. In other words, to a certain extent, one acts a part in a relatively cosmic drama—that is, one literally steps out of the world as it is into the world of some mythological system and for a while plays a role in that. In some very serious disturbances following the failure of dissociation, people fight out, with tremendous expenditures of energy, dramas virtually on a cosmic scale; for example, one of my patients at one time exhausted himself in the battle of the nuns and the fathers. Adjustment to the uncanny is doing this with a feeling that *you* do it instead of its being forced upon you by transcendental powers. A few people have had experiences in their developmental years of meeting situations actually characterized by these extremely disquieting and extraordinarily repelling uncanny emotions, in which, for a while, they acted as if they were one of the demigods or the demidevils or what not, and got through it, and so from then on knew more about life on the far side of it.[2]

The Schizophrenic Way of Life and Possible Outcomes

All things connected with dissociated systems are risky. The act of dissociation is perhaps the most magnificently complex performance of human personality, and it is certainly the riskiest way of dealing with any of the very major motivations in life. Even in adolescence and preadolescence—as the very high schizophrenia rate of these eras indicates—the risks are anything but nominal. And after these developmental thresholds have been passed, continuing risks—that is, if there are major systems in dissociation—are really pretty ominous.

But let me now discuss the dramatic manifestations of risk—that is, the disasters that come from having major systems in dissociation, or major components of motivational systems in dissociation. These disastrous failures are most likely to occur in the age group from fourteen to twenty-seven, roughly. Of the very, very risky things that can happen, perhaps the least disastrous in outcome is the 'displacement,' with very serious disturbance of consciousness, of the conventional personified self by behavior patterns, and so on, concerned with the dissociated pattern. This is the real fugue. One may come out of the fugue in a very sad state indeed; or the fugue may suddenly clear up after possibly a year and a half's duration, and one then seems to be all right. Fugues occurring in this adolescent era are quite frequently not as successful as some of the so-called hysterical fugues, in which a person who is not really crooked embezzles a lot of money and wakes up in a strange city with an assumed personality.

[2] [*Editors' note:* In another lecture, in 1945, Sullivan described the "adjustment to the uncanny" as follows: "After an uncanny experience there then supervenes a total state of personality, one might say, in which one says, 'Well, this is it; for good or evil, for better or worse, it is so.' And this acceptance of something—even though one cannot think of it, cannot analyze it—as being so, to be survived or not as the case may be, is what I mean by the peculiar expression, adjustment to the uncanny."]

The fugue might be called a very massive change of personality. Another, somewhat less massive, disturbance of personality is what I call the eruption into awareness of *abhorrent cravings.* In my view the term "craving" doesn't need the adjective "abhorrent," but I wish to indicate by this term the entrance into personal awareness of increasingly-intense-because-unsatisfied longings to engage in something which is abhorrent—that is, the picturing of engaging in it is attended by uncanny emotion such as horror, dread, loathing, or the like. The classic instance of this eruption of cravings is the eruption of 'homosexual' desires—desires to participate in what the patient feels, classically and outstandingly, to be homosexual performances. I think I can illustrate this, perhaps without misleading you too badly, by mentioning one of my patients, an only boy with five sisters, who had led as sheltered a life as that situation would permit. Shortly after getting into uniform in World War II he was prowling around Washington, and was gathered up by a very well-dressed and charming dentist, who took him to his office and performed what is called fellatio on this boy. The boy felt, I presume, a mild adjustment to the uncanny, and went his way, perhaps in some fashion rewarded. But the next day he quite absent-mindedly walked back to the immediate proximity of the dentist's office, that being in some ways, you see, an untroubled fugue—whereupon, finding himself so very near what had happened the day before, he was no longer able to exclude from awareness the fact that he would like to continue to undergo these experiences. This is a classical instance of an abhorrent craving in that it was entirely intolerable to him. The day before it had been a kind of new experience, but when it burst upon him in this way, it was attended by all sorts of revulsions and a feeling that it would be infrahuman, and what not, to have such interests. And he arrived at the hospital shortly afterward in what is called schizophrenic disturbance.

The eruption of abhorrent cravings may or may not precipitate immediately a change for the much worse, but in a good many cases fugues or the eruption of abhorrent cravings in the adolescent days soon precipitate a state which is so completely disorganizing that it may be called, with certain reservations, *panic*. I think it very rarely approximates the panic which occurs when something that one has utterly trusted collapses—the sort of mixture of terror and absolutely blindly disorganized inactivity, which one sometimes hears of in theater fires, and so on. Panic does not lead to action; panic leads to nothing. One is disorganized. Terror usually follows panic, and terror very often includes blind frantic activities which can be very destructive to oneself or others. The panic that quite often is the outcome of fugue or the eruption of abhorrent cravings is a very brief complete disorganization. In this case, the most significant of the things which are disorganized is the structure of one's beliefs and convictions as to the guarantees and securities and dependable properties of the universe in which one is living. And the far side of these panicky instances may be anything from terror to great religious exaltation. In any case, the personality is partly torn from its moorings and has moved from what was actually its developmental level into a state which we call the schizophrenic way of life.

In the schizophrenic state, very early types of referential process occur within clear awareness, to the profound mystification of the person concerned. And since many of these referential processes are literally historically identical with the composition of the not-me components in personality, their presence is attended by uncanny emotions, sometimes dreadfully strong. These referential processes seem so bizarre to people who have not had them that the schizophrenic way of life is often described as unpsychological and completely beyond understanding. The justification for such reckless language is that those schizophrenic processes which we encounter represent attempts on the sufferer's part to communicate types of processes that most of us ceased to have within clear awareness by the time that we were two-and-a-half. There is a possibility that a dissociated system which has broken cover in this way can only very briefly continue to be free from being greatly complicated by what remains of the security apparatus, the self-system; and this possibility completes the picture of why the schizophrenic illnesses give one a feeling of the utter futility of human thought to understand what is going on. If the eventualities of a fugue, or the eventualities of the eruption of abhorrent cravings, are followed by experience which is able to terminate the association of a major part of the particular motivational system with these uncanny emotions, and associate it with the main trends of personality development, then we would have achieved the integration of a previously dissociated motivational system with the rest of the personality; and there would then be none of this dreadful spectacle of the schizophrenic way of life, with its exceedingly ominous probable outcomes. People can actually suffer recurrent—and they can recur as frequently as several times an hour—waves of schizophrenic process, or seem actually to remain continuously in schizophrenic process for a matter of years, and quite suddenly effect a reintegration of personality, make a very quick recovery, and go on for the rest of their life with no major disturbances.

But a great many of the people who get involved in schizophrenic disturbance proceed through it to one of two very unfortunate outcomes. One we call the paranoid maladjustment, in which sundry elements of blame and guilt in the personality are attached to other people round about, with such disastrous effects on the possibility of intimacy and simple relation with anybody in the environment that there is no way back. In the other outcome, people literally disintegrate so much under the force of horror in this schizophrenic business that they become examples of something scarcely noticed in the developmental years—namely, relatively satisfactory preoccupation with the simple pleasures of the zones of interaction provoked by one's own manipulations, which seems to be about the essence of what we call the hebephrenic change, or the hebephrenic dilapidation of personality. These illnesses are not to be regarded, according to my light, as part of schizophrenia, but as very unfortunate outcomes of schizophrenic episodes; and they are not so successful but that for many, many years after these unfortunate outcomes have been instituted, episodes of schizophrenic processes may still occur. That is not always the case; some people make stable paranoid maladjustments which are singularly free from schizophrenic processes, which actually insure them from occasions where they will have schizophrenic processes. And I am sure that some people dilapidate in such a fashion that they are very little troubled by schizophrenic processes. But a great many of the people who have undergone these very unfortunate developments have not solved life to the point where they can be happy though psychotic.

CHAPTER

20

Sleep, Dreams, and Myths *

Sleep as Relief from Security Operations

IN DISCUSSING the comparatively neglected topic of sleep, dreams, myths, and the related disorders of living, I shall refer to sleep only briefly. It is a phase of living which is very important indeed, in that—aside from all the biological factors involved—it is the part of life in which we are almost by definition relieved from the necessity of maintaining security. In other words, while we are asleep, we have a comparative dearth of security operations, because the movement into the state of sleep in itself requires a situation more or less routinely known to be free from dangers to one's self-esteem. When anxiety is severe, sleep is practically impossible, although as one gets tired enough, the need for sleep becomes impossible to fight off; under those conditions, sleep is cut up into very brief periods of deep sleep and relatively long stages of very light sleep, which are hard to tell objectively from waking. In certain other situations, deep sleep tends to be an insidious incident in periods of such light sleep that the patient not uncommonly reports that he has not slept at all; although there does not seem to be any obvious danger to one's self-esteem or any very striking sources of anxiety in such situations, on deeper study it is found that something characterized by anxiety does exist in the realm of reverie processes, such as dealing with difficult people, or the like. I used to have a fairly critical feeling about patients who reported that they had had no sleep and were utterly exhausted,

* [*Editors' note:* The illustrative material from myths that Sullivan has used in this lecture has not been changed, although the stories are not in precise agreement with the legends and stories that we know: for instance, the published version of Mark Twain's *The Mysterious Stranger* has a different setting, characters, and events.]

when it was perfectly obvious, from the report of dispassionate observers, that they had slept a good part of the night; I thought that this was some type of substitutive operation which should be dealt with as such. But on one occasion when I was aroused regularly at brief intervals throughout the night, I discovered that the very expense of maintaining the processes of preparing myself for being aroused, and of trying to avoid all the processes thereunto pertaining that would tend to waste time in my getting back to sleep, amounted actually to my sleeping so superficially most of the time that I did not enjoy relief from security operations, relief from processes all too closely related to the stressful aspects of waking life. I began very rapidly then to understand why people who, during a night, have never fallen profoundly asleep nor stayed asleep as long as they needed to—though they may have slept, at intervals, a total of even five, six, or seven hours—are inclined to think that they haven't had any sleep at all, and, in fact, have certainly not derived any benefit from what they have had.

As I have said, the functional importance of sleep, from the psychiatric standpoint, is that there is a very great relaxation of security operations. As a result of this, many unsatisfied needs from the day, and unsatisfied components of the needs satisfied during the day—which cannot be satisfied in waking life because of the anxiety and security operations associated with them—are satisfied, insofar as may be, by covert operations, symbolic devices, which occur in sleep. This is difficult to demonstrate directly but is a fairly probable inference made on the basis of the state of people when they are denied sleep; in such a situation, a person's previous handling of unwelcome, disapproved motivations, and so on, deteriorates fairly rapidly, with serious impairment of his apparent mental health.

Although I have suggested that security operations are inconspicuous in sleep and that the sleep situation is actually defined by the possibility of relaxing self-system functions, I have not said that the self-system is absolutely relaxed, or that it has no effect whatever. Evidences of its actual state of functional activity are perhaps most vividly demonstrated in the relatively frequent occurrence of the onset of schizophrenia during sleep. Quite a number of people who are tense and extremely uncomfortable while awake, have a frightful nightmare, one night, which they cannot awake from, even though they objectively 'wake up'; and not very long after that such people become unquestionably schizophrenic throughout their apparent waking life. Now, that which awakens one from certain covert operations in sleep must be, clearly, a manifestation of the self-system. In other words, we maintain our dissociations, despite recurrent periods of sleep, by maintaining continued alertness, continued vigilance of the dissociative apparatus in the self-system. As a derivative of that, it may be said that the more of personality which exists in dissociation, the less restful and more troubled will be the person's sleep. Thus, depth of sleep is in a certain sense really a direct, simple function of the extent to which the activity of the self-system can be abandoned for a certain part of the twenty-four hours; and when powerful motivational systems are dissociated, it is impossible to abandon enough of the self-system function so that one can have deep and restful sleep.

The Significance of Dreams in Psychotherapy

I now want to present the comparatively direct evidence for my statement that sleep is a period of life during which covert operations deal with the unsatisfied needs which waking life does not take care of, although my evidence is pretty far from the kind obtained with a caliper or a measuring telescope in the natural sciences. The best evidence is in the shape of the reports of remembered dreams. I believe most of us will agree that we dream, and that we remember something of what we have dreamed on certain occasions. But what we can recall of dreaming is never any too adequate, unless the dream is very brief and marked by tremendous emotion. My point is that there is an impassable barrier between covert operations when one is asleep and covert operations and reports of them when one is awake. If the barrier is passable at all, it is only by the use of such techniques as hypnosis, which are so complex as to produce data no more reliable than the recalled dream, so that in essence the barrier *is* impassable. In other words, for the purposes of my theory, one never, under any circumstances, deals directly with dreams. It is simply impossible. What one deals with in psychiatry, and actually in a great many other aspects of life, are recollections pertaining to dreams; how closely, how adequately these recollections approximate the actual dreams is an insoluble problem, because as far as I know there is no way to develop a reasonable conviction of one-to-one correspondence between recollections of dreams and dreams themselves.

Many of us probably have had the experience of having a dream of the night before so much in mind that we just had to tell somebody what we recollected of it. This feeling of urgency about reporting and discussing a dream is the mark that these covert operations are of very material importance in keeping us going as social beings in human society. An important part of intensive psychotherapy consists in recognizing that if a patient, without encouragement, recalls something that has occurred in the sleep component of his current living and is impelled to report it, then that is a valid and important part of his relation with the psychiatrist. In intensive psychotherapy there need never be any question of what actually was dreamed; but the psychiatrist can have many reasonable questions about the completeness of the report and its communicative value. I have heard accounts of dreams which impressed me as definitely truncated, as very highly improbable accounts of what had happened. In many accounts of dreams there are areas that are as foggy and uncommunicative as are many of the statements of persons utilizing substitutive processes in reporting on their current living. At those points in a reported dream where the psychiatrist has a definite feeling of improbability or of unnecessary obscurity, there is no reason in the world why he should not make the same efforts to obtain completeness and to clear up obscurities as he would for an account of the patient's waking life. I do not mean by this that one person will be able to follow lucidly another person's dream; such an expectancy is at best a very pleasant delusion. But when a psychiatrist feels that he is hearing, in the report of a dream, an obscured account of living—perhaps so obscured that it is impossible to distinguish whether one of the critical figures in this account of living was a man or a woman, a wolf or a bear—I think that there is no reason against inquiry, and that there is much benefit to be derived from clarifying whether the dreamer really cannot make any discrimination between these relatively dissimilar possibilities. Establishing such a point is important, for such lack of discrimination is a valid, presumably important, part of a person's current living. The psychiatrist's merely accepting without question the unclarity of a person's report of a dream is very much like merely accepting the general unclarity of every obsessional neurotic—it means that the psychiatrist will never quite discover what is being discussed, but will just go on in a comparatively useful semisocial relationship.

In the intensive study of personality, the psychiatrist works with these curious survivals from the dream life, which is always cut off from the waking life. In most of the dreams that the patient feels more or less compelled to report, one frequently encounters massive evidences of security operations that have gone into action on awakening. Although the fragments of these dreams which are reported might be very helpful if they could be preserved in meaningful detail, they have quite insidiously and unwittingly been woven into great textures of dramatic action in which everything which met the real utility of the dream has been almost hopelessly confounded into what Freud called secondary elaborations. But these elaborations are actually interventions of the self-system which simply foredoom the possibility of using these reports meaningfully. Certain other dreams that the psychiatrist hears have as their most obvious characteristic the fact that they are rather simple statements of dramatic action; they are very vivid, very strongly colored, very succinct statements of something. In some of these simple statements which occur at the most critical times in a person's life, there is some strong feeling, although that feeling may be as vague as a mere feeling of urgency and importance connected with the dream. For instance, a person may come to his friend or his therapist, more or less preoccupied with the necessity of reporting the dream; but as he reports the dream, he is swept into the feeling of the dream, which may be terror or any of the uncanny emotions such as dread. That particular experience I have to mention, not because it is frequent, but because it is of such dangerous importance that it's very sad for a psychiatrist not to realize what a critical situation has suddenly shown up in his office.

In some particularly unfortunate people, we discover that from very early in life something has apparently been going terribly wrong in the part of their life which is partitioned to sleep—that is, they have night terrors. Night terrors sometimes show up in very early childhood—conceivably in very late infancy—and can continue, so far as I know, indefinitely, although with any increase in competence at being a person, night terror usually passes over into nightmares. The term, night terror, applies to the situation in which one awakens from some utterly unknown events in practically primordial terror; in this state, one is on the border of complete disintegration of personality—in other words, there are almost no evidences of any particular competence and one is almost disorganized, since one is actually in a state of panic. By the time the personality has pulled itself together to the point where anything like interpersonal relations could be manifested, the curtain has descended—that is, there has been a separation from consciousness of any trace of what was going on at the time of the primordial terror. Thus night terrors are empty in terms of any recollection of what they were about. Night terror is distinguished from nightmare by the fact that the content in night terror is more completely obliterated, since night terror appears very early when the process of becoming a person is terribly threatened. But nightmare—dreadful dreams, with recollectable content—represents a grave emergency in personality at a time when the personality is more competent to deal with it; that is, the personality can make use of interpersonal relations in a curious attempt to validate the nature of the threat, or to overcome the terrible isolation and loneliness connected with the threat.

Some of you will recall having had occasionally an extremely unpleasant dream which awakened you, but did not awaken you completely; in other words, it moved you from deep sleep to very light sleep. The evidence of your still being in light sleep is that while you have every feeling of being awake, and certainly have perfect freedom of voluntary motion—which is rather strikingly curtailed in anything like deep sleep—you cannot get what you know to be reality to behave. In this connection, I will mention fragments of two or three dreams which come to my mind. One was a dream which I had to undergo very early in my study of schizophrenia, in order to realize that I had some grave barriers to the task which the gods had brought me. To give some background on this dream, I should say that in my very early childhood it was discovered that I was so repelled by spiders that the body of a dead spider put at the top of the stairs would discourage my ambulatory efforts, which had previously often resulted in my falling downstairs. Now, of course, if one considers that the spider is a mother symbol, and that this occurred around the age of two-and-a-half to four, one can picture what profound problems I had in repressing my hostility to the mother, or something of the sort. But I prefer to say, simply, that I didn't like spiders, and I disliked them so much that I wouldn't pass one. As the years rolled by, I never got fond of spiders. I haven't very much objection to most living things, but I have never appreciated spiders and other predatory creatures of that kind, and I fear I never shall. I had the following dream at the time when it became possible, finally, for me really to start on an intensive study of schizophrenia, partly by my own efforts and largely by accident; and I had decided on this study and all the arrangements were satisfactory. You all recall the geometric designs that spiders weave on grass, and that show up in the country when the dew's on the ground. My dream started with a great series of these beautiful geometric patterns, each strand being very nicely midway between the one in front of it and the one behind it, and so on—quite a remarkable textile, and incidentally I am noticeably interested in textiles. Then the textile pattern became a tunnel reaching backward after the fashion of the tunnel-web spiders, and then the spider began to approach. And as the spider approached, it grew and grew into truly stupendous and utterly horrendous proportions. And I awakened extremely shaken and was unable to obliterate the spider, which continued to be a dark spot on the sheet which I knew perfectly well would re-expand into the spider if I tried to go to sleep. So instead, I got up and smoked a cigarette and looked out the window and one thing and another, and came back and inspected the sheet, and the spot was gone. So I concluded that it was safe to go back to bed. Now, I'm not going to tell you all about what that meant, because only God knows what I dreamed; I've just told you what I recalled. I'm trying to stress the hang-over, the utter intrusion into sensory perception, which required the shaking off of the last vestige of sleep process, the definite reassertion of me and mine, Washington, and what not, in order to prevent the thing from going on. Fortunately, with some assistance, I guessed what might be the case, and thus escaped certain handicaps for the study of schizophrenia. I might add that spiders thereupon disappeared forever from my sleep—so far as I know.

To go on to another dream: At one time I had a really marvelous assistant—one of those people without any particular formal education whose gifts and life experience had produced the sort of person who automatically reassured terrified people. He possessed no suitable hooks that panicky young schizophrenics could use to hang their terror on, and he reflected in many other ways the naturally estimable personality structure that would be required for dealing with schizophrenics. In those days there was a great deal I didn't know about the risks attendant on dealing with human personality, and this young man rapidly became not only my left hand, but, I suppose, most of my left upper extremity. After the pattern of the-good-if-they-do-not-die-young, he became of great interest to a bitterly paranoid woman. Thanks to the eternal vigilance which we do preserve, however blindly, he was worried about this relationship, and talked to me about it. And I talked to him and talked to her, and counseled delay, because she seemed to be suffering frightfully from his very casual heterosexual life away from her, and I thought that such worries would grow if they were legitimatized, and so on. And also I didn't want him upset—he was too valuable. Whereupon he dreamed a dream. Some of you may have been in the environment of Baltimore and have seen Loch Raven. Loch Raven is one of those monolithic concrete dams which produce very beautiful artificial lakes behind them. And this monolithic dam is quite impressive—very high, with a wide sluiceway. This dream is set at the foot of the Loch Raven dam. There is an island, very small, very green—a lovely island—not far from the shore, on which this assistant of mine and I are walking, engaged in conversation. He gazes up at the dam and sees his fiancée at the top of it, and is not particularly distracted in his conversation with me. Then he observes that the area of water between the island and the shore, over which we had stepped, is rapidly widening. He awakens in terror, finding himself leaping out of bed into a pool of moonlight in the bedroom.[1]

The two illustrations I've given—and studiously refrained from interpreting—show how a good deal of waking activity—that is, activity we ordinarily associate with being awake—can actually carry into it surviving referential processes from the period of sleep, and that these processes take precedence over the capacity to actually perceive reality. Thus when a psychiatrist hears a patient report a dream and the patient is thoroughly undone by the reappearance of the uncanny emotion or the terror associated with the dream, the psychiatrist has to assume that he is seeing in this very situation grave peril to the maintenance of full awareness while one is nominally awake; in other words, the psychiatrist is literally seeing a mild schizophrenic episode right there in the office. In the same way, any of us who have difficulties in asserting our knowledge of reality on awakening from certain types of unpleasant dreams are, at least for a few minutes, living in a world completely of a piece with the world in which schizophrenics live for hours. In the practice of psychiatry, it is really up to the psychiatrist to observe the imminence of any such very serious upheaval of personality, and then to do something besides listening and preparing to hear free association in pursuit of the latent content. It is not possible here to do more than suggest what should be done in this kind of situation. But I will say that when the patient's anxiety is becoming, in the reporting of a dream, utterly unmanageable and very dangerous for the continuity of useful work, the psychiatrist should intervene. Intervention in this situation is but a special instance of intervention whenever the patient experiences such anxiety. Thus the psychiatrist should treat reported dreams, I believe, in the same way that he treats everything else that seems to be extremely significant: the psychiatrist reflects back to the person what has seemed to him to be the significant

[1] One might compare here somnambulistic performances in which people have complete freedom of locomotion—that is, complete control of their skeletal musculature and so on—but cannot discover what they were doing when they crawled around in their sleep, are completely cut off, in the act of being awakened, from whatever was going on, and, in fact, sometimes go back to bed with only accidental observers knowing anything about it.

statement, stripped of all the little personal details, confusions, and obscurities which often protect significant statements, and then sees if it provokes any thought in the mind of the patient.

To give an example: An obsessional neurotic, who is reporting on a highly significant difficulty he is having in living, will usually tell the psychiatrist different instances of much the same thing for perhaps six weeks. The instances gradually become somewhat clearer to the psychiatrist—that is, he can finally guess what the devil's really being reported. He can't possibly do it the first time because the patient deletes, through security operations, everything that would improve the psychiatrist's grasp on the subject. The patient has not lied; but he has neglected to report anything that would be highly provocative of the psychiatrist's grasping what's being reported. After the psychiatrist has delimited the area of the patient's careful deletions so that he can finally catch on to what's probably being reported, he can then say, "Well, is it that you are telling me that you did so-and-so and the other person did so-and-so?" Whereupon, with considerable anxiety the patient says, "Yes," and the psychiatrist has something to work on. I believe that it's the same with the dream, except that it doesn't take so long. The psychiatrist clears up as much as he can of what is irrelevant and obscuring in the reported dream, presents what he seems to hear in terms of a dramatic picture of some important problem of the patient's, and then propounds the riddle: "What does that bring to mind?" And if the psychiatrist has been good at it, it often brings something very significant from the patient.

For example, for many, many months in working with a schizoid obsessional patient, I heard data of how vaguely annoying and depressing his mother had been for several years past. His father was a hellion, to put it mildly, and we didn't have so much difficulty understanding what father did. But about all mother did was somehow to depress and annoy him, discourage him vaguely. Now this patient dreamed of a Dutch windmill. It was a very beautiful scene, with a carefully cared-for lawn leading up to the horizon on which this beautiful Dutch windmill revolved in the breeze. Suddenly he was within the windmill. And there everything was wrack and ruin, with rust inches deep; it was perfectly obvious that the windmill hadn't moved in years. And when the patient had finished reporting his dream, I was able to pick out the significant details successfully—one of those occasional fortunate instances. I said, "That is, beautiful, active on the outside—utterly dead and decayed within. Does it provoke anything?" He said, "My God, my mother." That was his trouble, you see. The mother had become a sort of zombi—unutterably crushed by the burdens that had been imposed on her. She was simply a sort of weary phonograph offering cultural platitudes, without any thought of what they did to anybody or what they meant. Though she was still showing signs of life, everything had died within. We made fairly rapid progress in getting some lucidity about the mother. You will note that I have not discussed the latent content of the dream; but in psychotherapy, as I've come to consider it, one is occupied chiefly in benefiting the patient.

Myths: Dreams That Satisfy the Needs of Many

The types of operations which are recalled, however imperfectly, from sleep are not limited in importance to the purpose they serve in the life pattern of the person who reports them. Some of them not only seem to serve some purpose for the person who had the dream, but come so near to dealing with general problems that they become incorporated into the culture as myths. And to understand the higher level of referential processes which we have named parataxic, there is perhaps no better approach than the study of highly significant dreams and myths which have held considerable force over perhaps centuries, certainly over the stretch of culture eras. And so I am going to mention a few of these myths. I would like to remind you that you will find very little here that is simply and directly explicit statement of fact, since I am now dealing with material that is inferential about parataxic processes in living.

The oldest myth that comes to my mind in this connection is that of Balaam and his ass. Quite recently I came in contact with this survival from the prehistory of the Western culture—that is, the Jewish culture—and I had an experience with it which is perhaps worth taking a little time on. During his long fatal illness, my beloved friend Sapir was reading the Bible in Aramaic and he encountered the myth of Balaam and his ass. He recounted it to me, and it annoyed me, and I made some unpleasant comment as I very often do when I am annoyed. The myth is something like this: Balaam was a very fine character indeed, one of the outstanding merchants and benefactors in a city which was under attack from certain 'barbarians' over the mountains. The city didn't seem to get very far with the 'barbarians,' and so finally Balaam was sent as an emissary—Balaam himself. And he mounted his ass and fared forth toward the mountains. And at a certain point the ass balked, and Balaam spoke gently to the ass, but the ass continued to balk. And so he beat the ass. And then the ass spoke—and this is the sort of thing that annoys me in dreams or myths—and said to Balaam, "Balaam, Balaam, why beatest thou me? Have I not always been thy faithful servant, responsive to your slightest request, patient under your increasing weight, and one thing and another?" Balaam was ashamed because of what the ass presented to him; and as he felt this shame, the scales fell from his eyes and he discovered an angel with a sword standing in the path in front of him, which accounted for the ass's balking. And, as I say, this myth annoyed me; but while I was waiting for a bus later that evening, it occurred to me that way back in this shadowy period some Jewish scholar had presented one of his dreams in this shape, and that it was a very simple statement of the relationship between our proud self-consciousness and our contact with life as a going concern. Balaam and his ass might well be human personality, and only the proud self-respect-pursuing part of personality would overlook the imminent danger—the whole personality would not. The psychiatrist finds unnumbered instances in his work in which people cling, with a certain tense franticness, to certain idealizations of life which get them into a great deal of trouble; but the intensity with which they cling indicates that the ass—the deeper, older part of personality—knows the thing isn't true, knows it isn't so. For the psychiatrist to be taken in by the intensity with which these ideals are presented is merely to fit into the chronic illness of the patient. If the psychiatrist observes the peculiar path in life which the patient is taking—in that the patient gives lip-service and a frantic amount of conscious attention to the ideal, and carefully vitiates it through other interpersonal performances —the psychiatrist will often discover that the patient is living by standards which were inculcated in childhood but which he knows from other experiences are not valid. But since the patient can't formulate what he knows, he goes on in the same old way.

I would like to refer only briefly to the subject of personal myths; many of us have such myths which we can be led to tell when we are tight enough or feeling friendly enough. For example, I sometimes tell the myth of the Stack family, which interests at least me.[2]

I shall now mention a myth which was borrowed from Northwestern European culture by the great musical genius, Wagner, and woven into the "Nibelung Ring"; the myth is of course the Rheingold. The Rheingold represented transcendental power that could be utilized by man. It was protected rather carefully by various beings from falling into the hands of any man, because the Rheingold when seized conferred such terrible powers on its stealers. Moreover, it should be noted that seizing the Rheingold brought doom, the doom being foretold by the weary earth-goddess, Erda. This myth illustrates a practically universal feeling, in all times and among all people, that to seize transcendental power may well be evil.

I am reminded of a story which is very much closer to us than the origins of Balaam and his ass or the Nibelung saga. It is Mark Twain's *The Mysterious Stranger*. After he had finished writing the story, he was moved to suppress it, stipulating that it not be published till after his death. I believe the scene is laid in a very beautiful Swiss village where everybody has known each other for generations. There was almost no evil in this community. Among the estimable young was a fine young boy greatly cherished in the community and with many friends. And this little country hero was out walking, basking in the natural beauties one morning, when he met another very lovely young man—a stranger. This

[2] [*Editors' note:* Sullivan has made scattered references to the legend of his mother's family throughout his published and unpublished writings. In one footnote, he says, for instance: ". . . consider an only surviving child of a proudly professional maternal family not yet recovered from the reduction in status that attended on grandfather's emigration—among the mythological ancestors of which is the West Wind, the horse who runs with the Earth into the future. . . ." "Towards a Psychiatry of Peoples," *Psychiatry* (1948) 11: p. 109.]

stranger seemed to be quite as attractive as our hero, who was a paragon of Swiss virtues. Our hero asked him his name, and he said, "My name is Satan." That startled our hero, so he said, "Well, not the Satan that—" "Oh, no, no, a remote relative, perhaps a second cousin." Well, Satan was taken to the bosom of the youthful community. He excelled in all sports, but also in appropriate humility, and the rest; in fact, he was an enormous addition to the community. Both young and old admired him.

One day, one of the other boys got caught in a whirlpool in one of the mountain rivers, and it was impossible to rescue him. Our hero, who was standing on the bank with Satan and suffering with the impending disaster, said aloud, "I would give almost anything to save John." And Satan said, "What!" And our hero said, "Yes, yes, I'd do anything to save him." And Satan said, "You wish to save him?" And our hero did. The stream suddenly dried up. The boy, of course, walked ashore. Then the account goes on for some time, during which, by a terrible inevitability, the rescued boy comes to a dreadful end, which wrings the heart of everyone ever so much more than would have his sudden death in the whirlpool. But two or three times more, our hero in the midst of his anxiety, terror, and grief over impending disaster expressed his mental state in such a way that Satan, this accommodating new friend, could realize what he wished. Each time Satan was astounded, but each time Satan intervened; and always dreadful, horrible, unutterable consequences flowed from this intervention of human wishes, not through Satan's action, just through the tedious interrelation of events. That myth, as written by Mark Twain, has passed into a certain decline; perhaps it is not hard to guess why. For there is a great distinction between what this myth says of life and of the evils of transcendental power at the disposal of man, and that which is said in the Nibelung myth of the Rheingold and in many other myths to be found in the lore of peoples.

Let me say in brief that both the myth and the dream represent a relatively valid parataxic operation for the relief of insoluble problems of living. In the myth, the problems concern many people, and it is this fact which keeps the myth going and refines and polishes it as the generations roll it around. The dream has that function for a person in an immediate situation; but insofar as he remembers it and communicates it, he is seeking validation with someone else. The schizophrenic illness, the living by the schizophrenic way, is the situation into which one falls when, for a variety of reasons, the intense handicaps of living are so great that they must be dealt with during a large part of one's waking life in this same dream-myth sort of way. Insofar as schizophrenic content, reported dreams, or personal myth are stripped of some decoration in the telling and thus undergo to some extent the general process of consensual validation, the dreamer, the schizophrenic, or the myth-maker has some awareness of aspects of his life problems that have hitherto been utterly prohibited from such awareness by security operation. In these terms, such content can be dealt with in therapy; but to deal with it on the basis that one can convert dreams or myths into consensually valid statements by intellectual operations seems to me such a misunderstanding—such a complete missing of the point of how we got along before we had consensually valid formulae—that I don't know how one can take it seriously. People who feel that they should analyze either a dream or schizophrenic content into what it stands for, seem to me to be in exactly the state of mind of the person who says to a child of two-and-a-half, "You ought to show more respect for your mother because God on Mount Sinai said to Moses, 'Honor thy father and thy mother.'" There are limits to what is practical and practicable. I do believe that the reporting of dreams can be very significant in intensive psychotherapy as long as the patient is not encouraged to waste time by whatever he can build up about his night life; but the importance of dreams lies in that which they obscurely deal with, which the psychiatrist may or may not be able to elicit. Obsessional ideas and schizophrenic content, and so on, are important in the same way, although the less troubled an obsessional is, the less important the content. In all these cases, the psychiatrist is dealing with the type of referential operation which is *not* in the syntaxic mode, and one merely stultifies himself, to my way of thinking, by trying to make this kind of report syntaxic. The fact that it is not syntaxic in no sense alters its validity and importance for the work.

CHAPTER

21

The Later Manifestations of Mental Disorder: Matters Paranoid and Paranoiac*

As I have already noted, failure to achieve late adolescence is the last blow to a great many warped, inadequately developed personalities with low self-esteem. And the usual solution in chronological maturity is to cover over one's chronic defect in self-esteem by disparaging others—a solution which is used by all of us in varying degrees.

Tributary Developmental Difficulties

In childhood, the deviations begin which, unless modified in the subsequent developmental eras, may result in disastrous mental disorder in later life. With the beginning of the emphasis on cooperation, the child undergoes the experience of fear when he does not live up to the required behavior, and the complex anxiety derivatives of shame and guilt are inculcated. Thus the child is presumed to deserve or require punishment at times, and this punishment takes the form of the infliction of pain, which may be accompanied by anxiety. As a result, the child often has to make

* [*Editors' note:* Through p. 348 of this chapter, we have had to rely largely on the Notebook, since no recording of the lecture itself was made. In order to provide the continuity of Sullivan's thinking, we have put into sentence form the topical outline given in his Notebook and expanded this on the basis of related material given elsewhere in this book. Beginning with the section on the Wish-Fulfilling Fantasy, the chapter is from a recorded lecture.]

complex discriminations of authority situations, so that the ability to conceal things from the authoritative figures and to deceive them becomes a necessity which is implemented by the authority-carrying figures themselves. As a part of this comes the development of precautionary techniques and propitiatory activities such as verbal 'excusing,' often with the evolution of techniques for the maintenance of 'social distance.'

A great many children learn that anger will aggravate the situation and they develop instead *resentment;* and resentment has very important covert aspects. Sometimes even the resentment has to be concealed in childhood, and this gradually results in a self-system process which precludes one's knowing his resentment. Again, I have commented on the fact that the manifesting of the need for tenderness toward the significant people around one often leads to one's being disadvantaged, made anxious, made fun of, and so on. And in this way the groundwork is laid for the malevolent attitude toward life in general, in which other people are viewed as enemies, which is the greatest disaster that happens in childhood, in that it may represent a great handicap for profitable experience in the subsequent stages of development.

In the juvenile era, the need for compeers brings about the threat of ostracism. There is a difference in background, abilities, in speed of maturation, and so on, which helps to set up the in-groups and the out-groups. And under this segregating influence, a great many juveniles feel ostracized and suffer a loss of self-esteem. Most people have had in the juvenile period an exceedingly bitter experience with their compeers to which the term "fear of ostracism" might be justifiably applied—the fear of being accepted by no one of those whom one must have as models for learning how to be human. In this era also there is the learning of disparagement, with the possibility for chronic defect in one's self-esteem. This disparagement has its beginning for the most part in influence exerted by the parental group, who teach the juvenile to notice the shortcomings of others. And this necessity of maintaining self-esteem by pulling down the standing of others, if uncorrected in subsequent developmental eras, has unfortunate later outcomes. In the juvenile era this kind of security operation literally and importantly interferes with adequate appraisal of personal worth. Since one has to protect his feeling of self-esteem by noting how unworthy everybody else is, this fails to provide any convincing data on one's having personal worth; one begins to think, "I am not as bad as the other swine."

But one hates one's 'weaknesses'—one's feeling of shame and guilt, one's loneliness—particularly if one believes in the doctrine of the transcendental will. It is clear that a very great number of people suffer from the illusion of voluntary choice and its attendant consequences of transcendentally conditioned guilt and self-blame; and the transcendental element is the supernatural character of the will, whether it is recognized as such or not.

Security Operations for Maintaining Selective Inattention

In some instances, these difficulties, as I have already noted, are remedied at the thresholds of the subsequent developmental eras. But sometimes there is failure to profit from experience. Even though there may be many actual opportunities, various security operations interfere with observation and analysis, and thus prevent the profit one might gain from experience.

We have already discussed the tedious miracle of selective inattention, which is, more than any other of the inappropriate and inadequate performances of life, the classic means by which we do not profit from experience which falls within the areas of our particular handicap. Since the identification of areas of selective inattention is an important part of the therapeutic intervention, I would like now to set up certain gross classifications of security operations which help to maintain selective inattention and which have their beginnings in childhood. For the areas of selective inattention are, like Balaam's ass, actually fields of experience. And these difficulties in living, as I have already mentioned, begin in childhood.

The first security operation for the maintenance of selective inattention is found in the dramatizations of roles which a person *knows to be false*. In other words, these spurious subpersonalities are more or less clearly assumed. Such a person adopts patterns of behaving *as if* he were someone else, although he privately knows he is not. Even though this often overtaxes his abilities, he must ignore his errors, lest he 'give himself away' completely.

Second, a person may use parataxic me-you patterns [1] which are incongruous with the actual interpersonal situation; and in this instance he has no clear realization of the multiple "personalities" involved and of the instability of his behavior. In this connection, we shall presently consider the esteemed psychiatric term "projection."

Third, a person may use substitutive processes running the gamut from 'deliberately' talking about something else, in the sense of changing the subject; through unwitting shifts of 'communicative set,' which can be very subtle (this has possible bearing on states called "excitement," in which people show extreme distractibility, staying on no particular topic for any length of time); to the utmost absorption in intense preoccupation with covert processes. The wish-fulfilling fantasy, which I shall presently discuss, is an example of the last of these substitutive processes. Preoccupation with covert processes may be with or without behavior which is, or borders on being, wholly inexplicable. But when the intense absorption spills over into speech, the speech is clearly uncommunicative. To illustrate these substitutive processes, I shall presently discuss hypochondriacal preoccupations and self-pity.

And, finally, there are transient or enduring "transformations of personality"—and remember that personality is here defined as the *relatively* enduring pattern of one's characteristic interpersonal relations. We have already discussed the malevolent transformation in childhood, in which one acts unpleasantly when one needs tenderness. We have also touched on the more transient transformation under the topic of fugue. We shall have more to say on transformation of personality with respect to the massive transfer of blame, or *paranoid transformation.*

Jealousy and Envy

Before going further, let me discriminate my meaning of the terms, jealousy and envy, which are often tossed around as synonyms. There is a fundamental difference in the felt components of

[1] [*Editors' note:* For a discussion of "me-you" patterns, see Patrick Mullahy, "A Theory of Interpersonal Relations and the Evolution of Personality," in *Conceptions of Modern Psychiatry.*]

envy and jealousy; and there is also a fundamental difference in the interpersonal situation in which these processes occur, for envy occurs in a two-group, with perhaps a subsidiary two-group made up of the person suffering envy and his auditor, while jealousy always appears in a relationship involving a group of three or more. I define envy, which is more widespread in our social organization than jealousy, as pertaining to personal attachments or attributes. It is a substitutive activity in which one contemplates the unfortunate results of someone else's having something that one does not have. And envy does not cease to be envy when it passes from objects to attributes of another human being, for envy may be an active realization that one is not good enough, compared with someone else. Although it involves primarily a two-group situation, one of the two may be a more-or-less mythological person.

Jealousy, on the other hand, never concerns a two-group situation. It is invariably a very complex, painful process involving a group of three or more persons, one or more of whom may be absolutely fantasied. Jealousy is much more poignant and devastating than envy; in contrast with envy, it does not concern itself with an attribute or an attachment, but, rather, involves a great complex field of interpersonal relations. While data are hard to get, apparently jealousy occurs frequently in adolescence, and frequently with real or fancied lustful involvement with someone else. In such cases, the jealous person has a deep conviction of his own inadequacy and unworthiness in participation in lustful involvement, along with the conviction that his partner and the third person could do much better.

Jealousy in malevolent situations often assumes delusional proportions, in which the person tends more or less insidiously to become inaccessible to remedial experience by being secretive and, later, by supplementary processes which make any factual data ineffective. Jealousy becomes properly termed paranoid when the sufferer "sees" that the second person in the threesome—the link—is doing things to make him jealous out of pure malice.

The "Wish-Fulfilling Fantasy"

I would like now to discuss the expression, "wish-fulfilling fantasy," which is, I suppose, still very fashionable. Now, there are, unquestionably, quite witting covert processes which go on in human beings, and there are, undoubtedly, many circumstances in which one, over a long period of time, derives some satisfaction, or freedom from severe anxiety, as a result of these witting covert processes. This is entirely in contradistinction to the type of process that goes on in sleep, or goes on in those waking states of abstraction when one doesn't know what one is thinking of —states to which such terms as "brown study" have been applied. In certain instances, these prolonged witting covert processes, or reverie processes, represent, beyond any shadow of doubt, a partial satisfaction of needs. And among these, the simplest of all are of a compensatory character, with awareness, ranging from vague to clear, of the felt need which is being satisfied by the reverie process. But these quite witting processes include some components which are less witting. Let us say, for example, that after having been rebuffed by a very charming woman met at a cocktail party, one sits at home having a drink later that evening, entertaining a fantasy that is quite the contrary of rebuff by this same charming woman. Even in a reverie of such a simple compensatory character, there are apt to be, in the actual content of the reverie processes, evidences of processes which are *not* simply the need which the fantasy principally satisfies. Furthermore, in a good many so-called wish-fulfilling fantasies, the principal motivating force is not primarily the satisfaction of a need, but is something pertaining to security, or freedom from anxiety. All of you have experienced classical instances of this. For example, let us say that somebody at a party makes a bright and perhaps disconcerting remark to you; later, while you are driving home, you think up the perfect response; this response, unhappily, has to be discharged in your reverie process since it comes after the situation has passed into history. Thus a great many of these so-called conscious reverie processes exist for the discharge of hostility and other disjunctive motivation, and for the relief of anxiety. And not at all infrequently, in the more unhappy type of person, a great deal of the so-called wish-fulfilling fantasy is actually of a very complex compensatory character, arising in various ways from chronic low self-esteem and self-blame.

When reverie processes of this 'witting-fantasy' sort are reported to the psychiatrist, he should carefully study them in order to determine to what extent they are 'mere' partial satisfactions, and to what extent they include elements of foreseeing—in other words, to what extent they are prospective reverie, tending to improve what one does in the next similar situation. Furthermore, the psychiatrist should determine what elements in the reverie are not really understood by the person who has the reverie, and the extent to which these elements reflect aspects of personality of which the patient is relatively unaware.[2]

Customarily Low Self-Esteem

I now want to touch upon a phenomenon that is described rather widely in the psychiatric literature and in the conversation of psychiatrists as "feelings of inferiority." I believe that this phenomenon can better be described as the experience of customarily low self-esteem—that is, the person's personification of himself is not very estimable by comparison with his personifications of significant other people. By low self-esteem, I do not mean accurate self-esteem in a person who has, indeed, had very few opportunities, or perhaps has limited abilities; low self-esteem is the outcome of certain unfortunate experiences. Now if one customarily entertains a low opinion of oneself, a great handicap is imposed on the manifestation of what I call *conjunctive motivations*. By this

[2] Thus the psychiatrist should think twice before too glibly dismissing something reported by the patient as "mere wish-fulfilling fantasy." For it is practically impossible for one to be entirely free from intervention of the self-system—even though one is just entertaining himself with daydreams. The element of partial satisfaction of genuine needs, the element of self-system function—the minimizing or avoiding of anxiety—the actual discharge of hostile disjunctive impulses which are in part anxiety, and the very complex processes necessary for the maintaining of dissociation—all these may be fairly easily discoverable in the structure of fantasies. Yet the psychiatrist often acts as if fantasies were some minor misdemeanor of the patient, or discusses them with colleagues as if they were silly little evidences of immaturity. Sometimes one of these fantasies is actually a manifestation of foresight—an analysis and planning of situations and study of possibilities in case similar situations appear in the future. In such cases it is particularly bad for the psychiatrist to practically denounce the fantasy to the patient as an instance of something not quite respectable. Thus I believe that talking with patients and colleagues about "wish-fulfilling fantasy" is misleading rather than helpful, and actually tends to limit the clarity of the psychiatrist's own thought.

term I refer to those impulses which integrate situations in which needs can be satisfied and security enhanced. The great classic example of conjunctive motivation is love, which, however rare in itself, has its great root tendencies in the many impulses which make up the need for intimacy. But customarily low self-esteem makes it difficult indeed for the carrier person to manifest conjunctive motivation—to find himself comfortably able to manifest good feeling toward another person.

People who have customarily low self-esteem may minimize their anxiety by concealments and social isolation, may channel their anxiety and disjunctive motivations in interpersonal relations by exploitative attitudes and substitutive processes, or may manifest them in dissociative processes.

Concealments and Social Isolation

Many of the people who have this customarily low self-esteem minimize their anxiety by the use of sundry concealments, one extreme of which is *actual* social isolation. In any event, there is usually some degree of social isolation, for these people are unapproachable excepting on certain bases stipulated by them. Perhaps the crudest instance of this is found in the person who conceals by elaborate fictions which have become practically true—that is, the person who uses them has become so accustomed to them and so skillful in their indication or expression that he scarcely doubts them himself. As a general rule, then, a person with customarily low self-esteem has some form or degree of social isolation—that is, some degree of limitations or stipulations on his contact with others.

Exploitative Attitudes

Another aspect of these people with customarily low self-esteem is that anxiety and other disjunctive motivations—many of which, such as hatred, are derivatives of anxiety—tend to be channeled, in interpersonal relations, in a number of ways that are not perfectly obvious. Since conjunctive—that is, tender, friendly—relations with significant others are very difficult for these people, many of them have a *direct exploitative attitude*, to which psychiatric slang has attached the term "passive dependency." Here again, instead of merely making ourselves comfortable by using the words, let us try to think what it would feel like to *live* such a thing. What happens is that a person who has a low opinion of himself develops a relatively suave way of manifesting, if not inferiority to significant people, at least such blatant hints of inferiority that he becomes more or less an object of philanthropic concern on the part of the other person. This represents the development of considerable skill in interpersonal relations—sometimes remarkable skill—although the actual motivation concerned in these interpersonal relations is all relatively unfriendly. Now, since people with chronically low self-esteem are involved in these situations, the situations are apt to be somewhat unpleasant and complex for the other people involved—particularly if the other people are prone to find themselves in relationships in which domineering and vassalizing their fellows is their source of security. Under those circumstances, the passive-dependent people fall very readily into the orbit of these others, and all concerned do a great deal for one another without any particular satisfaction.

More puzzling for the psychiatrist is the *indirect exploitative attitude* for channeling disjunctive motivations, in which this almost explicit admission of inferiority does not appear. Instead, there is a sort of continuous offer that one can be found to be dependent. It suggests to me the expression "come-on"; one offers, but one does not quite deliver. One cannot bear to be regarded as dependent—and this is the reason for the indirection; a person has to have some complications in the business to save what self-esteem he has. In this connection a theory of personality and interpersonal relations has appeared, in the literature of the recent past, that is built up, in striking part, on the notion of masochism; I don't now keep up with all competing theories, so this one may have been laid away in its grave—I would hope so. I think there's probably nothing in the notion of masochism except foggy thinking. Masochism was, I believe, brought over the horizon of psychiatric thought in intimate companionship with another notion, called sadism. And in those estimable days, it was all very simple: People who liked to be hurt, as well as to be engaged in lustful sports, were masochists; and those who liked to hurt the partner, as well as engage in lustful sports, were sadists. But after the habit of a fungus the thing grew and got all sorts of places. And masochism has finally, I think, been attenuated to such a point that if a person keeps quiet while somebody else is talking, it could be called the manifestation of a masochistic tendency. In any event, there is a large number of people who appear to go to rather extraordinary lengths to get themselves imposed on, abused, humiliated, and what not; but as you get further data, you discover that this quite often pays—in other words, they get things they want. And the things that everybody wants are satisfaction and security from anxiety. Thus these people who get themselves abused and so on are indirectly getting the other people involved in doing something useful in exchange.

Another aspect of the indirect exploitative attitude might be termed "preying on sympathy." Actually this way of channeling disjunctive motivation approaches the substitutive activities, which I shall discuss next, and may indeed often be confused with them. Preying on sympathy, as an indirect exploitative attitude, is manifested in a development of interpersonal technique by which, no matter whether the person has done something rather exceptional or has made a very dreary flop, he has to get some audience to feel sorry that he was laboring under such handicaps. This group includes people who after having said, "Good morning," begin to rattle off a long list of current minor disasters and worries that have crushed their spirits completely, simply in the expectation that you will show sympathetic understanding of their woe—whereupon they look for the next person. This is, I suppose, indirect exploitation at its most highly symbolic level; it doesn't seem to be much of anything else. Of course, this preying on sympathy can also serve the much more practical purposes of tying your hands so that you can't criticize the person for something that is really detrimental to you and your interests; and there the indirect exploitative attitude is quite clear.

Substitutive Processes

But it is not always meaningful, in thinking of interpersonal difficulties, to describe such behavior as "preying on sympathy." For instance, it may not be self-evident whether the behavior has anything indirectly exploitative in it or whether it is a part of this vast body of complex performances which we call substitute activity; it is particularly difficult to make this distinction in dealing with a stranger. Substitute activity, in contrast to indirect exploitative attitudes, is not addressed primarily to an audience; instead it is addressed primarily to avoiding certain conscious clarity about one's own situation, one's own motivations, and so on. When this is the case, the apparent "preying on sympathy" actually touches more upon a preoccupation which, for want of a better term, I shall call "self-pity." And this preoccupation is actually in the realm of substitutive processes. It is important to distinguish between two kinds of self-pity in trying to clarify one's thoughts about what sort of problem one has on one's hands. It may be a massive preoccupation—an extraordinary facility at filling up time, in reverie or in conversation, with long series of thoughts which wind up with the speaker practically in tears about how wretchedly he is treated by fate. Or it may be a concomitant of only certain situations in a relatively limited field. People with massive preoccupation—and this is one of the fields of my greatest defeats in therapy—meet almost all interpersonal situations in which they feel inferior to the other person by looking for anything that can be utilized in building up one of these long trains of covert or conversational processes which serve to show what a woebegone and very unhappily used person the speaker is. But in the second group, although the preoccupation is substitutive in the sense that it obliterates something costly to self-esteem, the preoccupation is in a particular context, and does not represent a very unhappy way of life. For example, I sometimes say and feel very deeply that my lectures have not gone very well or been very clear because I was too tired. In any event, preoccupations with one's misfortune which represent pure substitution for something much more disturbing are legion. But it is the psychiatrist's job, when such a preoccupation comes along, to discriminate whether it is exploitative or substitutive—to figure out, to put it crudely, whether he is being put on the spot to do something for the other person, or whether this is a process by which the other person is keeping off the spot with himself. In other words, the substitutive processes are primarily addressed to minimizing or avoiding anxiety, whereas the more exploitative techniques are ways of getting what one wants but feels one could not get on one's face value.

This element of self-pity is within calling distance of a group of substitutive activities which I have already mentioned—that enormously popular business of entertaining envy. Envy perhaps is in no sense self-pity, but certainly it is substitutive activity. It is called out in all sorts and kinds of situations where the person with customarily low self-esteem is disturbed. And it saves one from invidious comparisons which would be anything but uplifting to one's self-regard.

Now, beyond these preoccupations I have mentioned, there are the hypochondriacal preoccupations, a field of substitutive activities which ordinarily channel the anxiety and other unfriendly or disjunctive motivations that are more or less characteristic of people who have chronically low self-esteem—although sometimes they can serve even conjunctive impulses. Hypochondriacal preoccupations, which is the traditional term for great preoccupation with one's health or with the operation of certain parts of one's somatic apparatus, are not devices for preying on sympathy; curiously enough, there are some people who show hypochondriacal preoccupations only in the face of the other person's strong friendly motivation. These preoccupations are a very special group of substitute activities which are to be understood on the basis of one's personifying oneself as customarily handicapped. They are not to be understood as preoccupation with one's health in the sense of always wondering if one might catch a cold, or something of that kind; they are much more specific. For example, I know a very distinguished man who travels a great deal, always equipped with a fair-sized suitcase containing drugs enough to put a country general practitioner to shame in terms of preparation for any form of illness that man might fall heir to. While I am, needless to say, being extravagant, it sometimes seems to me that my friend carries preparations for practically any eventuality from smallpox to pregnancy; and among them he carries treatments for a large series of weaknesses, illnesses, and disabilities which he *has*. He's a very efficient person, by the way; I love to think what he'd be if he did not have all this really dangerous substitute activity going on in him. But time and again, on occasions when I was perhaps within gunshot of being bored, I've seen him suddenly become preoccupied and hurry away; and I know just what he does: he goes home and treats the malady which showed signs of becoming active under the same circumstances in which I became bored. My friend is an unusual instance, however, because the hypochondriacal person ordinarily doesn't manifest extraordinary gifts, broad interests, or anything of that kind. He is, on the other hand, capable of very deep preoccupation with his pulse rate, which is not taken as such, of course, but as evidence of serious risks surrounding the heart; he can give a tremendous amount of attention to his digestive tract, a preoccupation which I think is much more common; and—this is indeterminately common—he is capable of very deep preoccupation with sensations, or the absence of sensations, in the urogenital tract.

Thus in these deep, absorbing preoccupations, in which one loses practically all touch with things outside of oneself short of fire, there is great centering of conscious referential process on tiny little signs, often grossly and dreadfully misinterpreted, of something going on somewhere in the somatic organization of the body. Perhaps an illustration would serve to clarify what I am discussing here. A good many young men who have had very unfortunate experience, who are intensely socially isolated, and who are about to have a schizophrenic episode, show a particular type of hypochondriacal preoccupation with their genitals. This preoccupation has the following substance to it: When one is tense, the urinary bladder wall is tense, which in turn makes for high pressure against the internal urethral sphincter. If then the person is distracted, it is quite possible for the internal sphincter to relax according to the general pattern of getting ready for action. That permits a drop of urine to escape from the bladder into the prostatic urethra, which produces a distinct urgency to urinate. But it is quite possible that this sequence of events may not be completed in the person who has the particular type of hypochondriacal preoccupation with the genitals which I am discussing. So although the drop of urine escapes into the prostatic urethra, the person goes on into new tensions which somewhat distract him from the necessity to urinate. A little while later, the person becomes entirely absorbed in the, to him, awful experience of having seminal fluids sneaking out through the penis; in fact, he may actually inspect the penis, and he may then see a very little visible, palpable moisture at the meatus of the penis. To him, here is proof that he is losing vitality—for semen can take on remarkable symbolic importance. And this was all because he was too distracted and too preoccupied to notice that he might have urinated. Now, this situation gets wound up to the point where it practically becomes a vicious circle: the person is constantly anxious about this loss of vitality by way of the semen; and he loses it any time he's distracted by contact with anybody else or by any idea and so on, because at that time the internal sphincter is apt to relax a little bit; so the drop of urine gets in the prostatic urethra and then gets metamorphosed by this profound preoccupation with further loss of semen. Now this is an instance of hypochondriacal preoccupation which has been of such great interest to me that I've taken the trouble to figure out how a great many instances of it happen. Let me assure you that it is no more complex in its structure than a great many other hypochondriacal preoccupations with which certain desperately unhappy people can occupy practically their whole waking life.

I now want to discuss the special instance in which social isolation is combined with these hypochondriacal interests, in which case the latter are an important part of the dissociative system within the self-system. In this connection, one must remember that in addition to a motivational system which is dissociated—completely cut off from representation within awareness—there is also a complex system composed of dissociative processes which *maintain* this dissociation. In other words, one cannot maintain a dissociation without having a lot of precautionary apparatus, and so on, in the self-system to avoid any sudden crashing of the dissociation. These hypochondriacal interests quite often are part of the dissociative system, in which case one would expect these interests to become extreme and absorbing whenever the interpersonal relation is such that something in dissociation tends to become active. This is often strikingly demonstrable in the group of young men I have just mentioned. It is one of the classical occasions on which the careless psychiatrist might say that the patient 'blocked.' In other words, as a conversation between the psychiatrist and the patient moves into a region which might, by some accident, stir a dissociated tendency in the patient, then the patient becomes profoundly preoccupied with the fact that he is now losing a little more vitality. But since this thought is always fringed with the possibility of uncanny emotion, he doesn't tell the psychiatrist about it. And in any case, the patient feels that it is profoundly irrelevant to what he was talking about. All this is accompanied by such unpleasant emotion and has such preoccupying power that whatever he was talking about is as completely lost as if it had been erased. The psychiatrist has to start all over again, and if he and the patient can get to the same place at which blocking first occurred, blocking will probably occur again at that place. Of course, it is unlikely that they can get to the same point, because the patient will be already warned and will block as soon as that progression barely gets started.

"Being Taken Advantage Of"

The subject that I now want to discuss may seem to be quite removed from what I have just discussed, but actually it is quite closely related. The experience that I will describe is ordinarily called "being taken advantage of." This is probably within the experience of everyone, and very sadly and frequently within the experience of some people. Some of the less significant instances of this experience are, for example, being cheated or outwitted in the realm of real property. But the instances which I am concerned with here occur when someone takes advantage of you in such a way as to lead you to expose a weakness; as a result of this exposure, you suffer real or fantasied ridicule and have a feeling of being humiliated. I am quite sure that most of you can recall at least one person, in your more distant past life, who would now and then, as if by malice aforethought, entrap you into doing or saying something for which he then ridiculed you. In adult life, you may still find yourself occasionally in such situations; but now you probably have so much presence, so much caution and social distance, that the nearest you come to following the earlier pattern is that you wonder if the other person is ridiculing you; at least that's the ordinary attenuation.

A discussion of real or fancied ridicule seems a good place to embark on a discussion of "projection." When we get to the point of wondering whether people are admiring us or ridiculing us, we may have some little difficulty in distinguishing between that situation and what is usually meant by projection. But first I want to comment on the loose use of the term, projection. To begin with, we project in all interpersonal relations. We attempt to foresee action; we foresee it as the activity of embodied others; and that in itself is projection. Thus foresight applies in those situations in which you have put your worst foot forward and you think that the person who led you into the situation will now tell others about it with joy. But the term projection, as it is often used in psychiatry, seems to mean—if it means anything—that we project the wrong thing; for example, when I'm thinking very well of you, you 'project' upon me malice, hatred, and contempt! Well, that's nice—for certain late-evening-alcoholic psychiatric discussions. What I want to stress is that the degree to which foresight can be good, adequate, and appropriate, and the degree to which it can be far beside the point, is a matter which varies in everyone, from occasion to occasion, on such bases as what motivational complex is at work in the one person, what motivational complex is at work in the other, how tired the one or the other is, and, literally, what the recent past has been. I have already suggested the degree to which people with chronically low self-esteem anticipate unfavorable opinions in others; and I do not think that the mechanism of projection accounts for much of anything.

The Failure of Dissociation

I now want to consider a particularly important situation which arises as a special instance in these people with chronically low self-esteem who have advantage taken of them. And this is the situation in which the weakness which is so revealed actually includes some evidences of a dissociative system in the personality concerned. And, in these instances, the experience of being led to reveal one's weakness is, briefly or permanently, attended by some measure of the uncanny emotions—awe, dread, loathing, and horror. These emotions are, in many ways, the nearest that anybody comes to the reality of dissociated components in his personality, unless a person plunges into the sort of waking bad dream of schizophrenia. These, then, are instances of momentary representation within awareness, or of more durable representation within awareness, of the not-me phase of personality, which I can scarcely say is ordinarily personified, but which under certain unfortunate circumstances *can* now become personified. As I have noted briefly before, these situations may be accompanied either by such fascination that the person, despite dreadful feelings, cannot seem to avoid being entangled with this unpleasant person who has taken advantage of him; or else by revulsion, which is an extreme avoidance coupled with an uncanny feeling, so powerful and intense that the person is in the unhappy position of wondering what on earth could have made this particular affair so repulsive—which, in itself, is an unhappy addition to one's self-awareness. Or these situations may be accompanied by the still more chilling *awful suspicion* by which one really begins to build up structures of probability—or improbability—which become more and more uncanny.

And here we approach the experience of *jealousy*. Now jealousy may either be not particularly uncanny; or it may be what older psychiatrists call "delusional jealousy." Its form of manifestation is, in a large measure, determined by the extent to which dissociated systems are involved in its occurrence. That is to say, according to my experience with patients, jealousy is colored by uncanny emotion to the extent that dissociated systems are involved. And the more uncanny—that is, the more pathological—and the more marked the jealousy, the more fantastic one or two of the three people concerned will prove to be. This fantastic character is a complex function of the defense which the self-system exercises against the appearance of dissociated motivation; and insofar as that defense has to be vigorous, the dissociative distortions become striking.

Beyond fascination, significant revulsion, and awful suspicion, the next stage—in this unhappy concomitant of one's having been led unfairly to reveal one's weakness which happens to have something to do with a dissociative system—is the occurrence of what I will call *full-fledged "autochthonous" ideas*. Now, this tedious old word refers to a content of thought, a matter in mind, which seems literally to have come from outside one, as if put there—that is, one has no feeling of ownership or parentage. Thus while the self-system excludes from awareness clear evidences of a dissociated motivational system, that which is dissociated is represented in awareness by some group of ideas or thoughts which are marked uncannily with utter foreignness—they have nothing to do with oneself. And they really have nothing to do with oneself except that they are a kind of compromise.

The next step in this unhappy process is the actual occurrence of *hallucinations*, which with astonishing frequency are auditory. The occurrence of hallucinations means not only that one has something in mind which seems foreign and imposed from outside, but that one experiences events which are uncanny—one hears something which is strongly colored with a feeling of awe, dread, horror, loathing, or something of that kind. The hallucination has, so far as I know, every indication of being a perfectly valid experience, except that it is uncanny. And whether the hallucination needs any external source or not is perfectly irrelevant—in fact, the question is one of the most tedious topics of psychiatric drivel.

The Paranoid Transformation of Personality

Although hallucinations do not necessarily usher in schizophrenic episodes, they very frequently do so. And I would now like to discuss briefly what happens when the schizophrenic episode has occurred, followed—often quite promptly—by what I call a paranoid transformation of personality. In these situations, it is now impossible to maintain reasonable dissociation of previously dissociated tendencies in one's personality which are still, in terms of the personified self, *apart*. As a result, that which was dissociated, and which was in a certain meaningful sense related to the not-me, is now definitely *personified* as not-me—that is, as *others*. And the others carry blame for that which had previously had to be maintained in dissociation as an intolerable aspect of one's own personal possibilities.

Now, at the beginning of this transformation, the only impression one has is of a person in the grip of horror, of uncanny devastation which makes everyone threatening beyond belief. But if the person is not utterly crushed by the process, he can begin rather rapidly to elaborate personifications of evil creatures. And in this process of personifying the specific evil, the transformation begins to move fast, since it's wonderfully successful in one respect: it begins to put on these others—people who are outside of him, his enemies—everything which he has clearly formulated in himself as defect, blamable weakness, and so on. Thus as the process goes on, he begins to wash his hands of all those real and fancied unfortunate aspects of his own personality which he has suffered for up to this time. Under those circumstances, needless to say, he arrives at a state which is pretty hard to remedy—by categorical name, a paranoid state. If the schizophrenic prelude is very inconspicuous—in which case, I might add, the development may be in some ways a little more ominous—the beginning phase of the paranoid state has a curious relationship with what I call moments of 'illumination.' These occur when, by extremely fortunate circumstance, one actually sees, to a considerable extent, a real situation that he had been selectively inattending to previously, so that he is really better oriented. But far more common than these fortunate illuminations is the onrushing of this paranoid transformation of personality—the transfer of blame—in which the person suddenly 'sees it all.' The beginning of this process comes literally as a sudden insight into some suspicion and it comes with a blaze of horror. The suspicion may have hovered around before the sudden insight, and may have been marked by a little uncanniness; but with the insight, one has started living in a world in which not-me has become personified, very active, and very absorptive of one's weaknesses.

Now, the thing that ties all this together is that in some people there is an interweaving and alternation of hypochondriacal preoccupations and paranoid interpersonal relations. Intense hypochondriacal preoccupations often usher in disasters which can emerge from schizophrenia as paranoid transformations. At certain times, in the course of the paranoid way of existence, there can be a recession of all this fearing of enemies and seeing plots, and so on, in favor of a profound preoccupation with disorder of the bodily function—with the idea of disastrous things going on.[3] This

[3] It is interesting to note that hypochondriacal preoccupation is not preoccupation with healthy function, as the hebephrenic deterioration seems to be.

alternation—which many of us have encountered, for it's not too uncommon—is of very considerable importance in suggesting the reality underlying the conceptual structure of not-me.

I think that I can hint at the processes concerned in this interweaving of hypochondriacal preoccupations and paranoid states by mentioning the only very markedly paranoid schizophrenic whom I ever brought to what I felt might imply ultimate recovery. This boy, as he began to really clear up after a very extensive paranoid schizophrenic illness, still complained of his throat. His throat bothered him terribly. It was very difficult to quite discover what symptoms accompanied it, but there was no shadow of doubt that he was profoundly preoccupied with his throat. I sent him to a laryngologist who was both very skillful and quite sympathetic to the problems of psychiatry. The boy's throat was examined very carefully, and at the same time he was given a fine anatomical textbook and was permitted to look at it and to notice how neatly his throat coincided with the skillfully colored anatomical picture. And he went away very deeply touched; it had been a very successful adventure. But the next time I saw him, he came into the office and said, "Look, Doctor, I don't care anything about what ails my throat; I want something cut out."

PART IV

Towards a Psychiatry of Peoples

CHAPTER 22*

PSYCHIATRY has come to mean something to a great many people, but, for our purpose, it must be defined. There is a meaning of psychiatry which makes it an art or body of empirical practices pertaining to the treatment or prevention of mental disorder. This meaning of psychiatry is irrelevant, here. Psychiatry, as here to be discussed, is a science and its related technology. The science of psychiatry has been nurtured by work with the mentally ailing, has grown in the milieu of hospital and clinic, but is no more a science of mental illness than geography is a science of Western Europe.

The mentally ill are particular instances of people living among others in localities of more or less uniform culture. The science that has grown from preoccupation with these mentally disordered ways of living has naturally to become a science of living under the conditions which prevail in the given social order. I believe that this statement is simply axiomatic, but it does not imply that a particular psychiatric scientist need concern himself with any and all aspects of man's life in society.

A physicist may usefully concentrate his scientific efforts on particular aspects of the phenomena anciently called *light*. His results, so far as they are good physics, will be meaningful throughout physics. They may be more richly meaningful in, for example, the region of wave motion than in that of gravitation; but here one may recall the confirmation of Einstein's anticipation that light would be found to 'bend' in traversing a gravitational field.

The general science of psychiatry seems to me to cover much

* [*Editors' note:* This chapter is mainly taken from "Towards a Psychiatry of Peoples" (*Psychiatry* 11:105–116). Beginning with the section headed "Whence the Urgency," there appears an excerpt from "Remobilization for Enduring Peace and Social Progress" (*Psychiatry* 10:239–252; p. 244). Most of the chapter has also been reprinted in *Tensions That Cause Wars*, edited by Hadley Cantril (Univ. of Ill. Press, 1950).]

the same field as that which is studied by social psychology, because scientific psychiatry has to be defined as the study of interpersonal relations, and this in the end calls for the use of the kind of conceptual framework that we now call *field theory*. From such a standpoint, personality is taken to be hypothetical. That which can be studied is the pattern of processes which characterize the interaction of personalities in particular recurrent situations or fields which 'include' the observer. Since any one participant observer can study but a finite number of these situations or fields, which, in turn, will be anything but representative of the whole variegated world of human life, not all of the personality of the observer will be revealed and 'what he comes to know about himself' will always be somewhat incomplete and variously contingent on poorly defined or actually unnoticed factors. Generalizations which he can make about "the other fellow" cannot but be even more incomplete and contingent.

The observer, the instrument used in assembling the data of psychiatry, is, then, seen to be an only imperfectly understood tool, some of the results of the use of which may be quite misleading. This conclusion might be taken to forbid any effort toward developing a scientific psychiatry, much less a psychiatry of everyone everywhere in the world. It certainly forbids any conceit about the present state of psychiatry, but one may well notice that every science has been—and, less obviously, still is—in the same position. One may note, also, that ignorance of the principles of the internal-combustion engine has not prevented the expert driving of automobiles, although it might prove costly to anyone who substituted a high explosive for gasoline fuel because he was in a hurry.

Bear with me now in an attempt to outline a position in general psychiatry from which I shall presently undertake to make some temporarily valid generalizations of world scope. What anyone can observe and analyze becomes ultimately a matter of *tensions* and *energy transformations*, many of the latter being obvious *actions*, but many others of which are obscure activities that go on, as we say, in the mind.

What anyone can discover by investigating his past is that the *patterns* of tensions and energy transformations which make up his living are, to a truly astonishing extent, matters of his education for living in a particular expected society. If he is clever, he can also notice inadequacies in his educators' expectations; he finds that he is not any too well-prepared for living in the groups in which he has come to be involved.

If he is philosophically inclined and historic minded, he is apt to conclude that this very element of being ill-prepared has characterized people in every period of expanding world contacts and ensuing accelerated social change.

If he is interested in psychiatry, he is almost certain to come to consider the role of *foresight* in determining the adequacy and appropriateness of the energy transformations, his overt and covert activity, with respect to the actual demands of the situations in which he finds himself involved with significant others.

I touch here on what I believe is the most remarkable of human characteristics, the importance exercised by often but vaguely formulated aspirations, anticipations, and expectations which can be summed up in the term, foresight, the manifest influence of which makes the near future a thoroughly real factor in explaining human events. I hope that you will resist the idea that something clearly teleological is being introduced here: I am saying that, *circumstances not interfering*, man the person lives with his past, the present, and the neighboring future all clearly relevant in explaining his thought and action; and the near future is influential to a degree nowhere else remotely approached among the species of the living.

Note that I have said "circumstances not interfering." It is from study of the interferences which reduce, or otherwise modify, the functional activity of foresight that a great deal of light has been thrown on the nature of man as revealed in his doings with others.

We assume that all biological tensions arise from the course of events "inside" and/or "outside" the gross spatial limits of the organism. Human tensions are no exception to this, but one of their congeries—one very important kind of tension—ensues from a kind of events the experiencing of which is almost unique to the human being.

With this single important exception, tensions can be regarded as needs for particular energy transformations which will dissipate the tension, often with an accompanying change of "mental state," a change of awareness, to which we can apply the general term *satisfaction.*

Thus the particular tension the felt component of which we call *hunger* is pleasantly satisfied by activity which includes the taking of food. Our hunger is *not* the tension, the tension is not merely a "mental state," a phenomenon within awareness, nor is it entirely "within" us in any simple space-time sense. But for practical purposes, I may usually trust this particular once-familiar "mental state" to coincide perfectly with my need for food, and "make up my mind to eat," or "decide to go to dinner," or entertain within awareness some other 'thought' which sounds as if something quite powerful named "I" is directing something else, "myself," to do something about "my being hungry" with reasonable certainty that I shall feel more comfortable, when the performance has been finished.

Whatever pomp and circumstance may go on "in one's head," the need for food reaches into the past in which it has arisen, and on the basis of which its felt component can be said to have 'meaning,' and it reaches into the future in which its tension can be foreseen to have been relieved by appropriate action in proper circumstances.

We share most, if not all, of this large congeries of recurrent needs with a good many other species of the living—even including our recurrent need for contact with others, often felt as *loneliness,* which is paralleled in the gregarious animals.

The single other great congeries of recurrent tensions, some grasp on the nature of which is simply fundamental to understanding human life, is probably restricted to man and some of the creatures which he has domesticated. It arises not from the impact of physicochemical and biological events directly connected with keeping alive and reproducing the species, but from the impact of people. The felt component of any of this congeries of tensions includes the experience of *anxiety;* action which *avoids* or *relieves* any of these tensions is experienced as continued or enhanced *self-respect* or *self-esteem,* significantly different from what is ordinarily meant by self-satisfaction. All the factors entering into the vicissitudes of self-esteem, excepting only man's innate capacity for being anxious, are wholly a matter of past experience with people, the given interpersonal situation, and foresight of what will happen.

There is nothing I can conceive in the way of interpersonal action about which one could not be trained to be anxious, so that if such an action is foreseen one feels anxious, and if it occurs one's self-esteem is reduced. The realm of this congeries of tensions is the area of one's *training for life* at the hands of significant others, and of how much or little one has been able to synthesize out of these training experiences.

One cannot be trained by others in advance of certain biological events; namely, the maturation of appropriate capabilities of man the underlying animal. Training efforts exerted before this time are undergone as something very different from what was "intended" and, if they have any effect, exert thoroughly unfortunate influence on the future development of the victim.[1] This biologically ordained serial maturation of capabilities underlies the currently entertained scheme of stages in human development [infancy, childhood, the juvenile era, preadolescence, early adolescence, and late adolescence to maturity]. . . . Let me discuss the implication of the idea of developmental stages. When, and only when, maturation of capacities has occurred, experience of a valuable kind can occur. *If it does not occur*, if experience is definitely unsuited to providing competence for living with others, at this particular level of development, the probabilities of future adequate and appropriate interpersonal relations are definitely *and specifically* reduced. The reduction of probability is specifically related to the forms of competence which are customarily developed under favorable circumstances in the course of this particular stage.

Seen from this viewpoint, not the earlier stages only, but each and every stage, is equally important in its own right, in the unfolding of possibilities for interpersonal relations, in the progression from birth toward mature competence for life in a fully human world. It is often true that severe warp incurred, say, in

[1] They generally contribute to the not-me component of personality, the source of the tension in interpersonal fields elsewhere described as the experience of uncanny emotions—awe, dread, loathing, and horror—felt components of the most strongly disjunctive force of which we have knowledge.

childhood interferes so seriously with the course of events in the succeeding juvenile era that the constructive effects of living with compeers, and under school and other nonfamily authorities, are meager. It also happens, and not infrequently, that quite serious warp from childhood is all but corrected by good fortune early in the juvenile era, so that its residual traces are observable only under circumstances of "intense emotion," severe "fatigue," anoxemia, hypoglycemia, or alcoholic and related "decerebration." [2]

In the course of intensive, guided psychotherapy one may observe, in many instances, a condensed, relatively vicarious, remedying of deficiencies in developmental experience, and this seems to be a successful way of consolidating favorable change in the patient's interpersonal relations.

Thus unremedied misfortune in the preadolescent phase leaves one at a lifelong disadvantage in dealing with important strangers of the same sex. *When this pattern of discomfort has been made clear* by participant observation 'with' the patient, the latter will often develop a belated, transient, preadolescence. Some previously guarded contact will deepen into a very warm friendship; the satisfactions and security of the "buddy" become overwhelmingly important to the patient and his current activities are largely directed to promoting them. At the same time, any strong motivation in the patient-physician relationship is in abeyance, as if he had lost any particular interest in the work. Then, presently, the 'outside' attachment loses intensity and a favorably changed patient is again at work with the psychiatrist, tracking down the ramifications of the disability from which he is now recovering.

This illustrates the meaning of isophilic in my triad: the autophilic, the isophilic, and the heterophilic are those persons, respectively, who can manifest in their interpersonal relations the pattern of field forces properly called *love* for no one, for a person of one's own sex, or for persons of one's own and of the other sex. The ability to love is a factor in the patterning of genital, sexual, behavior; but it is only one of three factors which must be considered in order to 'make sense' of what goes on in that con-

[2] Even in these 'reduced' states, the peculiarities of interpersonal relations can sometimes be seen to be a movement as if to remedy ancient deficiencies of experience.

nection. In this culture, many people show the ability to love in advance of the occurrence of puberty. Many others have yet to evolve the ability to love long after a relatively active sexual life of one kind or another has been established.

Much more important, for my present purpose, is the import of the illustration as an example of 'curative' processes in interpersonal fields. It is from prolonged consideration of psychotherapeutic "successes" and "failures"—and of possibilities for increasing the proportion and speeding the achievement of the former—that I have come to feel sure that we may depend on everyone's drive toward more adequate and appropriate ways of living; in a word, toward improved mental health, *if* an improved ability to foresee the future can offer a fair prospect of becoming contented. That "if" is a big one when one has been 'out of life' for years in a hospital for the mentally disordered, when one is advanced in years, or when the prospect appears to entail giving up sources of prestige and income which one's current, however troubled, life is providing.

The often great difficulty encountered in achieving improved ability to live with significant others is considered to arise, then, not from a deficiency of tendency but from something else; something which manifests itself as an equilibrating factor in living, whether the living be fortunate or unfortunate; namely, the extensive organization of experience within personality which I have called the *self-system.*

I think it will suffice for my present purpose to say that anything which would seriously disturb the equilibrium, any event which tends to bring about a basic change in an *established pattern* of dealing with others, sets up the tension of anxiety and calls out activities for its relief. This tension and the activities required for its reduction or relief—which we call *security operations* because they can be said to be addressed to maintaining a feeling of safety in the esteem reflected to one from the other person concerned—always interfere with whatever other tensions and energy transformations they happen to coincide with.

This in no way denies the usefulness of security operations. They are often quite successful in protecting one's self-esteem. Without them, life in an increasingly incoherent social organization would be exceedingly difficult or impossible for most people. We, the people of these United States, in particular, would quite certainly exterminate ourselves before we could devise and disseminate adequate substitutes for our now ubiquitous security processes.

Let us be very clear about the fact that anxiety and security operations are an absolutely necessary part of human life as long as the past is more important in preparing the young for life than is the reasonably foreseeable future.

But for all their indispensable utility to each and every one of us, in these days, security operations are a powerful brake on personal and on human progress—as I can perhaps indicate by referring to a particular one of them which is very frequently to be observed.

I shall use as an example the process called *selective inattention*, something very different indeed from mere negligent oversight. By selective inattention we fail to recognize the actual import of a good many things we see, hear, think, do, and say, not because there is anything the matter with our zones of interaction with others but because the process of inferential analysis is opposed by the self-system. Clear recognition of the implications of matters to which we are selectively inattentive would call for basic change in an established pattern of dealing with the sort of interpersonal situation concerned; would make us either more, or in some cases less, competent, but in any case *different* from the way we now conceive ourself to be. Good observation and analysis of a mass of incidents selectively overlooked would expand the self-system, which usually controls the contents of awareness and the scope of the referential processes that are fully useful in *communicating* with others. The ever iterated miracle of selective inattention explains the faith we have in unnumbered prejudicial verbalisms, "rationalizations," about ourself and others and half explains the characterization of the Bourbon as one who never forgets anything and never learns anything.

While there is some reason to believe that a sufficient degree of novelty will always call out a disjunctive force the felt component of which we know as *fear*, a very great many otherwise illuminating observations, of by no means intimidating novelty and difference, fail entirely to inform us about the world we live in because of the equilibrating influence of the self-system—the tree that all too frequently reflects the way the twig was bent in the developmental years.

The extension of psychiatric theory beyond the confines of the familiar into the world of "foreigners" whose ways of life are alien to us calls for a sharp discrimination between fear and the various manifestations of anxiety and self-system activity, especially those of irrational *dislikes*, *aversions*, and *revulsions*, and the today so widespread *distrust of others*.

Current theory makes *hate* the characteristic of interpersonal situations in which the people concerned recurrently and frequently 'provoke anxiety in each other,' yet 'cannot break up the situation' because of some conjunctive forces which hold them together. If the conjunctive force acts entirely outside of awareness, uncanny *fascination*, with moments of revulsion or loathing, may appear. If the integrating forces are not very strong; if the situation is 'not very important,' the milder manifestations of 'more or less concealed,' "actually unjustified," dislike and distrust are shown. The "actually unjustified" means that a consensually valid statement of adequate grounds for the dislike or distrust cannot be formulated. The unpleasant 'emotion' arises from something more than what either person could readily come to know about the situation.

Let me illustrate the meaning of these terms by some thoroughly crude examples. A couple make what certainly is a marriage of great convenience. Friends of each notice with increasing discomfort that husband and wife seem more and more bent on humiliating each other in the presence of the friends. This illustrates an increasingly hateful integration.

A mother, taking over the care of her first-born from the nurse, is greatly upset—feels faint, looks pale, trembles severely, and is bathed with perspiration—on first encountering soiled diapers. She is undergoing the uncanny variant on the much more commonplace *disgust*, either of which is mostly a matter of her training for life.

Another mother discovers her fifteen-month-old child holding his obviously "excited" genital. She is filled with a shuddering 'emotion' not unrelated to the fascination *and* horror many people encounter when first thinking about witches' sabbaths, Voodoo rites, or other folk encounters with personified Sexual Evil. Parenthetically, the infant by empathy is filled with the most primitive anxiety, almost as paralyzing and as uninformative as a blow on the head from a hammer; but if the mother's 'reaction' does not change by virtue of habituation or "insight," he will gradually catch on to enough of what happens to come to the juvenile era a person who shows *primitive genital phobia*—a more or less contentless aversion to action or thought about "touching himself" in the perineum; often with a lively, if unwelcome, hope that he may be "touched" by others, and perhaps "touch" them in turn; after which actual experience he would come to "dislike" and avoid them, or, more unhappily, suffer recurrent deeply disturbing revulsion after each of a series of "conflictful" repetitions.

I can perhaps now proceed to the thesis of this paper; namely, that while no one can now be adequately equipped for a greatly significant inquiry into the fundamental "facts of life" of everyone, everywhere, there are many possibilities of greatly constructive efforts in this direction—if, and only if, instead of plunging into the field recklessly "hoping for the best," one prefaces one's attempt with a careful survey of one's assets and liabilities for participant observation.

Every constructive effort of the psychiatrist, today, is a strategy of interpersonal field operations which (1) seeks to map the areas of disjunctive force that block the efficient collaboration of the patient and others, and (2) seeks to expand the patient's awareness so that this unnecessary blockage can be brought to an end.

For a psychiatry of peoples, we must follow the selfsame strategy applied to significant groupings of people—families, communities, political entities, regional organizations, world blocs—and seek to map the interventions of disjunctive force which block the integration of the group with other groups in pursuit of the common welfare; and seek out the characteristics of each group's culture or subculture, and the methods used to impose it on the young, which perpetuate the restrictions of freedom for constructive growth.

The master tactics for a psychiatrist's work with a handicapped person consist in (1) elucidating the actual situations in which unfortunate action is currently shown repeatedly, so that the disorder-pattern may become clear; (2) discovering the less obvious ramifications of this inadequate and inappropriate way of life throughout other phases of the present and the near future, including the doctor-patient relationship and the patient's expectations about it; and (3) with the problem of inadequate development now clearly formulated, utilizing his human abilities to explore its origins in his experience with significant people of the past.

It must be noted that an identical distortion of living common to doctor and patient makes this type of inquiry, at the best, very difficult. Neither is able to 'see' the troublesome patterns, and both are inclined to relate the difficulties to the unhappy peculiarities of the other people concerned in their less fortunate interpersonal relations. Each respects the parallel limitation in the other, and their mutual effort is apt to be concentrated on irrelevant or immaterial problems, until they both become more discouraged or still more firmly deceived about life.

For a psychiatry of peoples, these tactical requirements of good therapy—which is also good research—have to be expanded into (1) a preliminary discovery of the actual major patterns of tensions and energy transformations which characterize more adequate and appropriate living in that group; this is a background for noticing the exceptions—the incidents of mental disorder among these folk—uninformed study of which would be misleading; (2) a parallel development of skill at rectifying the effects of limitations in our own developmental background; in order (3) that it may become possible to observe better the factors that actually resist any tendency to extend the integrations of our subject-persons, so that they would include representatives of other groups relatively alien to them—a pilot test of which is the integration with ourself—and (4) thus to find real problems in the foresight of intergroup living which can be tracked down to their origins in our subject-people's education for life.

There is good reason to believe that all this is not impossible. These world-psychiatric inquiries are not at bottom particularly different from the already mentioned, all too common, instances where doctor and patient suffer approximately *the same* disorders in living. Let me say a word about the way in which one may proceed to reduce the handicap of such a situation, at the same time pointing to the answer to an oft-heard question: "What can I do to help myself?"

My conception of anxiety is in point here. While we may be unaware, at least temporarily, of milder degrees of any one of the other tensions connected with living, we are never unaware of anxiety at the very time that it occurs. The awareness can be, and very often is, fleeting, especially when an appropriate security operation is called out. The awareness can be most variously characterized from person to person, even from incident to incident, excepting only that it is always unpleasant. At the moment that anxiety occurs, one becomes aware of something unpleasant; but whether this seems to be a mere realization that all is not going so well, or a noticing of some disturbance in the activity or postural tone in one of the zones of interaction—a change in one's 'facial expression' or in one's voice, as examples—a feeling of tightening up in some group of skeletal muscles, a disturbance of the action of one's heart, a discomfort in one's belly, a realization that one has begun to sweat; as I say, whether it be one of these or yet another variety of symptoms, one is always at least momentarily aware that one has become uncomfortable, or more acutely uncomfortable, as the case may be.

No matter what may have followed upon this awareness of diminished feeling of well-being, there was the awareness. It best serves in ordinary interpersonal relations to "pay as little attention to it as one can," and to "forget it." But if one is intent on refining oneself as an instrument of participant observation, it is necessary to pay the greatest attention, at least retrospectively, to these fleeting movements of anxiety. They are the telltales which show increased activity of the self-system in the interpersonal field of the moment concerned.

They mark the point in the course of events at which something disjunctive, something that tends to pull away from the other fellow, has first appeared or has suddenly increased. They signal a change from relatively uncomplicated movement toward a presumptively common goal to a protecting of one's self-esteem, with a definite *complicating* of the interpersonal action.

To the extent that one can retrospectively observe the exact situation in which one's anxiety was called out, one may be able to infer the corresponding pattern of difficulty in dealing with others. As these patterns are usually a matter of past training or its absence, detecting them is seldom an easy matter, but, I repeat, it is by no means impossible—unless there is an actual *dissociation* in one's personality system, in which case there will be prohibitively great difficulty in recalling anything significant about the actual situation which evoked the anxiety.

Two things more remain to be said about this, shall I say, self-observation of disjunctive processes in interpersonal relations.

Anxiety appears not only as awareness of itself but also in the experience of some *complex* 'emotions' into which it has been elaborated by specific early training. I cannot say what all these are, but I can use names for a few of them which should 'open the mind' to their nature: embarrassment, shame, humiliation, guilt, and chagrin. The circumstances under which these unpleasant 'emotions' occur are particularly hard to observe accurately and to subject to the retrospective analysis which is apt to be most rewarding.

A group of security operations born of experience which has gone into the development of these complex unpleasant 'emotions' is equally hard for one to observe and analyze. These are the movements of thought and the actions by which we, as it were, impute to, or seek to provoke in, the other fellow feelings like embarrassment, shame, humiliation, guilt, or chagrin. It is peculiarly difficult to observe retrospectively and to subject to analysis the exact circumstances under which we are moved to act as if the other person "should be ashamed of himself," is "stupid," or is guilty of anything from a breach of good taste to a mortal sin. These interpersonal movements which put the other fellow at a disadvantage on the basis of a low relative personal worth are extremely troublesome elements in living and very great handicaps to investigating strange people.

Disparaging and derogatory thought and action that make one feel "better" than the other person concerned, that expand one's self-esteem, as it were, at his cost, are always to be suspected of arising from anxiety. These processes are far removed from a judicious inquiry into one's relative personal skill in living. They do not reflect a good use of observation and analysis but rather indicate a low self-esteem in the person who uses them. The quicker one comes to a low opinion of another, other things being equal, the poorer is one's secret view of one's own worth in the field of the disparagement.

It is rather easy to correct interferences in participant observation of another which arise from one's true superiorities to him. It is quite otherwise with the baleful effects of one's secret doubts and uncertainties. We are apt to be most severely critical of others when they are thought to be showing an instance of something of which we ourselves are secretly ashamed, and which we hope we are concealing.

This must suffice as an indication of the more pervasive of the often unnoticed interferences with participant observation with representatives of somewhat unfamiliar background. I need scarcely discuss the role of linguistic difficulties or that of sheer ignorance of the culture patterns to which remarks make reference. These latter are actually only somewhat more striking instances of similar interferences in getting acquainted with any stranger.

Progress toward a psychiatry of peoples is to be expected from efforts expended along two lines of investigation: (1) an improving grasp on the significant patterns—and on the pattern of patterns—of living around the world; and (2) the uncovering of significant details in the sundry courses of personality development by which the people of each different social organization come to manifest more or less adequate and appropriate behavior, in their given social setting.

Each of these lines of investigation is a necessary supplement to the other. The first, which may be taken to pertain more to the interests and techniques of the cultural anthropologist, cannot be pushed very far, very securely, without data from the second. The second can scarcely produce meaningful data unless it is informed by the provisional hypotheses of the former. The two provide indispensable checks upon each other, without which neither can proceed noticeably without running into increasing uncertainty.

The theory of interpersonal relations lays great stress on the method of participant observation, and relegates data obtained by other methods to, at most, a secondary importance. This in turn implies that skill in the face-to-face, or person-to-person, *psychiatric interview* is of fundamental importance.

While the value of interchange by use of the mediate channels of communication—correspondence, publications, radio, speaking films—may be very great, especially if the people concerned have already become fairly well acquainted with each other as a result of previous face-to-face exchange, it must be remembered that communication in the psychiatric interview is by no means solely a matter of exchanging verbal contexts, but is rather the development of an exquisitely complex pattern of field processes which *imply* important conclusions about the people concerned.

This is scarcely the place for a discussion of current views about what one can learn about the theory and practice of psychiatric interviewing; I wish chiefly to emphasize the *instrumental* character of the interviewing psychiatrist and the critical importance of his being free to observe—and subsequently analyze—as many as possible of his performances as a dynamic center in the field patterns that make up the interview.

Everything that can be said about good psychiatric interviewing is relevant to the directly interpersonal aspects of any work in the direction of a psychiatry of peoples. Every safeguard useful in avoiding erroneous conclusions about 'the other fellow' becomes newly important when the barriers of linguistic and other cultural uncertainties are in the way.

Inquiries into the alien ways of educating the young must be oriented with close regard to *biological time* as it is reflected in the serial maturation of capacities; to *social time* as it is reflected in the series of formulable expectations concerning what the young will 'know how to behave about' from stage to stage of their development; and to the exact *chronology* of presumptively educative efforts brought to bear on the young.

The spread of variations in each of these three fields is of great importance in understanding the people and their relationships, which make up any community. Consider, for example, the effect of delayed puberty on the adequacy and appropriateness of subsequent behavior in many a youth in any of our urban areas. Consider, again, the effects on the living of the outstandingly bright boy from a small town when he enters a great metropolitan university. And, finally, consider the probable effects of early training in venereal prophylaxis in contrast with that of suppression of information in this field.

It is by virtue of an ever better grasp on the significant patterns in these series of events that we help patients to help themselves, at the same time becoming better and better informed about the factors which govern the possibilities of interpersonal action. To the extent that we have useful approximations to an understanding of the actual processes of personality development which have ensued in the people with whom we deal, we become able to 'make sense' of what seems to be going on. This must be the case, whether one is a stranger in Malaya or host to a visiting Malay.

Whence the Urgency

In a world in which time is of the essence, in which we can scarcely defer great constructive changes until we shall have raised a new generation to political power, the most searching scrutiny of the dynamics of favorable change in personality becomes utterly imperative. Even if time were not of the essence, the imperative would be much the same, for we cannot "jump a generation" and *training for life as it is becoming* begins in, and reaches very far forward from, the primary group of the home. The less of parents' work that has to be corrected, the quicker man moves ahead. The surer our aid to parents in preparing their young for life, the more geometrically expanding will be the resulting good to the greater number.

I think it is no longer wise or expedient to talk and think *as if* the great majority of chronologically adult people, here or elsewhere, will ever become well-informed about a great deal that is acutely vitally important to them.

I think that we must recognize explicitly that universal literacy and complete "freedom of information" *in themselves* offer no solution to any of the imperative problems of the times. . . . Freedom of information is meaningless unless it is used for a purpose, namely, to promote the peace and well-being of humanity.

Can anyone who is experienced in dealing with others doubt that it is ever so much easier to replace one prejudice with another than it is to bring about informed judgment? Do we not actually have this in mind when we express ourselves to the so-called laity? Or perhaps better put: *should* we not have this in mind? Consider, for instance, the effects, detectable even in some psychiatrists' homes, of disseminating information about the evil effects of parental mismanagement. Some considerable number of parents now suffer such uncertainty about "frustrating" and "fixating" and "making dependent" and the like that they themselves need psychiatric help and their offspring will certainly require it. We do not seem to have done too good a job of public education in this vital area. Perhaps our information was not adequate; perhaps, on the other hand, it was not so bad but we used it badly.

I hold that it is self-evident that a very great many chronologically adult people must act on faith with respect to almost every field of living. The great hope for the future lies not in attempting to change this fact but in so reducing the effectiveness of certain vicious elements in current faiths that the young who grow up under the influence of these elders will have much greater freedom to observe and to understand and to foresee correctly than had their parents and teachers and the others under whose authority their abilities for interpersonal relations were molded.

The achievement of this exceedingly desirable goal is anything but easy and foolproof. The thinking-out of constructive, functionally coherent, revisions of any one of the major cultures of the world, so that the personal imperatives which derive from it —whether in the obscure, very early inculcated, patterns of *conscience* or the subsequently acquired, less recondite, patterns of acceptable rationalizations and potent verbalisms—shall be less restrictive on understanding and more permissive of social progress; that, truly, is a task to which unnumbered groups of the skillful may well apply themselves.

There will remain the intimidating task of implementing the better, once it shall have been designed; but for the first time in the history of man, there is world-wide, if often most unhappy, realization of the necessity, and at the same time a set of administrative agencies clearly charged with the responsibility. I say to you with the utmost seriousness of which I am capable that this is no time to excuse yourself from paying the debt you and yours owe the social order with some such facile verbalism as "Nothing will come of it; it can't be done." Begin; and let it be said of you, if there is any more history, that you labored nobly in the measure of man in the twentieth century of the scientific, Western world.

Index

HARRY STACK SULLIVAN, M.D.

Conceptions of Modern Psychiatry

The First William Alanson White Memorial Lectures

With a Foreword by the Author
and a Critical Appraisal of the
Theory by PATRICK MULLAHY

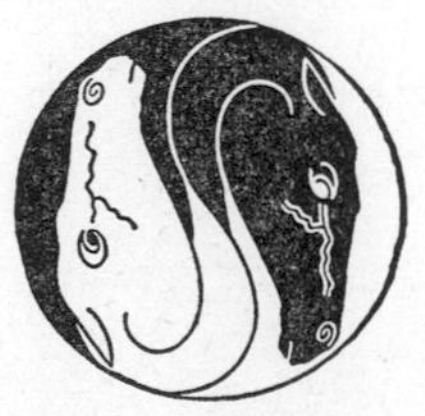

W · W · NORTON & COMPANY · INC · *New York*

SECOND EDITION

PRINTED IN THE UNITED STATES OF AMERICA

Contents

▾

Preface to the Second Edition

THIS NEW edition of Sullivan's 1939 lectures on *Conceptions of Modern Psychiatry* marks the fifth time that these lectures have been reprinted, but the first time that they have ever appeared on a book publisher's list. The story of how these lectures came to be written down, printed in a journal, reprinted as a sort of makeshift book, and reprinted again and again—all simply because people had heard of them by word-of-mouth and wanted them—is a tribute to the contagion of the ideas themselves.

In 1939, the William Alanson White Memorial Lectures were inaugurated by the White Psychiatric Foundation, and Sullivan was asked to give the first series of lectures. The series consisted of the five lectures in this book, which were given to a small audience in the U. S. Interior Department auditorium in Washington. Immediately there was an influx of requests for copies of the lectures, and Sullivan hastily prepared the transcriptions of the lectures for inclusion in the February 1940 issue of PSYCHIATRY, the Journal which he edited for 12 years. In the following months and years, requests for this issue of the Journal kept coming in, and finally the stock was exhausted. In 1947, the Board of Trustees of the Foundation authorized a small reprinting of the lectures for the use of students. Sullivan himself was somewhat reluctant. He felt that the first three lectures were "grossly inadequate," as he put it; but he gave his permission, since by then he was deep in a heavy teaching and training program, and did not know when he would have time to revise them. The reprints were yellow, because the Journal is printed on yellow paper, and the printer had a supply of it on hand. At the last minute, someone had the idea that the reprint should have a hard cover to make it more durable.

The subsequent story of this yellow reprint in the hard cover which was intended for students is remarkable even in the commercial publishing world. For in five years, it had sold over 13,000 copies. It had gone to countries all over the world. It was being used as a textbook in social science departments in several universities. The first indication of what to expect came when, in the summer of 1947, several months after its publication, Lloyd Frankenberg published a review of it in the *New York Times Book Review*. It was given modest space, and Frankenberg pointed out that it was a difficult book to read. But the review had about it the magic of the book—the excitement of Sullivan's ideas and personality. And that summer, the entire administrative staff of the Foundation wrapped and mailed books, hundreds of them, carrying sacks of them out to the mail box every night. Thus the reprint for students had turned into a book.

At the time that the reprints were made, the Foundation decided to include a critique of Sullivan's theories by Patrick Mullahy, which had been published as an article in PSYCHIATRY in May 1945. This article, which appears in the back of this book with a few changes, was one of the very first comprehensive evaluations of Sullivan's work, and was in great demand by students. Mr. Mullahy has since written extensively and brilliantly on Sullivan's ideas, but this 1945 article remains a classic explanation of these lectures.

As the only book of Sullivan's writings published during his lifetime, this book has a certain historical significance. But it is by no means a fossil. The challenge of its ideas, as evidenced by the feeling of excitement with which each new reader "discovers" it, makes it indeed a new book for an ever-growing audience.

DEXTER M. BULLARD, *President*,
The William Alanson White Psychiatric Foundation

Foreword

THIS SERIES OF five lectures, of which only the last two were expanded to reasonable proportions before publication, has had to serve as the available statement of my theoretical position while a four-year collaboration with the faculty of the Washington School of Psychiatry was testing and refining the theory and developing some technical innovations in intensive psychotherapy which are implicit in it.

This collaboration has included a series of 248 lecture-discussions at Chestnut Lodge, 66 seminars on clinical research, 57 teaching seminars, and almost 2,000 supervising conferences concerned with treatment or the training of candidates for a career in intensive psychotherapy, in addition to eight courses of lectures given in the regular curriculum of instruction.

Continuing close contact with the practical problem and theoretical preoccupations of twenty colleagues has done much to clarify and make communicable the views derived from 15 years of research with schizoid and obsessional people in a quarter century of practice.

The here reprinted lectures fail of close correspondence with my current views in the following more significant respects.

The theory of *anxiety*, its bearing on personality development, and its crucial importance in observing and influencing interpersonal relations, is not adequately stated. The developmental history of the *self-dynamism* is, therefore, left relatively unclear, its functional activity in *selective inattention* and in other peculiarities of interpersonal relations is not set forth, and the concept of *dissociation* comes to have undue importance as an explanatory principle. Mr. Mullahy's analysis will help to correct this inadequacy.

These lectures are nowhere else as open to criticism as in their sketch of the *developmental history of interpersonal relations.* Here certainly one of Mr. Philip Sapir's many valuable criticisms of these lectures—"nothing can justify condensing two paragraphs into one sentence"—applies with peculiar force. Five lectures averaging two hours in length here 'cover' all psychiatry. In the current series of 34 School lectures, *infancy* as a phase in the human animal's becoming a person is not finished by the twelfth hour.

It is in the structure of inferences about the first few years of life that one finds the key to formulating the otherwise baffling complexities of later stages of interpersonal relations which are brought into being by the combination of serially matured potentialities, experience, and the function of *recall* and *foresight* in the sundry interpersonal situations through which we live. In this connection, also, Mr. Mullahy's analysis adds something, but could scarcely communicate views which are but now at last becoming systematic.

Psychiatry as it is—the preoccupation of extant psychiatric specialists—is not science nor art but confusion. In defining it as the study of interpersonal relations, I sought to segregate from everything else a disciplinary field in which operational methods could be applied with great practical benefits. This made psychiatry the probable locus of another evolving discipline, one of the social sciences, namely, *social psychology.* Both seek an adequate statement of living, including every instance of relative success or failure that is open to participant observation. The scientific psychiatrist would know wherein and wherefore his patient fails and whither his remedial efforts could reasonably be expected to lead an improved facility for living.

This psychiatry was scarcely to be learned by administering the affairs of patients in custodial hospitals for the mentally disordered, nor by effecting a consensus of uninformed prejudice with patients in private practice. Needless to say, it would scarcely evolve from "treating" people with metrazol, electroshock or ablative brain surgery. It required great technical refinement of the psychiatrist as a participant observer interacting with his patients in the context of life as it has to be lived. From this, the psychiatrist must inevitably gain information about living; his patient, in some instances, all that he needs for continuing favorable change.

Because the psychiatrist is always dealing with living—partly adequate, partly unfortunate, but always simply human—the terms of his scientific language might well be refined from the common speech by chief virtue of which he and his patient have acquired some skill at communicating. The terms of scientific psychiatry would then be misunderstood by the uninitiate, as what terms are not? The absurdity of much meaningless discourse might be more easily discovered, with great saving of something other than "face."

Gordon Allport and H. S. Odbert some years ago listed 17,953 words used to indicate alleged qualities of human *individuality*. Mr. Mullahy has some pithy comment on my disaffection for people's "individuality" as an interest of the psychiatrist. That his discussion is germane is attested by a great variety of misunderstandings in this connection. I have inveighed against "the delusion of unique individuality" and referred to personality as the hypothetical entity which we posit to account for interpersonal relations. I do not believe that this denies anyone "a personality"; it serves its purpose if it warns anyone that I never expect to *know* all about his personality—and am as certain as can be that he too will always share my ignorance in that regard.

Personality, I now define in the particularist sense as *the relatively enduring pattern of recurrent interpersonal situations which characterize a human life*. The term, *pattern*, in this statement is to be taken to mean *the envelope of all insignificant differences*. *Significant* differences in to-be-recurrent interpersonal relations occur, at times, when personality changes.

Some of these changes are relatively invariant, marking important phases in the progress from birth towards maturity. Some of them are by no means universal and may represent peculiarly fortunate incidents, incidents of so-called serious mental disorder, or of recovery therefrom.

That there are particular human lives, each with a unique career line, I no more deny than do I the fact that I am a particular person who has a particular dog. I can say with Bridgman that "I act in two modes—my public mode . . . and in the private mode [in which] I feel my inviolable isolation from my fellows. . . ." So doubtless does my dog; the transformations of energy which he manifests in living his canine life often transcend being-my-dog in the culturally patterned world of dogs and people which is his life space. He doubtless acts much more frequently in the private mode than could I think that I do, and I doubtless act much less frequently in the private mode than it is easy to think that I do. The immutably private in my dog and in me escapes and will always escape the methods of science, however absorbing I may once have found the latter.

Without digressing on the value of the comparative approach in formulating noncultural and especially nonlanguage aspects of living, I seek here to stress the central fact that the true or absolute individuality of a person is always beyond scientific grasp and invariably much less significant in the person's living than he has been taught to believe.

Individual differences, especially those which are principally matters of language and customs in people from widely separate parts of the world, may be extremely impressive and may present great handicap to discovering the significant differences in relative adequacy and appropriateness of action in interpersonal relations, which constitute extraordinary success, average living, or mental disorder.

The therapist or the research psychiatrist, however, participates intelligently in interpersonal relations with his confrere only to the extent that these handicaps are successfully overcome or evaded and finds opportunity to gain skill in this particular in his dealings with any stranger.

HARRY STACK SULLIVAN

31 December 1946

Conceptions of Modern Psychiatry

LECTURE I

Basic Conceptions

In the preface to his autobiography,[1] Dr. White remarked "when we look about us and see the confusion that the world is in at the present moment, see the antagonisms that are loosed by national rivalries and realize the possibilities of war, of disaster, of death, which they conceivably may entail, then realize that all of these results hang upon the way in which mental factors are evaluated and the powers of mind are utilized, we must come to the conclusion that we cannot overemphasize the importance of this field of interest."

Rather than attempt some expression of the honor which this occasion brings to me, let me take these words of one of the pioneers of modern psychiatry as my text and proceed with what is bound to prove too great a task for adequate performance. A definitive expression of the conceptions inhering in modern psychiatry would be a task indeed. I shall attempt in this series of lectures little more than an outline of the field of thought within which there are insights that seem destined to illuminate some age-old and many future problems of living, of the relations of man to man, perhaps even of peoples to peoples.

For those of you who are not too familiar with the thinking

[1] *William Alanson White: The Autobiography of a Purpose;* Garden City, N. Y.; Doubleday, Doran and Co., 1938 (xix and 293 pp.). The next paragraph in the preface expresses the author's qualified belief "that the average medical man is, by and large, about as thoroughly lacking in information as to the significance of mental factors in relation to disease as is the average layman."

of psychiatrists, I might suggest something of the diversity of their views by mentioning three sorts of psychiatrists: those to whom all mental processes are but epiphenomena; those to whom mental disorders signify biological—or spiritual—inferiority; and, happily, those who accept the mental as a scientifically valid, if largely unexplored, field.

Quite beyond diversity of views, however, our discipline has two chief bodies of meaning. One reaches back clearly to the Hippocratic school of medicine, among the writings of which there are excellent psychiatric contributions. This part of psychiatry—this definition of the psychiatric field, if you please—I have elsewhere described as the art of observing and perhaps influencing the course of mental disorders.[2] It was overwhelmed in the recession from the Classic Period and had its renaissance with Pinel—1745 to 1826—as physician to the Bicêtre in 1793. In those days, people who were the victims of serious mental disorders were treated in rather barbarous fashion, only occasionally being as fortunate in this regard as were those imprisoned for crime. He eliminated the chains and shackles, the brutal handling, exsanguination, and drugging. As Director of the Salpetriere, from 1795, he evolved a remarkably modern system of psychiatric institutional care, which was fortunately perpetuated by his most distinguished student, and successor, Esquirol—1772 to 1840.[3]

[2] Psychiatry. *Encyclopædia of the Social Sciences;* New York, Macmillan (1934) 12:578–580.

[3] A history of culture would have as its most significant part a history of ideas and information about man's constitution, functional activity, and communal existence with his natural, biological and personal environment. This would be the history of "human nature." These and the following remarks are no more than a laying of the pen-point on paper for writing such a history. The appended references are but an iota in the alphabet of psychiatric history. Given opportunity, one should certainly read Semelaigne, René, *Aliénistes et Philanthropes;* Paris, Steinheil, 1912 (4 and 548 pp.).

See Pinel, Phillippe, *Traité médico-philosophique sur l'aliénation mentale ou la manie* [2 ed.]; Paris, Brosson, 1809 (xxxii and 496 pp.), and *Nosographie philosophique* [6 ed.]; Paris, Brosson, 1818 (3 volumes). See also Esquirol, Jean-Etienne Dominique, *Des maladies mentales considérées sous les rapports médical, hygiénique et médico-légal;* Paris, Baillière, 1838 (2 volumes)—

The second body of meaning of psychiatry—the alternative definition of the psychiatric field—is coeval with man as a social being. In the shadows before prehistory, as man began to take on the social habit of life, the germs of this discipline must have sprouted. As man appears clearly in history, it showed itself in the performances of his medicine men and magicians, his seers and prophets and sages. They observed their fellows with unusual clarity and elaborated wisdom from experience to the end of leadership, guidance, and the cure of disorders of living.

This broader aspect of psychiatry would include the narrower medical aspect and, if I mistake not, in time to come the medical aspect must expand to the full breadth of human psychiatry. However, of this, more anon.

The medical man of the Hippocratic era was a skillful observer, and, since Paracelsus, this tradition has been renewed in the Western world. The course of development of modern medicine ran through anatomical and then pathological studies, with increasing concentration on the cellular structure of living tissues—and recently on the biochemical and biophysical aspects of the tissue and cell function. While there arose a class of medical practitioners who tended to exemplify the finest sort of physician, the vast increase of medical information led presently to increasing specialization of interest, and diagnostic

Esquirol, Jules-Etienne Dominique, *Mental Maladies. A Treatise on Insanity* [tr. from the French, with additions, by E. K. Hunt, M.D.]; Philadelphia, Lea and Blanchard, 1845 (xviii and 496 pp.).

Esquirol may be called the father of modern psychiatry, for Pinel, while spurning materialistic philosophy, looked chiefly to physiological formulations and taught that mental disorders were the results of heredity and stresses and excesses in living. Esquirol's observations directed his thinking much more towards explanations in psychological or psychobiological terms.

It is to be noted that Johannes Weyer, a sixteenth century psychiatrist—author of *De Præstigiis Dæmonum* published in 1566—is considered by Gregory Zilboorg to be the father of scientific psychiatry. He refers its moral awakening to Weyer; its humanistic, to Pinel. See his *The Medical Man and the Witch During the Renaissance* [The Hideyo Noguchi Lectures]; Baltimore, The Johns Hopkins Press, 1935 (x and 215 pp.); also Binz, Carl, *Doktor Johann Weyer;* Bonn, Mareus, 1885, to which Zilboorg refers.

and therapeutic practice. The physician to the ailing patient tended to fade out and give way to the medical expert dealing with the disease which interested him.

Again in retrospect, in the days of Pinel, there lived Pierre Jean George Cabanis—1774 to 1838—a medical scientist who came to hold that all mental functions were functions of the brain.[4] Franz Joseph Gall—1758 to 1828—meanwhile having devoted some years to the study of the brain, came to understand something of cerebral localizations of motor functions, and reported on his work to the Institute of France. The great comparative anatomist, Georges Cuvier—1769 to 1832—and Pinel were members of the Institute's committee. The phrenological buncombe which was mixed with Gall's scientific work led to an unfavorable reception.

Pierre Flourens—1794 to 1867—about the same time was experimenting on localized damages to the brain with observations of the animal's subsequent loss of functions. This pioneer neurophysiologist is entitled to high honor, for he perceived clearly the total-function aspect of the central nervous system in contradistinction to those more localized phenomena which were soon—prefaced by Marshall Hall, 1790 to 1857, who evolved in 1833 the conception of reflex action—to influence the psychological formulations throughout the era of the mechanistic philosophies, and to underwrite the mésalliance of medical psychiatry with neurology which persists in many quarters to this day. A great figure in this was Hughlings Jackson—1834 to 1911—who progressed from the study of epileptic phenomena to the formulation of rather simple cerebro-mechanical explanations of many of our most complex performances in relations with others. Henry Head—b. 1861—may be said to have reopened the field,[5] although the neuro-

[4] The remark is attributed to Cabanis that the brain secretes thought as the liver secretes bile. See his *Rapports du physique et du moral de l'homme*; Paris, Bureau de la Bibliothèque choisie, 1830 (2 vols. 405 and 430 pp.).

[5] Head, Henry, *Aphasia and Kindred Disorders of Speech*; Cambridge, The University Press, 1926 (Vol. 1:xiv and 549 pp.).

physiologists had already destroyed the neat structure of reflexology.[6] We may rest secure in the knowledge that much is yet to be learned concerning the central nervous system.

The mésalliance of neurology and psychiatry has by no means been dissolved. The emergency of the World War brought us *neuropsychiatrists*, and a cultural factor, the aversion to mental disorder which is the linear descendant of belief in demoniacal possession and witchcraft, still makes it more certainly respectable to be treated by a neurologist for a "nervous breakdown" than to consult a psychiatrist about one's difficulties in living. The euphemism covers superstition and protects conceit: both are powerful checks on the progress not alone of psychiatry, but of civilization as a whole.

Processes in the central nervous system, in the other nervous systems, and in the autacoid dynamism, have importance in explaining *some* of the conditions of behavior, human or infrahuman. We have to look to the broader aspects of psychiatry for light on some other indispensable conditions of human behavior.[7] And we have a great deal to learn in both fields.

In the enlightenment, the broader field of psychiatric interest evolved in directions which took many of its students far from medical preoccupations. It became the conviction of many that the study of man in the group would be productive of information valuable in government and in promoting the

[6] See, in particular, among many relevant contributions: Bard, Philip, On Emotional Expression after Decortication with Some Remarks on Certain Theoretical Views. *Psychol. Rev.* (1934) 41:309–329 and 424–449. Rioch, David McK. and Brenner, Charles, Experiments on the Corpus Striatum and Rhinencephalon. *J. Comp. Neurol.* (1938) 68:491–507. Rioch, David McK., Certain Aspects of the Behavior of Decorticated Cats. PSYCHIATRY (1938) 1:339–345. Rioch, David McK., Neurophysiology of the Corpus Striatum and Globus Pallidus. PSYCHIATRY (1940) 3:119–139. See, also, Bard, Philip, Central Nervous Mechanisms for Emotional Behavior Patterns in Animals. *Research Publications of the Association for Research in Nervous and Mental Diseases*, 19:190–218.

[7] My own interest in those types of explanations which Adolf Meyer has so aptly termed "neurologizing tautology," I owe to a conversation with Gilbert Horrax, the neurosurgeon, shortly after the World War. His comments on the sequelæ, and the lack of sequelæ, of serious cerebral wounds was most illuminating.

common weal. The social sciences thus developed techniques for studying, and allegedly studying, group behavior, factors making for mass performances, and specialized aspects of man's social life. Only recently have there appeared social scientists who are interested in the data of medical psychiatry, and still more recently psychiatrists who are interested in such fields as cultural anthropology and sociology. While I had something to do with starting the latter rapprochement, the appearance of this trend towards a complete psychiatry depended primarily on three great figures who appeared in the later years of the Nineteenth Century—Sigmund Freud, Adolf Meyer, and William Alanson White.[8]

Freud—1856 to 1939—and Josef Breuer—1842 to 1925—published in 1895, *Studien über Hysterie* in which they indicated that hysterical symptoms arose from extra-conscious mental processes, the energy of which was diverted or converted into a personally meaningless disorder of function. Freud presently invented the free-associational technique for reintegrating *repressed* material, evolved the psychoanalytic instinct-theory, and drew attention to what he called the *transference.* His *Traumdeutung* was published in 1900, and by 1905, he had formulated the *libido* theory and the doctrine of the *Œdipus complex*, as the most important conflict in the growth of the child, and the problem, failure to solve which leads to "neurosis." There followed the evolution of psychoanalysis as *depth-psychology* with dynamic, economic, and topographical points of view; and the postulation of a *Todestrieb*, or death-instinct.

It is with the first fruits of Freud's genius that we shall con-

[8] Listings of recent significant persons must express personal convictions as to the probable appraisal of their work by scholars yet to come. Compare for example, Stanley Cobb's statement ". . . . of the six major contributors to psychiatry in the last twenty-five years (Kraepelin, Freud, Sherrington, Pavlov, Wagner von Jauregg, and Cannon), three are physiologists"; a footnote to his "Problems in Cerebral Anatomy and Physiology" in *The Problem of Mental Disorder;* N. Y. and London, McGraw-Hill, 1934 (x and 388 pp.). Dr. Cobb is of the opinion that "no sound psychologist doubts that the brain is the organ of the mind."

cern ourselves. The phenomena appearing in prolonged free-associational interviews, with the study of the transference-distortions that accompany—or precede—the verbal material, together provide a bridge across those discontinuities which had hitherto prevented the formulation of a comprehensive psychology of mental content. Freud revealed the experiential origin of specific limitations of personal awareness. By this achievement, he cleared the way for the scientific study of people, in contradistinction to mind, or society, or brain, or glands.[9]

"It is manifestly impossible to formulate all the difficulties of human adaptation in biological terms, in psychological terms, or in sociological terms; or, for that matter, in a meaningful blend of any or all of these. The psychobiology of Adolf Meyer—b. 1866—is the most distinguished recent effort to find a new locus for problems, a new level of reality and knowledge, and new conceptual tools. Meyer recognizes the hierarchies of organization and proceeds from a consideration of organismic integrating factors . . . . to bridge the gap between biology and psychiatry by the concept of *mentation*, a peculiarly effective integrating activity by the use of symbols and meanings." Meyer finally emancipated psychology from its medieval heritage. Himself a most competent neurologist and neuropathologist, he denied the usefulness of preoccupation with neural analogies. He indicated that it is by a superordination of physiology by means of the integrating functions and particularly by means of the use of symbols as tools that man was able to develop, on the one hand, his grasp on reality, and on the other, his remarkable problems in dealing with his personal reality and the reality of others around him.[10]

The genius of William Alanson White—1870 to 1937—

[9] See Intuition, Reason, and Faith: An Editorial. PSYCHIATRY (1939) 2:129–132 from which the quotation that follows is taken.

[10] The bibliography of Meyer is published in a special number of *Archives of Neurology and Psychiatry* (1937) 37:725–751. For an exposition closely related to his views and often in his own language, see Muncie, Wendell, *Psychobiology and Psychiatry;* St. Louis, Mosby, 1939 (739 pp.).

was of amazing scope. The particular contribution which I would stress here is his perception that this psychiatry, now principally centered on mentation and the utilization of symbols, very convenient and effective devices for dealing with very complex entities and relations in the world—that this science, which had begun to grasp the realities of the troubles of living, was a science not only qualified to deal with the mentally ill, but a science having vast relevance in human affairs, touching I know not how many fields of human endeavor and human problems; in fact, a fundamental discipline for all those fields that deal with the performance of man, whether in health or in illness or in those vast congeries of twilight states which the individual regards as health but society might well regard as illness.

There was effected in Dr. White's vision the first synthesis of the two great trends of psychiatric meaning—the medical discipline concerned with human ills, and the other great body of observational techniques, formulations, hypotheses and experiments which are included in all those efforts to understand social situations and to deal with social problems as they have appeared in the history of man.

This synthesis is not yet complete. The next, I trust, great step in its emergence came with the realization that the field of psychiatry is neither the mentally sick individual, nor the successful and unsuccessful processes that may be observed in groups and that can be studied in detached objectivity. Psychiatry, instead, is the study of processes that involve or go on between people. The field of psychiatry is the field of interpersonal relations, under any and all circumstances in which these relations exist. It was seen that *a personality* can never be isolated from the complex of interpersonal relations in which the person lives and has his being.[11]

[11] Sullivan, Harry Stack, Socio-Psychiatric Research: Its Implications for the Schizophrenia Problem and for Mental Hygiene. *Amer. J. Psychiatry* (1931) 10[o.s. 87]:977–991.

Let me suggest to you a few of the problems that we encounter by mentioning that our ordinary relation between an object and a percept has as a generally overlooked but none the less necessary link the act of perceiving. There is the object: emanations from it in the form of light waves, odors, sounds and so on impinge on our sense organs. They send certain specific impulses to a more central organ in which this group of impulses is connected with more or less related impulses which we experienced in our historic past. And out of this blend, this instantaneous comparison in the central nervous system and related tissue, there arises in our mind a conviction that we are observing, say, an orange, or something of that kind; on the one hand, the object, eternally separated from us by the act of perceiving it, and, on the other, the percept in our mind.

Now, when it comes to the matter of perceiving another person, not only is there the object, this other person, and the perception of the emanations from that person—appearances transmitted by light rays, indices transmitted by sound waves, meanings transmitted by statements, implications transmitted in the whole act of communicating—but also the distorting and confusing and complicating factor of our past experience with other people who looked like this, who sounded like this, who made those statements, who had certain implications that happen to be irrelevant here, and so on. In other words, the central synthesis of acquaintance, the percept in our mind, concerning another person is fabulously more complicated than is the case with non-personal reality.

So complex is this synthesis that it is practically impossible to elaborate techniques by which we can make our objective contact with another individual reasonably good. His performances in a situation, what he says and does; and, with increased uncertainty, what he says as to what is going on *in* him: these we can observe scientifically. We can improve our techniques for participant observation in an interpersonal situation in which we are integrated with our subject-person. This is evidently *the* procedure of psychiatry. I urge it as implying the root-premise of psychiatric methodology.

The unique individuality of the other fellow need never concern us as scientists. It is a great thing in our wives and our children. They have, however, æsthetic and other values that are outside of science; when it comes to science, let us confine ourselves to something at which we have some chance of success. We can study the phenomena that go on between the observer and the observed in the situation created by the observer participating with the observed. I hold that this is the subject matter of psychiatry; some rather remarkable results have already come from its definition.

It must be understood that the performances of a person in interpersonal relations include not only acts, including speech, but also the subject matter of certain remarks. If I say to you, "This is a beautiful room," while it may not possess quite the validity of *your* opinion that it is a beautiful room, still it may be accepted as highly probably my opinion of the room. It is the type of indirect communication of a subjective phenomenon which gives the, if you please, lunatic fringe to psychiatry even in its much more refined state.

Human performances, the subject of our study, including revery processes and thought, are susceptible of a two-part classification which is based on the end states, the end conditions toward which these processes are obviously moving, or which our prevision has reached. In other words, now and then you set out to start for somewhere. You preview the steps which will be necessary to get there and we can foresee the whole process on the basis of your reaching that place.

The most general basis on which interpersonal phenomena, interpersonal acts, may be classified, is one which separates the sought end states into the group which we call satisfactions and those which we call security or the maintenance of security. Satisfactions in this specialized sense are all those end states which are rather closely connected with the bodily organization of man. Thus the desire for food and drink leads to certain performances which are in this category. The desire for sleep leads to such performances. The state of being which is marked by the presence of lust is in this group; and finally, as the most middling example, the state of being which we call loneliness. All these states lead to activity which is the pursuit of satisfaction.

On the other hand, the pursuit of security pertains rather more closely to man's cultural equipment than to his bodily organization. By "cultural" I mean what the anthropologist means—all that which is man-made, which survives as monument to preexistent man, that is the cultural. And as I say, all those movements, actions, speech, thoughts, reveries and so on which pertain more to the culture which has been imbedded in a particular individual than to the organization of his tissues and glands, is apt to belong in this classification of the pursuit of security.

The thing which many people if they were quite honest with themselves would say that they were after when they are showing a process of this type is prestige, and one of my long-acquainted colleagues, Harold D. Lasswell, a political scientist, worked out a statement for this field in three terms: security, income, and deference. All these pertain to the culture, to the social institutions, traditions, customs, and the like, under which we live, to our social order rather than to the peculiar properties of our bodily or somatic organizations.

This second class, the pursuit of security, may be regarded as consisting of ubiquitous artifacts—again in the anthropological sense, man-made—evolved by the cultural conditioning or training; that is, education of the impulses or drives which underlie the first class. In other words, given our biological equipment—we are bound to need food and water and so on—certain conditioning influences can be brought to bear on the needs for satisfaction. And the cultural conditioning gives rise to the second group, the second great class of interpersonal phenomena, the pursuit of security.

To follow this line of thought profitably, however, one must look closely at this conception of conditioning, and one must consider especially the states characterized by the feeling of ability or power. This is ordinarily much more important in the human being than are the impulses resulting from a feeling of hunger, or thirst, and the fully developed feeling of lust comes so very late in biological maturation that it is scarcely a good source for conditioning.

We seem to be born, however, with something of this power motive in us. An oft-told story beautifully illustrates the early appearance of what I am discussing as the motive toward the manifestation of power or ability. The infant seeing for the first time the full moon, reaches for it. Nothing transpires. He utters a few goos and nothing transpires; then he starts to cry in rage, and the whole household is upset. But he does not get the moon, and the moon becomes 'marked' unattainable.

This is an instance of the frustration of the manifestation of power; one has failed at something which you might say one expects oneself to be able to achieve—not that the infant does much thinking, but the course of events indicates the application of increasingly complex techniques in the effort to achieve the object.

The full development of personality along the lines of security is chiefly founded on the infant's discovery of his powerlessness to achieve certain desired end states with the tools, the instrumentalities, which are at his disposal. From the disappointments in the very early stages of life outside the womb—in which all things were given—comes the beginning of this vast development of actions, thoughts, foresights, and so on, which are calculated to protect one from a feeling of insecurity and helplessness in the situation which confronts one. This accultural evolution begins thus, and when it succeeds, when one evolves successfully along this line, then one respects oneself, and as one respects oneself so one can respect others. That is one of the peculiarities of human personality that can always be depended on. If there is a valid and real attitude toward the self, that attitude will manifest as valid and real toward others. It is not that as ye judge so shall ye be judged, but as you judge yourself so shall you judge others; strange but true so far as I know, and with no exception.

The infant has as perhaps his mightiest tool the cry. The cry is a performance of the oral apparatus, the lips, mouth, throat, cheeks, vocal cords, intercostal muscles, and diaphragm. From this cry is evolved a great collection of most powerful tools which man uses in the development of his security with his fellow man. I refer to language behavior, operations including words.

Originally the infant's magical tool for all sorts of purposes, all too many of us still use vocal behavior as our principal adaptive device; and while none of you, of course, would do this, you must all know some people who can do in words practically anything and who have a curious faith that having said the right thing, all else is forgiven them. In other words, they are a little more like the infant than we are; they figure that a series of articulate noises turns any trick. We have, of course, learned that many other acts, performances, and foresights are necessary for success in living. None the less, denied our language behavior and the implicit revery processes that reach their final formulations in words, we would be terribly reduced in our competence and materially diminished in our security in dealing with other people.

At this point, I wish to say that if this series of lectures is to be reasonably successful, it will finally have demonstrated that there is nothing unique in the phenomena of the gravest functional illness. The most peculiar behavior of the acutely schizophrenic patient, I hope to demonstrate, is made up of interpersonal processes with which each one of us is or historically has been familiar. Far the greater part of the performances, the interpersonal processes, of the psychotic patient are exactly of a piece with processes which we manifest some time every twenty-four hours. Some of the psychotic performances seem very peculiar indeed, and, as I surmised in 1924,[12] for the explanation and familiarization of these performances, we have to look to the interpersonal relations of the infant, to the first eighteen months or so of life after birth. In most general terms, we are all much more simply human than otherwise, be we happy and successful, contented and detached, miserable and mentally disordered, or whatever.

To return to the epoch of infancy, first let me state that this is the period of maturation, of experimentation, of empathic 'observation,' and of autistic invention in the realm of power. Two of these terms may need some explanation.

From birth it is demonstrable that the infant shows a curious relationship or connection with the significant adult, ordinarily the mother. If the mother, for example, hated the pregnancy and deplores the child, it is a pediatric commonplace that there are feeding difficulties, unending feeding difficulties, with the child. If a mother, otherwise deeply attached to the infant, is seriously disturbed by some intercurrent event around nursing time, is frightened by something or worried about something around the time of nursing, then on that occasion there will be feeding difficulty or the infant has indigestion. All in all we know that there is an emotional linkage between the infant and the significant adult.

[12] See discussion of "Primitive Mentality and the Racial Unconscious," *Amer. J. Psychiatry* (1925) 4:671. The matter in point is illustrated, for example, by Ribble, Margarethe A., Clinical Studies of Instinctive Reactions in New Born Babies. *Amer. J. Psychiatry* (1938) 95:149–158. Note the stupor reaction following defeat of the infant's efforts at sucking—pp. 154–157. See, then, Sullivan, Harry Stack, The Oral Complex. *Psychoanalytic Rev.* (1925) 12:31–38 and, the same, Erogenous Maturation. *Psychoanalytic Rev.* (1926) 13:1–15. Note also Hadley, Ernest E., The Psychoanalytic Clarification of Personality Types. *Amer. J. Psychiatry* (1938) 94:1417–1430; in particular, pp. 1424–1425. Some observations in this connection were reported at the 1938 meeting of the Association for Research in Nervous and Mental Diseases; McGraw, Myrtle B., *Research Publications* 19:244–246.

Empathy is the term that we use to refer to the peculiar emotional linkage that subtends the relationship of the infant with other significant people—the mother or the nurse. Long before there are signs of any understanding of emotional expression, there is evidence of this emotional contagion or communion. This feature of the infant-mother configuration is of great importance for an understanding of the acculturation or cultural conditioning to which I have referred.

We do not know much about the fate of empathy in the developmental history of people in general. There are indications that it endures throughout life, at least in some people. There are few unmistakable instances of its function in most of us, however, in our later years; I find it convenient to assume that the time of its great importance is later infancy and early childhood—perhaps age six to twenty-seven months. So much for empathy.

The other strange term in our statement about the epoch of infancy is *autistic*, an adjective by which we indicate a primary, unsocialized, unacculturated state of symbol activity, and later states pertaining more to this primary condition than to the conspicuously effective consensually validated symbol activities of more mature personality. The meaning of the autistic will become clearer in my discussion of language.

We see our infant, then, expanding as a personality through the exercise of ability or power. We see him using the magic tool of the cry. We now see him acquiring another tool, which in turn also becomes magical. I refer here to his expression of satisfaction. It is biological for the infant when nourished to show certain expressive movements which we call the satisfaction-response, and it is probably biological for the parent concerned to be delighted to see these things. Due to the empathic linkage, this, the reaction of the parent to the satisfaction-response of the infant, communicates good feeling to the infant and thus he learns that this response has power. Actually, this may be taken to be the primitive root of human generosity, the satisfaction in giving satisfaction and pleasure: another thing learned by some people in infancy.

I shall pass infancy now, to return presently to one aspect of it. As soon as the infant has picked up a vocal trick, saying perhaps "ma" and getting a tremendous response from the significant adult, without any idea of precisely what has happened but catching on the second time it happens, as soon as the rudiments of language habits have appeared, we say that infancy as a state of personality development has ceased and that the young one has become a child.

Childhood includes a rapid acculturation, but not alone in the basic acquisition of language, which is itself an enormous cultural entity. By this I mean that in childhood the peculiar mindlessness of the infant which seems to be assumed by most parents passes off and they begin to regard the little one as in need of training, as being justifiably an object of education; and what they train the child in consists of select excerpts from the cultural heritage, from that surviving of past people, incorporated in the personality of the parent. This includes such things as habits of cleanliness—which are of extremely good repute in the Western culture—and a great many other things. And along with all this acculturation, toilet habits, eating habits, and so on and so forth, there proceeds the learning of the language as a tool for communication.

The ability to make articulate noises and the ability to pick phonemal stations in vocal sound—that is, the peculiar ones of a continuum of sounds which are used in the forming of words, which varies, incidentally, from language to language —the ability, as I say, to learn phonemes,[13] to connect them

[13] The *phoneme* is a particular zone or station in the continuum of audible vibrations around which the use of a particular language has established meaning for the identification of verbal intention. A phoneme is more than a particular number of cycles per second of vibration; it is a family of such particular c.p.s. plus overtones, etc. The K sounds in *can, cool, keep, come* are of one phoneme. The phoneme is the linguistic unit of the person's speech; the *diaphone* is the corresponding term for the approximate phonemal coin-

into syllables and words, is inborn. That is given in the human organism. The original usage of these phonemal stations, syllables, words, however, is magical, as witness the "ma" and as witness, for example, any of you who have a child who has been promised on a certain birthday a pony. As you listen to the child talk about the pony you realize perhaps sadly that twenty-five years from now when he talks about ponies, pony will not have a thousandth of the richness of personal meaning that pony has for him now. The word of the child is autistic, it has a highly individual meaning, and the process of learning language habits consists to a great extent, once one has got a vocabulary, in getting a meaning to each particular term which is useful in communication. None of us succeeds completely in this; some of us do not succeed noticeably.

Along with learning of language, the child is experiencing many restraints on the freedom which it had enjoyed up till now. Restraints have to be used in the teaching of some of the personal habits that the culture requires everyone should show, and from these restraints there comes the evolution of the self system—an extremely important part of the personality—with a brand-new tool, a tool so important that I must give you its technical name, which unhappily coincides with a word of common speech which may mean to you anything. I refer to *anxiety*.

With the appearance of the self system or the self dynamism, the child picks up a new piece of equipment which we technically call anxiety. Of the very unpleasant experiences which the infant can have we may say that there are generically two, pain and fear. Now comes the third.

cidences that make up intelligible speech. See Sapir, Edward, *Language, An Introduction to the Study of Speech;* New York, Harcourt, Brace, 1921, reprinted 1929 (vii and 258 pp.); Sound Patterns in Language. *Language* (1925) 1:37–51; Dialect. *Encyclopædia of the Social Sciences;* New York, Macmillan (1931) 5:123–126; Language. *The same* (1933) 9:155–169; La Réalité Psychologiques des Phonèmes. *Journal de Psychologie* (1933) 30:247–265. A selected bibliography of this great linguist and cultural anthropologist appears in PSYCHIATRY (1938) 1:154–157.

It is necessary in the modification of activity in the interest of power in interpersonal relations, including revery and elementary constructive revery—that is, thought—that one focus, as it were, one's interest into certain fields that work. It is in learning this process that the self is evolved and the instrumentality of anxiety comes into being.

As one proceeds into childhood, disapproval, dissatisfaction with one's performances becomes more and more the tool of the significant adult in educating the infant in the folk ways, the tradition, the culture in which he is expected to live. This disapproval is felt by the child through the same empathic linkage which has been so conspicuous in infancy. Gradually he comes to perceive disapproving expressions of the mother, let us say; gradually he comes to understand disapproving statements; but before this perception and understanding he has felt the disapproval which he was not able to comprehend through the ordinary sensory channels.

This process, coupled with the prohibitions and the privations that he must suffer in his education, sets off the experiences that he has in this education and gives them a peculiar coloring of discomfort, neither pain nor fear but discomfort of another kind. Along with these experiences there go in all well regulated homes and schools a group of rewards and approbations for successes. These, needless to say, are not accompanied by this particular type of discomfort, and when that discomfort is present and something is done which leads to approbation, then this peculiar discomfort is assuaged and disappears. The peculiar discomfort is the basis of what we ultimately refer to as anxiety.

The self dynamism is built up out of this experience of approbation and disapproval, of reward and punishment. The peculiarity of the self dynamism is that as it grows it functions, in accordance with its state of development, right from the start. As it develops, it becomes more and more related to a microscope in its function. Since the approbation of the important person is very valuable, since disapprobation denies satisfaction and gives anxiety, the self becomes extremely important. It permits a minute focus on those performances of the child which are the cause of approbation and disapprobation, but, very much like a microscope, it interferes with noticing the rest of the world. When you are staring through your microscope, you don't see much except what comes through that channel. So with the self dynamism. It has a tendency to focus attention on performances with the significant other person which get approbation or disfavor. And that peculiarity, closely connected with anxiety, persists thenceforth through life. It comes about that the self, that to which we refer when we say "I," is the only thing which has alertness, which notices what goes on, and, needless to say, notices what goes on in its own field. The rest of the personality gets along outside of awareness. Its impulses, its performances, are not noted.

Not only does the self become the custodian of awareness, but when anything spectacular happens that is not welcome to the self, not sympathetic to the self dynamism, anxiety appears, almost as if anxiety finally became the instrument by which the self maintained its isolation within the personality.

Needless to say, the self is extremely important in psychiatry and in everyday life. Not only does anxiety function to discipline attention, but it gradually restricts personal awareness. The facilitations and deprivations by the parents and significant others are the source of the material which is built into the self dynamism. Out of all that happens to the infant and child, only this 'marked' experience is incorporated into the self, because through the control of personal awareness the self itself from the beginning facilitates and restricts its further growth. In other words, it is self-perpetuating, if you please, tends very strongly to maintain the direction and characteristics which it was given in infancy and childhood.

For the expression of all things in the personality other than those which were approved and disapproved by the parent and other significant persons, the self refuses awareness, so to speak. It does not accord awareness, it does not notice; and these impulses, desires, and needs come to exist disassociated from the self, or *dissociated*. When they are expressed, their expression is not noticed by the person.

Our awareness of our performances, and our awareness of the performances of others are permanently restricted to a part of all that goes on and the structure and character of that part is determined by our early training; its limitation is maintained year after year by our experiencing anxiety whenever we tend to overstep the margin.

Needless to say, limitations and peculiarities of the self may interfere with the pursuit of biologically necessary satisfactions. When this happens, the person is to that extent mentally ill. Similarly, they may interfere with security, and to that extent also the person is mentally ill.

The self may be said to be made up of reflected appraisals. If these were chiefly derogatory, as in the case of an unwanted child who was never loved, of a child who has fallen into the hands of foster parents who have no real interest in him as a child; as I say, if the self dynamism is made up of experience which is chiefly derogatory, then the self dynamism will itself be chiefly derogatory. It will facilitate hostile, disparaging appraisals of other people and it will entertain disparaging and hostile appraisals of itself.

As I have said, the peculiarity exists that one can find in others only that which is in the self. And so the unhappy child who grows up without love will have a self dynamism which shows great capacity for finding fault with others and, by the same token, with himself. That low opinions of oneself are seldom expressed with simple frankness can also be explained.

So difficult is the maintenance of a feeling of security among his fellows for anyone who has come to have a hostile-derogatory self, that the low self-appreciation must be excluded from direct communication. A person who shrewdly attacks the prestige of sundry other people can scarcely add to each such performance a statement to the effect that he knows, because he has the same fault or defect. At the same time, we know that that which is in the self is not dissociated from the self; in other words, if it shows in the witting performances towards others, it is within the limits of personal awareness and not outside, resisted, so to say, by anxiety.

The relative silence about the low self-appraisal is achieved in part by the clamor of derogating others, in part by preoccupation with implicit revery processes that dramatize the opposite of one's defects, or protest one's rights, or otherwise manifest indirectly one's feeling of unworthiness and inferiority.

Let us rest this matter here for the time being, and review what has been said. We have seen something of the origin and organization of the self and of its marked tendency to stabilize the course of its development. We have seen that if, for example, it is a self which arose through derogatory experience, hostility toward the child, disapproval, dissatisfaction with the child, then this self more or less like a microscope tends to preclude one's learning anything better, to cause one's continuing to feel a sort of limitation in oneself, and while this can not be expressed clearly, while the child or the adult that came from the child does not express openly self-depreciatory trends, he does have a depreciatory attitude toward everyone else, and this really represents a depreciatory attitude toward the self.

The stabilizing influence of past experience is due to the fact that when it is incorporated in the organization of the self, the structure of the self dynamism, it precludes the experience of anything corrective, anything that would be strikingly different. The direction of growth in the self is maintained by the control exercised over personal awareness and by the circumscribing of experience by anxiety when anything quite different from one's prevailing attitude tends to be noticed.

We have seen how the self can be a derogatory and a hateful system, in which case the self will inhibit any experience of friendliness, of positive attitude toward other persons, and thus continue to go on derogatory, hostile, negative, in its attitude toward others.

This selective exclusion of experience which leads to one's being occupied with or noticing only the hostile unfriendly aspect of living not only is manifested in one's attitude toward others, but also is represented in the attitude toward the self. No matter how well the outward manifestations of self-contempt may be disguised, we may be assured that they are there. We see here the explanation of one of the greatest mysteries of human life, how some unfortunate people carry on in the face of apparently overwhelming difficulties, whereas other people are crushed by comparatively insignificant events, contemplate suicide, perhaps actually attempt it.

This is to be understood on the basis not of the particular 'objective' events which bring about the circumstance of success under great hardship or self-destruction; it is to be understood on the basis of the experience which is the foundation of the self system, the organization of experience reflected to one from the significant people around one—which determines the personal characteristics of those events. In no other fashion can we explain the enormous discrepancy between people's reactions to comparable life situations.

Every one of you knows of circumstances in which people encounter things which you would regard as too much to be borne, yet they go on with a certain measure of cheerfulness and optimism; whereas other people who, so far as you can see, have every advantage, have much to look forward to, meet some, to you, rather trifling rebuff, become depressed, and may actually destroy themselves.

The practice of suicide is a strange ingredient of culture. So far as we know, there is nothing remotely approaching it in the infrahuman primates or any of the lower animals. It is distinctly a human performance, and to some a very mystifying one. It is to be understood in many cases, if not in all, by realizing the force of the dictum which I have offered to the effect that the attitude manifested toward others reflects faithfully the attitude which must be manifested toward oneself. It is merely a question, then, of when a derogatory and hostile attitude, ordinarily directed toward the outer world, is directed with full force toward the self.

I do not need to tell you in this connection how hatefully conceived and executed many suicides really are, if you have taken the trouble to study any instance of this event. This, of course, does not get into the newspaper accounts, but if you know a family situation in which such an event has occurred you will be impressed with the fact that the self-destruction had an evil effect, and may well have been calculated to have a prolonged evil effect on some other people. This is literally a miracle of the dissociation which education gives us, by which our impulse to live—our grasp on the always numerous and largely unpredictable future possibilities—by which the optimism that makes us look toward the unpredictable with hope shall, in these people, be vanquished entirely by a hateful combination of impulses which leads to destroying oneself in order to strike at some other person.

The act of suicide at the moment is again becoming fashionable. When I say that it is becoming fashionable, I do not refer to some index, some statistical sign, which means that out of 100,000 such and such number have this year destroyed themselves. I refer to the fact which has been seen repeatedly during so brief a compass as my own lifetime, that, regardless of economic factors and other indices of the gross movements in the population and in the affairs of the people, the frequency of suicide periodically—or aperiodically—mounts rapidly and then declines. It is common human experience that suicide is much more often contemplated than it is attempted. It appears that to think of destroying oneself, to follow a train of revery in which one's death is a feature, is not at all unusual; certainly in many people it is not at all unusual, although, parenthetically, in some people it would be very strange indeed.

The revery in which self-destruction is, for our purpose, the theme, does not stop with the contemplation of self-destruction. It goes on. Self-destruction, therefore, is not the goal of this revery process, of this daydream, this private symbolic operation, if you please. Something else is the goal. A quite frank report of some of these reveries shows that while one may start out meditating on how worthless life is, how gladly one would be rid of it and all, one drifts from there to contemplations of what the situation in regard to other people would be after the act.

This is the sort of revery which is not uncommon. It very often discharges the suicidal impulse. One thinks about it to oneself, which we call having a revery, and then one drops it. One drops it because the revery process, after the fashion of revery processes, is a constructive movement, calculated to discover the probable effects of an event or the probably successful ways of achieving an end. From that standpoint the rumination on self-destruction, thought through, is seen not to be a means of obtaining any desire.

The revery studies danger, personal probabilities, with, as an unwitting goal, a goal that is not noticed by the person who is entertaining the suicidal fantasy, the prevention of this very act of self-destruction. The prevention of the hostile-destructive act is the unwitting goal, the unnoticed goal, of the revery process. Suicidal reveries are not as a rule fantasies with, as an end, the destruction of oneself; they are reveries in which one actually considers consequences and reaches the decision, if you please, that self-destruction would not achieve the object concerned. It would follow that that object is the exteriorization of an hostile, derogatory attitude which one has acquired in infancy and childhood, particularly childhood, which one has continued to entertain because of the focussing effect of the self system, and to manifest toward other people.

Almost incidentally the having of this suicidal revery resolves the situation which provokes the impulse to self-destruction. Then one drifts into reverie processes that lead to constructive, or at least much less destructive, ends.

More illuminating in the same connection is the unsuccessful attempt at suicide. To call your attention to a group of processes that are concerned in many of these attempts, I shall tell a story from my own experience which has, so far as I know, nothing to do with suicide.

Once upon a time I was able to enjoy my pleasure in horseback riding, and on a certain occasion, under certain unamusing circumstances which I must suppress because their recital would reduce the solemnity of this occasion, I fell from a horse. Of course, as I could tell it, the horse threw me; but in any case I ceased to be on the back of the horse and contacted the earth with considerable violence, such that I fractured a jaw.

Prior to this accident I had been somewhat given to jumping horses. Subsequent to the accident, for over a year and a half, I made no successful jumps. I invariably pulled the horse off as we approached the hurdle, to my great embarrassment and very considerable loss of prestige. It none the less happened inevitably, and it was only after about a year and a half that I succeeded in so 'controlling' my motor apparatus that I and the horse could get over a hurdle again.

The story is told to illustrate the vanquishing of my desire for prestige and my satisfaction in such things well done by something which was quite exterior to my control. In all it was me, but when I say it was me I mean that it most emphatically was not my self. My self was all set to resume jumping horses with the pleasure that comes from it and that special expansive satisfaction that attends doing something about which many people are somewhat hesitant and which not too many people do quite well. Not any need of security on my part in the sense that I have expressed here, nor any lack of need for the satisfaction that comes from this particular type of sport; neither of these groups of impulses had anything to do with my pulling the horse away from the jump. Something else had to do with that, something of which I had no vivid awareness and over which I certainly had nothing of what is ordinarily meant by control. My will, to drop into the archaic language, was too weak to control some base impulse in me that thwarted the horse and me.

We have here an instance of a part of personality working in dissociation, but working very powerfully, more powerfully than all the motives that are channelled through the self.

Many of the attempted suicides which prove such dramatic failures that we are inclined to suspect the honesty and reality of the attempt are of much the same order as my failure to jump the horse. The act has been contemplated carefully and the motivation is there. So far as the person is aware there is no room for doubt but that he will now destroy himself. But something 'stupid' is done so that the act fails and he does not die.

This is not by any means as often a fraudulent dramatic attempt to do something which one doesn't intend to do for the purpose of coercing someone else as it is the intervention of the dissociated part of personality, the part of the personality that has been growing up under great handicap in contradistinction to the experience to which the self is receptive. In the particular instance which I have stressed so much, where the individual experience as incorporated in the self has been almost entirely derogatory and hateful, you will realize that the dissociated part consists of the experience of human warmth and friendliness. It is this part of personality, this group of processes, which intervenes to prevent a fatal issue of the impulse.

It is almost cavalier to rest with such fleeting reference to the extra-self—at that, almost as an addendum to a consideration of suicide. If, however, you have finally seen the dichotomous character of these hypothetical personalities of ours—how that which is excluded from awareness by virtue of the directing influence of the self dynamism, must be quite different in some essential aspects from that which is incorporated in and manifests as the self—you can see why we seem so individuated, and yet can be, to quote myself, much more simply human than otherwise.

LECTURE
II

The Human Organism and Its Necessary Environment

It has been suggested that a consideration of the meaning of psychiatry could carry us from the dimmest past through the work of innumerable people, with almost as many contradictory views—sometimes self-contradictory views—as there were workers. So also would a survey of the history of the meaning of man spread before us an ineffably wearisome account of circuitous progress in the face of stupendous obstacles created by man. As in the first case, so here we would come finally to a present view which is anything but universally accepted.

In the dreary progression, if our wits are not bemused, we would observe many views that represent what we now know that man is *not.* Man is not a creature of instinct—the view of Aristotle and of William McDougall; of transcendental powers between or among which he may choose his allegiance—the medieval view rather sympathetic to Otto Rank; of logic and its categorical opposite—Bacon and in a way Alfred Adler and Alfred Korzybski; of the evolution of social intellect—Compte and some mental hygienists; of racial fitness—de Gobineau and Fuhrer Hitler; of a conflict of society and one's instincts—Freud; or of a racial unconscious—Jung.

As we survey the present, we can see four significant conceptions. For the general biologist, man is the most complexly integrated organism thus far evolved. For the psychobiologist, man is an individual organism the total-function of which is mentally integrated life. For the social psychologist, man is the human animal transformed by social experience into a human being. For the psychiatrist as a student of interpersonal relations, man is the tangible substrate of human life.

These definitions grow progressively more complex in scope. Let us consider the beginning of anyone, the fecundated ovum in the uterus. This cell manifests the basic categories of biological process. The cell carries almost stupifying potentialities. It exists as a demonstrable entity. It lives, however, and starts the realization of its potentialities, not as a unit organism surrounded by a suitable environment. It lives communally *with* the environment. Physico-chemical factors, substances, plentiful in the uterine environment flow into the cell. They undergo changes while they are within the describable cell-area. They return presently as other physico-chemical factors, to the environment. The cell dies if the continuous exchange is interrupted. Progressive changes depend utterly on the communion; retrogressive changes appear swiftly on its restriction.

From a relative position in time and space, the environment flows through the living cell, becoming of its very life in the process; and the cell flows and grows through the environment, establishing in this process its particular career-line as an organism. It is artificial, an abstraction, to say that the cell is one thing and the environment another. The two entities thus postulated refer to some unitary thing in which organism and environment are indissolubly bound—so long as life continues.

In the cell-medium complex one can observe much that is marvelous. There are factors of organization, including polarity and dynamic gradients, which establish an oral and an aboral end in the expanding cell mass, which gradually evolves the fœtus, ready for birth.

Before there are any elaborate differentiations of tissue, however; before in fact there has been a single division of the fertile cell, there is organization in the cell-medium complex such that a vital balance is maintained in the more purely organismic part of the complex. True, a change in the maternal blood may prove too great for the successful maintenance of this balance, and the complex disintegrates, the ovum dies. Quite marked changes in the medium, however, do not disturb the optimum conditions in the cell-medium complex, due to functional activity of the region to which we refer as the cell wall. This region performs the function for which the fœtus will ultimately be provided with elaborate organizations of tissues; in fact, duplicate organizations of whole systems.

Biologically, then, an organism is a self-perpetuating organization of the physico-chemical world which manifests life by functional activity in the complex. It is easy to think that the organism is an entity that can be removed from the complex, and some color is given this erroneous view by virtue of the storage capacity that is part of the vital organization.

The process of birth would seem to a naive observer to cut off the infant from the maternal—placental—medium and project him into the medium of the outer world. The communion with the physico-chemical environment has in fact to be maintained with but a short-term interruption—during which the oxygen and other necessary substances stored in the fœtus are all that prevent death. Breathing must begin promptly. It is essential also that coverings be supplied to prevent loss of heat. Nursing cannot long be delayed.

The infant is born in far too immature a state to live by its own functional activity, unaided by interventions from others. This is quite different from the guinea pig, which has been described as born in its old age.[14] It reflects a fundamental fac-

[14] Tilney, Frederick, and Casamajor, Louis, Myelinology as Applied to the Study of Behavior. *Arch. Neurol. and Psychiat.* (1924) 12:1–66. Note, also, Hooker, Davenport, Fetal Behavior. *Publications of the Association for Research in Nervous and Mental Diseases* 19:237–243; and the relevant part of Conel, J. Leroy, The Brain Structure of the Newborn Infant. . . . *The same,* 19:247–255.

tor that makes civilization possible—the long stretch of post-natal life required by the human young for the attainment of independent competence to live. As growth and maturation proceed acculturation is inevitable, because in the earliest stages, the infant is cared for by people, and modified by this personal element in the environment. The course of existence from fecundation of the ovum may be said to be: parasitic, new born (animal), then infantile (human). The change from new born to infantile is less dramatic than its predecessor, but it is a very great change indeed; and also entails a change of medium implying a change of functional activity in a complex of changing organization.

Almost from birth, the infant begins to attend to movements and objects about him.[15] Several of Peterson's infants looked at him and followed his movements with their eyes as early as the seventh day after birth. There is no room for doubt as to the significance attached to the object which satisfies the hunger and thirst of the infant, and we may safely infer that the *mothering one* is the first vivid perception of a person relatively independent of the infant's own vague entity.

I surmise that a part of her, the nipple, provides the first of all vividly meaningful symbols—a vaguely demarcated "complex-image" or protoconcept with very wide reference. The clarification of the nipple as borne by another person instead of its being a relatively unmanageable part of one's own cosmic entity is the first step in shrinking to life size. Outer objects of a more neutral sort—that do not satisfy physico-chemical needs directly—come gradually to mark off the limits of one's private world, and so to establish the reality of the relatively manageable as against the wholly independent.

[15] See Peterson, Frederick, The Beginnings of Mind in the New Born. *Bulletin of the Lying-in Hospital of the City of New York* (1910) 7:99–122. In this paper, the work of Adolf Kussmaul (1859), Alfred Genzmer (1873), and Traugott Kroner (1882) on infants in maternity hospitals is summarized, and new observations on 1060 babies—some premature—are reported. Special sense responsivenesses were determined in from 31 to 78 infants within the first six hours after delivery.

We learn in infancy that objects which our distance receptors, our eyes and ears for example, encounter, are of a quite different order of relationship from things which our tactile or our gustatory receptors encounter. That which one has in one's mouth so that one can taste it, while it may be regurgitated to the distress of everyone, is still in a very different relationship than is the full moon which one encounters through one's eye but can in no sense manage.

This difference of relationship to objects is an important category for organizing one's knowledge about the world. We organize our acquaintance with the world in order to maintain necessary or pleasant functional activity within the world with which, whether the objects be manageable or unmanageable, remote or immediate, one has to maintain communal existence —however unwittingly.

I have spoken of the functional interaction, in infancy and childhood, of the significant other person, the mother, as a source of satisfaction, as an agency of acculturation, and finally as a source of anxiety and insecurity in the development of social habits which is the basis of development of the self system. Let us now attend, particularly, to the mediate channels of acculturation, in particular the products of the printer's art.

In this culture all children fairly early encounter pictures. Many of them have picture books, as they are called. Picture books often have a little printed matter in them, and gradually the child learns to read. Remembering what was said before as to the autistic, the highly personal meaning of everything to the young child, we can best illustrate the process of consensual validation by referring to what goes on when, for example, the young child learns that a certain colored or black and white pattern in a book is "kitty," although, of course, there is also "kitty" who runs around and occasionally scratches one.

I am sure no child who can learn has not noticed an enormous discrepancy between this immobile representation in the book which, perhaps, resembles one of the momentary states that kitty has been in on some occasion. I am certain that every child knows that there is something very strange in this printed representation being so closely connected with the same word that seems to cover adequately the troublesome, amusing, and very active pet. Yet, because of unnumbered, sometimes subtle, sometimes crude experiences with the carrier of culture, the parent, the child finally comes to accept as valid and useful a reference to the picture as "kitty" and to the creature as "kitty."

The child thus learns some of the more complicated implications of a symbol in contradistinction to the actuality to which the symbol refers, which is its referent; in other words, the distinction between the symbol and that which is symbolized. This occurs, however, before verbal formulation is possible.

From the picture book and the spoken word in this culture one progresses to the printed word and finally discovers that the combination of signs, c-a-t, includes "kitty" in some miraculous fashion, and that it always works. There is nothing like consistent experience to impress one with the validity of an idea. So one comes to a point where printed words, with or without consensually valid meaning, come to be very important in one's growth of acquaintance with the world.

There was first the visually and otherwise impressive pet, which was called "kitty" (an associated vocalization); then came the picture of the kitten; now comes the generic *c a t* which includes kitty, picture of kitten, a kitten doll, and alley cats seen from the windows. And all this is learnt so easily that —since no one troubles to point it out—there is no lucid understanding of the sundry types of reality and reference that are being experienced. Familiarity breeds indifference, in this case. The possibilities for confusion in handling the various kinds of symbols, naturally, remain quite considerable.

Let me now suggest something of the wide spread of significance in speech as speech, rather than as spoken words and sentences. Some of you may recall from childhood the experience of first encountering a person whose dialect was not the accustomed one. Or, perhaps, you may recall the first hearing of a conversation in a foreign tongue.

If some such experience is recaptured, let us compare it with the general experience of children with strangers. When the stranger speaks in the accustomed dialect—quite aside from the extensive significance of other non-verbal factors in everyone's speech—the insecurity felt by the child is diminished. The familiar diaphonic progressions convey some reassurance as to the *naturalness* of the stranger. He is not some awesome creature from the autistic world blended out of dreams and longings and tales of wonder that one has been told.

This unity in one's dialect-group, which presently spreads to include one's language-group, is by no means restricted to the era of childhood. Many Americans who go to Europe and move among peoples in the use of whose tongue they are not competent, show the same factor in the attitudes that they manifest. The people whom they encounter are not invested with as complete a set of human traits as are even the more obnoxious of our acquaintances at home. These foreigners are not quite human. One feels emancipated correspondingly from some or many of the restraints that govern one in life at home. One does odd things—sometimes durably regrettable things—that have never occurred to one before. There is an attenuation of our conventional inhibition because we do not recognize these strangers as fully human and do not accord them the same critical attitudes towards us that we have accustomed ourselves to live with.

The solidarity creating power of a common tongue is most important. This factor comes gradually to manifest itself, also, in the matter of the printed word.

That which is printed is ordinarily directed to a larger and less specific audience than is the spoken word.[16] It almost neces-

[16] The written expression of any language must be recognized to be more

sarily conveys some feeling of impersonality, of larger than tete-a-tete situations. Correspondingly, it usually tends to expand one's feeling of acquaintance with the world—the world of behavior, of opinion, of geographical facts. This function of the printed page is what I meant by mediate acculturation: the accession of cultural factors not directly from a significant person who manifests them, but through the instrumentality of narrative and reading.[17]

We come now to the juvenile era, in which the use of this mediate channel is very important. Childhood, for our purpose, is marked off from the juvenile era by the appearance of an urgent need for compeers with whom to have one's existence. By "compeers" I mean people who are on our level, and have generically similar attitudes toward authoritative figures,

---

or less *a different* language than is the same tongue, used in vocal speech. The "inner speech" of more elaborated revery processes is still a different language. The degrees of difference of these three categories of verbal symbol operations vary from person to person. See: Sapir's Language; *Encyclopædia of the Social Sciences* (1933) 9:155–169, already cited; also Newman, Stanley S., Personal Symbolism in Language Patterns. PSYCHIATRY (1939) 2:177–184 and Vigotsky, L. S., Thought and Speech [translation of Chapter VII of his 1934 monograph on Language and Thought, by Drs. Helen Kogan, Eugenia Hanfmann, and Jacob Kasanin]. PSYCHIATRY (1939) 2:29–52.

[17] The processes of acculturation are rich, largely unexplored, fields for research. In the last few years, a new *mediate* channel has appeared in the shape of the radio. The person who speaks over the wireless is addressing a presumptively great number of people. His speech—all the more because of existing rules as to submitting "script" in advance—tends to approximate the written rather than the spoken version of the language. If he is at all expert, however, his voice communicates the impression *not* of someone reading something aloud *but of a rounded personality talking to one*. In this fact, there lies a field of investigation of very great importance. The study of the personalizations of the radio speaker, as they appear in persons who habitually listen to him, is a certainly fruitful approach to an understanding of the nonverbal communicative aspects of the voice.

American radio research seems quite indifferent to this problem. See, however, Pear, T. H., *Voice and Personality;* London, Chapman and Hall, 1931 (ix and 247 pp.) and Allport, Gordon W. and Cantril, Hadley, Judging Personality from the Voice. *J. Soc. Psychology* (1934) 5:37–55. The accuracy of judging personality from the voice is not, of course, the point of my discussion. By discovering what sort of personalizations the voice may evoke, by seeking out the factors in voice and in hearer that are concerned in this, we may finally come to some understanding of the voice as a uniquely important factor in interpersonal relations.

activities, and the like. This marks the beginning of the juvenile era, the great developments in which are the talents for cooperation, competition and compromise.

But before we have done with the developmental epoch of childhood, let me recall to you the biological fact of communal existence. If one scrutinizes the performances of any child, it will be evident that the child as a creature is existing in communal existence in or with an environment now importantly cultural in its composition. The cultural entities, so to speak, are part of the necessary environment. The human being requires the world of culture, cannot live *and be human* except in communal existence with it. The world of culture is, however, clearly manifest only in human behavior and thought. Other people are, therefore, an indispensable part of the environment of the human organism. This is absolutely true in the earlier phases of personality development. The factor of fantasy may cloud this issue in later stages, as in fact, it may be observed to do at the end of the epoch of childhood in the case of isolated children.

The era of childhood ends with the maturation of a need for compeers. The child manifests a shift from contentment in an environment of authoritarian adults and the more or less personalized pets, toys and other objects, towards an environment of persons significantly *like* him. If playmates are available, his integrations with them show new meaningfulness. If there are no playmates, the child's revery processes create imaginary playmates. In brief, the child proceeds into the *juvenile era* of personality development by virtue of a new tendency towards cooperation, to doing things in accommodation to the personality of others. Along with this budding ability to play with other children, there goes a learning of those performances which we call competition and compromise.

In the juvenile era, in this culture, school is the great new arena for experience. If one's parents have been reasonably wise, one is somewhat prepared for what one encounters. If that was not the case, one is apt to have a very hard time, for one's compeers are not yet come to possess sympathy and forbearance. Quite the contrary, they are having enough problems of their own, enough new thwartings and humiliations, to be very unpleasant to the luckless juvenile who has recourse to inappropriate magic from childhood—tears, tantrums, telling mamma, or the like.

School brings new experience in adjusting oneself to authority. We may assume that one has evolved techniques for handling one's parents with only a modicum of pain. Now come other adults who have to be managed. One discovers quite suddenly that parents are by no means the worst people in the world; that parents, whatever their faults, take one rather more seriously than do teachers and older boys and girls. One finds that tried and trusted symbol operations—speech, gesture, excuses, promises—are no longer effective. Autistic fringes begin to stand out as barriers to communication. Mediate and immediate acculturation proceed apace. The world begins to spread, the horizons move off. One begins to see that there is a great deal which one had not previously suspected.

The interpersonal factors between teacher and the pupil in this school situation may work good or may work evil effects on the growth of personality. Where, for example, there has been an eccentric parent, let us say for example a person of extreme puritanical rigidity, a teacher may give the first clue to the child that this is not the ubiquitous attitude of people, of important people, to life. The child, at first—because novel experience is very difficult to get within the focus of the self—may feel that the teacher is some queer kind of dangerous inferior creature, the sort of person with whom one's parents would not associate. Still gradually, gradually, because other children who are now important put up with this, take it for granted, seem to think that it is perfectly natural; because of this powerful support or validation of the novelty, the self may expand somewhat. This is always a difficult achievement; but the self may come as it were to doubt certain of the harsh puritanical restrictions which have been incorporated in it, and while perhaps they do not disappear and in times of stress throughout life may manifest themselves clearly, still the experience of the school may head the self dynamism in another direction which will make for much greater opportunity for contented living, for mental health.

On the other hand, harsh, cruel teachers—and there are certain people teaching school who enjoy the discomfiture of their charges—may affect the child from a happy home who has been taught to expect friendliness and a receptive and inquiring attitude, may teach him gradually by reiterated pain and humiliation, that the world into which he has moved is an unfriendly and cruel world, and may start revery processes in him the goal of which is to return to the home from which he has unhappily been expelled, apparently for no reason other than that he had gotten older. In this, a very considerable evil has been done because the character of these reveries is regressive. They seek to go back, and this child may indicate this regressive, retreating-into-the-past tendency by regretting that he has grown older, by wishing that he was younger again.

This regressive tendency is a great evil because development still has a very long way to go. If at the very beginning of the more specialized socialization of personality which the juvenile era, according to its limits, initiates, there is this strong reverse, this powerful rebuff, this cutting off of satisfactions or undermining of security, in the mind's eye the child turns backward, he seeks to avoid the future, to escape experience which would teach how to live with one's fellows. This example may suffice to emphasize the effect on the growth of personality of the interpersonal factors which exist between teacher and pupil. Even as this is true, it is also true that barring extraordinary situations—all too frequent before school entry—the effect is neither very bad nor very good. By and large it is useful.

Besides contacts with the school personnel there is the playground situation with other children, the bully, and so on, perhaps with a supervisor of playgrounds, a useful addition in many situations. Also, there is another side of the school situation; namely, the reaction of the home to the rumors of what goes on in school. This, too, can work good and evil. And then there is the attitude of the home toward the compeers, these others who have now become so significant in the development of personality.

With this briefest of indications I shall leave this prolonged and tremendously important era and go on to the next era of personality development.

Around the age of eight and one-half, nine and one-half to twelve, in this culture, there comes what I once called the quiet miracle of preadolescence. Quiet because there is nothing dramatic or exciting about its appearance; there is no sudden change by which one has ceased to be a juvenile and has become a preadolescent. In fact, everything is rather gradual, flows out of the past through the present into the future in personality performance, however dramatic somebody else's story of it may sound. I say "miracle" of preadolescence because now for the first time from birth, we might say even from conception, there is a movement from what we might, after traditional usage, call egocentricity, toward a fully social state.

Up to this time there have been *no* instances in which some other person approximated to the subject person, the child, the juvenile, the affectional significance which the child or juvenile had for himself. Those of you who have children know your children love you, know how thoughtful they are of you, how very foresightful they are for your comfort and happiness. The student of personality who has nothing at stake but observed phenomena is, however, unable to listen with complete conviction to your accounts. He will, instead, wonder as to what particular devices, training or conditioning you have used to bring about this to you so satisfactory state. If he can get near enough to the child or the juvenile to hear what the child or juvenile can say of the situation with you, it will sound much less sentimentally perfect. It will suggest a realistic appreciation of a necessity and a human development of devices to meet the necessity. There will not be this sentimental glow of love, consideration, and so on, but rather that marvelous human thing, great adaptive possibilities applied successfully to a situation.

I suggest thus the egocentric character of personality up to the epoch of preadolescence. Adjustments made? Yes. Very subtle adjustments made? Yes. Great satisfactions to people who are interested in the child as a human? Yes. Great successes in school, great respect from the teacher, adoration of the teacher—all sorts of things which, on careful study, seem, however, to leave the child or the juvenile as the center of his processes, the thing that matters above everything to him.

This is exceedingly fortunate. The human race would have expired long centuries ago were it not so. A most thoughtful, considerate parent who would change this and who would bring about the miracle to which I am about to refer before its time would cripple his offspring, at least to the second generation. There are the most excellent reasons why true social orientation takes a long time coming. But it comes in preadolescence. The capacity to love in its initial form makes appearance as the mark that one has ceased to be juvenile and has become preadolescent. What this means in the outline of situations which it brings about is this: at this point the satisfactions and the security which are being experienced by someone else, some particular other person, begin to be as significant to the person as are his own satisfactions and security.

You have just heard a definition of the end state of love which, if you are not accustomed to this type of thinking, may seem to you a strange one. Let me repeat it, because it has certain objective validity which many other definitions might be found to lack. When the satisfaction or the security of another person becomes as significant to one as is one's own satisfaction or security, then the state of love exists. So far as I know, under no other circumstances is a state of love present, regardless of the popular usage of the word.

This state of affectional rapport—generically love—ordinarily occurs under restricted circumstances. In the beginning many factors must be present. Some of these may be called obvious likeness, parallel impulse, parallel physical development. These make for situations in which boys feel at ease with boys rather than with girls. This feeling of species identity or identification influences the feeling involved in the preadolescent change. The appearance of the capacity to love ordinarily first involves a member of one's own sex. The boy finds a chum who is a boy, the girl finds a chum who is a girl. When this has happened, there follows in its wake a great increase in the consensual validation of symbols, of symbol operations, and of information, data about life and the world.

This comes about as a fairly obvious consequence of the fact that the other fellow has now become highly significant to one. Whereas previously, one may have learned to say the right thing to one's companions, to do the right things, now these sayings and doings take on a very special significance. One's security is not imperilled by one's love object. One's satisfactions are facilitated by the love object. Therefore, naturally, for the first time one can begin to express oneself freely. If another person matters as much to you as do you yourself, it is quite possible to talk to this person as you have never talked to anyone before. The freedom which comes from this expanding of one's world of satisfaction and security to include two people, linked together by love, permits exchanges of nuances of meaning, permits investigations without fear of rebuff or humiliation, which greatly augments the consensual validation of all sorts of things, all in the end symbols that stand for—refer to, represent—states of being in the world.

In this period there begins the illumination of a real world community. As soon as one finds that all this vast autistic and somewhat validated structure to which one refers as one's mind, one's thoughts, one's personality, is really open to some comparing of notes, to some checking and counter-checking, one begins to feel human in a sense in which one has not previously felt human. One becomes more fully human in that one begins to appreciate the common humanity of people—there comes a new sympathy for the other fellow, whether he be present to the senses or mediated by rumors in the geography, or the like. In other words, the feeling of humanity is one of the aspects of the expansion of personality which comes in preadolescence. Learning at this stage begins to assume its true aspect of implementing the person in securing satisfactions and maintaining his security in interpersonal relations through the rest of life.

Previous to this time many people have learned for fun. Those were the bright pupils who very often satisfy the teacher perfectly, and the year after haven't the ghost of an idea of what the deuce it was all about. Or learning has been difficult, for rewards and punishments. It is only when the world expands as a tissue of persons and interpersonal relations which are meaningful that knowledge becomes truly significant, and learning becomes a serious attempt to implement oneself for one's future life.

It is true that some people arrive at preadolescence so crippled by 'educational' experience that this particular phenomenon in regard to learning may appear erratically, rather than uniformly. There are instances in our educational system in which the utility of the knowledge, of the learning, is so distorted that a field of information is permanently barred to any ordinary development of the personality. You will find, for example, a good many people who tell you that they are no good at mathematics. Now, it is true that mathematical genius seems to have something to do with germinal constitution. It appears in some imbeciles as well as in some people who are definitely geniuses. It runs in certain stocks, certain families, perhaps; that is, it is more abundant in them than in the population, generally. Germinal constitution is not, however, what is involved when a person tells you, "Oh, I am no good at mathematics." If you can establish a condition of sufficient confidence with this person and work back to the time when he encountered mathematics, usually in the teaching of arithmetic, you will learn that his security was grossly undermined in this process, that in some fashion or other he suffered so much pain, so much threat of anxiety, so much anxiety itself, that the whole field of intrinsically mathematical symbol operations has taken on a vague mark of anxiety. When he is confronted with a mathematical problem he experiences anxiety. He ordinarily avoids becoming involved in such problems, for this excellent reason.

When there is anxiety, it tends to exclude the situation that provoked it from awareness, and so the person made anxious by the mathematical problem tends to overlook certain commonplace, obvious aspects of the problem that are well within his grasp. The tendency is to move away from, rather than simply to grasp, the factors making up the situation presented to him.

The juvenile era often includes experience which dams certain fields of learning; the preadolescent expansion of consciousness and sympathy for a larger world of many relationships, many complexities and many people then tends to be blocked off from particular fields of knowledge. Otherwise one now begins to learn because knowledge is demonstrating its usefulness to oneself and one's friend.

One thus comes to an expansion of the necessary human environment that—with but one great interruption—goes on to the fullest development of the human organism. The interruption is the coming of genital sexuality. It may be well to review the path that we have been following, before we take up the era of adolescence, itself.

We have seen how the self comes into being as a dynamism to preserve the feeling of security. We have observed that it is built largely of personal symbolic elements learned in contact with other significant people. We have noted that the self comes to control awareness, to restrict one's consciousness of what is going on in one's situation very largely by the instrumentality of anxiety with, as a result, a dissociation from personal awareness of those tendencies of the personality which are not included or incorporated in the approved structure of the self.

The point is that the self is approved by significant others, that any tendencies of the personality that are not so approved, that are in fact strongly disapproved, are dissociated from personal awareness.

We saw that these dissociated tendencies, which do not cease to exist merely because they are excluded from the self, manifest themselves in actions, activities, of which the person himself remains quite unaware. The actions are unnoticed and the goals of the activities are things of which the person has no conscious knowledge.

This dissociation of components of the personality is not restricted to the pursuit of satisfaction. Some of the power processes which the infant and the child, perhaps even the juvenile, found effective also come under such stern disapproval at a later stage of personality that they, too, are dissociated, and from then on manifest outside of the awareness of the person himself.

They were tolerated by the significant personal environment for a time, as shown, for example, for the attitude that the infant has no particular mind, and, therefore, is justified in being wholly irresponsible about certain things; but when he gets to be a child these activities are no longer satisfactory, and under certain circumstances at least he must dissociate some of the power operations, magic performances, of infancy from his consciousness of performance as a child.

It may be that anything which is useful at one stage of personality development will be dissociated in the next stage unless the culture-carrying adults encourage its continued elaboration within the self. The elaboration of some drives, like these drives to maintain security and to manifest personal power, personal capacity, capability, importance, have reasonable chance of being elaborated, at least in the case of people who grow up in rather hygienic homes. Certain other tendencies are not so fortunate and are quite certain to suffer dissociation from the personal consciousness.

We may say, however, as a generality, that healthy development of personality is inversely proportionate to the amount, to the number, of tendencies which have come to exist in dissociation. Put in another way, if there is nothing dissociated, then whether one be a genius or an imbecile, it is quite certain that he will be mentally healthy. The precise meaning of this term "mentally healthy" will gradually appear.

If, on the other hand, a person be very talented but be required by his experience, by the significant people who bear on him at various stages in his development, to dissociate from his awareness a considerable number of powerful and durable motivational systems, then that person will be markedly exposed to mental disorder. He will inevitably be maladjusted in some of the situations through which his life must develop, and that maladjustment, due to the partition in his activity, will come about quite certainly, the partition being between those activities of which he is aware versus those which he does with no awareness.

Inverting the entire proposition, one might say that the larger the proportion of energy systems in a personality which act exterior to the awareness of the person, the greater the chances that he will meet some crisis in interpersonal relations in which he cannot act in the fashion which we call mental health.

The likelihood of an acute disturbance in some interpersonal relation is greatly increased by the presence of an important motivational system in dissociation.

We have considered the growing complexity of the human environment, which we pointed out was made up of not only the physico-chemical universe, which may be assumed to be present to all the living things, and the biological universe, plants and animals that are of some interest to us, but the personal and the cultural, the cultural manifesting itself through persons, but none the less being susceptible of abstract study, as is done by the cultural anthropologists. Culture in this sense we hold to include institutions like the government, the Department of the Interior, the church, the school, and so on; the forceful convictions as to right and wrong ways of living, the mores, as sociologists are wont to call them, the traditions of the family group, of the community, and the like, and the fashions which are in force at the particular time concerned.

These are the cultural entities which are highly significant in the human environment, and all of them have their being and their manifestation so far as any particular person is concerned in other people who are significant for one reason or another to him, originally the mother as the provider of all sorts of necessary protection and satisfaction; in childhood the parents and the home society, people who are frequently in the home and related by bonds of intimacy or hostility to the parent; in the juvenile era, the school, the school teacher and all that machinery, and to a certain extent one's play companions; and in preadolescence the chum and the people in whom the chum is interested.

We have seen how this personal environment is expanded by the mediate channels of communication, the telephone, the radio, and particularly the printed word.[18]

[18] We might illustrate the power of the press by commenting on its unintended effect of determining the fashions of suicide from time to time. Fashion is used advisedly. As I recall, I have lived through three periods in which self-destruction by way of bichloride poisoning enjoyed typical vogue. Bichloride poisoning is a horrible way of terminating life. The newspapers, without

We have considered the stage of personality development in which the other fellow, the chum, someone of the same sex and approximately the same age, becomes highly significant, and by this very fact acts as the final binding agency to connect the growing individual with the full force and control action of the cultural environment. One can follow certain autistic courses, certain individualized highly personal courses of development, giving lip service to the requirements of one social environment so long as nobody in that environment has more than instrumental meaning to one. One can for instance do homage to people who are afflicted with a sense of greatness without feeling any sympathy with what they regard as important. It pays; it gives something that is repaid with what one wants—satisfactions or security. But when somebody else begins to matter as much as I do, then what this other person values must receive some careful consideration from me. So it is in the preadolescent change that the great controlling power of the cultural, social, forces is finally inescapably written into the human personality.

We will presently discuss the phase of personal evolution which is the last step toward fully human estate, with respect for others as for oneself, with the dignity befitting the high achievement and with the freedom of personal initiative which

---

mentioning this, report, some time or other, that some more or less notable person has died of bichloride of mercury poisoning, self-administered. Shortly afterwards there are little squibs here and there in the newspapers to the effect that this and that person has died by bichloride. The fashion is spreading.

The most dreadfully satirical element of this particular fashion in poisoning lies in the peculiar deviltry of the drug. One is horribly ill. If one survives the first days of hellish agony, there comes a period of relative convalescence—during which all the patients I have seen were most repentant and strongly desirous of living. Then comes the third phase, during which one suffers unimaginable agonies, again for days. Then with awful inevitability, one finally dies.

The ephemeral printed word of the news sheet influences the style of suicide after the pattern of fashion change, and the growth and the decay of a fashion of destroying oneself, the grossest of misdirections of living, literally can be traced to the accounts of a, for the moment, new method, and to the gradual ennui that comes from multitudinous reports of the same thing.

is comfortably adapted to the circumstances which characterize the particular social order of which one is a part.

Before I can discuss the phase of adolescence it is necessary that I say something more about the impulses which underlie the pursuit of satisfaction and the protection or pursuit of the feeling of security. Many of you have doubtless noticed that thus far in a presentation which started with the statement that the study of individual personality did not seem to be within the field of science, the only thing that seems amenable to scientific approach being the actions in interpersonal situations; that which someone does with me, that can be observed, both by me and by some objective third person—what goes on in that person, the unique peculiarity of his personality, seems to escape any method of science—yet I have proceeded after this preamble for over two hours with such terms as tendency, impulse, goal, and so on, as if I had departed my own dogma and were discussing individual human personality as the subject of study.

We have finally come to the point where this convenient, this false unitary individualistic language becomes highly confusing instead of definitely indicative. By that I mean this, that while I have tried thus far to indicate by the use of the conventional individualistic language some of the considerations relevant to psychiatry, I can no longer continue in that course without apology and without reemphasizing my original position, because one cannot even seem to make sense, from here on, in the individualistic language of common speech and of the traditional psychology.

We have to realize that when we talk about an impulse that underlies the pursuit of satisfaction we are using a figure of speech that comes very naturally to us, by which we must be referring to something quite different. Let me try to express the more valid content of this instance of individualistic speech more lucidly and more accurately.

When we speak of impulse to such and such action, of

tendency to such and such behavior, of striving toward such and such goal, or use any of these words which sound as if you, a unit, have these things in you and as if they can be studied by and for themselves, we are talking, according to the structure of our language and the habits of common speech, about something which is observably manifested as action in a situation. The situation is not any old thing, it is you and someone else integrated in a particular fashion which can be converted in the alembic of speech into a statement that "A is striving toward so and so from B."

As soon as I say this, you realize that B is a very highly significant element in the situation. Many situations are integrated in which A wants deference from B, and B, mirabile dictu, wants deference from A. It looks as if there were something in A and something in B that happened to collide. But when one studies the situation in which A and B pursue, respectively, the aim of getting from the other person what he himself needs and what the other person needs, we find that it is not as simple as it looks. The *situation* is still the valid object of study, or rather that which we can observe; namely, the action which indicates the situation and the character of its integration.

The situation is integrated in such manner as to resolve itself after a change that is satisfactory or satisfaction giving, or tributary to security. This is the general statement of all interpersonal situations. They are integrated in such fashion that as processes—and you remember the living are always manifesting processes and you do not have static situations, nor static people—the situation is so integrated that what action there is in it can move to the discharge or resolution of some dynamic component in each of the people.

When that has happened, the situation is at least temporarily adjourned. It has ceased to be more than a memory and a potentiality for similar situations to occur. Following, however, what we have said about the impulses that are accompanied by awareness and those that are dissociated from the awareness of the person, you will see that many situations may be integrated among or between people such that both a witting impulse, a known impulse, an understood and recognized impulse, and a dissociated impulse, are involved.

I should illustrate this, for example, by having a person integrate a situation with another person in order to get a promotion. Let us say that he is subjected to a rigid interrogatory, not only to determine his qualifications and the justification for his promotion, but also to humiliate him very cruelly.

What have we here? In the old language of common speech you would say, "Well, he has to deal with a cruel or a sadistic superior." The "has to" is open to question. Whence the compulsion which requires at this time that he should take steps to get a promotion? That might be anything. It *may* be that he has to.

Yet, let us study the superior instead of this person whom we have just discussed. Let us observe that someone else in his organization wishes to be promoted. He is interrogated, but he is interrogated carefully, so that his self-respect will not be wounded, so that he will not be humiliated or hurt.

Let us say that neither gets the promotion. There is nothing in either situation as I have described them, which implies favorable or unfavorable action. But there is a difference in these two situations which have in common an administrative person. How do we understand this? We may understand this by saying that the first person, the one who was hurt and humiliated, manifested toward his superior certain actions which called out the superior's hostility and destructiveness, that the second person in the integration with the administrator prohibited, in some fashion, the manifestation of these durable traits of the administrator.

In the first case we may safely assume that the underling did not wittingly, did not to his knowledge or with his conscious awareness, provoke the cruel impulses in the administrator. In the second case we may say that the underling did not consciously prohibit those impulses in the superior. But both situations were multiply determined. There was the acknowledged, the known, the consciously evidenced desire for progress, for improvement in one's life situation in both the applicants. There was in the first case a willingness to undergo pain, humiliation, and so on; in the second case there was some dangerous hostility which it was well to let sleep. This is a crude, perhaps not too convincing, illustration of a situation integrated by the consciously accepted motives within awareness and other impulses more or less incongruent to them.[19]

You will realize that it is very difficult for a person to feel secure and self-respecting if he knows that he carries in himself impulses which cause him to be humiliated or otherwise made to suffer by anybody in authority. And you will also, such of you as have any trace of this not too rare impulse, know that one seldom is clearly and unblushingly aware of the fact that he is rather dangerous when he is hurt. These things have been dissociated from the self in the process of development to the state, in our example, of our underlings before they apply to the superior.

Now let us consider preadolescence in connection with that type of self organization in which the predominating attitude toward others is hate. Such a state does not necessarily preclude a development to preadolescence. It may be a great handicap. It often leads to experience which does prevent development

[19] Even in so sketchy an imaginary situation as that described, multiple possibilities as to the dissociated impulses appear. In the first case, for example, the administrator may have used the applicant as a convenient foil for expressing attitudes called out by some third person, in the immediate past. In the second case, the administrator's cruel-sadistic impulse may have been inhibited from any expression by some feature of the applicant's personality which attracted him powerfully. If we have applicant Number One follow Number Two, under these circumstances, the inhibiting of the cruel-sadistic impulse towards Number Two will provide a reinforcement for its (invited) expression towards Number One. There are several other possibilities; the actual dynamics of any real situation depend on a large but finite group of factors and can be discovered by investigating the actual historic courses of patterning that have resulted in the manifest behavior of persons concerned.

to preadolescence. But it does not always do so, and quite often people whose attitude toward others is almost uniformly derogatory, whose attitude toward the self is hostile, do get on to preadolescence, and in preadolescence undergo what I have called the quiet miracle of developing the capacity of love. Someone else begins to be as significant as oneself.

What do we see in these situations? What do we see of the no longer acceptable hateful attitude in so far as it pertains to the love object? We see the evidences of a recent dissociation; in the midst of rather effective *toward* performances there will come some untoward acts of hostility to the person newly elevated to an equality of importance with oneself.

These acts are ordinary mysteries. They mystify the person who manifests them, despite the fact that such acts were about all that he manifested until, say, two months ago. Now it comes to him as shocking, he cannot understand why he does it. It has been dropped out of the realm of awareness, but it has been dropped so recently and after such a great body of experience that dissociation is not complete. It is in the anteroom, you might say, on the way out. One can remember that it is not as novel as it seems, and, therefore, one may well develop a plausible perplexity about it.[20]

We touch here on a situation that is clearly in the realm of personal problems, of mental disorder in contradistinction to the progression which we call mental health. Preadolescence to a considerable degree and adolescence to a high degree, are the epochs in which warp of development in earlier stages manifests itself as severe handicap. I shall, for this reason, postpone the discussion of adolescence to the next lecture, con-

[20] *Rationalizing* is the technical word for this misuse of reasoning which, in some people, amounts to their major nuisance value in society. All the things they do that don't happen to receive just the right response from the other fellow are "explained," and they are always explained plausibly, although few indeed of us know why we make particular social mistakes. If I were asked at a moment of weariness, "What is the outstanding characteristic of the human being?", I believe I would say, "His plausibility."

cluding tonight with a reconsideration of the communal environment of the preadolescent era.

Preadolescence is usually spent in school and at home. Parents are still people of significance, but their merits and demerits have been fairly well appraised. This does not mean that from henceforth they are to be accorded a simple, realistic status. Quite the contrary; the adolescent upheaval which is impending will bring with it a revaluation of everyone, parents included. The preadolescent frames of reference are, at least in our culture, about the clearest and most workable ones that we have. They do not include lust as a complicating and distorting factor—generally, a confusing and misleading element. Love is new and uncomplicated. The parental complex is viewed from this new angle and, while there may still be aspects which do not make sense, the appraisal is often more valid than is the view which will be adopted some five or six years hence.

The relatively uncomplicated experience of love is entirely ennobling. Sympathy flows from it. Tolerance as a respect for people—not as an intellectual detachment from prejudice —follows it like a bright shadow. Authoritarian figures in the home and elsewhere are recast as of good intention, however stupid and uninformed.

A remedy has at last been found for many thwartings and humiliations, for sundry prohibitions. One looks about one at one's compeers, without sentimentality but with a feeling that they have come naturally by their assets and deficiencies.

A new form of participation develops, in part from sympathy and understanding, in part from awe at the newly expanded world. The preadolescent evolves the practice of *collaboration*, a valid functional activity as a person in a personal situation. This is a great step forward from cooperation—*I* play according to the rules of the game, to preserve *my* prestige and feeling of superiority and merit. When we collaborate, it is a matter of *we*. The achievement is no longer a personal success; it is a group performance—no more the leader's than the led.

In this brief phase of preadolescence, the world as known gains depth of meaning from the new appraisal of the people who compose it. The world as rumored is a wonderful place; the quest of Sir Lancelot rises from the mists of faëry to all but a pattern of life to be lived. Experiences reported from excursions away from home carry a coloring of friendly wonder. The future is constructed in relatively noble terms by the reveries that prepare for tomorrow and that assuage disappointment, take the humdrum out of monotonous tasks.

The imaginary people of preadolescent fantasy may seem to us insubstantial; the imaginary play of the preadolescent may seem but old, romantic folklore crudely adjusted to the spirit of the times. The illusions that transmute his companions —if they be illusions—may seem to us but certain of an early end, a disillusionment. But whatever his people, real, illusory or frankly imagined, may be, they are not mean. Whatever his daydreams with his chum, whatever his private fantasies, they are not base. And as to his valuations of others, here we may take pause and reflect that it may be we who see "as through a glass, darkly."

These young folk are grossly inexperienced. They are often grossly misinformed as to the motives that are prominent in adult life around them. But I surmise that after the measure of their experience, they see remarkably clearly. Also, I believe that for a great majority of our people, preadolescence is the nearest that they come to untroubled human life—that from then on the stresses of life distort them to inferior caricatures of what they might have been.

LECTURE
III

Developmental Syndromes

WE SHALL now consider the phase of personality development which is the last stage on the road to the fully human estate. Once successfully negotiated, the person comes forth with self-respect adequate to almost any situation, with the respect for others that this competent self-respect entails, with the dignity that befits the high achievement of competent personality, and with the freedom of personal initiative that represents a comfortable adaptation of one's personal situation to the circumstances that characterize the social order of which one is a part.

The epochs that lead up to adolescence are closely if obscurely related to somatic maturation. Adolescence begins with the most spectacular maturation of all, the puberty change, with its swift alteration of physiological processes to the completion of bodily development. I still find virtue in dividing the epoch of adolescence into three eras: [21] early adolescence, from the first evidences of puberty to the completion of voice change; mid-adolescence, to the patterning of genital behavior; and late adolescence, to the establishment of durable situations

[21] This conception reaches back certainly as far as the *Sheppard Farewell Lectures* [to the staff of the Sheppard and Enoch Pratt Hospital] 12 Oct. to 9 Nov. 1929 (Privately circulated in mimeograph). The clarification of the stages had to await my emancipation from the residues of faculty-psychology, etc. I have not yet solved the problem of communicating in writing the special implications of the interpersonal view. If, on first reading, these lectures seem difficult *but* probably significant, may I bespeak a review—perhaps section by section—after the rough outlines of the whole have been apprehended.

of intimacy such that all the major integrating tendencies are freely manifested within awareness in the series of one's interpersonal relations.

The farther one moves from birth, the less relevant an absolute physiological chronology becomes. The epoch of adolescence is thus the least fixed by mere somatic duration. It varies from culture to culture, and its actual time of appearance in young people among us is very widely varied. Over the world, the puberty change would seem to occur from as early an age as eight to as late as the twenties. Among some 250 people whom I have studied more or less intensively, I have seen quite a few in whom the inception of adolescence was deferred to around the eighteenth year.

It is from the data of these patients that I have come to feel that environmental influences, cultural influences emanating from significant people, are the predominant factor in bringing about delays—and accelerations—in the later stages of personality development.

The data of these patients, in so far as they have been of American and Western European stock, certainly emphasize the significance of experience—remote and recent—connected with genital (sexual) behavior and the emotion of lust. I have to add a word of caution, here, for there are those among us psychiatrists who make of sex a nuclear explanatory concept of personality, or at least of personality disorder. This is an error from insufficiency of the data. The highly civilized Chinese of the pre-Christian era were not bowled over by sex. A number of the primitive peoples who have been studied by anthropologists are found to take sex rather in their stride. Even the American Negro crashes through adolescence with relative impunity—if he is of the lower classes.

The lurid twilight which invests sex in our culture is primarily a function of two factors. We still try to discourage pre-marital sexual performances; hold that abstinence is the moral course before marriage. And we discourage early marriage; in fact progressively widen the gap between the adolescent awakening of lust and the proper circumstances for marriage. These two factors work through many cultural conventions to make us the most sex-ridden people of whom I have any knowledge.

I think that it might be well at this point to indicate something of what this means by discussing an instance of maladjustment in adolescence. To do this, I must go a long way back from the problem as it presents itself, say, at age 15. To formulate any personal situation, one must almost certainly know a great deal about how it came into being. I shall then take a few minutes to sketch the picture of a boy to whom adolescence will be quite disastrous.

We will take him in the cradle, and here we will see him, after the fashion of all his predecessors, actively and pleasantly engaged in the exercise of such ability as he has discovered. He will perhaps not have kicked a slat out of the cradle, but he certainly will have poked all the slats of the cradle, he will have felt of nearly everything, including a great deal of himself, he may have put a good deal of himself in his mouth, or tried to, but in this business of exercising newly elaborated motor systems and gradually clarifying sensory feel, he will almost inevitably, since we make it a "him," have fallen upon a small protuberance in the groin, and in doing this he will have found it handy. It is suited to manipulation. It is astonishingly well located geometrically. A slight curve in the elbow puts it well within reach of the already nimble fingers.

So far nothing of any moment has occurred. But we will now have, let us say, the mother—fathers usually keep fairly far from the nursery—we will have the mother encounter this discovery of the infant, and we will make her a person who has been forced to organize the self on the basis of our more rigid puritanic tradition.

Under these circumstances, although in ordinary consciousness she is not wholly unaware of this anatomical peculiarity of the male, in her own infant she will feel that Satan is in the very near vicinity, that here is a manifestation of the bestial nature of man in the very act of erupting in her infant, and she will want to do something about it. She will wish to save this infant; Lord knows what awful visions unroll before her eyes as she witnesses this; but anyway the infant is badly upset by empathy, undergoes various somatic disturbances, and experiences what amounts to an acute and severe discomfort.

Infants are not afflicted by long, carefully formulated memories. To the infant whose discrimination of such things is nil, this discomfort does not attach to the manipulation of the little protuberance. Almost anything in the situation may be related to this feeling of discomfort so far as the infant is concerned. He has not learned.

This course of events is discovered again, perhaps the same day. The stress in the mother is terrific. The doctor is consulted, and we will say that the doctor is either very anxious to build up a good practice and surmises that this mother will bring him patients, or that he, too, knows no better; so he puts medical 'intelligence' or rumor that has come to him, to work. And so the infant has a mitten put on the hand and tied around the wrist.

Thus begins the emphasis in the infant's mind that something about this hand is connected with the recurrent feelings of acute and severe discomfort—the *anlage* of insecurity and later of anxiety.

Well, infants, like people, are ingenious. And the immobilization of, let us say, the right hand, does not effect the immobilization of the left. As the genital is handy, and as it has a slightly different sensation from the thumb, the nose, and so on, the event recurs. Again there is the great discomfort in the presence of the mother. Presently both hands may be tied at the side, and by that time even an infant begins to realize that it has something to do with the genital.

All animals tend to react with rage to immobilization, or to any thwarting or restraint which amounts generically to immobilization. To leap over months of struggle between the mother, aided by her medical adviser, and the infant's natural impulse to explore all his abilities and the limits of himself and the rest of the world; after months of struggle there has been impressed upon this infant a type of interest, a mark, if you please—an emotional mark—about the groin area which is so significant that when I was younger and more reckless about language, I called that state "primary genital phobia," which, being translated, is primary fear, irrational fear, of the genitals.

One does not fear something of no interest to one. Anything invested with fear must by definition, by the inherent character of our contact with the universe, be of interest to us. And, therefore, because of this taboo the child has interest, unusual interest, an utterly useless interest so far as the development of personality is concerned, attached to the penis.

As a child and as a juvenile he continues to have this interest. Why? Because this thing was precipitated in personality very early, very firmly. All the red flags of anxiety came to attach to it. Moreover, mamma is always watching. Where the devil has shown up once, you may confidently expect him to return —quite unlike lightning.

And so here we have a person who, long before the puberty changes, has come to have a considerable conflict of impulse pertaining to genital manipulation, a thing fully meaningful only years later; and a conscious center of interest in the genitals, but a negative one, in that they are to be left alone at any cost.

Of course, one is always waking up to discover that one has violated this regulation in one's sleep. Interest has some way or other gotten one to violate this taboo. One is horrified. One has the feeling, "Oh, the devil that is in me. Here I am, doing this worst of possible things in my sleep."

Such a person, having stumbled through preadolescence, let us say, carefully avoiding any physical intimacies with anybody, comes to adolescence. At adolescence the genital dynamism awakens. Experience begins to be colored by a new emotion, and one of singular emphasis, to which we apply the term, lust.[22] As hunger is generically a state of dissatisfaction which orients awareness towards the integration of nutritive—and related—situations chiefly affecting the oral zone of interaction, so lust is a state of dissatisfaction which orients awareness towards the tendency to integrate situations chiefly affecting the genital zone.

Even in our particular boy with the puritanical mother, lust swings his attention towards his penis as an instrument in social situations. Along with the coming of this impulse there appears a curiosity as to the stories about it which the social environment produces, and it gets to be frightfully troublesome. Being compelled to enter into interpersonal situations, and being subjected to powerful social pressure which makes it proper, right, respectable and decent for him to go with a girl, he now goes with a girl.

What, then, occurs? He comes presently to realize quite clearly that he is not acting as was expected. He may know what should be done, but cannot do it. He may have to inquire to discover what is the matter. The knowledge does not help him. Nor does his inability in any way relieve him of the driving lust. It does not resolve the activity of the genital dynamism. But it does put very serious kinks in his relations with a member of the other sex. He is doubly unsatisfied, and, in all likelihood more or less chronically anxious. The failure reflected to him from the companion also strikes at self-esteem

[22] I can picture the commotion to which this statement may provoke the more conforming of the psychoanalysts by recollecting a conversation had some ten years ago with Ives Hendrick—*Facts and Theories of Psychoanalysis* [2 ed.]; New York, Knopf, 1939 (xiv and 369 pp.)—in the course of which I remarked that I could not accept the *phallic* phase of development, as formulated by Freud.

and the feeling of personal competence and security. It is small wonder that things go from bad to worse with him.

Let us say that this boy about whom we are talking has had anxiety a number of times when he awoke to discover that he was violating the taboo that had been written into his personality. We have said that the instrumentality of anxiety is ordinarily sufficient to maintain in dissociation impulses which are entirely contradictory to the self dynamism, impulses which are entirely unsuited to the type of life for which the self-system has been organized.

What happens when the sexual impulses, the impulses to genital behavior, collide with the self system, as in our particular example? Under certain circumstances, the self is able to dissociate lust and the impulses to genital behavior. This can be achieved only by the development of new and elaborate "apparatus" in living. I make here but a crude and hurried touching on something which I will develop at greater length, presently. The point which I wish to emphasize now is that, late as it is in maturing, the genital lust dynamism is something that can be dissociated only at grave risk to effective living, and that in most people it cannot be dissociated at all. It will again and again, at whatever great expense to security, whatever suffering from anxiety, manifest itself.

When the genital drive is dissociated, what precisely do we observe? I shall use this rather uncommon situation to give new emphasis to the meaning of our interpersonal viewpoint. When we speak of drives, impulses, tendencies, we mean always tendencies to integrate situations that will be resolved in a particular significant fashion—often by activity chiefly pertaining to one of our zones of interaction with the environment, and activity chiefly that of one of our several dynamisms.

Without hoping to make clear in a small part of one lecture the greater than somatic character of these dynamisms, let me make a rather necessary digression to discuss the physiological substrate of the zones of interaction of the personality.

We say that the principal zones of interaction are as follows: the *oral*, the retinal, the auditory, the general tactile, the vestibulo-kinæsthetic, the *genital*, and the *anal*, or aboral.[23]

The zones of interaction are developed, elaborated, equipped for dealing with particular phases of the physico-chemical, biological, and interpersonal environment.

The oral zone is made up of a great deal of apparatus. It includes for practical purposes the respiratory apparatus and the food-taking apparatus, from which is evolved the speaking apparatus; so that this zone is very important indeed, and is utilized from the first moment of life to the last. It has special tactile equipment in the lips, in the mouth, and in the nasopharynx. It includes our two most purely chemical receptors, the gustatory sense, and the olfactory.

As I say, this oral zone may be considered as a unit, and while it is always reckless to speak of any part of a person as a unit, still the oral zone is at least a describable part of the person, and the function of the oral zone, in common with all of these zones of interaction, is probably awarded a certain amount of the vital energy, whether it is needed there or not. Given, let us say, twenty units of vital energy from the chemical changes going on in us, two units, perhaps, will be partitioned to this oral zone and will tend very strongly to be used in oral activity, which as you can conceive may be very highly variegated in later life, but in the beginning consists largely of breathing, sucking, and crying.

The retinal area of interaction brings us our most incredibly expanded integration with things not immediately within reach —the retinal receptor is the distance receptor par excellence, and with the aid of optical apparatus permits us to see over distances of a great many light years. Besides this, it is peculiarly related to things *within* reach, for its evolution is closely con-

[23] By the italics, I wish to set off the three zones the dynamisms of which are greatly varied from person to person because of the special cultural influences that are included in their organization and functional activity.

nected with dexterity, with our prehensile and manipulative skills shown primarily in the functional activity of the hands.

The auditory apparatus dealing with air vibrations, vibrations in fluid media, is also a distance receptor, but one of very slight ability compared with the retinal. Regardless of this comparative weakness in overcoming distance, it is the exceedingly important channel for word-learning, and is closely connected with speech—thus being involved with the oral dynamism, of which it might be considered a part. This fusion is not helpful, however, excepting that it shows the interdependence of the parts in the whole.

The general tactile receptors, on the other hand, are for immediate contact.

The kinæsthetic apparatus is involved with the activities of the muscles and joints, and locating ourselves in regard to the relevant geometry of space. It includes the equilibrium equipment.

The genital zone combines highly specialized tactile receptors and apparatus which could be put in the kinæsthetic class except that it pertains to involuntary muscles rather than to striated muscles, equipment connected with corpus spongiosum, the prostatic urethra, the motor elements in the seminal vesicles, and the prostate itself.

At the other end of the alimentary tract again around a muco-cutaneous juncture there is a highly specialized tactile apparatus, similar to that around the lips—conceivably necessary for the maintenance of safety of these delicate areas, there being special nutritional problems wherever the mucous membrane joins the skin.[24]

The oral, genital, and anal zones of interaction with the en-

[24] They are quite different types of tissue, the skin and mucous membrane, with different biochemical processes; the blood supply of the two is specifically different, and the junctures are unusually vulnerable because all this differentiated tissue is combined more or less along a line. Injuries of the muco-cutaneous junctures are troublesome, as all of you who have had cold sores or anal fissures must know.

vironment are greatly affected in the educational acculturation procedure. Many people have their olfactory abilities seriously reduced as a result of the distaste with which culture-carriers in authority treat interest in smells and acts of smelling on the part of the child.

The special tactile activity of the mouth is conditioned by peculiarities and restrictions about taking nourishment, sucking, and the like. The gustatory part is conditioned by prejudices about what is food and what is clean and proper to take into the mouth, and so on and so forth. We shall have more to say about this, presently.

The genital is so conditioned by the prejudices and beliefs of the parents that it is apt to be permanently impaired for its biological function, if not for all forms of interpersonal activity, and similarly, the anal zone is strongly conditioned by culture, in the teaching of our rather elaborate toilet habits.

The result of this strong invasion of culture into the physiology of the organism is very apt to be attended with phenomena of symbolic segregation of various parts of the body. If you are taught that you are a good boy when you do not put your thumb in your mouth, *not doing* so as a virtue begins to be mixed up with being a good boy; and when you are impressed with the cataclysmic character of manipulating your genital, the genital is apt to get invested with marks of danger to be avoided, and also mixed up in yourself, in the self dynamism; and tinkering around the lower end of one's alimentary tract is quite distracting to many parents, and one is apt to get to understand that that particular part of one's anatomy is to be treated only indirectly. You must have your hand wrapped in paper before you approach this part of the body, and that is apt to get itself invested with considerable interest in itself.

The oral zone is involved in such varied functions that it is perhaps the central trunk, the main stem for evolutions of the self. It is fortunate that the excrementary orifice does not get so much significance. Now and then, however, it gets rather remarkable significance. What with the parents' interest in cleanliness and the general American conviction that regularity of bowel action is vital—and the delicate organization of the infant, anyway, so that one can't ignore its bowel action completely—quite often this zone is used in interaction with the parents to express hostility and resentment which usually takes the form of extraordinary interferences with the excrementary function. Biologically things are so keyed that when the rectum is pretty well engorged, its emptying is automatic. That does not do at all among civilized people who wear clothes, and late in infancy or early in childhood quite often the parents have to cudgel their brains, and sometimes the child, a great deal to overcome his *excessive* control of the sphincters. In other words, he refuses to accommodate. Having had his excrementary function thoroughly acculturated, he simply improves on example, you might say, and outdoes this highly desirable learning, and that causes consternation in the environment—thus proving that it is an instrument of power.

The cry was originally the powerful tool of the infant. All too frequently the constipation becomes the powerful tool of the child. The parents have gotten used to listening to him talk and he does not get very much that way, but clamping down on the sphincters at the lower end of the alimentary tract gets action—lots of action, lots of attention, and, thereby, begins to take on significance in this important matter of power, which is so woven into the self dynamism as to be in one way the explanation of the self's existence. One of the great elements in the feeling of security is the conviction that one has power enough in an interpersonal situation: One can feel 'in control' of the situation.

Let us now return to the question, What do we observe in our young man. He is free from awareness of lust, he does not wittingly enter any situation with the purpose of having something genital happen. What do we perceive? We perceive that this man is hounded by the accidents by which he finds himself involved with the wrong type of person. What does this mean? It means that the power of this integrating tendency is such that even though it works entirely outside of his awareness, it works, and works conspicuously, and while he believes that he has become interested in a young lady, has sought her company and has finally got himself noticed so that he can discuss calculus with her, the facts which determine that situation are very much more on the side of the genital lust motive than they are on the intellectual pursuit of calculus. But it is only of the latter that he can be aware, and so he is constantly having difficulties in his interpersonal relations.

The girl has regarded his 'approach' as quite subtle—but he never arrives. She may give him a helping hand, but he somehow overlooks or misinterprets it. If she makes the best of a bad job and they actually discuss calculus problems; even then—as under any other circumstance—he leaves unsatisfied, with a feeling that things have not worked well. That night, he awakens wet with perspiration, from a dream in which he has been kissing and fondling this girl's breasts—and has just bitten one and swallowed the nipple!

And here we must digress again from our young man, and consider the psychiatrist's views of sleep and dreams. I have asserted that psychiatry is the study of interpersonal relations. What are the interpersonal relations of one who is asleep? It is true that most people have a relatively short period each night of what we call *deep* sleep, in which there are no evidences of anything personal at work. Most of the time that one is asleep, however, one is engaged in a peculiar kind of interpersonal activity. Now and then the sleeper is awakened by a dream. If you were to ask why he awoke, he might say that he had been frightened by the dream. He may have had a dream attended by terror, or horror, or a danger that grew so threatening that, almost as if by force, he suspended sleep. He woke up, he says, to reassure himself. Perhaps this was not too successful; when wide awake—according to his judgment—the shadows of the dream hung on. The familiar furnishings of the bedroom did not appear. The bureau persisted in being a menacing object. Perhaps he had to rise from bed and walk around before he was again quite at home in his bedroom, quite free from the threat of a resumption of the dream did he but fall asleep again.

Now these are phenomena of dreams, you say. And what are dreams? Dreams are interpersonal phenomena in which the other fellow is wholly illusory, wholly fantastic, a projection, if you please, of certain constructive impulses, or of certain destructiveness, or of certain genital motivations, or something of that kind.

Dreams, we have to assume, are for the purpose of maintaining sleep, and the fact that they fail now and then is not any reflection on the utility and efficacy of dreams, but is an index to the gravity of the situation with which the person is confronted. If one awakes from a terror dream, it is quite certain that one's life situation is treacherous. If one awakes with inexplicable anxiety, it is quite certain that one's life situation includes plenty of cause for anxiety. The fact that he knows nothing about what he dreamed is a suggestion, not an inevitable index, but a strong suggestion that the problem is in the field of something dissociated from the self system, or by the self system, as you will.

This tells us something about dreams. It is quite possible that minor integrating tendencies dissociated from the awareness often discharge themselves predominantly during sleep, and, therefore, the dream-work not only protects the incident of sleep but also helps to maintain adjustment and mental health despite dissociation.

Our boy, in whom the genital lust dynamism is involved in conflict—and some components of which are dissociated—has horrible disturbances of sleep. Either he commits sins in his sleep and awakens feeling ruined, all tired out, or he commits these sins and wakens feeling fine, which again is a sin. More often than that, however, he has no clear sexual dreams.

He has dreams in which he commits atrocious crimes, like his dream of cannibalistic incorporation of the girl's nipple.

How does this come about? Clearly in sleep, in dreams, impulses which in waking life are dissociated make their appearance and play out dramas of interpersonal relations with more or less purely fictitious people. This suggests that in sleep the force which maintains the dissociation in waking life is enfeebled. We say that as the self system was evolved primarily for the maintenance of interpersonal security, since sleep is impossible unless some distinct measure of security exists, it is only natural that the self dynamism might be somewhat in abeyance, somewhat weaker in its manifestations, in sleep, when by definition we will have no contact with a real person—and you will remember that the self was derived from very real people.

Even though this is true, only rather strikingly healthy people have rather explicit, quite simply meaningful, perhaps quite simply constructive, dreams. Most people dream things which, as they recall them on awakening, are fantastic and meaningless.

Some of this is due to the transition from sleep to wakening. The transition from a state of being asleep with some remembered dreams to the state of being awake is a great change in consciousness. One can dream in the most illogical, perhaps, literally in a ruleless, way. When we are conscious, however, we are more or less completely under the sway of the processes of consensually valid communicative thinking that we have had to learn. Therefore, in the very act of changing from one stage of consciousness to another, where different frames of reference are applied, many details of the dream are just too intricate to be fitted into the waking consciousness and they disappear or they get themselves simplified. There is a real barrier in this very transition of consciousness that makes us somewhat obscure in our relation to that which went on when we were asleep.

Besides that, while the self is relatively dormant in sleep it does not disappear, it is a perduring aspect of personality and the dissociated impulses must, by fantastic means in many cases, follow a principle which is very strikingly manifested in the waking life in many of the mental disorders; the character of the interpersonal phenomena which are manifested in sleep is often regressive in the sense that it is of an earlier stage of development.

I have tried to suggest to you that the awareness of the infant is of a very diffuse and unspecified kind. We may, therefore, say that the maximum regression of prehending processes is to a sort of an amorphous universe in which one has one's being—doubtless, a fairly early infantile mental state. If there were necessity, one could revert in dreams to that sort of attack upon one's problems. Seemingly quite insignificant changes in this vague sort of center-of-the-universe picture might mean very great things at the adult day-consciousness level.

Regression is not usually anything like so deep. There is no necessity for such profound recessions. One can drop back from too disturbing a clarity as to what is going on to a time in one's past when any such disturbing clarity had not been comprehended, and actions could go on then which adultly, in our waking state, would mean the satisfaction of a tendency, but which, as we recall the dream, just seem to be sort of childish.

Also, much is made in dreams of a process familiar to the children of many a home. Take the case of the boy caught getting into the jam. And mother says, "Willie, I told you not to touch that jam," and Willie says, "I didn't touch the jam; my hand did."

Also, in dreams one may show some displacing of feeling, and that again is an ancient habit. For example, when one is angry at the teacher who has quite unjustly punished one for somebody else's act, one does not show it, if one is wise and well controlled, but on the way home one can raise hob with some other schoolboy. The affect, you might say, has been carried for a while and deposited on a less dangerous object. And so in dreams, feeling may be moved around so that it does not focus too keenly the alertness on what is actually the case.

These processes occur to enable one to avoid the disturbing anxiety or the feeling of insecurity which will suspend sleep. They usually become notable in the period of adolescence when the problems of adaptation to others become pressing. Let me now proceed to a consideration of adolescents and chronologically adult people as we encounter them.

When we seek to formulate the syndromes [25] of maladjustment or mental disorder we have to consider two fields of data, two somewhat remarkable separate universes of phenomenal completeness, the—to use old-fashioned words—world of the subjective, and the world of the objective.

What does this person, this patient if you please, notice, and what else is there to be noticed by the ideally unhampered observer? The subjective, that which the person himself notices, has always to be communicated to the observer. We have been ingenious in devising apparatus and in refining observational techniques which show that the subject person, the patient, is experiencing something. Thus, for example, we may put a person in the circuit of a very delicate galvanometer, notice the resistance that his skin interposes to the passage of an electric current, and find that when certain stimuli are presented there is an abrupt change in this electrical resistance. It falls rapidly, many thousands of ohms, and we know that this change in skin resistance is intimately, if not absolutely, associated with some change in the integration of the person. Or

[25] The term *syndrome,* literally a concourse or concurrence, means a pattern of phenomena—signs and symptoms—which is frequently encountered, and the abstracting of which from the flux of events is presumed to be based on a valid insight into human life. It is much to be preferred in psychiatry to the term, *disease. Mental disorder* may be used, if mental refers to those aspects of living that are manifested in behavior and thought.

we may, with less refinement, have a way of counting the number of breaths which a person takes per minute, and we find that at a certain time this rate of breathing is markedly augmented. We know that at certain times a person stops breathing for a measurable interval. There is a brief inhibition of the impulses which make for breathing. We know that these phenomena mean that something has happened in our patient. And we know, if we have sufficiently refined our own instruments—in this case, our hearing—that there are times in which the tone of the voice loses its rich quality and becomes flat, monotonous as it were, and we know again that this, the moment that it occurs, represents the particular timing of some event in the configuration involving the person.

But all these ingenious instrumental expansions of our senses in interaction with people, and all the acuity which we can develop from long contact with people, tells us only that something has happened. When it comes to testing the validity of our notion as to what has happened our only recourse is to listen for a long time to the reports of the patient as to what seems to him to be going on.

When we do this, we find some very interesting correlations; of a thousand people we find that 942, for example, report that when we said so and so, they experienced so and so. And the instruments in the meanwhile recorded a shift in the resistance of the skin and a change in the breath rhythm. But when it comes to discovering what that person experienced subjectively, what meaning the situation had for him, we have only the report, the attempt to communicate by the use of words and gestures to us, of something that is extraordinarily private.

The facts are that it is only by the skilful use of our most specialized tool of communication that we can seem to overcome the privacy of these so personal worlds. By responsive speech we are able to bridge the gap with inferences of high probability as to what is actually the case.

You may remember in the first hour that I suggested to you

that our perceptions of the physical universe are always separated from that physical universe by the act of perceiving. I went on to say that in the realm of interpersonal relations, the mediation between the personal situation outside us, namely, our idea of that personal situation, is much more complex. We again recur here to this point and suggest that the best that speech—by far our most refined instrument of communication, a tool for relating ourselves meaningfully to another person—can bring about is an understanding of the other person which has high probability of correctness.

High probability of correctness is very different, indeed, from absolute certainty. The moment that one introduces the concept of probability one realizes that it may approach one hundred per cent as a limit, but that it never gets to that limit; that it may approach zero as a limit, but it is never quite that low. Probability is always uncertainty, but it is sometimes very little uncertainty and sometimes very great uncertainty, and to understand the other fellow in his most intimate relationship with us, the best we can achieve is a partial understanding of what is going on. If we are wise and clever, this may have high probability of being correct.

Now the syndromes which are most useful in the diagnosis of personal situations, come more and more clearly to appear to be statements of the past, the momentary present, and the future of the career of the person who is our subject. The career that we are discussing is made up of the events which have connected, now connect, and will presently connect him with the lives of other persons.[26]

[26] The term *diagnosis*—literally a discrimination, and medically a deciding as to the character of the situation before one—is in the study of personality inextricably involved with *prognosis*—literally a foreknowing—the formulation of the probable outcome. Kraepelin's famous classification of the functional psychoses had an all but absolute prognostic slant. Current internal medical diagnosis is more inclined to consider the multiplicity of events that *may* influence the outcome—thus tending to set diagnosis apart from prognosis. Personality problems involve an even greater number of unpredictable factors than do most problems of internal medicine. The use of statistical ex-

These useful syndromes are different from the category of mental and nervous diseases which are taught to the medical student even to this day. They are perhaps somewhat more like the statements about this and that one which are heard in the privacy of the home, among intimate friends. The point we make here is that the ancient preoccupation of psychiatrists was a diagnosis of mental disorder, which had every now and then to be revised. From this field, the interest has moved on to considerations of how people could be classified. All that is out of sympathy with the central view of this series of lectures, to the effect that the subject of psychiatry is the study of interpersonal relations. Dementia præcox, schizophrenia, neurasthenia—these things are the privilege of the person who has them, in blissful separation from any suggestion of the social communality. The symptoms are ordinarily discussed as if they are static characteristics of a thing, very different indeed from statements about "How does Mr. A. act with Mr. B.?" "What goes on in the situation integrated between Mr. A. and Mr. B.?"

As I say, as one shifts the emphasis in psychiatry from the study of alleged personalities with alleged disorders to that which beyond any doubt is scientifically accessible; namely, what goes on in the situation with this person, then this panoply of neurasthenia, dementia præcox, anxiety neuroses, and so on, fade out of the picture. The picture becomes somewhat simpler and at times much more complex.

It becomes somewhat simpler in that one is relieved of the necessity of maintaining a God-like objectivity as if literally from an ivory tower. It becomes much more complex because one really has to notice what is going on and to derive some

perience as a basis for prognostic formulations is, therefore, a very dubious performance.

It is well-known among physicians that all persons suffering tuberculous meningitis die. A patient at the Sheppard and Enoch Pratt Hospital, so diagnosed by three outstanding internists—and confirmed by the laboratory—recovered. The internists became unhappy about their diagnosis. The patient has been doing well for ten years.

inferences at to the past, the present and the future of the career-line from these participantly observed events.

If I say neurasthenia is a condition characterized by pain in the neck, great readiness for fatigue, and preoccupation with fancied disorders, often of the genitals, which cannot be explained on any organic basis, the medical man feels that he has been told something useful to him. If I say that as a student of personality I cannot find any virtue in the conception, neurasthenia, that is another matter, much less satisfying.

The person who has an acute belly-ache followed by a feeling of extreme sickness, great anxiety, fear of death, and so on, calls the family physician, who takes his temperature and a blood specimen, pokes him around, hits some very tender spots in the abdomen and says, "Johnny, you have appendicitis." Johnny is greatly relieved to hear this word "appendicitis." It is not entirely a matter of verbal magic, if you please. When the doctor says, "Oh, this is appendicitis," this indicates that the doctor knows what he is talking about. Even if the patient is very much worried, here is the doctor, representative of medical science, who regards the thing much as he regards the weather—it is clearly not anything to be much excited about.

The new viewpoint of psychiatry teaches us that we cannot parallel the performances implied in the medical diagnosis, and, however enthusiastic the patient or his relatives may be about having a scientific name for the trouble, we must discontinue the finalist performances by which, for example, we have been classifying large groups of our fellows who are chronic inhabitants of mental hospitals. They are there. Something is the matter with them, but we should no longer feel happy because we have applied a label to them.

The first group of our syndromes pertain to the relatively uninterrupted career-lines of people; the second group, to more or less clearly episodic changes in direction. The first group, therefore, appear to be diagnoses of personality; the second, of disorders of personality. Actually, the first group refer to degrees of development and the second to a blend of the developmental factors with the vicissitudes of the person in his communal existence with others.

We have seen how the culture in which we chance to live comes finally to have great prescriptive power over our thoughts and behavior, not only because other people, the carriers of the culture, thwart, humiliate, punish and reward us, and facilitate our securing satisfaction and maintaining a sense of personal security, but finally in preadolescence and adolescence because some of these other people become highly significant to us.

Our first syndrome is made up of phenomena which appear at first sight to contradict these considerations. There are people among us whose integration of interpersonal situations is chiefly characterized by lack of duration. These people live through a great number of fugitive, fleeting, involvements with other people—and even with the more tangible of the institutions of the particular society in which they have their being. They are disappointing to everyone who is interested in them. They are themselves always disappointed in other people—but this does not make them bitter, nor does it excite them to inquiry as to what may be the matter. Without troubling to think it out, they exemplify the saying that all the world is queer, except . . . . They move through life giving many of the appearances of human beings; they just miss being human—and they do not lack fluency in verbal behavior. They almost always say the right thing. They often say it well. But it signifies very little.

The striking things about these people are their inability to profit from what we would consider to be their experience, and their disregard for the future. The intelligence factor is not involved. They experience life differently from others and their insight into reality is correspondingly different. Not only is it different, but it is far more imperfect than the average.

Here and now may be grasped quite well. The past is vague and the future is of no real interest.

These are the non-integrative, the so-called *psychopathic*, personalities [27] who are superlative in social nuisance value and of great theoretical interest for psychiatry. This latter interest arises from their peculiarly qualified insight into their personal reality—and that of others—which implies an extraordinary peculiarity of their self dynamism. It is so difficult and disconcerting to deal with them that but little valuable data has been accumulated.[28] I believe that the first essential in a research in this field is the application of the techniques used in the study of anthropoids. This will give us useful clues towards the elucidation of language behavior in the psychopath, and thus we may come to unravel their relatively vestigial self.

Secondly, in these syndromes, we come upon the *self-absorbed*, or fantastic person. To those of you who are given to reading about psychoanalysis, this is the person whose relations with others and with the more objective institutions of society are shot through with "wishful thinking"—for me, a difficult concept.

The prototype of these people is to be sought in early childhood. To make this clear, I must say something as to the prehension [29] and perception of significant people, as we conceive

[27] Comment on two patients of the category appears in Regression: . . . *State Hospital Quart.* (1926) 11:208–217, 387–394, and 651–668. The (1925) view expressed in footnote 13 is in part erroneous. An "unconsciously determined inability to profit from experience" is now seen to be equivalent to *biological* defect. The factors of personality exterior to awareness do not arrange difficulties of this sort; the self dynamism is the 'part' that interferes.

[28] Kraepelin classified psychopathic personalities under seven rubrics: the excitable; the unstable; the impulsive; the egocentric; the liars and swindlers; the antisocial; and the quarrelsome. Eugen Kahn—*Psychopathic Personalities* [tr. by H. F. Dunbar]; New Haven, Yale University Press, 1931 (521 pp.)—has a most elaborate classification, some of which doubtless pertains to the people whom I am discussing. See in particular, Partridge, George E., Current Conception of Psychopathic Personality. *Amer. J. Psychiatry* (1930) 10[o.s. 87]:53–99. See, also, Henderson, David K., *Psychopathic States;* New York, Norton, 1939 (178 pp.); and Partridge, George E., A Study of 50 Cases of Psychopathic Personality. *Amer. J. Psychiatry* (1928) 7[o.s. 84]:953–973.

[29] To prehend is to have potential information or misinformation about

them to develop in infancy. The nipple is probably first prehended as a part of one's vague cosmic entity. It gradually stands out as an attribute of the Good Mother. There gradually evolves another complexus of impressions which—because of the empathic linkage—is the Bad Mother. Objectively, to us, the person concerned is the mother; to the infant, these are two vaguely limited but entirely distinct people. The discrimination of the Good Mother pattern of events and the Bad Mother pattern of events constitutes a primary bifurcation of interpersonal experience, evidences of which persist in most people, throughout life.

In later infancy there is a synthesis of experience which dulls this primary discrimination and gradually evolves an adequate perception of the mother as a person who is sometimes good—giving satisfactions and security—and sometimes bad. The fantasies of childhood show, however, that the earlier formulations have not disintegrated. For that matter, many of the puzzling excesses in the child's emotional reactions arise from the continuance of these dynamic factors. But for practical purposes, the child has learnt that mother is not as good as was the lost Good Mother, nor as bad as the other one. There is loss and gain.

The loss, being a privation, is more vivid than is the gain. I believe that we can safely read back into these early times, the usual ways of dealing with irreparable losses of this kind; and if so, we may feel sure that constructive fantasy appears only after mere representative fantasy has worn itself out. The child fogs the undesirable aspects of mother with recollections of the Good Mother; thus reinstating security and satisfaction enough to sleep in peace and to remedy slights and frustrations. This gradually fades from waking life, as better adaptations to the more real mother are invented. It probably persists in the preliminary stages of falling asleep.

something; to perceive is to have information or misinformation in or readily accessible to awareness.

In people who show our self-absorbed type of performances, however, the element of representative fantasy continues as a major ingredient of life. All sorts of interpersonal prehensions are fogged into what is called 'wishful' distortions or misinformation about people. These people have no grey; everything tends to be black *or* white. Their friends are simply wonderful people. People whom they dislike are just simply impossible. Their "love" is melodramatic to a degree that confounds its object—excepting the object be another self-absorbed person. Together, by a sustained miracle of accommodating—or ignoring—the individualistic misconceptions of each other, two of these folk can have quite a good time. With the rest of us, however, they are apt to be disappointed, wounded, misunderstood. And we, if we care to study the processes at work, cannot but marvel at the failure of learning which has left their capacity for fantastic, self-centered, illusion so utterly unaffected by a life-long series of educative events. These people integrate situations with foggy embodiments projected upon us from their fantasies about themselves.

Let us now look at a type of organization which represents less blandly a cosmic centering in the person concerned. We shall call this syndrome of characteristics that of the *incorrigible* person, choosing this none too satisfactory term for the reason that these people have actively evaded or resisted the educative influences that in more fortunate people lead to a more practical organization of the self dynamism. I may suggest their characteristics by saying that they integrate more durable situations only with people whom they regard as their inferiors. Towards all others, their basic attitude is hostile, unfriendly, or morose and forbidding. It is clear that these people have a grave defect in the field of security; often inculcated by a parent who just would not be satisfied with the child.

The syndrome makes clear appearance in the juvenile development. These young folk cannot progress to the stage of give-and-take, of competition and self-satisfying compromise.

The incorrigible person does not attack the really strong. He has failed in the most significant of efforts to overcome dissatisfaction with him. The scar of this failure remains and he is forewarned from contests that might renew the pain. Authority—paradigmatic of the disapproving parent—is anathema to him, but to smooth-working, competent, authority he interposes no objection. To authority that is exercised with any uncertainty, any irrational contradictions, any 'stupidity,' the incorrigible person is intolerant and intolerable. If he is intelligent, he shows a genius for finding defects in the exercise of social controls, and for making trouble about it. He is a thorn in the side of teachers. From school, he proceeds into the larger world, to put "stuffed shirts" where they belong.

The fourth syndrome that I shall present you is the *negativistic* person. These are the people, to keep to our earlier figure, who have no black or white, but only grey. They are in many ways antithetic to the self-absorbed person; their selves are organized on the basis of appraisals that make them insignificant—until their constructive fantasy hit upon negation as a device for forcing notice if not approval. If mother says "It's time for little Willie to go to bed" and little Willie goes; that is one thing. It may be but one of unnumbered brushings of little Willie out of the way. If now, instead of going to bed, little Willie says "No" and reinforces his non-cooperation with all means at his disposal, his significance in his world may become at least briefly, very great.

I shall not digress to consider various reactions to the child's negation: the submersion in "sweetness and light," the submission to tantrums, and so on and so forth. I wish rather to indicate the typical negativistic syndrome which has its origin in the discovery that it is better to be a problem child than a mere necessary evil.

Insecurity in the negativistic is met with an assertion of refusal. If such a person feels any tendency towards minimizing him or taking him for granted, he resists a suggestion, or refutes a statement, or differs with an opinion, or in some other nugatory way accentuates his significance in the interpersonal situation. If he is keenly insecure, he may be simply uncooperative in everything, to such an extent that the other fellow can but go away.

The negativistic way of life is apt to be highly educative, and it thus comes about that many prevailingly negativistic people get to be quite expert in some field—even that of conciliation. Being highly competent, it is no longer necessary to feel insecure in situations in which they are recognized as the expert, and their long experience with divergent views comes in handy.

It was necessary for me to present the negativistic category before mentioning a syndrome of the interpersonal phenomena which is in many ways a super-incorrigibility, and in some ways a super-negativism. This, our fifth syndrome, I shall call that of *the stammerer*. These people make use of vocal behavior—or misbehavior—not for communication but for defiance and domination. They have discovered a magic of articulate sounds that really works. By demonstrating their inability to produce a word—and to desist from effort at producing it—they immobilize the other person and arrest the flow of process in the world. This is a power operation of no mean proportions. It represents a grave disorder of development at the time when sheerly magic operations were being abandoned and the consensual validation of verbal behavior was beginning. The disorder of speech is but one of several striking phenomena in this syndrome, about which, however, I shall say no more at this point.

It is to be noted that these first five of our syndromes are of early origin in the development of personality. They all come from the time of predominantly autistic verbal behavior. They are deviations of growth that are not chiefly a result of verbal communication between parent and child, teacher and pupil. They occur before the mediate acculturation of the juvenile era, which includes, among many other important accomplishments, the learning of things through the written and printed form of the language; and in particular, learning about legendary people who embody ideals, mores, and norms of the particular culture-complex.

One learns, for example, of Hans Brinker's feats. We learn of him through the mediation of speech, but he becomes an immediate ingredient of our thinking. We do not expect to meet him, as we did Uncle Herbert; but he is just as significant. He more or less adequately represents, perhaps by his very abstractness, his purely traditional existence, traits of character that are praiseworthy. As something greater and less than life, Hans Brinker becomes a denizen of the self.

The syndromes that present distortions of development after this spread of acculturation are of a greater complexity than are the first five. I shall present them in the order of complexity, which is naturally the order of developmental stage chiefly concerned in each.

The sixth syndrome may be called the *ambition-ridden* personality. These people have to use everyone with whom they are integrated. If you are no good for advancing his interest, the ambition-ridden person can find someone who is, with whom to enjoy whatever other satisfaction he had been having in your company. Some of them are scrupulous about some ideals, some of them are almost wholly unscrupulous. Some are clever at avoiding dangerous competition; some have to compete with everybody. Your personal experience will fill in this picture, for there is no dearth of these folk among us.

We come to a seventh syndrome, the *asocial.* Please note that the term is asocial, not antisocial. Antisocial is a nuisance-word which carries a penumbra of confusion: it is used indiscriminately to refer to the asocial, the incorrigible, and the psychopathic. The asocial are by no manner of means brigands, criminals, or people who are always rude without provocation. Many asocial people are among the more delightful folks I have known. They are the people whose integrations with others are assumed by them to be of no special moment *to* the other person, and to be of the duration of his convenience only. Some of them show considerable error of judgment as to the other fellow's convenience, being as we say, so sensitive that they are put off by quite insignificant things and withdraw long before one would lose them. Some of them are quite obtuse and drift along with us long after we have been discouraged as to the possibility of intimacy with them.

They may be thought to be extraordinarily lacking in self-esteem, and in one way this is quite correct. They often esteem themselves, quite properly, quite highly—many of them are competent people. But they have not grasped the possibility that they themselves may be valued, cherished, by others. All that category of experience is missing from their self dynamism. The approvals which are incorporated are chiefly the products of mediate acculturation, and not of direct early experience. It is not strange, therefore, that these people often have highly formulated and rigidly held ideals of behavior. This does not exempt them from loneliness, and many of them have no difficulty in overlooking shortcomings in themselves and others with whom they have relations.

For an eighth syndrome, we may consider the *inadequate person*, including under this rubric all those people who integrate situations of dependency with others, and the people who derive their feeling of personal significance from identification with some extravagantly over-valued 'cause.' Some of these people have been obedient children of a dominating parent. They go on through life needing a strong person to make decisions for them. Some of them learned their helplessness and clinging-vine adaptation from a parental example. Some of them took over a justifying invalidism from a similar source.

A ninth syndrome may be named the *homosexual*, although this term has accumulated so great a freight of misunderstanding that I could wish for something less ambiguous. These are the people whose earlier experience has erected a barrier to integrations with persons of the other sex. The barrier may be relative or absolute. It may be highly specific in regard of the type of situation concerned, or it may be quite general—as in the 'woman hater' who really dislikes the presence of any woman. We would say that his barrier was absolute and general in its effect. We encounter men who preferred to play with girls, in the juvenile era, and whose most enjoyable companionship is still with women but who cannot integrate sexual situations with them. We encounter men who have no use for women except for integrating sexual situations with them—and, believe me, these situations include nothing of love. I need not say that parallel deviations appear in women, though the cultural definitions of rôle adds and subtracts features from the phenomena that we encounter.

Some of these people, in preadolescence or later, learn to integrate sexual situations with persons of their own sex. Some of these are relations of love, and are stable and durable. Some are devoid of love and are very transient. Some are relations of hatred, durable or otherwise as the determining circumstances dictate.

Many of these people discharge their lustful impulses by self-manipulation, with or without explicit fantasy of another person. Some of them depend chiefly on processes that go on in sleep. A marginal group follows the heterosexual pattern of genital behavior with women of a particularly highly differentiated type, and some of these integrations are relationships of love, and wholly durable.

Our tenth syndrome, the last that I shall indicate, is really a congeries of syndromes, but it has enough of consistency to merit its title of the *chronically adolescent.* These are the people who never find the right love object. Some of them are driven by lust, and go on seeking the right person, always disappointed with anyone who has been available. Some of them become cynical and adopt lustful performances as an ideal indoor sport. Some of them are celibate, withdrawn from genital behavior, and—as I said earlier—in real danger as to personal stability. They all pursue the ideal and they find it not.

These are some of the more outstanding diagnostic syndromes which appear in the series of interpersonal relations through which one passes. They tell us of the past and permit shrewd guesses—predictions of high probability—as to the future integrations which the person will show. More significant for the clinical practice of psychiatry, they provide the meaning for otherwise mystifying episodes that occur in the lives of those who experience mental disorder. For the broader aspects of psychiatry, they are reference-frames for understanding what will and what will not work, in connection with a particular person.

LECTURE

IV

Explanatory Conceptions

It has been said that the history of mankind depicts a spiral progress; the course of events returns at increasing interval to the neighborhood of the starting point.[30] There is more than a little evidence in favor of such a view regarding the history of each person's ideas, and from this I must hope for justification for taking you back now to yet another sojourn along the coordinate of individual physiology. I have now to point out that the pursuit of satisfactions and the maintenance of security—the great motors of human behavior and thought—have physiological substrates that must be considered in any attempt at explaining states of mental disorder or maladjustment.

The rôle of muscle tissue in adjustment is rather obvious when the moving of material objects is concerned. Muscles contract and do work in moving the bones and the tissues they support. That is rudimentary. But what of the continuing tension or *tonus* of each muscle? Some muscles are never completely relaxed; most muscles are in a state of considerable tonus throughout our periods of deepest sleep. Moreover, this tonus

[30] C. Delisle Burns—*The Horizon of Experience;* New York, Norton, 1936 (372 pp.)—shows a table of the rhythm of development of the Western civilization: new horizons, 800–400 B.C.; Greek-Roman System, 400 B.C.–A.D. 400; new horizons [the Dark Ages], A.D. 400–800; Medieval System, A.D. 800–1400; new horizons, A.D. 1400–1600; Renaissance System A.D. 1600–1900; and new horizons, A.D. 1900–. He remarks that the rate of rhythm seems to become shorter. "But the Renaissance System, with which we are familiar, is really only a continuance of the Medieval, as the Roman was of the Greek. The only breakdown as great as ours was that of A.D. 400–800, the Dark Ages."

changes rather generally throughout the major muscular systems of the body, without direct relationship to demands for work and movement. A person who is tense—has rather high tone in the skeletal musculature—on laughing in amusement, undergoes a swift and general reduction of this tonus. A person who is engaged in friendly conversation, unexpectedly severely criticized, undergoes a rapid increase in the tone of most of the skeletal muscles. This clearly has something to do with one's feeling of comfort and discomfort.

The facts seem to indicate that tonic changes in the unstriped, involuntary, muscles of the viscera—the internal organs of the body—are, from birth onward, intimately related to the experiencing of desires, needs for satisfaction. Heightened tone of the stomach wall is called out by depletion of our chemical supplies, and the occurrence of vigorous contractions in these tense muscles gives rise to the 'pangs of hunger.' The taking of food—the ingestion of which probably leads to a release of nutritive substance stored in the liver—promptly relieves the excess tone and the contractions quiet down to the churning of the stomach contents. Hunger, in a way of speaking, is from the first influx of food, more a matter of the oral dynamism than of the stomach. In infants, at least, once this dynamism has discharged itself, alertness disappears, vigilance is withdrawn from circumambient reality, and sleep supervenes. Throughout life the pursuit of satisfactions is physiologically provoked by increased tone in some unstriped muscles; and the securing of the satisfactions is a relaxation of this tone, with a tendency towards the diminution of attention, alertness, and vigilance, and an approach to sleep.

In this satisfaction-securing behavior, the striped, skeletal, muscles are of relatively instrumental value. They do what is necessary and then relax. This picture is adequate for the earlier phases of untroubled infancy. It is no longer relevant when acculturation has come to include prohibitions and disapprovals.

When the infant begins to need security—primarily a security from noxious emotional states empathized from the personal environment—the skeletal muscles take on a new function. The oral dynamism has been the channel for performances needed to appease hunger—and pain and other discomforts. It may be presumed that its function in emitting the cry has been quite automatic. This may not have worked too well, and delayed response to the cry may be one of the first experiences that tend to focus alertness. But in any case, the oral dynamism is not now effective in securing relief from the discomfort set up by empathy; on some occasions, it is simply ineffectual, and on other occasions, its activity is accompanied by increase of the empathized discomfort. This leads gradually to a differentiation of empathized from other discomforts, and to the *inhibition* of the cry as a universal tool. The inhibiting of a complex pattern of behavior is not as simple as was its automatic initiation. Some of the movements are cut off, but the increase of tone in the appropriate muscles may not be inhibited. The experience of empathized hostility, or unfriendly prohibition, or, as it later comes to be observed, a forbidding gesture, becomes colored by and associated with heightened tone in some striped muscles—at first those concerned with the cry.

The course of acculturation, in so far as it pertains to toilet habits, is also a learning to suffer increasing tension in the bladder and rectum, and to resist the automatic relaxation of the sphincter muscles concerned in retaining the urine and feces. Failures in this are often accompanied by empathized discomfort, and success is often the occasion of empathized comfort—which is added to the satisfaction from relief of the tension.

The whole course of acculturation is replete with forbidding gestures and indications of approval. The forbidding gestures—scowls, frowns, expressions of embarrassments, certain tones of voice, certain variations in enunciation, for example—inspire a feeling of insecurity and the self comes into being in learning to avoid the acts which provoke them—and in performing the acts which bring about approval or, at least, cause no disapproval. The parents' and other older people's "patterns of behavior-toward-a-child are generally far from simple; their restraints and facilitations of behavior are usually much less adequate than is the case in their interpersonal relations with compeers. All too generally they inculcate a great deal that is incoherent and incapable of unitary integration. Almost universally they encourage the continuance of autistic-magical processes in the field of speech behavior—'You are a naughty boy; say that you are sorry,' for example, includes being-naughty as an addition to conceptual 'me' that has its real basis in empathized hostile-disapproving attitudes of the authoritarian individual, with somatic heightenings of muscle tonus; while saying-I-am-sorry comes to have the power of reducing or dissipating the hostile-disapproving attitude, without in any way undoing the activity which comes presently to be seen to be the exciting cause for the disapproval. When one considers how much of this sort of thing almost every child experiences, it does not seem so peculiar (or inevitable) that, while some considerable proportion of our people develop aptitudes for manipulating machinery and scientific concepts in a practical way, very few people show much 'sense' in interpersonal relations, and almost everyone deals with other people with a wonderful blend of magic, illusions, and incoherent irrelevancy. Childhood is the incubator of man's evil genius for rationalizing, a special aspect of the delusion of unique individuality which is necessitated by the peculiar limitations of conceptual 'me' and 'you' as a governor of one's perceptions, a reference frame that determines the accessibility of one's experience to awareness."

"One has information only to the extent that one has tended to communicate one's states of being, one's experience."

"Much of the child's life goes on without any necessity for

alertness. Needs call out adjustive movements and achieve satisfactions without particular attention from the authorities, and therefore without implicit or explicit communicative processes. They tend to be unnoticed, to remain outside of the realm of information and misinformation, outside of the growing elaboration of conceptual 'me' and 'you.' These adjustive performances are a part of the experience of the organism, are a part of the growth process, and contribute, like all other experience, to the refinement and differentiation of behavior of the individual. But they are a part of experience the memory of which is not readily accessible to subsequent states of awareness. As one proceeds toward adulthood one's more lucid states of consciousness tend more and more completely to be concerned with experiences definitely involving the conceptual 'me' and 'you'—experiences about which there has been at least a tendency to communicate. It is usual to be able to recall a great deal of one's experience of which one was clearly aware at the time it occurred; it generally requires a special set of circumstances, a peculiarly characterized interpersonal situation, to provoke the mnemonic reproduction of previously unnoticed experience." [31]

The psychiatrist, as he listens to his informant, "must realize that he is participating in speech behavior that pertains chiefly to the conceptual 'me' and 'you,' with corresponding manifestation of the factors that have distorted and continue to complicate the interpersonal relations of the subject personality. As one who speaks, he is keenly aware that he is using linguistic processes in a configuration in which the hearer enters most significantly into the outcome of the attempt at communication.

"In the interpersonal contexts through which the writer has passed, it is recurrently necessary to dissipate the importance

[31] Sullivan, Harry Stack. A Note on the Implications of Psychiatry . . . for Investigations in the Social Sciences. *Amer. J. Sociol.* (1937) 42:848–861. The quotations that follow are also from this paper.

of statements allegedly indicative of various aspects of reality, but actually far too complex to accomplish anything more than self-deception of the speaker. Some insight has developed as to the function performed by uncommunicative, unintelligible, and misleading statements in allegedly communicative interpersonal contexts. These have been observed to occur when the integration is *parataxic;* [32] that is, when, besides the interpersonal situation as defined within the awareness of the speaker, there is a concomitant interpersonal situation quite different as to its principal integrating tendencies, of which the speaker is more or less completely unaware.

"Besides the two-group integrated of psychiatrist and subject there is in the parataxic situations also an illusory two-group integrated of psychiatrist-distorted-to-accommodate-a-special-'you'-pattern and subject-reliving-an-earlier-unresolved - integration - and - manifesting - the - corresponding - special-'me'-pattern. The shift of communicative processes from one to another of these concomitant integrations may be frequent or only occasional; in any case, the alertness of the speaker is usually sufficient to insure the weaving of word patterns and other linguistic elements into grammatical speech. There, therefore, ensues an apparently coherent discussion, and one usually rather clearly addressed to the hearer." [33]

This is a succinct expression of the theory; I wish now to expand various of its terms. The performances of a person arise from a complex of factors, and our observation of these performances is influenced by our own previous experience. When we talk professionally with a person—whom I shall now call 'the patient'—the speech behavior occurs in a situation including the two of us and an indefinite and shifting group of illu-

[32] This term, I believe, was first utilized in a psychiatric sense by Dom Thomas V. Moore, M.D., The Parataxes. *Psychoanalytic Rev.* (1921) 7:252–283.

[33] This conception is made much more explicit in *Psychiatry: Introduction to the Study of Interpersonal Relations* Chapter I. The Data of Psychiatry. PSYCHIATRY (1938) 1:121–134.

sions and impressions as to each other. The patient, newly come to me, is strongly influenced by his impression as to what a psychiatrist is like, and by statements told him about me. If he observes no surprising discrepancy between his expectation and the person he finds, he will proceed on these implicit assumptions. I cannot know what they are, but I must discover them as best I can. Otherwise, I shall have little or no valid basis for observing the interpersonal processes and formulating an impression of the complexities in them which constitute his maladjustment or mental disorder.

It is often useful to inquire as to what brought him to me; who advised it, and for what purpose. If he comes from someone well-known to me, I may have a shrewd guess as to what was said about me. That is by no means a knowledge of the expectation created in the patient—the elements of his previous experience and his relationship with the referring person are complicating factors. If, however, he says "Dr. A. said that I had schizophrenia and that you were the person to cure me of it," I have certain surmises which can be tested almost at once. I surmise that his term, schizophrenia, is almost entirely autistic; I surmise either that Dr. A. is misquoted as to the 'cure,' or that Dr. A. produced a dubious impression as to his honesty. This last surmise arises from the fact that I know that Dr. A. does not believe that a schizophrenic state can progress to recovery.

One can now go on to uncovering the *noticed* difficulties of the patient in his relations with others. The autistic term, 'schizophrenia,' may be a useful fixed point in the shifting field of our discourse. Its appearance preceded our integration and connects the present with the time before consulting Dr. A. I seek an impression of that time by inquiring as to what took the patient to see Dr. A. Let us suppose that he replies "My father took me; he thought something was the matter with me." I then inquire "And what made him think so?" The patient states that he does not know, but "Father said I was acting funny; I know I didn't want to go out of the house." Had there been any marked change here; did his dislike for leaving the house appear suddenly? He guesses so, he hated to have people stare at him, so he stayed at home. Why did people stare at him? He does not know—and is obviously keenly uncomfortable. Were they acquaintances or strangers? He rather morosely says he does not know. I comment, looking at him, that I see no reason why people should stare at him. In most cases, at this point, he will either show relief from tension or show suspicion of my good faith.

The manner in which my remarks are made may perhaps be suggested if I state certain of the preconceptions that underlie the psychiatric interview. First, the patient is a stranger and is to be treated as a stranger. There is every reason for his being here; but there is no reason whatever for presuming on any friendly or unfriendly attitude. He comes to an alleged expert whose expertness is to show itself, if at all, *in uncovering the processes at work in the patient's relations with others*—not in omniscience, omnipotence, magical reassurance, persuasion, or exhortation.

Secondly, the interrogation proceeds in so far as possible from a given point in a direction easy for the patient to follow. If he cannot foresee the direction of inquiry, his responses lose known orientation and become relatively uninterpretable. If, on foreseeing the direction, there are shifts in his bodily tensions, their source is not wholly private. Consider, in our example, the substitution of "Did people stare at you," or "What made you think that people were staring at you," for the question "Why did people stare at you." The first is thoroughly disconcerting, thoroughly disorganizing to the direction of inquiry. Suppose I ask you your age, and, having been told, ask if it is so, or why you think it is so. The patient has clearly shown his belief—or his intention that I shall understand—that people stared at him. I am in no position to contradict this, even if I wished to do so. Moreover, he is probably in no condition to yield his conviction, or his intention that I shall share it.

It is not by any means just a misapprehension on his part, to be brushed aside by some feeble conversational magic. The father probably wore out his patience in just such attempts at "reasoning" with his son. Also, the disruption of our directed inquiry would put us back at the beginning, if in fact it did not awaken grave suspicions in him about me.

A third preconception underlying the interrogation is to the effect that little can be learned as to 'what manner of man is this' by direct questioning. If I ask a person if he believes in evolution, he is apt to answer generically 'Yes,' 'No,' or 'What?'. This tells me nothing. If he elaborates his answer, I *may* catch on to—develop insight into—what the term, evolution, means to him, and as to the complicating beliefs that he also entertains. The result, in dealing with a stranger, is much more certainly obtained by other devices; namely, the synthesis of indicative statements that have been made by him in highly personal references, rather than in discussion of abstract concepts. By and large, one's beliefs in abstract concepts are far from guiding principles in interpersonal relations. Consider the widespread belief in forgiving offenses and injuries, and the parallel faith in the magic of apology.

Many of the positive statements volunteered by an informant require testing by an inquiry into his supporting ideation. Our patient may say, "People stare at me because I am so ugly." If I find him remarkably unattractive in appearance, I may be inclined to accept this as an unfortunate idea based on all too real a foundation. Suppose, however, that I am true to my presupposition; without denial or affirmation, seek to uncover the patient's views as to his personal appearance; and learn that, to him, his significant ugliness consists in a change that has recently taken place in his mouth, such that his lips have become Negroid. This matters; my reference-frame for pulchritude is simply irrelevant.

A fourth preconception is the general dynamic view of interpersonal relations. Nothing is static, everything changes—

changes in velocity or changes in organization. In the psychiatric interview, we expect, we desire, and we must if possible quickly perceive, changes in the organization of the interpersonal situation. This is additional to the changes in direction and the speed of interpersonal processes. The organization of the situation changes as some of the parataxic elements change. The possibility of such a change appeared, for example, when I said to our patient that I saw no reason for people's staring at him. He grew less tense—his security increased—because I enfeebled a shadowy conviction that I was experiencing the alleged factor making for staring. Or he grew suspicious—more tense and less secure—because a conviction appeared to the effect that I was trying to deceive him. The situation was simplified in the first case; complicated in the second.

A fifth preconception may be illustrated at this point. One assumes that everyone is much more simply human than unique, and that no matter what ails the patient, he is *mostly* a person like the psychiatrist. This implies that a great many of the techniques of interpersonal performance continue to be just as applicable here as elsewhere. I am not pleased by the shift of our situation towards greater complexity. I 'discourage' the suspiciousness of me, not by some omniscient "aha! so you now distrust me," but by showing irritation. The discouraging is really our old friend, the forbidding gesture, which communicates more in a moment than any bright remarks would in an hour; with the great advantage that it does not require formulation by the patient—he does not have to 'think'. The irritation is communicated by a change of voice. I ask in a less neutral and somewhat unfriendly manner "Perhaps you can say something about it [the staring]?" If this fails, we are at an impasse in this attempt. One then picks up a new line of approach.

Another preconception is to the effect that, in an indefinite field, one accommodates to the apparent prevailing tendencies.

When, in other words, my patient will say nothing further about the cause of the staring and is obviously unfriendly, I accept the fact that this line of inquiry is for the present ended. I have been defeated in an inquiry and it is important that I avoid any irrational performance called out by the rebuff. I do not retire with an Olympian "Oh, very well; it is of no moment." I do not punish with some "Well, it's your loss, if you can't talk." I do not fold my psychic hands in mute acceptance of a juvenile 'the patient will not cooperate.' I have shown irritation in an effort to disintegrate the new hostile parataxis. I take up another line of inquiry, but I hold the expression of irritation until we are moving along a new line—until there is a simple human reason for changing.[34]

The seventh and last of the preconceptions which I shall mention bears directly on the growth of information about oneself—or *in* one's self dynamism. In general, one cannot accomplish good by increasing a patient's anxiety. Any question, and in particular, any explanatory statement—interpretation—that arouses anxiety is apt to prove worse than useless. At the same time, we must come to formulations that are of rather high probability. This means that the patient must obtain new insight into himself, for otherwise the psychiatrist has no confirmation of his surmises and they are therapeutically quite useless.

The preconception to which I am leading is this: personality tends towards the state that we call mental health or interpersonal adjustive success, handicaps by way of acculturation notwithstanding. The basic direction of the organism is forward. Regardless of the warp incorporated in the self, the psychiatrist, given sufficient insight and skill, may expect favorable changes to ensue from his study of the patient's situation. The disappointing outcomes and the difficulty encountered in successful

[34] The patient, too, knows that I am more simply human and like him than different. He has experienced innumerable impostures and has been 'taken in' by many of them; but his like everyone's efforts at communication imply the conviction of similarity, and the less this conviction is strained, the better.

therapy are referable to the culture-conditioned selves concerned—the patient's self, the psychiatrist's self, and the other selves that are significant in the course of the therapeutic situation. Some people are ill-equipped for life by defect of ability—particularly the intelligence factor. If now they have been trained to expect some day to be President, the maladjustment which they present may be prohibitively difficult of attack—primarily because of difficulty of communication, and of elaborating information. Some people have been educated and otherwise acculturated for life in a social order that has swiftly undergone profound change after they had reached chronological adulthood. For these, there may no longer be enough probable lifetime for the great reorganization that is necessitated by the new order. Somewhat parallel to this is the case of the person who for years has lived a simplified existence as a patient in an institution for the mentally disordered. For many of these, the social order has changed so much, while they were out of touch with it, that the reintegration from regressive change is discouraged. But these are exceptional situations, far from the case of most people who seek psychiatric help, and far indeed from the case of those who might benefit from the wider utilization of psychiatry.[35]

Having again said something of handicaps arising from or otherwise related to acculturation, it may be wise at this point to remind you that acculturation is necessary for the human estate. Growth implies incorporation of chemical substances

[35] To minimize their misunderstanding this conception, let me recast it—as far as possible—in the terms used by (Freudian) psychoanalysts. This conception denies categorically the possibility of a death instinct. Excepting in so far as cultural conditioning may lead indirectly to injury or destruction of the person, it questions any explanation of phenomena in terms of a drive towards self-destruction. It states that only the energy of the Id impulses is available for maintaining the therapeutic situation and for overcoming the difficulties encountered in therapy—the 'resistance' and the 'repetition compulsion.'

Therapeutic results are the expansion of the self dynamism and the simplification of living which results from this. I shall not attempt to express this in terms of the Ego and the Super-ego. I have not found these conceptions useful in formulating problems.

for the somatic organization, and of cultural entities for the personality. Deficiencies in either field may be disastrous. Noxious entities may be incorporated from either field. The body, at birth, has some capacity for selective relationship with environing physico-chemical entities; this capacity is, however, tenuous and increases greatly during infancy and childhood. The personality also, in the beginning, may be presumed to have certain limiting capacities. We have seen how the self comes presently to govern its own growth. Some people grow up in environments deficient in iodine, and, therefore, are distorted in the fashion that we call cretinism. Some people grow up in environments the other people of which are deficient in self-respect, and, therefore, are distorted in the fashion that I have called hateful. But certain chemicals are necessary for the continuance of life itself, and some culture is necessary for the appearance of humanness. Deficiencies and incongruities in acculturation are the handicaps, not acculturation itself.

To carry this parallelism a bit further; as a person seeks within varying limits to correct deficiencies in diet, so also one seeks for experience which will correct his deficiencies in acculturation. This is another way of saying that there is a tendency to achieve mental health.

Also, as the evil effects of dietary deficiencies appear so insidiously that they often remain undiagnosed until some intercurrent disorder brings them to light, so too the evils of personality handicap are usually revealed by a crisis in living, which in turn constitutes an episode of mental disorder.

It is my purpose now to develop in rudimentary outline the more significant of the syndromes which are seen in these episodes. The first syndrome to which I shall refer may come as something of a surprise. It is the episode of "love."

This "*love*" is an effect of culture patterns that still have great force; that, four generations ago, could scarcely be escaped unless one were of extraordinary ability or remarkable ugliness. These patterns bear with the greatest force upon the young. There is no end of talk about love, the movies are full of it, the newspapers recount varied facets of these situations, romantic fiction arises almost exclusively from it, and all the other boys and girls seem to be involved in it. Yet only the preadolescent and the adolescent have matured the capacity to love. Those who, regardless of chronological age, are not yet that mature, cannot experience it. Under social pressure, however, they do their best to conform and go through the motions of falling in love. As their need for security is great, the performance is as dramatically convincing as possible—to themselves and to others. Their demonstrations of emotion, occasionally knowingly fraudulent but often also self-deceptive, may be spectacular, quite beyond the real thing.

I can best illustrate the differences between "love" and love by recounting an extreme instance from the group of schizophrenics. A young man goes one night to the movies, alone, as usual. He often does this when he finds he cannot "concentrate" on his studies—in which he is doing less and less satisfactory work. He often falls asleep over his books but even with nine or ten hours of sleep, he awakens less and less rested. Sleeping is becoming his major activity; he can't seem to get enough of it. Yet he can't put the books aside and just go to bed; he knows he is not doing good work—and he is very ambitious to be a success. The movie is better than just chucking the book, and it is about the only thing he can do, at night, except an occasional solitary walk. He has long since given up his efforts to be one of the boys, to play games and converse with others. They don't seem to find him interesting; in fact, some of them have made fun of him, quite openly. At least, he is pretty sure that this happened, and that none of them have much respect for him—but he does not think about that if he can help it.

This particular evening, as the platinum-blonde heroine is revealed to the ecstatic audience in a moment of ingenuous helplessness. something happens to our boy. He has an 'electric' feeling; he is jolted out of his all too usual gloomy calm; he realizes that here is the Perfect Woman. He is in "love."

He sits through a second showing of the film, aflame with mounting excitement. He goes out and walks the streets—walks, in fact, far out into the country. Dawn finds him writing a letter to his love. He may or may not mail it. If he does entrust it to the mailbox, in all likelihood the postman ultimately brings him a photograph—straight from Hollywood. But in any case, his life is changed. The gloom is gone. He is warmed by an inner fire. He spends long hours in fantasy about the dear one. Studies cease to have any relevance. And the people who were once sources of self-abasement, are now of no moment whatever. They wonder what has happened to him; he does not notice them at all. The 'affair' may go on for months—as our boy moves on to the schizophrenic dénouement. All the reality of the love-object is photographic. He has no need even for the sloppy 'details' of her life distributed to the hungry world in the movie journals. Everything is provided by his revery processes; other people's views would garble his private perfection.

There are many variations on this theme of the fantastic love affair. Sometimes, the unwitting object is a classmate. Sometimes, as the revery grows and grows, the luckless youth is driven to reveal the state of affairs—to the astonishment, chagrin, and sometimes horror, of the girl. The events that then transpire do his tenuous self-esteem no good whatever and the psychosis, the severe mental disorder, frequently makes itself manifest in his performances immediately after the shock of the misunderstanding.

These are extreme examples, of a piece, however, with all the episodes of "love." That many of them go on to marriage is not surprising. That this is an important source of income and deference for psychiatrists also follows. The related patterns of our culture succeed all too frequently in coupling ill-assorted young people in what proves to be a singularly frustrating and unhappy relationship which sometimes leads to homicide; fairly frequently, to suicide; and increasingly often, to divorce, the damaged-goods situation, and the long tedium of alimony. There are also the children of these psychiatrically impossible marriages, pregnancy being one of the devices to which the interpersonally wretched often have recourse.

Let us now turn to another of these episodes which is related to the dynamism of grief. Grief is the way by which we detach our integrating tendencies from a lost significant person. It is as if our ability for integrating situations with fantastic persons would endanger our survival in the case of the death or other removal of anyone highly significant to one. We see this in "*grief*," chronic mourning, in which the survivor remains preoccupied with the departed one and carries on a semblance of life centered in the lost one, who still subsists and is functionally effective all the more ideally as a companion or lover because he is now but an illusion of the survivor.

Only superficially related to grief and mourning is the type of episode that we call *depression*. Depression is not a dynamism for the health-preserving release of integrative bonds which connect one to another. It is a chiefly destructive process. It cuts off impulses to integrate constructive situations with others. Only destructive situations are maintained, and these are extremely stereotyped. There is even a change in the physiology such that vital processes are slowed down and movements, particularly those of the large joints, are much reduced in speed and in frequency. The depressed person is preoccupied with a circle of ideas about evil, hopelessness, destruction, and damnation: "I am a great sinner; God has forsaken me; I am horribly punished; I have committed the unpardonable sin; I have lost my soul; I have destroyed my family; I am a great sinner," and so forth. The circle can be repeated day in and day out. It is all that the patient has to say; facial expression, sighs and groans make up the rest of the communicative activity.

Another form of episode is in some unclear fashion closely related to depression, although its signs and symptoms are in most particulars the very opposite. I refer here to *manic* and *hypomanic* states, in which there is a great outburst of fleeting impulses to integrate situations with others, a great variety of these abbreviated integrations, a great volubility—usually of low communicative effect, however, because there is great distractibility of the attention and what is called "flight of ideas"—and a corresponding acceleration of the physiological processes and increase in movements, particularly those of the large joints. The manic person is preoccupied with nothing; it is as if his attention shifted as frequently as possible, without rhyme or reason excepting the availability of some new distraction.

Depressed states frequently follow on states of manic excitement, perhaps after an interlude of approximately conventional behavior. The depressed episode may be the first; the manic, the following. The series, depression-excitement or excitement-normality-depression, once started, may go on for years. The people who show these types of disturbance in living often have a history of wide swings in their mood. One learns that they have been easily elated or begloomed; their mood has been mercurial. Moreover, to a noticeable if not to a statistically validated degree, they tend to be of a particular type of somatic organization; the body-build which Stockard termed *the lateral.* I have regarded these states as the manifestation of a peculiarity of the bodily constitution, but without any great conviction. It may, however, be noted that cocaine intoxication, in certain people, gives something of the hypomanic picture; and that mild poisoning with some other drugs —luminal, for example—produces some of the symptoms of depression.

It is easy to establish the fact of the serial order of manic and depressive states in the career-line of some people and, therefore, an entity called the *manic-depressive psychosis* is included in psychiatric diagnosis. There are many instances of disorder that do not closely approximate the manifestations of this entity, yet resemble it. These patients are often identified as suffering from a psychosis *allied to* the manic-depressive. Moreover, the pictures of the hypomanic state and states of depression have been generalized in attenuated form, so that some psychiatrists teach that the entity or group of allied entities, manic-depressive psychosis, includes certain "mild" states. A mild depression is often diagnosed to exist when a patient suffers a considerable diminution of energy and initiative, extending over a period from weeks to months in duration—yet is allegedly physically sound. A mild depression is sometimes diagnosed on the basis of physical complaints—weakness, debility, insomnia, vague to marked discomfort in the head, belly, or cardiac region—when no "organic" basis for the symptoms is discovered. Another diagnosis for this last mentioned picture is that of *neurasthenia*.

These diagnostic fringes to the manic-depressive entity require consideration from two standpoints. They give a very considerable leeway for psychiatric diagnostic prejudice to operate comfortably. They provide a convenient common ground for general medicine and psychiatry, in which common ground we may be certain about very little. The mild depression is diagnosed negatively, by the failure to demonstrate physiological factors making up a state of organic disease. In my opinion, this failure is, more often than not, the result of inadequacy of investigation. Many of the "mild depressions" and "neurasthenias" are deficiency states, malnutrition, and states of chronic intoxication. Insidiously developed ill-health is attended by increasing inertia, feelings of inadequacy and vague ailment. These attending symptoms have repercussions in the interpersonal performances, which in turn contribute signs and symptoms to the psychiatric picture.

The uncertainty and confusion of diagnosis reflected in these remarks is a strong argument for reformulating all diagnostic syndromes in terms of interpersonal processes. I shall not undertake to present a syndrome of interpersonal phenomena which would constitute a valid identification of manic-depressive psychosis. Instead, I shall speak of the *reactive depression*, another rubric in the accepted psychiatric classification. If one encounters a series of misfortunes and becomes depressed, after the pattern above described, this is presumed to be a much less serious mental disorder than is the obscurely initiated depression of the manic-depressive disorder. This, like a great many troublesome errors, seems rather obviously to stand to reason. If one should in the midst of a delightful experience, burst into tears, one is as certainly out of the ordinary as is one who does *not* weep at the loss of a parent. In either case, one has a lot to explain in order to maintain one's prestige and self-respect. This explaining—very generally rationalizing, appealing to mutually accepted prejudice—is perhaps the really significant factor in the relative seriousness of the alleged two kinds of depression. A person who has undergone a severe depression *which he cannot (understand or) rationalize* and which he and others certainly cannot forget, is by that very set of interpersonal factors made permanently insecure. If, on the other hand, he and his friends see as self-evident the "cause" of the depression, then there is a way of integrating the experience into the self without loss of prestige and uncertainty about his social and personal future.

Memory and recall deserve a word at this juncture. I have a theory of memory which has grown out of psychiatric experience, but which has not yet been formulated rigorously. Memory is the relatively enduring record of all the momentary states of the organismic configuration. In less abstract language, living beings *fix*, somewhere and somehow, meaningful traces of everything they live through, not as 'perceptions' or 'states of excitation of the cortex' or the like, but rather as the pattern of how the organism-and-significant-environment existed at the moment. I shall remember this moment as it exists, with all its implications past, present, and future—most of these implications having been present as tensional elements, and not as formulated statements. Let me illustrate: there is the spatial orientation—this beautiful and acoustically excellent auditorium; the rostrum, the microphone and its related system which tonight seems to be unmonitored, the audience as a certain amazingly large number of people, a friend who is deaf in the ear nearest me, the stenotype reporter, and many and many another detail of the geometric and local geographic situation —coupled with the *most significant* first experience of the related spatial orientation at the start of the first lecture in this series. There is the temporal orientation along several significant lines; the night after our unusually timed Thanksgiving, the 'place' of the moment in the exposition that I had planned for this lecture; the 'place' of the moment in a prehended durability of the lumped attention of the audience and their tolerance for my presentation; the 'place' in the attention-tolerance of certain more personally significant members of the audience; and various other details. There is the orientation in terms of my personal career-line; the lucidity of my formulation, the adequacy of its verbal expression—or rather, verbal indication, for one has no time to be exact and precise, if one is to cover these topics without exhausting the auditors—the effect on this moment of gaps in the earlier presentations, the 'coming' ideas that should grow out of this, its relation to the hoped-for success of the whole as an organization of all these statements and indications in terms of changes in the general audience, and new insights in the more personally significant auditors—including, very significantly, myself. I have mentioned these orientations without reference to the zones of interaction that are involved. I have omitted reference to the patterns of kinæsthetic and related data that exist in me, in connection with them. I can but invite your attention to the complex pattern of vocal—sound productive and sound receptive—past and future verbal and other voice-communicative processes concerned, and the effective or partially ineffectual and unfortunate function of these patterns in terms of what makes up this moment in each of you. I will only mention as yet other coördinates of the present moment, states of my visceral and skeletal musculature as terms in relative satisfaction or dissatisfaction with the momentary situation and with the accomplished and the potential performances of the whole lecture, the series of lectures, and with events before and to follow on the lecture. These are some of the items that may be abstracted from the momentary state of the organism—of a vast series of which one's memory is composed.

Recall is the functional activity of this organization of all of one's organismic past. Recall is vividly manifest in many of the details just presented. This auditorium is a recurrent, temporally durable item in my life. I *know* it. Awakening here after having been carried in, sleeping, I would *recognize* it because its traces in my memory would readily connect with the experience that I was undergoing. The aspect of recall that is not quite so obvious, however, is fully as important. The recall and recognition that I have mentioned occur within awareness. What of the activity which adapts me to the microphone? I do not wander out of its range. I maintain—with occasional error—a level of amplified speech which will serve my purpose. The memory of reverberation in this room this evening—appraised carefully in the first few moments—as it affects me through the auditory zone is operating smoothly, except when my fatigue or irritation at an inadequacy of communication disturbs the integration of the lecture-situation. This recall functions for the most part outside of my awareness. There are many phenomena of recall that represent its functioning entirely beyond the awareness of the person concerned. In other words, memory and recall are not restricted to the self. Recollection, recognition of and through recall, is another matter.

We do not consider disorders of memory, but only disorders of recall and its subdivision, recollection. It may occur to you that elderly people and those who suffer the injuries of cerebral arteriosclerosis are said to have defects or disorders of memory. The manifestations are of two orders. Relatively recent events are reputedly beyond recollection by the aged, while their memory of distant times is remarkable. To point to the explanation of this let me suggest that each of you may recall the first occasion on which you wore clothes of adult style; very few of you can recall in detail the last twenty times that you dressed. Recurring performances tend to become relatively automatic with a minimum of distinguishing characterization; if the actual demand in a situation includes the necessity for recalling the events of a given forenoon, the act and circumstances of dressing on that particular morning will recur. The recall will now meet a need, contribute to an adaptation. Otherwise, it is not forthcoming.

Difficulties of recall that arise from or are at least connected with disturbances of the brain may or may not carry with them a feeling of incompleteness, a sense of discomfort and inadequacy. This is also the case with the malfunction of recall which arises from fatigue, malnutrition and intoxication, and with that which is the result of multiple integration of one's situation—often experienced as a *conflict of motives*. The brain, particularly the cerebrum, neopallium, is the ultimate integrating apparatus of the organism; it serves the self system and the rest of the personality, and may be presumed—but not proven—to be almost exclusively concerned in the phenomenology of awareness. The central nervous system is also the most probable site of the principal factors of memory in the higher animals.[36]

[36] For the reason, primarily, that integrative representation of the historic momentary states of the organism may be presumed to occur here. One must not lose track of the "profiting from experience" which characterizes at least the whole of the animal kingdom—we are but beginning a comparable exploration of the vegetable world. Monocellular organisms show some phenomena of learning. The memory function may, therefore, be regarded as one of the aspects of (animal) life. Differentiation and specialization of functional activity culminates in the architectonically almost incredibly complex

If one cannot recall the name of an acquaintance, it may be because of fatigue which narrows the field of awareness; of intoxication or deficiency in nutritive substances, which impair the efficiency of organismic function; or of so-called psychical causes—factors in the immediate situation such as hostility to the acquaintance as a person (integrant) in the present situation, so that his presence is to an extent deleted or rendered merely potential by the defect of recall. It may be a particular instance of a general tendency to 'forget' all ordinal data. It may be a particular instance of a general tendency to forget names of people; this expressing a persistent characteristic of one's personality.[37]

The most astonishing of the disorders of recall are the *amnesias* which we encounter most frequently in self-absorbed people who have met insuperable difficulties in living. These folk live rather as if the world were a stage on which each performs, assisted by shadowy figures, for a shadowy audience including one luminously real person, the actor. It is not so strange, therefore, if, to them, recollections lack the brash reality to which the rest of us are accustomed; if they, instead, have a varying measure of uncertainty, so that some recollections of events have a rather dream-like or may-have-happened character. *Hysteria,* the mental disorder to which the self-absorbed are peculiarly liable, is the distortion of interpersonal relations which results from extensive amnesias. Let me indicate something of it by an imaginary instance. We have a

human central nervous system. Parallel with this goes a vast discrimination of the relevant factors in life-situations, and complexity of factorial integrations. This makes the central nervous system a very significant 'organ of mind' but not *the* organ of mind. Mind is a word referring to the organism, not to artificially separated parts.

[37] Let me point out, with these six of an indefinitely large number of explanatory hypotheses, the absurdity of *precocious interpretation.* There are some people who unhesitatingly express as the correct interpretation of a stranger's act, the one of several possible explanatory hypotheses which occurs to them. The interpretation is valid as a datum of magic omniscient performance useful in understanding the interpreter in his complex interpersonal situation. It may have very little to do with the person whose action is allegedly interpreted.

self-absorbed young man who finds himself married to a fiercely puritanical woman. He plays out the antiphony to her zeal very well, as long as speech serves the purpose. But he has need for sexual satisfactions in which she is wholly non-coöperative. We shall have him rebuffed one night; we shall have him roll over, turn his face to the wall, and think "This woman is driving me crazy with her damned morality." He falls asleep. He awakens with a cry; he clutches his wife in an excess of fear; he quivers, he stammers, he leaps about, he tears his hair, he beats his forehead. She calls a doctor. The doctor finds tachycardia—a fast pulse. The patient has a 'violent pain in his heart,' breaks out in a 'cold sweat,' rolls on the floor in pain and terror. A sedative is provided; he is lulled into quiet in bed; sleep finally supervenes. The most strenuous interrogation, during or after his attack, will uncover nothing of recollection of the thought that staged the drama. If by some transcendental magic a psychiatrist could ask "Did you not, before falling asleep last night, have the thought that your wife's morality is driving you crazy?," the patient may honestly—and indignantly—answer "Never; preposterous!" The most for which one might hope is that, afterwards, after the psychiatrist has left, our young man might recall the question and think "Now, that is queer, I do seem to recall thinking something about my wife, before I fell asleep." The attacks recur. They continue to be utterly inexplicable to the patient. The little detail, the preliminary thought which provoked the drama, is buried in amnesia. The fact that the doctor's comment about rapid pulse preceded the heart pains is also missing; the event cannot be recalled. These elements of memory are *repressed;* that is, they have lost their connection with the recollectable series of events. But both can be recalled in the peculiar situation which we call hypnosis.[38]

[38] Also, in hypnosis, anything else that suits the physician or other hypnotist can be "recalled," whether it happened or not—unless the hypnotist is careful to use no leading questions and give no other cues as to the "information" that he is expecting.

The dramatic 'maladies' of the hysteric are most varied. They include *anæsthesias*, losses of special senses. They include *paralyses*, loss of function of muscle-bone complexes. They include *visceral disturbances*—of the circulation, respiration, the gastric and the rectal function, the activity of the bladder, and of the genital apparatus. The "mild shell-shock"—attacks of disabling tremor—which was so dangerously contagious near the front line in the World War was hysterical. Many cases of "heart disease" have hysterical elements. Chronic coughs, some asthmatic conditions, and certain susceptibilities to "colds" are hysterical. There is hysterical indigestion, frequently complicated with diarrhœa. Frequent or difficult micturition may be hysterical, as are many cases of precocious orgasm. As a boy in grammar school, I had an illuminating experience with the hysterical possibilities. Having mixed a little red ink with a glass full of water, I was approached by a girl whom I disliked chiefly because of her remarkable cupidity. She had to know what it was; I said it was wine, and she had to have a drink of it. She thereon became most embarrassingly drunk. For fear of what might happen after the recess, I explained what it was. She thereon became poisoned. Not only did she defeat my efforts on her behalf for a half an hour, but then required the teacher's aid in surviving.

The hysterical interpersonal situation includes special disablements of a relatively clearly idea-born character which permit the securing of satisfactions or the protection of security without awareness of this meaning of the performances. Whether it is the highly moral person who makes sexual advances to a companion under cover of light sleep, or the "loving" person who revenges himself for any slight or thwarting by presently having an attack which makes life miserable for the other, the principle is the same. The other fellow is inhibited from attacking one's prestige or denying one's satisfactions by virtue of the complicating factor—the special state of light sleep, "One is not responsible for what happens in one's sleep"; or the attack, "You surely don't blame me for being sick."

Let us now look at quite a different type of performance, also often including signs and symptoms of physical disease. These patients, the *obsessional states*, too, have a variety of bodily ailments but their physical disorders are not simple tools in their interpersonal relations. They are supplements or aids in the maintenance of parataxic integrations. They do not protect prestige from easy attack, nor do they directly facilitate satisfactions. Often enough, they interfere seriously with bodily health, and thus undermine one's security and diminish the possibility of satisfactions. A frequent obsessional disability is the 'tense belly' with pylorospasm, hyperacidity, and sometimes gastric ulceration. There is usually a spastic constipation, with or without phases of diarrhœa. There may instead be cardiovascular phenomena, particularly hypertension. The patients are methodic, ritualistic, punctilious. The dietary restrictions imposed on them by well-meaning physicians may be carried out with such thoroughness as to induce malnutrition and deficiency disorders.

Interpersonal situations including an obsessional person are characterized by obscure power operations directed to the maintenance of control over everything that happens. I once had a patient, a good artist, who, however, hated to market his works. He lived in a two-story house and, one day, in coming downstairs, en route to a dealer's, was seized with the thought that he might fling himself over the rail and gravely injure or kill himself. The thought paralyzed further progression. He crept back to his studio and called his wife. He told her the awful experience . . . . To make a long story short, it was not long before his "fear of stairs" had immured him on the second floor. His wife, a rather domineering woman, was reduced to going for his commissions, delivering his work to the galleries, and bringing his food upstairs to him. He continued to do good work, but the necessities from his "fear" grew and grew until the wife was driven to call in a psychiatrist. He made rather prompt recovery—on the second floor of a mental hospital, with little but good, routine, institutional regimen. That is, he reverted to a simply quite obsessional condition, free from the disabling special fear of stairs. The wife thought he was basically improved.

I cannot leave the impression that mere pressure of circumstances will usually remedy the obsessional state. Perhaps it would, if we could carry the principle far enough in the right directions. The facts are not too encouraging, however, for obsessional states under threat of failure in their obscure power operations, often shift to even more grave disorder of living, as I shall presently illustrate. We have to expand their awareness as to the activities in which they are engaged, but this is extraordinarily difficult and usually fantastically time-consuming. The trouble arises from a very early, if not a lifelong, condition of profound insecurity. This has been made endurable by the perpetuation and refinement of personal magic, lineally descended from the late infantile and early verbal stages of personality development. These people cannot be comfortable as to their personal worth and as to the favorable attitude of others towards them. They have an abiding contempt for themselves, usually much more vividly manifested as an obscure to obvious contempt for others. The low level of self-esteem is concealed—very successfully concealed, in many cases—by the rôle of a powerful but subtle magician. The quiet grandeur of many of these patients is simply too staggering to occur to other people. A companion may, in temper, say "You always have to be right, don't you?" He does not realize that he has made a simple factual observation; the obsessional person is quietly omniscient and omnipotent. It has to be done in a subtle fashion; in the face of inescapable demonstration of error, he says "Of course; you are quite right." If you could prevent any such utterance, he would be terribly upset by the error. Instead, he passes grandly on, having by verbal magic reduced the situation to insignificance. When the state is severe, one can tell an obsessional person nothing; one can, however, provide data from which the information presently springs to the person's mind. I say to such patients, on particularly suitable occasions: "Quite often, when a person experiences such and such a series of events, it means such and such a motivation." This is usually, being offered with all humility, received politely and dismissed from attention while we go on with something important. Days to months later, the patient develops a surmise that there might be such a relationship. This is satisfactory; if he attempted to agree with me in the first place, my statement would have been metamorphosed in the process, if not in fact dissolved into sheer verbal fog. *He* has to be the one who knows, discovers, effects. My rôle, to match his ideal, would be that of one who 'only stands and waits'—a sort of admiring slave who never shows any unmistakable sign either of enslavement or freedom.

Sometimes the obsessional person is a tragic figure moving majestically through an awful world of inferior and malevolent people. Sometimes he is a great Christ-like figure who undergoes tortures in trying to "arrange" things as they have to be for his peace of mind, without interfering with anyone—in these cases, other people get nothing they want out of their integrations with the obsessional person. In the former case, they suffer and are provoked to cause suffering. Usually, any interference with the obsessional "arrangements" leads to withdrawal to an extremely detached, morose, or hurt position. Often, one cannot interfere, short of physical violence. This is typical of functional speech-disorder, in which, I am sure, the stutterer would follow one a mile rather than release one from waiting for the successful "arrangement" of the situation so that the word can be said.

The obsessional state is classically a state in which there is great activity of thought. The interpersonal relations are never simple, never free from great parataxic distortion, and they can be very strikingly illusory—particularly, of the Me-and-Myself type. These people are always "trying to make themselves" do this or that, or be this or that which is regarded as desirable —which they "ought" to do or be. One of them, told repeatedly in a series of consultative interviews that his fear of blushing could not be overcome by any effort of will, was nevertheless compelled each time to say "Don't you think I ought to stop thinking about myself so much." When they are relatively comfortable, they are often self-consciously observing their performances. As one of them put it, there are mental states like "Behold me, making my guests comfortable," "I am really being very agreeable," and so on.

These patients do not lack the drive toward mental health, but the growth of their awareness is wonderfully complicated. They notice and can report many an incident fraught with great possibilities of insight, but the report is so confounded with parataxic views as to what the other person was doing, that the hearer also is led astray. Under stress, they can overlook almost anything, or warp it unrecognizably to fit their determination as to what the situation must be. In this process, they often come to suffer severe visceral disturbances which take on the appearance of primary physical disease.

The son of a hateful, domineering, self-centered and self-seeking, ultrapenurious mother, and of a charmingly unreasonable and henpecked father, after a good many more obviously "suitable" contacts, married a woman some fifteen years his senior. The wife was a lady of great social charm, of broad interests, a philanthropist. She had been respected by his mother, and had herself always treated him in a definitely maternal way, very kindly. They had been acquainted for years. It was rather difficult to recall just how it had culminated in marriage; perhaps it was a result of the death of the patient's father, or merely of the son's realization that he was growing rather old. There had been some rather severe misgivings, and the consummation of the marriage was thoroughly unsatisfactory.

From the very beginning, there was a great disparity as to physical endearments. The wife was not interested at all. The man, however, could not adapt himself to this and often made endearing gestures—which were greeted with a tolerance that had obviously diminished over the years. The patient did not tell me this; it became evident as data accumulated. I learned also that, some years before consulting me, the patient had developed a gastric ulcer which had finally perforated, with grave hemorrhage. The patient volunteered the information that he had felt indifferent as to the outcome of treatment, at that time; quite willing, in fact, to die. The ulcer had healed, but there were still many symptoms of gastro-intestinal spasticity; diet and other hygienic requirements had to be followed quite rigidly. Despite meticulous care of himself, the patient still suffered quite a few attacks of gastro-intestinal disorder.

We worked intensively to clear up the severe obsessional state which he suffered. In about a hundred interviews, we came to a point at which it was possible to demonstrate, despite any power operations that the patient could muster, that the domestic life had long since come to include an unvarying manifest dislike of the patient by his wife. It was evident that she respected him; in fact, she did very well in maintaining appearances and in otherwise facilitating his career. But she clearly detested physical intimacy—and he was still, after fifteen years of discouraging, actively seeking it. As the patient came to recall clearly some of the unnumbered occasions on which he had pressed for some demonstration of pleasure in physical contact, always to be rebuffed—for some years, now, quite brutally—always withdrawing with concealed hurt and a "resolute effort" to put it out of his mind by considering how fine a person his wife was, how desirable a home they had, what standing they had in the community, and so forth, and so on; I say, as all this finally became clear and undisguised, it also became clear that on equally innumerable occasions he must have been filled with rage—of which he was only now beginning to be aware.

With the acceptance in awareness of the hopeless campaign to win over the wife to demonstrative behavior, the rebuffs, and the supplementary procedures by which he had been able to overlook his helplessness and avoid profiting from the recurrent humiliation, he became clear also about the rage and hatred that he experienced. The great "love" and contentment faded away and the couple came to live on a much less mutually provocative and painful basis. The gastro-intestinal spasticity correspondingly faded out of the picture and the patient finally 'recovered' from the disorder of alimentary function.

A number of rather parallel instances of spastic belly has led me to say that if one has to swallow resentment, one may be sure that it will give one indigestion. This may do as an allusion; what of the theory which underlies the occurrences? If you will devote all your attention, the next time you are suddenly angered, to noticing the movements and changes of tension that occur in your body, a clue may appear. You will notice a rather extensive group of phenomena; a suspension of exhalation of the breath, a change in tone of the facial muscles, a tension which may be referred to the diaphragm, and a tightening of the muscles of the abdominal wall. These phenomena are rather clearly represented in awareness. Changes in the distribution of the blood, changes in the rate of impalpable perspiration, and changes in the visceral tone will have no such vivid representation. Let us now suppose that, while you are made angry, this emotion and the situation factors pertaining to it arise from a dissociated tendency. Under this circumstance, the first group of changes, those well-represented in awareness, can scarcely be manifested in clear form. They would, so to speak, give the show away—or be involved in a rapidly developing attack of anxiety, which would complicate the experience beyond recognition. The group of substitutive processes which includes the obsessional states makes one, in general, proof against anxiety attacks under any but extraordinary circumstances. In patients belonging in this group, therefore, the skeletal and other clearly represented changes of tension and movement which accompany the working of dissociated systems are not manifested, and the changes of visceral tension (and movement) are markedly exaggerated—as if to drain off the excitation which would ordinarily effect the recognizable changes.

Besides this factor of drainage of "expressive" excitation into the visceral area, there is also the factor of duration of the unresolved situation. If one is aware that one is angry, in most cases one does something at least in fantasy, which tends to resolve the situation and discharge the impulse. If it is wise to inhibit all direct expression of anger, one can still have an imaginary situation in which, certain items being different, one can tell one's superior precisely what one thinks of him, even of his maternal parent. One feels better after this; the visceral resonance of the inhibited emotion is resolved. Consider now, however, the case of our patient—who went off smarting with rebuff and "told himself" what a fine wife he had. This clearly extends rather than resolves the somatic states connected with rage at his thwarting.

Some of us would be able to dispose of the emotional hangover and its visceral disturbances in sleep, by way of a dream. I surmise that it is only by this type of relief that patients in the group of substitutive disorders are able to live. But what one observes in them is something quite peculiar: their dreams are but obscurely related to the dissociated systems; the structure of the personality, the organization of self and non-self, is such that *no* clear representation is possible. Even at the time when by virtue of the inherent character of sleep itself, the person must feel relatively secure, the anxiety factor in the self dynamism is still effective. Clearly, even in sleep, the obsessional patient is not securing a fair return in repose and restitution for the time spent. Just as we saw our patient withdraw from rebuff with more or less concealed hurt—which means skeletal tension—which prohibits immediate relaxation; so also we expect to find that he needs a good deal of sleep, sleeps rather lightly, and is not too well rested in the morning, because security operations involving the self have also been going on during the night. This, the aspects of the problem which involve the self, is in addition to the effects of visceral tension, spasms and cramps, by which many an hour's repose is cancelled.

We have spent some time on these physical or at least bodily disorders of the obsessional patient. You must not suppose, however, that these patients have much to say about their symptoms. The contrary is the case; they are in fact often ashamed of being ill, and would be embarrassed by sympathy. They do not *use* their illness directly to achieve unacknowledged goals, as does the hysterical person. They are not preoccupied with their physical ill-health as are the *hypochondriacal* people. These latter, correspondingly, are much less obviously engaged in magical power operations in interpersonal situations than are the obsessional people. It is as if the hypochondriacal patient had abandoned the field of interpersonal relations as a source of security, excepting in one particular. He has to communicate data as to his symptoms; the illness, so to speak, becomes the presenting aspect of his personality. His interpersonal relations are chiefly influenced by the need to discuss the illness; he always gets around to it in any conversation; it is often about the only topic in which he has interest enough to sustain the effort of talking.

It might be thought that the hypochondriacal person, like the hysterical, is preying on sympathy. This also is not the case. It may be pleasanter to discuss one's ailments with a sympathetic, or at least an apparently attentive, listener; but discussed they must be, whether to a person obviously annoyed and bored, or even to a person who is delighted to hear of the suffering. This is one of the most illuminating features of the hypochondriacal state. The physical ailment, bizarrely enough, is a means for augmenting security in interpersonal relations. Without it, the patient would feel abased, inferior, and without any merit for the consideration of others. It is as if the source of chronic unworthiness which is obliterated as a subject of awareness by the obsessional routine, with concomitant disorders of tension and motility, is handled in hypochondriacal people on the level of obsession *with* the somatic symptoms and thinking about them. The source itself, however, being in the structure of the self dynamism—being a product of acculturation—is interpersonal in its origin and in its manifestations. Just as the obsessional person strives to overcome the promptings of this felt unworthiness by magical power over others; so does the hypochondriacal, by engaging others in discussion of the malady. Neither can withdraw from the world of people—even though, in their most aggravated states, the people concerned become highly illusory.

There is another of these substitutive states in which not the body but the world is treated as ailing. The *algolagnic* people seem to enjoy suffering, and passing it on to others. They have an astigmatic slant on life such that its unpleasant aspects are all that concern them. One of them, on his first trip abroad, rode on the "Coronation Scot" from Glasgow to London. He read a detective story throughout the journey, only thrice glancing out of the window. Finding himself observed, he remarked to his companion "Isn't the landscape boring." Asked as to the book in which he had seemed to be absorbed, he said that it was very tiresome. He mentioned in retrospect that the English trains were bad; the food, tasteless; the money entirely beyond his understanding. In brief, everything he noticed—or was observed to notice—was bad, wrong, or positively distressing. A grim possibility could be found behind any piece of good news; a high probability of evil lurked in every promise. Although an artist of great talent, he did practically no work because he was so distracted with the suffering caused him by life—with the suffering of his family, in case he could not find anything himself to suffer at the moment. These people, too, have to have a hearer; our particular artist had married a somewhat handicapped woman chiefly, I believe, to be sure of an audience.

Next in this series of substitutive states is the case of the *paranoid* individual. These folk regard themselves as the victims of specific, "deliberate," injury by other people. They are, in short, persecuted. The only durable integrations in which they are involved are situations in which they feel that the other person is doing them an injury. If they are seriously disordered, the others in their interpersonal relations tend to be highly illusory, often personalized abstract groups—the Masons, the Catholics, the Jews, or the Nazis, for example. Anyone in whom they are moved to be interested is soon discovered to be an agent of the persecuting agency—albeit sometimes an involuntary one.

People suffering the paranoid states can generally be provoked into expressing *ideas of grandeur*. Paranoid states are said to be characterized by ideas of persecution and of grandeur. This is somewhat misleading, because all substitutive processes include an extravagantly superior formulation of the self—for the good reason that they are all complex processes to overcome or at least obliterate from awareness an irremediable sense of inferiority, unworthiness, and incapacity to awaken positive attitudes in others. If one's efforts in this direction take the form of being persecuted, it is only natural that the rationalizing of this extraordinary state of affairs calls for some rather amazing explanatory beliefs. To have a whole group of people bent on one's injury or destruction may well be convincing evidence that one is a person of considerable importance. To document such an idea, one may have to go back a long way to the time in life when certainty was difficult or impossible. It thus comes about that many of them believe that they are not children of their alleged parents. They were exchanged, adopted, kidnapped. Their real parents are people of great importance, indeed. It is all part of some plot which they have finally discovered. It was a long time before they suspected, but finally they saw it all—and it explains a great many things that previously had mystified them.[39]

The paranoid, the algolagnic, the hypochondriacal, and the obsessional states are probably different patterns of much the same maladjustive processes. Patients manifest various blends of the four and some patients definitely alternate between one or another of them. Some hypochondriacal people become paranoid, and vice versa; and there may be more than one such transformation.

The processes which are woven into these four types of episodes are briefly, as follows. The early experience produced a prevailing negative self. There was not enough approbation. The negative attitude has interfered with the securing of interpersonal satisfactions. The projected low appraisal of suitable people has minimized every opportunity. The feeling of personal inferiority and unworthiness—which has to be concealed but is not thereby improved—has applied even in comparison with the already derogated others. The unsatisfied state, also more or less clearly represented in awareness—often as loneliness—is at times intolerable. Failure after failure undermines the vestiges of security which come from revery processes of a forward-looking type. They lose their utility, and a state bordering on despair supervenes.

The conviction grows that one is not fully capable of being human, and the intolerable insecurity that this entails deletes what is left of adaptive effort. One ceases to make positive or negative movements towards others. Random, relatively purposeless, restlessness becomes the expression of unsatisfied longings; sleep is disturbed and fatigue phenomena appear. The processes making for consensual validations are entirely sus-

[39] Persons who recall such fantasies need not be alarmed. They occur much more often in the early years than do paranoid developments in the later.

pended. Autistic features become more and more evident in one's reveries. The reveries themselves are regressive; they are oriented to constructive purpose, but the orientation takes the direction of a search in the past. One goes back as it were, over the course of one's development, seeking for a time in one's life which was satisfactory. In this regression, one always comes to something that is experienced as a way to start over again. The regressive direction now changes. The autistically valid but consensually inassimilable pattern now unfolds as an episode of mental disorder; it initiates a relatively stable maladjustive progression in interpersonal relations.

Various degrees of awareness attend these dramatic changes of life-direction from a regression in the face of despair to a progression along the line of one of our syndromes. The person who is regressing in the realm of interpersonal relations, be he ever so withdrawn from integration with real people, is not out of the world. Events continue to impinge on him. Some of these events are provocative of the revery processes, the highly illusory interpersonal relations, that he manifests in the regressive course. One of them may strike off a vivid alertness, all the more impressive because of the narrowing of consciousness which is a phenomenon of fatigue. This impressive event, perceived in the setting of an earlier state of development, may unfold itself as the very cause of the forward movement. This is the case with the unhappy person who "suddenly sees it all" and emerges from regression into a quickly systematized paranoid state.

Awareness of the origin of the classical obsessional states is as vague as that of the paranoid is dramatic. Sometimes, it is true, a patient may recall, for example, that on setting out for a difficult visit, she suddenly felt weak and thought "What if I were to faint"—thereafter having a morbid fear, a *phobia*, of fainting. But the obsessional state with phobias is nearer to the hypochondriacal, and the first intrusions of the magic which comes to characterize the classical maladjustment are seldom within the patient's ability for recall. Correspondingly, the evolution of the obsessional maladjustment is gradual. The patient becomes more and more of a magician—sometimes with occasional dramatic additions to the patterns of power operations.

I cannot leave this part of our subject without brief reference to a closely related life-pattern which, too, arises as the solution of a regressive change. It differs from the four that we have been discussing in that it is often quite successful as a way of life. I refer to the *sublimatory reformulations* of interpersonal relations. When there is severe conflict within awareness; when, for example, one ardently desires something the having of which one sternly disapproves; one cannot but regress to some earlier stage of development. This may, at first glance, seem none too self-evident. An example is certainly in order and, in our particular culture, a conflict situation involving sexual integrations would be among the most frequent. There are, however, other equally distressing states of sustained conflict, and I shall illustrate one of them before proceeding further with the topic.

We shall imagine a man of rigidly ethical upbringing, whose wife has developed what we call an involutional psychosis with decidedly paranoid coloring. For various reasons he resists psychiatric advice to the effect that she should be cared for in a mental hospital. He insists on caring for her in the home, where, despite competent nursing, he is available—at least, in the evenings—for integration in a decidedly destructive situation with her. She devotes considerable talent to making him utterly miserable. He discovers, partly through her promptings, a keen desire for her early death. This revolts him; he is horrified that he can entertain such thoughts about a person whom he certainly has loved, even though she is now greatly changed. Neither the desire for her prompt demise nor his abhorrence of his desiring it will yield; he is torn with conflict. The "death-wish" was at first attended by severe anxiety;

that is all past now and it has easy access to awareness. The conflict is clearly within the self.[40]

I shall not use this case of conflict to illustrate either the inevitable regressive changes or the sublimatory reformulation. Let me instead present the case of an imaginary young woman who, for reasons already suggested, is but imperfectly able to love a man. We shall have her marry much the sort of person as the husband whom we have just discussed, a somewhat remote, highly ethical, character who has attracted her all the more because he seems to have his sexual desires so very well under control. The consummation of the marriage will be quite unsatisfactory; throughout the years that they will have spent together, there will have been few instances of sexual intimacy. The wife early manifests a trait that is disturbing to the husband; she is intensely envious of other women and, as he discovers after giving singularly little cause, most irrationally jealous of him. We shall have her a prey to conflict between a powerful desire to engage in a life of easy virtue with many of the men she encounters, and a strong disapproval of anything the least 'free and easy' in a woman's attitude to a man. We shall see her withdrawing from social affairs as a regressive movement to reduce the force of this conflict, and we shall have her meet a clergyman of a particular, not too uncommon, type. He is of remarkable physical presence, great charm of manner to charming women, and much given to good works in which the people who have succumbed to his charm find a place. He is, of course, most circumspect in his relations with these people. This does not alter the fact that every

[40] The sketch of this case may well displease the psychiatrist skilled in the study of interpersonal relations. I have presented it as it is perceived by the husband. We know that he cannot have loved his wife in any realistic fashion; she would have loved him and could not have developed the involutional mental disorder. Correspondingly, we presume that the hostile-destructive impulse towards her is of no recent origin. It existed a long time in dissociation. Only the change in the wife's behavior to a frank and sustained torturing of him stirred it so powerfully that his self dynamism and anxiety were no longer able to maintain the dissociation.

woman with whom he deals comes quickly to feel that he is powerfully drawn to her, but under 'perfect self-control.' Our patient embarks, under his tutelage, in a truly astonishing career of practical philanthropy, looking after fallen women in the city slums. Her life is filled with this; her conflict all but disappears. She carries on with a minimum of contact with the good man who started it all; she lives in comparative peace with her husband and her women acquaintances.

This is an instance of the sublimatory reformulation of the impulses that expressed themselves in fantasies of prostitution. The motive is denied direct and complete resolution, but, in association with a *socially sanctioned* form of activity—the philanthropic work—is liberally if vicariously satisfied *in part*. This is the principle of sublimation: a motive which is involved in painful conflict is combined with a social (culturally provided) technique of life which disguises its most conflict-provoking aspect and usually provides some representation for the opposing motive in the conflict. The career thus brought into being is often pursued with all the more energy because it combines a disguised satisfaction with the achievement of personal security. In a word, sublimatory reformulations, when they work, work beautifully.

Our lady, now immersed in good work, may be somewhat of a bore. We may find her so 'concentrated' on her philanthropy that she is definitely a 'person with a cause' which is presented in and out of season with singular disrespect for other people's interests and avocations. There may seem to be something quite unrealistic about it, and one may be justified in wondering what would happen if it suddenly fell through. This is the price which is paid for sublimatory reformulations; they are ways out of a severe conflict, reflecting a disabling maladjustment of interpersonal relations, and they do not, in solving the conflict, greatly enhance the adaptive repertory. Unlike the obsessional, hypochondriacal, algolagnic, and paranoid states, the manifestations of sublimation in the specifically restricted field of the interpersonal relations are directly productive of prestige. Like any of the others, it presents a bar to the integration of situations of simple intimacy and complete satisfaction. It is, like all of the others, a power operation, but one peculiarly distinguished because the power-giving activity is endorsed by the culture. Its relationship to the others is shown by its combination with them, and by occasional alternations, in some people.

As another illustration, let me recite in briefest outline the case of a patient to whom I owe a glimpse of what may have been real *narcissism.* This term, so far as I know, originated in the early years of psychoanalysis, when certainly it was used to refer to a very dubious conception. The idea is that the infant is full of primary self-love, he has no object-love. I will not quarrel with the absence of object-love. The alleged primary narcissism, however, is not our concern; we look to "secondary narcissism" which—to quote one authority—is a retreat from object-love, so that one is compelled to seek pleasure in one's own attributes, fantasies, and so forth.[41] Anyway, as I encountered this veteran of the World War, in St. Elizabeths Hospital, he seemed as completely self-satisfied and self-absorbed as I can conceive mortal to be. He was unquestionably the product of a paranoid state, but the grandeur seemed to be complete, without evidences of his suffering persecutions. His end suggests to me that he had achieved that omnipotence so constantly pursued by the people that we are

[41] I take up the term, narcissism, only to condemn it. As formulated by Freud—in 1914, I believe—the conception underwent sundry modifications and, I surmise, came finally to be regretted by him. There is a certain cautious tentativeness in his later writings—not often enough the characteristic of his more ambitious followers—which makes for uncertainty as to just how greatly he had come to change his mind.

See, for a view sympathetic to my position, the scholarly "Selfishness and Self-Love" by Erich Fromm. PSYCHIATRY (1939) 2:507–523. A parallel view was expressed by Lewis B. Hill in an address, "The Treatment of the Psychotic Ego" before the Joint Session of The American Psychiatric Association with its Section on Psychoanalysis and The American Psychoanalytic Association, St. Louis, 6 May 1936.

discussing. One day while walking—in sublime detachment and completeness—with a party of patients, he leapt under a moving street car and was killed instantly. I believe that this impulse arose from a sudden defect of security, that he 'expected' to demonstrate his power to remain unscathed, and that there was no suicidal intention.

The history of this patient was something as follows. He was a sheep-herd in the Ozarks. One day, God spoke to him, told him of the war, directed him to enlist, and gave him assurances of his safety in this connection. The soldier repeatedly was decorated for valor. Only on demobilization was it noticed that he was psychotic. You will observe here, in this fragmentary outline, a paranoid sublimation, so to speak. What we encounter more frequently is a paranoid development as the outcome of failure in a sublimatory movement.

We can learn a good deal about the self dynamism from study of sublimatory reformulations that fail. In brief, they teach us that the escape from conflict by the reformulation is not an intellectual, 'voluntary,' performance. It happens in the way that the other substitutive processes take place. In a regressive state, it occurs to one that one might be interested in some particular form of activity. The idea 'grows on one.' Enthusiasm kindles. One moves forward again in the new interest. One has lost, or rapidly loses, anything but a memory —or an occasional exacerbation—of the impulses which stirred the severe conflict. The disappearance is, however, not without a trace. There are some peculiar new ingredients in the self dynamism, in the shape of more or less obscure taboos. These avoidances, which are frequently quite ritualistic, are based on situations which actually provoked the most troublesome instances of the conflict, in the days before the reformulation of life activity had taken place. It is rather as if the person arranges that the solution shall not be exposed to any very severe test, and is able to profit from experience in providing an unwitting protection. It was not possible to avoid the situations now avoided, until some components of the previously conflict-provoking motivation had been provided the socially approved mode of discharge. The taboo is an index of the impossibility of dissociating the motive, and an evidence that the reformulation *could* fail.

The relationship of the ritual avoidance in sublimation to the rituals and compulsive acts which are a part of many obsessional states amounts to a symbolic identity. The difference is one of degree, but degree of clarity of reference—in turn, an index of the depth of regression at which the solution was found. We do not shed much light on the situation by saying that a compulsive stepping on every third crack in the pavement is a ritual to avoid a situation like one in which one once had severe conflict. The meaning is shrouded by its origin in a deeply regressive state, when the representation of the conflict had lost resemblance to its 'objective reality.' If we demand of a person showing either the taboo of the sublimatory process or the compulsive act, an explanation of the why, we shall be told that it keeps his mind untroubled, or something to that general effect. This statement is fully responsive.

The compulsion to power operations and tests of—magic—strength in all obsessional people, to ritual acts and avoidances in some of them, to discussion of his symptoms by the hypochondriac, to expressions of derogation and suffering by the algolagnic, and to involvement with people who must be regarded as persecutors by the paranoid, are in every case to be regarded also as manifestations of the sort of solution found in sublimatory reformulation, *with the exception* that social approval is lacking. They are all complex processes, processes in parataxic integrations, which avoid painful conflict within awareness by virtue of resymbolization of the goals of the impulses that were disapproved as prejudicial to self-respect and security. All that can be accomplished by any therapeutically intended attack on the compulsively repetitious activity, under the most favorable circumstances, would be a renewal of the conflict.

It inheres in the nature of being human that one will relinquish, so to speak, a relative security and undergo anew a previously intolerable conflict within awareness *only* if one perceives a probability of speedy relief. If circumstances make a sublimatory reformulation ineffectual; as, for example, when a young person attempts the sublimation of all sexual motivation, so that the preoccupation with the new goals becomes more and more intense as conflict occurs; the course of events is often towards a paranoid excitement. By this I mean that the 'good works' are pressed ever more feverishly, with less and less judgment—less and less attention to consensually valid standards—and correspondingly increased feeling of frustration by others. There is apt to come a time when, from fatigue and recurring regressive movement, a paranoid state is substituted for the sublimatory one. I may be able to show something of the natural history of the substitutive processes by referring to a young man in the case of whom a swift unraveling of a residual compulsion was accomplished. This was a patient whom I had first seen some eleven years previously. I had found him suffering a severe obsessional state and had referred him to a psychiatrist for therapy. This had proceeded, on a meagre schedule of interviews, in the interval. At a time when the psychiatrist had been ill for nearly a year, and unable to see the patient, I acceded to his importuning and arranged for one interview an hour and a half long.

He told me that he was entirely recovered except for one symptom which still bothered him. He had still to throw away the part of his food that his fingers touched—I had not previously heard of this symptom. Please do not consider what follows either an adequate account of our interview, or an indication of the way to handle these patients. I said, after the complaint was heavily documented, that the symptom must have a history; that it expressed something akin to a notion that the hands were poisonous or otherwise contaminating. There followed what I consider to be the conventional movements to befog the issue. I pressed the point. The patient presently recalled—with many doubts as to its relevance—that as a boy, aged ten, he had developed a fear of being poisoned as a result of touching varnished wood. By dint of much urging, this idea was tracked down to its first remembered manifestation in connection with a bowling alley where he worked. He had then begun an excessive washing of the hands and an avoidance of that part of a slice of bread and the like which he had handled.

I insisted that such an explanation was inadequate, that while his account was good as far as it went, it omitted the really significant data. This sort of fear could not originate without an interpersonal root. There must be something that he had forgotten which involved a person, which would explain the fear of poisoning by the wood of the bowling alley. Could he think of anyone who might be concerned; of anything that had happened between him and someone else, before the appearance of the fear of poisoning. You must realize that I was operating in the field of a relationship created between us many years before, and occasionally renewed by my refusals of opportunities to see him, at intervals over the intervening years. In brief, the patient, under great pressure, recalled—with the usual doubts as to relevance, protest, as to why he should recall, and so forth—a boy with whom he worked in the bowling alley.

Under my insistence, he remembered that he had grown to be great friends with this boy; they had grown to be quite remarkably intimate; they had come to lie in each other's arms and to fondle each other, at times—he recalled someone discovering this, and telling him that it was wrong. He knows he never did it again. He agrees with me that the worry about touching the wood of the alleys appeared *after* he had been made to realize that there was something wrong with the intimacy with the other boy; after, in fact, he had stopped it. Because his therapist was not to see him for at least another six weeks, I made no effort to carry the explanation further. I did not ask as to the rôle of his hands in the happy intimacy with his friend, nor as to any physical basis for the idea of poisoning by way of the mouth.[42]

This example emphasizes, rather in the breach, my next point; namely, the course of events which is often initiated by a sudden failure of a sublimatory process.[43] Taking our young man who is assumed to have sublimated all recognized manifestations of lustful, genital, integrative tendencies, let us confront him suddenly with an extremely attractive and most forthright person who firmly believes that lust should be satisfied and that its satisfaction is unqualifiedly good—also, that he is attractive and suitable for genital integration. We shall presume that, in this uncompromising situation, he 'succumbs,' and enters, if not wholeheartedly, at least quite effectively into the integration. He has a shockingly good time. If the element of shock—postprandial, as it were—were not to materialize, he would be greatly benefited.[44] This, however, is not what

[42] Vague, or seemingly vague, ideas of poison—in our culture—have often to be related to autistic thinking about the semen. Poisons are *powerful* agents. Semen, the life-creating liquid ejaculated in sexual orgasm, is an ultra-powerful agent. Its ejaculation, in its fortissimo of unique sensation, is one of the sublime—if evil-marked—powers of one's organism. Power, lust, and the doctrines of sexual sin—related to the dark power of the body that overcomes the roseate, spiritual, and not in the given case quite adequate power of whatever is *not* the body—this is truly *something*. Coupled with all this not too distorted autistic thinking, go a variety of superstitions about *strength*. One loses one's manhood by "excessive" orgasm. Orgasm weakens one—a monstrosity grown from the observation that satisfactions induce repose and sleep. Loss of the semen produces or facilitates loss of the mind. And hundreds of other heinous outrages on troubled youth.

[43] Before I have left the topic of sublimatory reformulations, let me refer to the significant contributions: Chassell, Joseph, Vicissitudes of Sublimation. PSYCHIATRY (1938) 1:221–232; and Levey, Harry B., A Critique of the Theory of Sublimation. PSYCHIATRY (1939) 2:239–270, and A Theory Concerning Free Creation in the Inventive Arts, to be published in the May issue of PSYCHIATRY (1940) vol. 3.

[44] Here, again, the psychiatrist will recognize a defect in the presentation.

we wish to discuss. We shall assume that evil early experience has done its work, and that, as a result, the aftermath is self-recrimination and severe conflict. A good deal of his unhappy state of mind will get itself communicated to the partner, who will be distressed and repelled. Perhaps something will be said that makes him think that, not only has he done the wrong thing, but then made a fool of himself.

One of the courses of events subsequent to this is the rapid development of a state which I have called *ecstatic absorption.* The patient, as it were, makes a rapid regression to a state in which dream-like revery processes pertaining to a God-like condition solve the acute abasement. The recession is facilitated by his increasingly ineffectual attempts to remedy the interpersonal situation by conversational efforts that are becoming increasingly autistic and correspondingly puzzling to the sexual partner—or other significant persons to whom they are addressed. The state itself has its root-experiences in earlier performances connected with falling asleep when one was feeling very insecure. The increasing inutility of speech, the prehended disconcertment of the auditor, also has an effect in cutting off the attempts to maintain relations with actual people, and the patient—having perhaps become quite incoherent and completely incomprehensible—gives up all efforts to talk to anyone. His awareness is now that of a twilight state between waking and dreaming; his facial expression is that of absorption in ecstatic 'inner' experiences, and his behavior is peculiar to the degree that he no longer eats or sleeps, or tends to any of the routines of life.

Obviously, ecstatic absorption is a transitory state. Before I discuss its usual outcome, I shall present the picture of an-

Assuming a community of cultural background—our friend is at home, dealing with denizens of his culture-matrix, and not abroad among not-too-human beings—this lust-object that we have imagined is rather too good to be true. A person who found such a person as our young man attractive and suitable for genital integration *could not* be so healthy. A person who is integrated by sublimatory states is more motivated by power drives and/or hostility, than by simple, uncomplicated lust.

other development which may follow the sudden failure of sublimation. We shall return to our young man, a prey to self-recrimination and conflict. We shall have him, this time, leave the partner without any painful discussion; with, instead, some few hurried words of appreciation—which none the less strike her as reflecting an obscure but curious frame of mind. He will 'put the thought of his experience out of mind' by dint of preoccupation with something. The next night, he will sleep badly, perhaps tossing through the night harassed by unpleasant dreams. The next afternoon, as fatigue increases, he will be very restless and will take a long walk. He may set out for anywhere, but at some point, without warning, he will find that he is returning to see his sexual partner, that he is burning with desire to repeat the experience. And he will be terrified. *Panic*, or a state bordering on panic, supervenes.

Panic represents an acute failure of the dissociative power of the self. The mental state is best suggested by referring to a sort of experience which may have befallen anyone. If you have walked each day for years across a little bridge in the sidewalk, and it one morning yields under your feet, suddenly gives way and sinks a few inches, the eruption into awareness that accompanies this experience—a blend of extremely unpleasant visceral sensations with a boundless and practically contentless terror—*is* panic. All organized activity is lost. All thought is paralyzed. Panic is in fact disorganization of the personality. It arises from the utterly unforeseen failure of something completely trusted and vital for one's safety. Some essential aspect of the universe which one had long taken for granted, suddenly collapses; the disorganization that follows is probably the most appalling state that man can undergo. Panic, too, is a transitory state, and, unlike any of the maladaptive conditions I have discussed, a state wholly incompatible with life; it has nothing constructive or palliative about it.

The failure which is responsible for either ecstatic absorption or panic is not merely the collapse of a sublimatory reformulation. It is the failure of dissociations which were connected with, and made possible, the sublimation of the undissociated components of the sexual drives. It is important that one grasp precisely what is meant here, for there is a great deal of loose thinking about 'partial impulses' and 'components' of the broadly defined *libido* of Freud. To help in the clarification, let me revert to our woman who escaped prostitution fantasies by good works, at the behest of the attractive clergyman. It might look as if prostitution fantasies were a simple discharge by revery processes of a strong sexual drive. One often hears discussion of promiscuity, if not prostitution, as being the result of excessive lust. When, on inquiry, one discovers that the sexual partners of such a person are never very satisfactory; that promiscuous women are often frigid—have no orgasm; this simple explanation loses its force. In this culture, promiscuity is generally an outcome of dissociated, rather than of uninhibited, lust.

Our lady entertained fantasies of prostitution not because she simply lusted after many men, but because she had in dissociation a lust after women. She was of the homosexual personal syndrome, but whether by virtue of lack of any permissive acculturation, or of early experience which erected a strong barrier to integrations with members of her own sex, she had no awareness of the homosexual motivation. It existed in dissociation and, as is often the case under this particular circumstance, manifested chiefly in the complex relationship of jealousy. She had barriers which had prevented the evolution of satisfying genital situations with men; this culturally facilitated, however feeble, component had ready access to awareness; was, in fact, a part of the self dynamism. By utilizing its energy for the maintenance of heterosexual revery processes, which conflicted with her ideals of womanhood, a basic component in her self-respect, she none the less had a preoccupation which specifically facilitated the maintenance of the homosexual component in dissociation. Moreover, in this lesser conflict, she had an easy rationalization for any anxiety that she might experience in incipient homosexual integrations. She ran no risk of becoming aware of the dissociated motive, because she was fortified by the insecurity allegedly resulting from the prostitution fantasies. She had but to think "what would she think if she knew what goes on in my mind" to feel a sort of negative expansion of security—"She'll never suspect; I conceal it perfectly." The concealing passed as social necessity in connection with the fantasies; it served as an important attenuating, distance-producing, factor in the unnoted homosexual connection.

I can now point out the complexity of the sublimatory reformulations which are apt to fail in these dramatic and personally very dangerous fashions. The good works in which our lady found her calling kept her in intimate but socially detached contact with unfortunate women. To this extent, the sublimation of the heterosexual was a direct if attenuated satisfaction of the dissociated homosexual components of her genital drives. The social distance is defined by the culture and reinforced by a very necessary factor in the relationship which in a measure traverses the distance defined by social class; namely, the element of philanthropist doing good to others and being ennobled by the one-sided or one-way traffic in good. The nobility of the rôle makes difficult the appearance in consciousness of unworthy personal, physical, attractiveness. It can even be noticed, in abstract, 'objective,' fashion; in that case it had best be discussed with some compeer; this makes it less personal, a general and unimportant observation.

So, too, in the case of our young man, the evil effects of early experience did not merely necessitate a sublimatory reformulation of genital drives. There was also a barrier to women and the corresponding homosexual motivation existed in dissociation. It was the repercussion on the dissociating power of the self that made so dangerous the unpleasant aftermath of his unexpected sexual engagement. The ecstatic absorption is now seen to seek to accomplish a double function by isolating him from either woman or man. The panic appears clearly as the result of failure of all functional efficiency of the self dynamism. I can make the course of events somewhat clearer in the case of panic than in that of absorption; the end state may be almost identical.

Panic is disorganization. Personality reintegrates as swiftly as possible; often as a state of terror with extreme concentration of attention on escape from the poorly envisaged danger, and with every energy directed to flight. Unless something of this sort is possible, panic eventuates in circus movements, random activity, and finally incoördination of the skeletal muscles. In terror, the perception of the danger—the source of threat—is primitive, has the cosmic quality of the very early formulation of the Bad Mother. The whole world is threatening. Everyone is dangerous, hostile, and bent on one's destruction. There is no trace of coöperative, much less collaborative, attitude. The terror-stricken person is alone among deadly menaces, more or less blindly fighting for his survival against dreadful odds.

The extreme restriction of perception may be illustrated by reference to the frequent *delusionary* belief that one is being watched and followed. After panic has passed into terror, many patients believe themselves to be followed by people in automobiles. This comes about rather simply. All the cars that are noticed are behind one. As a car passes, it ceases to have any relevance whatever. It is no longer perceived. Therefore, no car passes one, and so long as there are cars behind one, and they stay behind one, it must be that they are menacing.

Even more disturbing than these errors of perception are the phenomena which arise from autonomous function of some zone of interaction, often the auditory apparatus.[45] Dissociated

[45] The auditory zone is intimately related to the oral zone, particularly in the coördinate function of communication. I have spoken of the partition of energy among the zones of interaction; the 'need to talk' and the need to hear are manifestations both of the tendency to enjoy any ability and of the bio-

impulses, when the self is functioning smoothly, discharge themselves in unnoticed acts. In people whose self integration is unstable, these acts may be a conspicuous part of behavior; in some cases, so prominent that consciousness is clouded at times to preserve security. These latter are the folk who engage in mediumistic and related performances, including automatic writing. In the state of *trance*, the medium may show speech behavior which is of considerable psychiatric interest. The voice-producing apparatus may shift in its pattern of function from the medium's waking speech to one or more markedly different speech patterns. A remarkable imitation of a deep-voiced man may be produced—as the voice of her "control"—not once but at intervals over years of a woman medium's life. The same medium may at times manifest two or more of these pseudo-personalities, by way of different patterns of vocalization, and maintain rather high consistency in these subsidiary patterns over months or years. I mention this to emphasize the degree to which the oral zone—supported by the auditory—can be taken over as it were, as the channel of behavior for dissociated systems.

In the phase of terror following panic which I am discussing, it is usually the auditory zone which becomes intermittently autonomous. The phenomenon of auditory or other *hallucinosis* represents the noticed activity of one of the zones of interaction as the expression of a dissociated system. One hears voices, spoken statements which pertain to the experiential structure of the dissociated integrating tendency. These hal-

---

logically inhering need to reduce tension by the expenditure of the supply of excitation.

David M. Levy has done invaluable pioneering work in this connection. See Fingersucking and Accessory Movements in Early Infancy: An Etiological Study. *Amer. J. Psychiatry* (1928) 7[o.s. 84]:881–918; Experiments on the Sucking Reflex and Social Behavior of Dogs. *Amer. J. Orthopsychiatry* (1934) 4:203–224; A Note on Pecking in Chickens. *Psychoanalytic Quart.* (1935) 4:612–613; and On Instinct-Satiation: An Experiment on the Pecking Behavior of Chickens. *J. General Psychol.* (1938) 18:327–348.

lucinated remarks carry with them many indications of the non-existent speaker's personality. The hallucinated utterances come rather quickly to be statements of particular illusory persons or personifications—God, the Devil, the President, one's deceased mother, and the like. The experience of hallucinosis is initially deeply disturbing. In patients who have suffered auditory hallucination for years, "the voices" may become commonplaces of life, of about the same importance as ordinary conversation.

It must be evident that the theory of hallucinosis is of much significance in psychiatry. To facilitate a grasp on the several types of process that are concerned, let me say something about the phenomena of the *tic*. Besides speech, we have gesture as a form of communicative behavior and, related to gesture, there are the postural changes, particularly of the face, by which we give more or less witting signs of emotional states. The tic is the autonomous activity of some part of this gestural or expressional apparatus, sometimes of a whole pattern—winking of an eye or the shrugging of a shoulder, for example—but often of but an uninterpretably small part of the pattern. Without any reason apparent to the person, but with some relationship to the interpersonal situation, the muscles concerned perform a personally meaningless action. There is awareness of the activity, but no perception of anything meaningful about it. The awareness of the movement can be absent; the person with a tic often becomes so accustomed to it that its occurrence is no longer noticed.

The automatism—tic, automatic writing, hallucination—is expressive of a dissociated tendency to integrate some particular interpersonal situation. Unlike our original presentation of entirely unnoticed behavior, however, these actions are—or may easily be—accessible to awareness. The difference is significant, but is one of degree rather than of kind. Thus, one can be led to notice manifestations of completely dissociated impulses, but one can not be led to perceive the meaning in them. Once having been led to notice them, they are much more apt to be noticed thereafter. In other words, they take on somewhat of the nature of the tic and other forms of automatism *within* awareness. The first directing of attention to one of them is almost invariably quite unpleasant, disconcerting or disturbing. Their subsequent intrusion upon awareness is also at least annoying. All this is quite exterior to their meaning, which, as I have said, cannot ordinarily be elucidated.

We have more than this inferential data if we reconsider the case of our young man who had to reject the part of his food which he had touched. In that case we were able to sketch the rough outlines of experience which had eventuated in the peculiarity of his behavior. The not very clearly formulated notion that his fingers were or might be contaminating was accessible to awareness. He was inclined to regard the habitual rejection of the pieces of bread that he had held as a symptom of his peculiar or abnormal mental state, his 'trouble.' He was led under strong situational pressure to retrace the evolution of the symptom—a very disquieting performance, beyond doubt. The sequence appears to have proceeded from malfeasance of his hands in lustful behavior with a chum, to a substitution *within awareness* of a fear that his hands would poison him as a result of touching the varnished wood at the place of employment, which gradually faded into an habitual but compulsive avoidance of food that he had touched—with the feeling that *other men noticed* the feeding peculiarity and might think he was funny or queer on that account. It is almost as if the final presenting state of awareness about the symptom had retained the second and last terms of a meaningful statement of his unsatisfied desires and had become puzzling and relatively undisturbing by deleting the first, third, and so on, terms of the statement. The particular tendency system under discussion was not fully dissociated from awareness. It was much nearer to clear representation than is the meaning of a tic. Yet nothing recognizably oral-genital had any longer any access at all.[46]

The relevant consideration is roughly the following. When a system of integrating tendencies includes so much energy that it cannot be dissociated—and conflict and anxiety continue—the self dynamism may achieve approximate security by a process of *resymbolization.* The conflict provokes a regressive process and the tendency system undergoes a backward shift along the line of its historic evolution. At some stage in the process, some of its most conflict-provoking components are reduced to elements that, projected in the more adult awareness, would be relatively general and non-specific in meaning. They are adopted as a troublesome, 'irrational' ingredient of life, a symptom, and *by timely appearance* they serve to ward off clear awareness, conflict, and severe anxiety. This is the general formula for compulsive acts, rituals, and taboos.

In the *schizophrenic state,* which we are considering as the sequel to panic, this relatively convenient solution of conflict by resymbolizing and substitution has failed and all that remains of security operations by the self dynamism is a disowning of the now far too meaningful symptoms. Schizophrenia

[46] It may seem that I take considerable liberty in suggesting that there was in this patient a dissociated, an imperfectly dissociated, system of tendencies to the utilization of the mouth in homosexual genital integrations. Consider the following excerpt from my fourth consultative interview with him, eleven years earlier. "To be absolutely frank and candid with you——when I was about six I committed the sin of sodomy——[meaning what?] Oh, God, Doctor, that is disgusting—I don't know just what to say, I can't express—you understand. [You know what you mean; am I supposed to be shocked?] Well, we were playing under the front porch of one of my friends—and a boy much older than either me or my friend—and he was urinating—and—I saw —his brother—take this other boy's penis in his mouth. Now, I didn't know what a horrible thing that was then—and the other boy was older than I—told me that there was nothing wrong with doing that—and committed that error —and that is something that I've been sorry for and would do anything—to wipe out that fact—but it's there. . . . . I haven't told anyone else that, but you and . . . . [his Father Confessor] as he put it, God had forgotten about that, and I ought to, as well."

The final remark indicates the substitution of unabsolvable 'guilt,' as one of the events along the experiential history of his symptom. The overscrupulous are one of the harassments of the clergy.

is a term meaning literally a fragmentation of the mind. The state is factually a splitting of the control of awareness. In all other conditions a monopoly of the self dynamism, awareness in schizophrenic states includes that which is in the self system and also that which attends the autonomous functional activity of the hallucinating zones of interaction. Put in other words, in nonschizophrenic states, awareness—at least awareness of personal meaning—of the situations in which one exists is restricted to integrations brought about by tendencies incorporated in the self dynamism. Nothing else but conflict and anxiety can be present in awareness. In schizophrenic states, on the other hand, a state of conflict has as it were been universalized, the conflict-provoking tendency systems being accorded independent personality with power greater than that of the self. Instead of anxiety, there is fear and often terror. So far as the self functions, the patient is engaged in (regressive) magic operations in an attempt to protect himself, to regain some measure of security in the face of mighty threats, portents, and performances in a world that has become wholly irrational and incomprehensible.

If I have made myself only moderately clear, thus far, you may be wondering why the schizophrenic person goes on suffering the terrifying experiences, when everything would be solved by accepting the dissociated tendencies into the self. This is a rather natural question, if one has lost hold of the interpersonal principle, and instead is thinking of the self as a thing and the dissociated as another thing, the two being the units which make a personality.[47] To 'accept a dissociated

[47] As the *ego*, the *super-ego*, and the *id* are sometimes understood by some psychoanalysts to be the three units—hydraulically, mechanically, topographically, or allegorically. I originally adopted the term, *dynamism*, to escape some of the dangers of slipping from a mechanistic analogy into a thinking about mechanism. This usage has spread somewhat, chiefly through the offices of Healy, William, Bronner, A. F., and Bowers, A. M., *The Structure and Meaning of Psychoanalysis as Related to Personality and Behavior;* New York, Knopf, 1930 (xx and 482 and xxiv pp.).

William V. Silverberg, in the introduction to a current study of The Jew

tendency system into the self' is tantamount to undergoing an extensive change in personality, implying a marked change in the sorts of interpersonal situations in which one will have one's being. Not only is there this element of great change, but also there is no possibility of foresight as to the direction and extent of the change. Finally, one could not foretell that this change will be tolerable; there is every prospect of its including serious conflict, for the self dynamism includes powerful tendency systems which are responsible for the character of the present life course. The metamorphosis is scarcely an attractive prospect, even theoretically. Practically, there is no such prospect; there is only the stable course of life in contrast with terrors and anxieties, easily referable to the unknown.

It comes about, therefore, that the schizophrenic person, even though he is aware—in the disowned, 'they,' fashion—of tendencies which manifestly involve him in rather durable integrations incongruous with his past experience and foreign to his at least dimly formulated career-line, cannot easily reintegrate a unitary awareness. Moreover, he cannot accept the manifestations disowned as the performances of others, of the "they" who communicate abuses and disturbing suggestions to him, who make him experience disagreeable and disgusting sensations, and who otherwise through the hallucinosis destroy his peace of mind, perplex and puzzle him, and by fatigue and other interferences reduce him to deeply regressed states of being. Everything in his 'personal awarenesses'—for he now has two—repudiates any suggestion that the experiences are not real, or that they arise from his unrecognized needs and desires.

If he has fortunate experience with the more real people whom he encounters in his disturbed state, the fury of the hallucinosis may decrease, the welter of delusional perceptions may diminish, and something approximating a stable maladjustment of a deeply regressive sort may supervene. The regression of

---

and His Fellowmen, has indicated that *ego, superego* and *id* must be understood as different *modes of functioning;* they make sense in no other way.

personality processes in these fairly quiescent states is such that the patient lives in a world and participates in interpersonal relations, all of which are dreamlike in varying degrees. As this is most clearly observable in the states which we call *schizophrenic perplexity*, I shall give an excerpt of an interview with such a patient. During the interview, the patient suddenly experienced a need to void urine. On his return to his room—where we were talking—the following took place.

"Well, I don't quite understand—what it means to go in there——to pass urine. It's your nature, I suppose, and. Well, for some reason or another, it's—it affects me very much—the —I don't know just how to explain—it affects me—well, just like—giving my—feelings away—to, say—you, instead of—this girl. [He drifts into drowsy preoccupation; is aroused, and presently continues with the following.] Yesterday afternoon—[Yes!] I was—in there—shooting some pool—[Continue!] I was in there shooting French——and——I—touches. What's-his-name puts the 3-ball in the pocket; and the 4-ball —(deep sigh)—and a—I touched the 4-ball, and no more than I did it, and I urinated some in my pants.——And—I'd like to see my girl—we—it was—If I understand it—in a certain way —I—suppose it was more or less this—being around here, and maybe I thought—Miss B.—I suppose she's French—[Miss B. is the black-haired nurse in charge of the ward, towards whom he lately has made some obscure sexual advances] or maybe the feelings—that everybody around here—I had sort of been in contact with and—anyway, as soon as I touched the 4-ball, I couldn't hold my urine.—And then,—after I had urinated, I—I started to write a letter—to the—girl I was talking about ['my girl'; a fantastic love-object]. I didn't write —I took it out and started to, but it was pitch dark in here, so I didn't bother. [Why didn't you turn on the light?]—I never thought about it."

This excerpt shows the classical schizophrenic *spread of meaning*. Matters which are utter commonplaces of life may be as it were dislocated from their place in the routine of living and elevated into focal awareness—with corresponding necessity to 'do something' about them, a start at which is to perceive their "meaning." This patient, having had a disturbingly sudden awareness that he must pass urine, is preoccupied with what the act means. This is no idle philosophizing. Patients who have come to trust one—part of the time—often ask questions like "What does it mean when you rub your nose?", or "What does it mean when people cross the right leg over the left?", or "What does it mean when a person sits down to the right of one?". The excerpt gives at least shadowy indication of what is responsible for the puzzlement as to the meaning of urinating. The patient progressed, through a phase of drowsy preoccupation from which the demand implied in my presence aroused him, to an obscure statement which might be translated: 'I have a tension which I think should be connected with my heterosexual love object. This need to urinate arises. I do so and the tension is gone; as if it had been connected with you instead of her.' He came to recount an incident which included involuntary urination. He was playing pool with some other male patient. He touched the 4-ball and as a schizophrenic result, urinated. The translation of his obscure remarks might run something as follows: 'I was growing tense in this game with what's-his-name and the 4-ball in some way associated itself with Miss B. and I touched it and the tension became overwhelming and I had an orgasm and I felt I'd better separate myself from this disturbing personal environment by renewing mediate contact with my girl.'

The excerpt is chiefly concerned with *regressive genital* activity. The pattern of action in the sexual orgasm of the male is a coördination of heightened tonus of the prostatic sphincter, secretory activity of the glands of Cowper, increased tone and finally emptying of the seminal vesicles into the prostatic urethra, synchronous emptying of the prostatic gland into the same area, and finally the occurrence of rhythmical expulsive contractions of the urethra. These latter are attended by keen sentience rather different from the sentience connected with the expulsion of the last few drops of urine—to accomplish which the prostatic urethra also contracts rhythmically. The difference again is more of degree than kind, and its extraordinary aspects are less the result of the complex processes that are coördinated, than of the sudden release of greatly heightened tone. The contractions of the urethra in orgasm are much more powerful than are those concerned in policing the urethra at the end of urination. But the history of the urethral component of the orgasm greatly antedates the occurrence of orgasm. In the dream-like regressed states, the emergence of a few drops of urine into the prostatic urethra—the event which underlies a strong urge to relieve oneself—sets off the emptying contractions, and the whole can be and often is perceived as a *sexual* phenomenon. These particular regressive changes often take incipiently schizophrenic patients to the medical man. The urologist who finds nothing the matter is all too traditional. The quack is yet another story.

Just a word more as to the indications of dream-like symbol operations which appear in the excerpt. These pertain to the impulses that have provoked conflict. There is the amazing significance of the 4-ball, its relation to French, to Miss B. who is mistaken to be French in origin, her significance as a relief from the pressure of the prevailingly male environment, factors making her unsatisfactory as an illusory sex-object, and the movement to be rid of the actual by absorption in the illusory integration with 'my girl'—a lady who in fact scarcely knew of the patient's existence.

Not only is much of the schizophrenic thinking identical with the symbol operations that are encountered ordinarily in sleep, but the disorder of speech communication in schizophrenia is also paralleled only in ordinary situations where conversation is being submerged by drowsiness or sleep. The schizophrenic peculiarities of speech are chiefly of two orders, called respectively *stereotypy* and the use of *neologisms*. In the first of these much the same thing is said repeatedly, as if it would function with relevance in many different connections. In the latter, new 'words' are created and used as if they were communicative. The two phenomena have in common the defect of consensual validation, the profound parataxic dislocation of the auditor to whom one hears oneself address remarks. In the stereotypy, there is an impractical concentration of meaning in the expression, somewhat the reverse of the extraordinary spread of meaning in happenings in the 'outer' world. In the neologism, a dream-like condensation of several meaningful elements has occurred without the patient's noticing it; as a result of which the new word seems utterly valid, regardless of its inadequate function in communication. Some of the meaning which has been conglomerated in the neologism comes from the tendencies that had provoked conflict, and the inadequate function of the neologism is, therefore, to some extent necessary and satisfactory in that it permits a degree of —autistic—expression without any resulting necessity for an exchange of intelligence—information—and the associated processes of consensual validation. This brings us close to the topic of insight, the bridge that will carry us over into a grasp of conceptions useful in the remedy of mental disorder.[48]

Before leaving the subject of schizophrenic states, we must look rather more closely at the onset and outcome of these grave developments. Before I can make myself entirely clear, however, I must explain to the medically trained members of the audience that my use of the term schizophrenic is not equivalent to a reference to *dementia præcox*. By this, I mean that my conception of schizophrenic states excludes a certain

[48] The fourth lecture of the series was given under the title "Explanatory and Therapeutic Conceptions." In revising the extensive material for publication, it seemed best to divide the subject. [*Editors' note:* Sullivan in his original series gave a fifth lecture on "Prospective Developments and Research." It appears at the end of Lecture V here in abbreviated form. He had planned to expand this later but never did.]

indefinitely large number of the patients who are lumped under Kraepelin's rubric, and under most modern revisions of it. At the 1929 meeting of the Association for Research in Mental and Nervous Diseases, I pointed out the great difference in outcome respectively of acute and of insidious onset of the disorder in superficially similar schizophrenic patients.[49] I did not then stress the differences which appeared in the interpersonal relations of most of the patients with insidious onset. I was still too preoccupied with the seemingly parallel—because inadequately observed and analyzed—outcome of some twenty odd per cent of all these patients, regardless of type of onset. This is the more difficult to justify, for Hadley had demonstrated in 1924, that the 'deterioration' of some chronic schizophrenics is anything but a disintegration of personality.[50] Moreover, I had observed several remarkable social recoveries in patients who had spent years in catatonic states, and had developed some ability for quickly arousing some patients who had been following an uninterruptedly downward course for several years.

In brief, I have come to the opinion that there are two unrelated syndromes confused under the rubric of *dementia præcox*, or—as it is often used synonymously—schizophrenia. One syndrome is the congeries of signs and symptoms pertaining to an organic, degenerative disease usually of insidious development. These patients are finally discovered to be psychotic, although no one can say how long the state has been develop-

[49] Sullivan, Harry Stack, The Relation of Onset to Outcome in Schizophrenia. *Schizophrenia (Dementia Præcox)*; Baltimore, Williams and Wilkins (1931) 10:111–118.

This paper summarizes the conclusions of a report to the Neuro-Psychiatric Section of the Baltimore City Medical Society, "Prognostic Implications of the Type of Onset in Schizophrenia," 6 March 1930. The further development of my views is the outcome of subsequent study of patients who showed the simpler substitutive maladjustments as a persistent state, with schizophrenic episodes at times of great situational stress.

[50] Hadley, Ernest E., Is the Prevailing Content of the Hebephrenic Dementia Præcox of an Anal Erotic Character? Report of Study in Hebephrenia, 2 June 1924. Unpublished.

ing. Their outlook is very poor—even, I surmise, under the treatments by partial decortication which now enjoy such vogue.[51] I am content that this syndrome be called *dementia præcox.*

The other syndrome is the one about which I am offering some data. It is primarily a disorder of living, not of the organic substrate. The person concerned becomes schizophrenic—as one episode in his career among others—for situational reasons and more or less abruptly. He may have had months or years of maladjustive living, of one or another of the sorts that I have mentioned. He may have seemed to himself to have been getting along all right, until a few days or weeks before the appearance of frank schizophrenic phenomena. In any case, he knows what has been happening to him. He has not gradually and inattentively drifted into a world of vague philosophizings in lieu of interpersonal relations, or a world of more or less pleasant fantasy quite like that of early childhood. He has come to where we find him by a course that has at times been fraught with fear, terror, or literal panic. At some particular time which he will never forget, the structure of his world was torn apart and dreadful, previously scarcely conceivable, events injected themselves. It may be that he soon finds a way in which to patch up a semblance of his previous living; like my patient who, having accidentally discharged a gun in the direction of a beloved uncle, underwent some days of mutism and refusal of food, but then became approximately as usual until he met rebuff in both sexual and security adjustments, whereupon a prolonged schizophrenic episode appeared. It may be that he

[51] I refer here to the Freeman lobotomy, the metrazol and camphor convulsive treatments, the electroshock, the block method, and so forth. These sundry procedures, to my way of thinking, produce 'beneficial' results by reducing the patient's capacity for being human. The philosophy is something to the effect that it is better to be a contented imbecile than a schizophrenic. If it were not for the fact that schizophrenics—in my sense—can and do recover; and that some extraordinarily gifted and, therefore, socially significant people suffer schizophrenic episodes; I would not feel so bitter about the therapeutic situation in general and the decortication treatments in particular.

finds a way of life such that the schizophrenic episode stands alone, only marking a turning point from which a not very changed career-line has proceeded successfully.[52]

One is definitely schizophrenic when the regression of one's security operations, enforced by parataxic interpersonal relations, actually menaces one's survival. Whether one shall continue to be typically schizophrenic or not is, I believe, wholly determined by situational factors. In other words, I hold that there are *no types* of schizophrenia, but only some rather typical courses of events that are to be observed in schizophrenic states. This view is widely at variance with the Kraepelinian psychiatry and its derivatives; at least four types are recognized in the standard classification. These are enumerated as catatonic, paranoid, hebephrenic, and simple. Some overlapping of these types has always been admitted. Lewis, who made something of a survey of current investigations, comments, for example, "Catatonic features may also occur occasionally, even periodically in some patients, during a lifetime course of hebephrenia, in fact the two reactions are so frequently combined that I prefer to call this class of disorders the 'catatonic-hebephrenic' group." [53]

[52] This constructive effect of schizophrenic disorder, on which I published a paper in 1924, was at the same time under study by Rev. Anton T. Boisen, at the Worcester (Mass.) State Hospital. For a statement of his matured judgments see *The Exploration of the Inner World: A Study of Mental Disorder and Religious Experience;* Chicago and New York, Willet, Clark, 1936 (xi and 322 pp.).

For a fairly comprehensive bibliography on the lumped disorders see Lewis, Nolan D. C., *Research in Dementia Præcox;* New York, National Committee for Mental Hygiene, 1936 (xi and 320 pp.). The most recent significant error arising from confusing the two syndromes appears in the work of Kurt Goldstein and his followers. See his *The Organism: A Holistic Approach to Biology;* New York, American Book, 1939 (xvii and 533 pp.) and The Significance of Special Mental Tests for Diagnosis and Prognosis in Schizophrenia. *Amer. J. Psychiatry* (1939) 96:575–588.

[53] "Research in Dementia Præcox" includes in its text many expressions of opinion that are equally illuminating as to the sad state of psychiatric thinking. The passage quoted—p. 36—is followed by reference to disorders initially of the 'paranoid type' that "seen a few weeks or months later . . . . [were] obviously hebephrenia. *As it is extremely unlikely that any mental disorder changes its type fundamentally*, this means that we have too little knowledge

If the course of one's interpersonal relations comes finally to a schizophrenic state, and this continues without complication, one manifests a pattern of peculiarities which may be called the *catatonic state*. The variation of details in the pattern of catatonic interpersonal relations is great. Its adequate delineation is, however, of no little importance, for the prospects of ultimate restitution to ordinary life continue to be relatively good only so long as the schizophrenic state is uncomplicated. I shall, therefore, attempt a further description, and supplement this by illustrating the changes that may be taken to indicate an unfortunate course.

In the catatonic state, the patient, as a self-conscious person, is profoundly preoccupied with regaining a feeling of security. The processes by which the self dynamism pursues this goal are of the sort rarely manifested after early childhood, except in sleep. Put somewhat more exactly, the integrations which manifest the self dynamism are like those in which a person under three years of age might be expected to be involved. The picture is complicated by the fact that an indefinitely great part of the relevant experience undergone by the patient over the years continues to be in evidence. These integrations include as other people, parataxic illusions after the pattern of the Good Mother, the Bad Mother, the Good Father, and the Bad Father. In so far as subsequent acculturation continues to be effective, it gives to these illusory people various attributes derived from religious beliefs and the particular mythology which the patient has absorbed. The goals of the integrations are security; the performances are almost exclusively power operations. The experience which the patient undergoes is of the most awesome, universal character; he seems to be living in the midst of struggle between personified cosmic forces of good and evil, surrounded by animistically enlivened natural

to enable us to make scientific differential diagnoses." The italics are mine. Note the absence of consensually validated thought in the pronouncement. All that is evident is the author's conviction that mental disorders have fundamental types.

objects which are engaged in ominous performances that it is terribly necessary—and impossible—to understand. He is buffeted about. He must make efforts. He is incapable of thought. The compelling directions that are given him are contradictory and incomprehensible. He clings to life by a thread. He finally thinks that he is dead; that this is the state after death; that he awaits resurrection or the salvation of his soul. Ancient myths of redemption and rebirth seem to reappear, not because the patient has tapped some racial unconscious, but because he has regressed to the state in which only an early type of abstract thinking can be active. He is dead but clearly is not through with life. The remnants of religious teachings appear as an explanation. He will be saved from the failures and faults of his past life. Then he will live again.

Acts and ideas reminiscent of the whole history of man's elaboration of magic and of religion appear in these catatonic states. The abysmal insecurity is the driving force. The deep regression of personality processes is the moulding influence.[54]

In the midst of this dreadful experience, the patient is beyond the commonplace acts by which we live. He takes no food or drink. He notices nothing of the emunctory processes. He does not talk. He does not recognize the personal meaning of other people's actions in his behalf. He may show little activity; may lie nude with eyes closed, mouth finally shut, hands clenched, most of the skeletal muscles in a state of tonic contraction. He may engage in strange, often rhythmical, movements. He may undergo sudden eruptions of excitement, occasionally pass from mute catatonic *stupor* into violent *excitement* with seemingly quite random activity. Other people may

[54] For more details about schizophrenic content, see Storch, Alfred, *The Primitive Archaic Forms of Inner Experiences and Thought in Schizophrenia* [Tr. by Clara Willard]; New York, Nervous and Mental Disease Publishing Co. 1924 (xii and 111 pp.). Reiss, Eduard, Über schizophrene Denkstörung. *Zeitschr. f. d. ges. Neurol. u Psychiat.* (1922) 78:479–487, discusses the relationship of catatonic to primitive (infantile) thought processes. Both authors are carried away by speculations which lack the sound foundations that will be provided by research into the ontogenetic beginnings of personality.

be harmed. He may kill himself. This, however, is all by misadventure. There is no personally oriented hostility nor self-destructive motivation.

Now, however, let us consider the case in which a personal orientation of the awesome phenomena *is* found. In other words, the patient, caught up in the spread of meaning, magic, and transcendental forces, suddenly 'understands' it all as the work of some other concrete person or persons. This is an ominous development in that the schizophrenic state is taking on a paranoid coloring. If the suffering of the patient is markedly diminished thereby, we shall observe the evolution of a *paranoid schizophrenic state*. These conditions are of relatively much less favorable outcome. They tend to be permanent distortions of the interpersonal relations, though the unpleasantness of the patient's experience gradually fades and a quite comfortable way of life may ultimately ensue.

The paranoid outcome of incipient or catatonic schizophrenic states is to be distinguished from a paranoid coloring of the onset of the psychosis. One has also to keep in mind that schizophrenic processes may erupt in the course of a chronic paranoid state which was previously relatively free from such processes. This case, too, requires special consideration. The estimation of probabilities as to outcome—and as to the proper limits of therapeutic approach—involves a nice appraisal of the actual course of events in which the patient has been involved.

Rather fugitive convictions that one is being subjected to persecutory or destructive influences are almost always incidents in the incipient schizophrenic state. The patient for a long time has felt unhappy over his inadequacies, has believed that others did not respect him, that they disliked his company and perhaps talked in a derogatory fashion about him. This has made him more and more seclusive. He has kept more and more to himself and has suffered increasingly from loneliness. In desperation, he may have put on a bold front and become somewhat exalted, or oddly jovial and overactive. As his processes of consensual validation are failing, his efforts in interpersonal relations can scarcely be other than increasingly unfortunate. He appears more and more preoccupied, inattentive, or given to puzzlement, misunderstanding, and misinterpretation. Interested and well-intending companions become convinced that something is wrong with him, that he does not know what he is doing. This is but natural, as his responses to questions are becoming more and more unintelligibly autistic. By this time, if he is still making some outward efforts at keeping in touch with others, he is certain to have received miscellaneous bits of advice, many of which have been warped into queer misunderstandings, some of which may have been carried out in a peculiar fashion, with even more disconcerting outcome. The patient sooner or later will have to withdraw from efforts to deal with his compeers. If he is living at home, he stays more and more indoors, often seeming to need the company of one of his parents yet becoming less and less communicative, perhaps more and more morose and unpleasant.

At this point, a definite persecutory formula is apt to erupt into the patient's awareness. His mother has been putting poison in his food; a friend is trying to make him homosexual; people are reading his mind and printing stories about him in the newspaper. With the expression of these persecutory thoughts, there may be an 'appropriate' emotion. On the other hand, the emotion may seem wholly 'inappropriate,' as when the patient, informing his mother that he believes she is poisoning him, grins with obvious embarrassment, and eats his meals thereafter, with outbursts of mirthless laughter; when, with tense and awkward excitement, the patient announces to an astounded friend that he is ready to submit to the other's sexual pleasure; or when, with what must be taken to be an obscurely angry helplessness, he tells an acquaintance that he has seen the piece in the evening paper. The *apparent* incongruity of expressed emotion and the related idea is most impressive; it is often taken to be pathognomonic of schizophrenic states, and theories of the disorder have been built around it.[55] I wonder that negative instances are so easily ignored, that the parallel in one's remembered dreams is overlooked, and that recollections of one's own behavior in awkward situations are not associated with this seemingly fundamental peculiarity of the schizophrenic.

The principal difference between the persecutory coloring of incipient and catatonic schizophrenic states on the one hand, and the ominous paranoid schizophrenic states, on the other, shows itself most obviously in connection with this 'inappropriate' emotional life. The parataxic complexity of the interpersonal relations of the catatonic state is such that very little indeed is manifested in a simple, conventional way. The appearance of any impulse is apt to be followed immediately by some negating impulse. In the act of expressing an idea, a whole series of contradictory or otherwise complicating ideas may occur. About the least that such a patient need expect is that only one pair of contradictory propositions shall be in mind at a time. It is not strange that patients are often 'blocked' in the act of speaking, nor that they often give up the struggle and become entirely mute. The stress of this sort of life is very great. For those whose personal history permits it, the elaboration of a paranoid distortion of the past, present, and future comes as a welcome relief. Instead of an exhausting and extremely embarrassing flow of belief and doubt, proof and dis-

[55] One reads of "disjunctures of affectivity," of "affect congruous with the patient's peculiar content which cannot be shared by the observer, or actual affective incongruity with the content of the moment." Whatever the latter cryptic statement means it seems to imply a separation of the 'observer' and the patient. In 1927, I reported the results of 23 months of intensive work with a patient previously diagnosed variously as *dementia præcox* simple type, paranoidal *dementia præcox,* and—at the Henry Phipps Psychiatric Clinic—schizophrenic reaction type with first catatonic and later paranoid features. That the patient was schizophrenic is beyond question; he was studied at the Sheppard and Enoch Pratt Hospital for some five years. This patient at one time or another in the course of our work, expressed well-nigh the gamut of human emotion, never in any instance that I studied with anything but a simple relation to the content in awareness at the time, or clearly evidenced as verging on awareness. *Publications of the Association for Research in Nervous and Mental Diseases* (1928) 5:141–158.

proof, and a blend of erratically shifting personalities involving each person with whom they are integrated, the paranoid systematization of experience is relatively firm and dependable. It is an improvement, so far as the security of the patient is concerned, not only on the catatonic state, but on the previous uncomfortable prepsychotic existence. Therein lies its most evil potentiality. It can lead to nothing conducive of personal development; quite the contrary. But it can and does give a pay-as-you-go security. The cost is an adoption of hate in the place of a never-quite-realized love. The result of this substitution of hate in place of love as the goal of interpersonal relations is the gradual disintegration of the patient. Before I develop this theme, however, let me remark that, once a persecuting person has been found, and a detailed retrospective account of the persecutory experience has been elaborated, the 'incongruity' of emotion in relation to ideas ceases to complicate the schizophrenic picture. There is rage (fighting fear), hatred (impotent fear), or an unwilling respect—perhaps progressing in this very order to, as the disintegration of the patient becomes marked, a final quite amiable vassalage.[56] The paranoid development, in contrast to the schizophrenic state, is a much simpler negative-destructive attitude to the persons involved in more or less intimate—significant—relations with the patient.

The differentiation of the paranoid development from the persecutory colorings of incipient and catatonic schizophrenic states is dependent on the appearance in the course of the schizophrenic phenomena of a retrospective and prospective falsification of experience pertaining to a person or a personified group. The falsifications are of a piece with those previously discussed in our consideration of paranoid substitutive

[56] As stated elsewhere, vassalage is used to refer to the more completely dependent-identification situations in which one of the people concerned seems to act as if he were the source of decisive impulses, while the other (or others) act as if they were but effector organizations for realizing these impulses. This sort of situation grades through limited dependency relations and restricted identification-attachments to lucid (consensually valid) subordinations to competent leadership or example. *Amer. J. Sociol.* (1939) 44:936.

states, plus the extremes of parataxic concomitance which the schizophrenic suffers. The term, *systematization*, is used in this connection. One systematizes a belief by suppressing all negative or doubt-provoking instances, and by bolstering an inherently inadequate account of one's experience with rationalizations in the service of an unrecognized purpose. If the rationalizations are feeble, the belief is said to be poorly systematized; if they are of the sort that would be apt to work with a jury of one's peers, the belief is rather well systematized.[57]

It must be evident that one's beliefs are not necessarily at all closely related to one's manifest interpersonal processes and that the transfer of blame for the results of one's inadequacies does not remove or reduce the manifestation of the tendencies concerned. It decreases the feeling of insecurity and to that extent contributes to the dissociating power of the self dynamism, and by this, it reduces the probability that powerful tendency systems will escape from dissociation and precipitate conflict, regressive change, and perhaps frank schizophrenic phenomena. A paranoid systematization is, therefore, markedly beneficial to the peace of mind of the person chiefly concerned, and its achievement in the course of a schizophrenic disorder is so great an improvement in security that it is seldom relinquished. I am of the opinion that only the most skilful of therapeutic approaches—or the most brutally direct and well-aimed of assaults on the self system—are apt to alter the balance of

[57] While dream-processes are too highly individuated to be apt to impress twelve of one's fellows, it is quite otherwise with rationalizations.

The psychiatrist has to be 'very realistic' about these twelve of one's fellows, for they may be the judges of whether or not he has committed *tort* or *felony* on the patient. Persons suffering paranoid states with minimal schizophrenic processes are often considered to be *sane* and entitled to all the freedom from interferences with personal liberty guaranteed by our government. There is an impressive number of homicides that have been committed by paranoid persons discharged from the custody of mental hospitals by juries of their peers. It is more than annoying that the victim is sometimes the very psychiatrist who had attempted to protect the community by resisting the writ of *habeas corpus*.

power in the direction of again receiving the dissociated tendencies into awareness, so that they may be worked over for good or ill. It is for this reason that the paranoid development in a schizophrenic state has to be regarded as of bad omen.

It might be interesting, at this point, to mention one of the extraordinary situations with which I have dealt. Dr. Paul Ewerhardt and I were some years ago confronted with the problem of diagnosing—with view to determining if a committing of his person or property was desirable—the mental state of an extraordinarily talented soldier of fortune. The father had extracted a promise from the patient that he would spend not more than three days in the Sheppard and Enoch Pratt Hospital, and 'coöperate' with the psychiatrist in discovering if he were of sound mind. We interrogated him for a three and a two hour period, the first day. We demonstrated nothing, even as we became convinced that the patient was suffering a paranoid state. The fact that he had been in the Secret Service of one Great Power, engaged in fomenting disorders among the alien subjects of another, made the task no easier. His work entitled him to believe that his life had been in danger—was still, for he had not retired from this work, but was visiting in the United States because, correctly or otherwise, he felt it had been wise to absent himself for a time from the scene of his operations.

He slept well the first night in the hospital and came fresh and enthusiastic to the interrogation the second forenoon. It, too, in about two and one-half hours, was wholly inconclusive. Dr. Ewerhardt had then to absent himself and I was tired enough of the patient's discourses to turn to other things for a while. In the late afternoon, however, he asked to see me. The exact reason for this, I shall never know.

On entering the office, and seeing me make it safe from eavesdropping, he drew me an odd diagram on a piece of paper. This, he explained, was the symbol of an association he enjoyed with a scientist with whom he had had casual contact on one occasion, abroad. I learned that these two people were about the most important people on earth. They exercised vast powers achieved by command over natural forces, through the instrumentality of hypnotism, and were soon to achieve what we now know as the ambition of Mr. Hitler, hegemony of the world. They were in constant communion, across the continent, by telepathy. Both were imperiled by a horde of secret agents who were all around us. In brief, the patient revealed a well-systematized paranoid state, with but incidental schizophrenic remnants in its structure. He revealed it because, he said, he had received an unmistakable command to do so immediately.

Before I leave the topic of paranoid developments, I shall pay some attention to one of our more venerable psychiatric terms; namely, *paranoia;* and the conception to which it pertains. According to the accepted definition, a person who suffers paranoia is mentally disordered in his reasoning, only. From the interpersonal viewpoint, this definition is absurd. What then of the traditional diagnosis of paranoia? Paranoia must be recognized to be an ideal construction, an abstraction from psychiatric experience. As such, to the extent that it is useful in organizing thought, formulating one's psychiatric observations, it is justifiable. The trouble has been that the ideal, artificial, and in fact impossible, character of the concept of paranoia has been overlooked. Paranoia, defined as an ideal pole in the field of paranoid states, immediately calls to mind as its antipole an equally ideal conception of *utter* schizophrenia. All patients in the large group of paranoid states may be located at some point between an ideal state of pure delusion without admixed autistic processes, and an ideal state in which nothing consensually valid exists. Neither of the polar states can have more than this relevance to psychiatry. It is already evident that the more paranoid a person may be, at a particular moment, the less schizophrenic are his interpersonal relations, and we shall presently see that it works the other way around.

The person diagnosed as a case of paranoia is an intellectually gifted individual whose systematizations make his self system impregnable to any disturbing influence emanating from the situation with the psychiatrist. It is not a case of his reason being disordered; quite the contrary, his reasoning is equal to divesting any communication of its power to stir dissociated tendencies and provoke conflict within awareness.

This does not mean that the more purely paranoid state is a comfortable way of life, a sort of eccentric state of mental health. The paranoid person must be integrated in paranoid interpersonal relations, otherwise the power of the dissociated tendencies comes to exceed the dissociating power of the self, with anxiety, conflict within awareness, or panic, and probable eruption of schizophrenic processes. Whether it is writing bitter and troublesome letters to his Congressman, or starting law-suits, or pestering psychiatrists, or intimidating neighbors; the paranoid person cannot merely repose in his persecutions and grandeur, but must show characteristic interpersonal activity.

I come now to the other unfortunate outcome of schizophrenic states, the *hebephrenic dilapidation*. This change may appear very early in the course of a schizophrenic state. It may occur as the termination of a prolonged catatonic state. It finally appears in any long-continued schizophrenic condition that has not tended markedly to recovery. After a term of years most of the patients who have suffered paranoid schizophrenic states become indistinguishable from the condition of those in whom the hebephrenic change appeared early. When it appears, the hebephrenic state is apt to prove permanent, although even this is not absolute—as demonstrated by the cure of one patient by Kempf, and the 'spontaneous' recovery of a few that I have studied.

The outstanding characteristics of the hebephrenic state, the signs ordinarily enumerated as its description, are a marked seclusiveness—avoidance of any companionship; a disintegration of language processes—the speech is described as scattered, incoherent, vague, unconnected, or showing poverty of ideas; a marked reduction of emotional rapport so that the patient gives the impression of dilapidation or impoverishment of the emotional aspects of life; and the following two kinds of disturbance of behavior. Occasionally, these patients, in most obscure contexts, perform strange, impulsive, and 'senseless' actions. They also, in any significant interpersonal context, show mannerisms. To these descriptive features, the statements are often added that these patients suffer vivid but changeable auditory and visual hallucinations, which may vary greatly in intensity from one period to another; and that they entertain changeable, fantastic, bizarre, or "silly" delusions. The Meyerian psychiatrists refer to an "empty dilapidation" of the habit patterns, with a "childish deterioration." A great deal is heard about the deterioration in which schizophrenic patients often come to spend the remainder of their lives, and I shall have a word to offer about it, later.

I wish now to deal particularly with the *mannerisms* of the hebephrenic patient. Mannerisms, hebephrenic or otherwise, come about by the stereotyping of a gesture or some other interpersonally significant pattern of movement. The activity becomes relatively rigid in the way it occurs, no longer delicately adaptable to the circumstances of the particular occasion. The person who is careful always to speak with an Oxford accent which the hearer finds tiresome is mannered in speech. His relatively rigid patterns of enunciation will affect one in a significantly different way than does the speech of a person long associated with people of the Oxonian dialectic peculiarities. The mannerism will be experienced as an irritating overcomplication, something stilted, artificial, or fraudulent. The usual tendency to suppress troublesome differences in conventional behavior is missing. There is rather an insistent effort as if to assert the particular presumptively prestigeful difference. We accommodate rather rapidly to the 'genuine' peculiarities of the stranger, but the nuisance value of mannerisms grows rather than fades.

While patients in the hebephrenic state often show extraordinarily mannered speech, may be peculiarly stilted in their utterances, and sometimes talk in a fashion that can scarcely fail to convey an element of inappropriate disdain for the hearer, these of their mannerisms are not of prime theoretical importance. Even their sometimes almost entirely stereotyped remarks and their often tedious use of neologisms are by no means pathognomonic. The mannerisms that are perhaps the most striking and significant features of the hebephrenic state appear in the field of nonvocal quasi-communicative gestures. I say quasi because the mannerism does not express anything that is accessible to the patient's awareness—it represents a dissociated impulse—and because the meaning is often obscured by the regressive character of the gesture.

We have already encountered this phenomenon in discussing the tic. We proceeded from that subject to further consideration of my patient who did not eat food that his fingers had touched, an avoidance which we might call a *symptomatic act.* The action was noticed by the patient, was regarded by him as a symptom of his trouble, and it stood for an imperfectly dissociated group of tendencies to integrate particular kinds of strongly disapproved interpersonal relations. If now we regard some few of the many peculiarities of behavior that may be observed in catatonic patients, the place of the term, mannerism, in this field of automatisms and relatively automatic action should become plain. A patient, for example, walked in a curious fashion, apparently as a result of extreme eversion of the feet. This postural peculiarity, on further study, was seen to be a necessary consequence of a persistent adduction of the buttocks. The history showed that he had suffered at one stage of the illness from cravings for pederasty; sensations in the anal zone associated with fear of attack and loathing of the idea of submitting to the procedure. With the development of the peculiarity in locomotion, the distress from these cravings faded out of the picture.

Another patient, when approached by anyone, closes his mouth in a peculiar fashion such that all the mucosa of the lips is pulled into the mouth, and the inverted lips are held between the teeth. This patient has thus been relieved of intense oral cravings, including the belief that his lips had grown thick like those of a Negro. I may remark here that great changes of persistent postural tone in the oral zone of interaction are one of the most frequently encountered phenomena in more promising catatonic patients. It is not uncommon to observe great differences in the amount of mucosa that is habitually everted, in each of the various phases through which the patient passes. Some patients show relatively persisting alterations of the mouth that are almost impossible to imitate, even briefly.

Catatonic patients may keep their fists so habitually clenched for such long periods that organic changes ensue, and the fingers cannot be extended unless the flexor tendons are lengthened by surgical operation.

Many catatonic mannerisms are much more subtle than these. One of my recovered patients, in the early phases of his catatonic state, distorted each 'g' in his writing. The lower loop was always so elongated that it crossed several lines of his script. Many of these patients show relatively persistent innovations in punctuation, capitalization, and even in spelling. This brings us close to the autistic neologisms, already discussed. Some at least of these may be catatonic mannerisms in speaking. We may now return to the quasi-communicative mannerisms of the hebephrenic patient,[58] and discuss the way

[58] The discussion of automatic acts should include comment on habitual movements. Some considerable number of people scratch the head, pick the nose, bore the ears, and the like, with only vestigial awareness of the performance—if they are alone or feel secure with the people present. Some schizophrenics actually rub off a strip of hair by persistently scratching the head. Many schizophrenics touch their heads very gingerly, or arrest a movement just before touching the scalp, often with peculiar movements of the face—which might be called a grimace. These performances may be called manner-

in which these differ from all the other superficially similar performances.

The remarkable thing about hebephrenic mannerisms is their meaning. Not only do they represent the autonomous activity of impulses dissociated from awareness, but they represent the activity of impulses that were once a part of the self dynamism, the dissociating system. In the hebephrenic state, what remains of the self system maintains more or less of a feeling of security by excluding from awareness various impulses which were a part of the prepsychotic self. These impulses had a part in the conflict and chaos of the catatonic state. They were then on the side of angels, opposed to the impulses the manifestations of which horrified or terrified the patient. Now, they themselves are in much the same relationship to the patient's awareness. If they tend strongly to integrate an interpersonal situation, the patient becomes acutely anxious, often becomes seriously disturbed, perhaps acutely hallucinated, excited, assaultive, and more or less randomly destructive.

The clue to this situation is to be found in close study of the hebephrenic way of life. The patient usually shows more ingenuity in avoiding personal attention from others than in anything else. His seclusiveness is no mere withdrawal from discouragement, humiliation, and feelings of being disliked. He avoids all semblances of intimacy with anyone because his peace of mind is seriously discomposed by even the most rudimentary relation with any real person. The people with whom he maintains protean interpersonal relations are animistic natural objects and other simulacra born of a very great recession of personal development. The regression may be so great that

---

isms, but are better considered to be schizophrenic distortions of habitual movements. See, as to the origin of some habitual movements, Levy, David M., Finger-sucking and Accessory Movements in Early Infancy; reference footnote 45, page 67. See also, Krout, Maurice H., A Preliminary Note on Some Obscure Symbolic Muscular Responses of Diagnostic Value in the Study of Normal Subjects. *Amer. J. Psychiatry* (1931) 11 [o.s. 88]:29–71.

very little exists in awareness except elaborations of sentience connected with the physiological processes of the patient's body. All that remains of acculturation and of integrative tendencies that once had high satisfaction value is in dissociation, expressing itself in the mannerisms, if at all. Real people endanger this state. They provoke the unwelcome integrative activity and they interfere with the activity by virtue of which the hebephrenic self is in its lowly measure secure.

I believe that the alleged emptiness of the hebephrenic is one manifestation of these security processes; the silliness, another. What little data I have from my own work with these patients seem wholly congruent with the findings of Hadley and of Kempf. The hebephrenic has shed the troublesome demands of living among people. He cannot escape the proximity of people, but he can, often in a sort of crudely humorous way, belittle them to his own level of existence—just so they leave him alone and do not stir up any of the past that has ceased to harass him.

On the wards of larger mental hospitals, one sometimes can listen in, as it were, to a 'conversation' between two of the dilapidated patients who have come to find each other's company inoffensive. The remarks of each are made with due regard for the principle that only one person should be speaking at a time. There may be considerable intonational coloring, as if, for example, questions were being asked and answered, or as if one had reminded the other of something astonishing to him. The remarks, however, have but the most remote, if any, connection with those of the other. Each is talking to himself, but is doing it in a sort of double solitaire played after the fashion of conventional language behavior.

The intrusion of someone to whom long habituation has not occurred, who moreover shows interest in the patient, and pays attention to anything said, is quite another matter. Mannerisms rather in abeyance during the 'conversation,' become conspicuous. There may be a forbidding display of anger. The patient may resentfully move away. If not, he will probably laugh in a 'silly' fashion, from time to time, and discourage the intruder by the incoherence and irrelevance of his utterances. The silliness, 'senseless grinning,' and the like, seem to be called out by obscene, belittling thoughts that occur to the patient. He is by no means devoid of humor, even if his 'refinement' is conspicuous by its absence. I think, also, that he is far from 'empty' of revery processes and practical thinking. His incentives are not at all adapted to our habitual mode of life; one of his chief concerns seems to be the preservation of the status quo, regardless of other people's pressure.

Here, again, my picture of hebephrenic dilapidation will not be complete without brief comments first, on the necessities that confront these patients, and then on the general pattern of their course. This state is not by any means one merely of contented vegetation to the accompaniment of primitive autistic reveries and the simplest of zonal satisfactions. Many patients in a hebephrenic state seem for long periods to be contented, if left alone. All of them may have episodes of extreme agitation and violence, the provoking circumstances of which are entirely obscure. They are all busily hallucinated at least part of the time, the 'voices' are usually accepted in good part, but under some circumstances become unpleasant and thoroughly disturbing. Many of the patients talk *with* the hallucinated voices, have long felt compelled to maintain amicable relations with the illusory "they" whom they hear, and have in fact sunk into the hebephrenic state in gradual relinquishment of any independent existence.

Whether, once this hebephrenic change has begun, the patient will continue to sink in the scale of personal evolution, or will come finally to a relatively stable condition, is, so far as I can determine, beyond early prediction. If the dilapidation progresses, the end-state of the patient is practically indistinguishable from that of the probably organic deterioration called *dementia præcox, simple type*. These patients undergo a progressive shrinkage of initiative, a disintegration of social habits, including communication, and a seeming evaporation of any interest in events impinging on them.

It has been demonstrated in a few cases of hebephrenic change that it is not irreversible. By great and well-directed effort, a patient has sometimes been brought back—by prolonged treatment with a stormy course—to the catatonic state or even to a measure of social rehabilitation. Therapeutic effort has sometimes been successful in relieving a hebephrenic patient of some particularly disturbing aspect of his problems, with improved institutional adjustment of the plateau type suggested above. On the other hand, attempts at therapy are often wholly ineffectual. After a patient has been out of contact with the ordinary courses of life for several years, it is often entirely impractical to expect more than an institutional adaptation to be possible for him.

Before I conclude this presentation of explanatory conceptions I must touch very briefly on the topic of the involutional states, after saying a few words about the *psychotic accompaniments* of various organic diseases and degenerations. An example may show a principle that is useful in this latter connection. *Paresis* is both a disintegration of the central nervous system as a result of its invasion by the microorganism causing syphilis, and also a mental disorder of more or less characterizable course—or courses. As the central integrating system is impaired, the interpersonal processes necessarily undergo changes. These changes include the altered attitudes of others as actually reflected to the patient and as distorted by the insidious changes affecting his integration of sentience and elaboration of information. The tendencies to stable maladjustment after the pattern determined by his career are clouded by the progressive organic change, and the paretic psychosis thus comes to be a blend of rather rapid disintegrative change with—most frequently—a grandiose expansiveness that becomes more and more boundlessly unreasonable. Almost any symptoms of interpersonal difficulties can appear as relatively transient phenemona in the picture.

Another important member of this group is the so-called *alcoholic psychosis.* The excessive use of liquor is not in the same class as is an infection. One usually drinks a long time before there are any demonstrable organic changes from chronic alcohol poisoning. Sometimes relatively non-personal factors intervene in an alcoholic career and precipitate the peculiar *delirium tremens.* The alcoholic psychosis, however, is not an acute internal medical problem. It is a rather characteristic deviation of the life course, determined by the patient's career among others, as it in turn has been altered by the specific effect on interpersonal relations of intoxicating amounts of liquor. The outcome is almost invariably a paranoid state with but little schizophrenic coloring. The delusions are very frequently centered around the emotion of jealousy with a conviction of the infidelity of the husband or wife.

Finally, quite frequently, in women around the time of the menopause and occasionally in men around the age of sixty, a so-called *involutional psychosis* may appear. These states are usually considered to be allied to the manic-depressive psychosis. I believe that this is not always the case in women and but seldom the case with men. The forms of the involutional illness are principally two: the agitated depression, which seems to be a depression with rather fixed schizophrenic features; and the *world-disaster psychosis*, essentially schizophrenic, and sometimes encountered in schizophrenic states occurring before age 25. As I can scarcely present enough of a picture of the schizophrenic state, I shall illustrate the world-disaster psychosis by a brief statement about such a 23 year old patient who made an excellent recovery.

This young man was deeply attached to his mother and very strictly disciplined by his father. He did well in school, took an interest in sports, and mixed well with other boys. After finishing high school and a brief special course, he secured a job away from home. This work was a seasonal position; the rest of the time he lived at home and worked on the farm. His father died suddenly of apoplexy, and the mental disorder began before the funeral. The following are selected quotations from our conferences.

"It is too late to do anything—I am worse now than I was when I came—I ate my stomach up and . . . . the real thing is I never believed in God—I believed, but I just kept putting it off, putting it off—I could have saved all this easily—I didn't do right—Everything is all gone now—I am not gone but—the whole earth is gone, almost. . . . . I won't see my mother any more. I am worse and worse. I keep going wrong all the time. Might as well have went to prison in the first [place], I would have been worse, I would have been better off. I am the worst sinner on earth. . . . ." Patient then explained that he had swallowed the filling out of an incisor tooth, as a result of which he had ruined his stomach, and was ruining the world. Said he now could not sleep at night; his room-mates called him disagreeable names all night long.

"I would have been all right if I had stayed at home. I was all right before I came up here [to the hospital]. Never will get back home now, will I? I wish I was back home. I can't get back home though. The world is coming to an end; that was caused by my coming here. [Swallowing the piece of tooth] caused me to eat up my stomach, insides; it ate itself up. I know that's what did it. I am worse than the Devil, ain't I? I haven't any feelings, hardly. . . . . I have brought crime on the world. I know it . . . . [The place where he worked] is all burned up . . . . I liked working in town. . . . . Dad said I ought to stay home and help him on the farm. . . . . The whole world is talking about me. Say I am the worst scoundrel. Dummy, small, bastard, yellow, dirt, and everything. . . . . Somebody dies every day on my account. People killing themselves all day long. The city is all tore up. . . . . I was a member of the church, took interest in everything, helped people. Just all at once I just got this stuff in my stomach and all over my hands and spread it through the air and that's how things started. The further I went the further it spread. Ought to have had better sense than to have come to a city. I couldn't tell you to save my life [what the stuff was]; I know it was some kind of stuff in my teeth. Just got nervous, kept sucking my teeth, and—ate my insides up. I haven't got any insides. They are inside there, but not in working order. I know when I eat it all goes to water, and everything. My bowels never move any more, since I left home . . . . if I lived, everyone else would get that. [If I] bury myself or starve myself for other people, it would be all right. . . . . There isn't anything in the world to eat. Everybody is starving to death and I just caused every bit of it myself. . . . . [The voices] call me 'bum' and all that. They call me every low name they could. . . . . I am losing weight all the time. The more I eat, why, the more people I send to hell. . . . . I am eating the Lord's body everytime I eat. . . . . The Lord said to me 'Well, you should live—you have got to die for the rest of the world'; and I didn't do it. . . . . Something is missing every day. . . . . [Today it is] some of my clothes. And I wasn't supposed to eat and I have been eating all the time [since being fed by the nasal tube, after refusing served meals]. Everything is gone, everything I own in the world is gone. I let the world come to an end. . . . . I was the one that was supposed to save the world, and I didn't do it. . . . . Every time I eat it gets colder all the time. . . . . I haven't any insides, any intestines. I haven't any lungs. I am dead, that's all, about dead. Should have starved myself. . . . . I am getting worse all the time, weaker. I ought to go home. Ought never to have come [to the hospital] at all. I think I'll—I think I'll go home. Should have been home long ago. . . . . I can go home now. . . . . Might as well go home, hadn't I? Don't do me any good to stay here; only doing harm to other people. People don't want me here. . . . I ought to go home. I know I should go home and tend to my own business. I know that people are suffering on my account [yawns]. I know I shouldn't eat, yet I keep on doing it."

When he was well advanced in reintegration of personality, this patient said: "I used to think I destroyed the world. I thought people were suffering on my account. . . . . Something on my mind caused it, probably my father's death. . . . . Felt afterwards maybe I could have been a better son to him, probably. My other brother was his favorite son. They used to get along good, but I never could get along with father; we'd work together and have a fuss. I had a pretty hard time with my father. He used to beat me, get a switch and whip me—for talking to him rather rough, or not doing something right, the way he wanted it done. It was mostly his disposition; that kind of a man, gruff, never explained anything. . . . . I used to tell him I was going away and never coming back any more. . . . . I would go to the city and after awhile he would write me to come home. I would go home, and it would be the same thing again. I would get more work done than the other brother, but he would get along better. He could take the car and go away if he wanted to. . . . . I used to go out and work and get giddy and sick . . . . especially in the hot sun; I used to almost have sun stroke at one time—about [the age of] 15, 16, 17—I was wearing long pants, I know. Always felt worried at home on the farm. Didn't like the work and didn't get along with father."

This young man was of a very strongly moral cast, and his psychosis was precipitated by the sudden—and shockingly welcome—death of his father. The involutional illness in the fifth, sixth, and seventh decades of life is frequently the outcome of a career of interpersonal frustration through the instrumentality of a rigid moral system acquired in the early years but energized in adolescence by the coming of lust. In many, if not in all of those who presently manifest this disorder, there has been throughout the adult years, an imperfect sublimatory handling of the more powerful integrating tendencies, with no instances of frank failure, but with many approaches thereto —and often, I believe, a sustained course of almost frankly meaningful revery processes which are entirely concealed from everyone else, and regarded as a secret vice. The psychosis is precipitated, in women, by realization that the time for fully meaningful sex life is at an end. In men, I surmise that the precipitating factor is the waning of illusions of potency. In other words, they too find that fantasy of full meaningful sex behavior after the established pattern is no longer possible. It is notable that the involutional disorder in men is almost always prefaced by an obscure gradual deterioration of physical health. Fairly frequently, there is a history of some disturbing event, such as loss of money, immediately before the health began to fail.

As a final contribution to the picture of schizophrenia, I shall here digress to illustrate the dramatic failure of the sort of career that might otherwise have terminated some years later in an involutional state. This is the case of a teacher whose work entailed an almost pastoral relation with adult students, mostly women. He was of impeccable virtue, but secretly he had for many years enjoyed a rather remarkable fantasy. He accompanied himself in his conferences with these students, with an illusory stallion who made most gloriously free with the women. As he entered the sixth decade of life, he passed swiftly into a state of utter terror—as the stallion broke loose from his 'imaginary' character, became real and autonomous, and even made free with the person of the teacher, himself. Admitted in a frantic excitement, with lurid hallucinosis, ideas of poisoning, utter refusal of food and drink, mutism, and continued catatonic activity, the patient rapidly exhausted his vitality and progressed into grave physical condition. Under treatment, however, he reintegrated a more adequate personal life which has kept him in comfortable circumstances for some fifteen years past.

The world-disaster psychosis is of no such abruptly self-disintegrating a character as was this psychosis of our teacher. It often first comes to notice by way of a panicky period on awakening during the night. The patient is more or less confused as to persons and objects in his environment, and convinced that something terrible is happening. Someone may be killing the family. The building may be afire. An earthquake, or an explosion, has happened. It is only after this acute disturbance passes that the more settled, preexistent content—such as bowel-change and world-disaster, a peculiarly frequent combination—rises to expression. The course of the disorder is deeply regressive, the behavior often manifests a great deal of hatred, and there is frequently a continuing preoccupation with the excrement, the patient becoming not only untidy but definitely coprophilic. The general type of nihilistic delusion is to the effect that the patient has destroyed everything, everyone, or at least the members of his family. The outlook for recovery is very poor.

The other type of involutional mental disorder, the *agitated depression*, occurs much more frequently. When fully developed, this is a picture of stereotyped depressive ideas, often of having committed the unpardonable sin—which cannot always be recalled—as a result of which the soul is lost and one is to be put to death. There is a recurrent or even a sustained state of apprehension, with wringing of the hands, moaning, groaning, and the utterance of woe—oh my God, oh my God, oh my God; and the like. The motor agitation may continue well into the night, so that the patient obtains but little sleep. There are apt to be ideas opposed to taking enough nourishment. The patients are often rather blindly resistive, yet given to clutching on to passers-by from whom reassurance is begged. Nothing of reassurance is possible. The patient becomes preoccupied the moment that she finds that one is not bringing her a message of doom. Fearing greatly that they will be killed, feeling that they are being or are about to be tortured, these patients are the most actively suicidal of all the mentally disordered.

I must bring to a close this sketch of the more important of our explanatory conceptions. I trust that, if nothing else has been accomplished, I have made clear that there are few fixed mental disorder entities; that instead far the greater number but manifest particular directions in which the field of interpersonal relations may be disturbed. The degree of disturbance in the case of any particular patient may become relatively unvarying; or, under stress of situational factors, may change from one relatively unvarying to another relatively persisting degree. Along the direction in which these disturbances can occur, we find it useful to formulate a series of definitions. These 'typical' states are naturally those points in the series at which many patients reach a relatively unvarying condition. There are other patients who do not approximate a 'type' but are somewhere in the series between two 'types.' The disturbances are ways of meeting the necessities of life as they are determined by one's history *and* the present interpersonal situation. The past conditions the particular events which precipitated the episode of mental disorder *and, with the foresight of the patient*, which is itself a function of the past, determines the type of disorder in interpersonal relations in which an equilibrium may be approximated. Events which alter the patient's anticipations of the future may open the way for a further development of the personality and a movement towards mental health. Other events may close these possibilities, so that the disturbed interpersonal relations are held as the only possible way to go on living. Suicide, intended or by misadventure, may end it all. Prolonged separation from more conventional life, and deep regression and disintegration of culturally conditioned interests and activities may fix the patient in the institutional setting, comfortably adapted to a rôle of some usefulness, or as a chronic nursing problem.

LECTURE V

Therapeutic Conceptions

THE PURPOSE of psychiatry is the understanding of living to the end that it may be facilitated. The goal may be viewed from the standpoint of treating mentally disordered patients. Even from this viewpoint, one cannot but realize that the social order itself is an important factor with which one must reckon in formulating therapeutic aims and the procedures for their realization. If the psychiatrist is able to maintain his perspective, he comes sooner or later to see that there is another perhaps even more significant standpoint from which to consider the ways and means by which the purpose of psychiatry can be achieved. I refer here to contemplating the social order, not merely as it sets the limits within which the patient's interpersonal relations may succeed, but rather as the mediate source from which spring his problems which are themselves signs of difficulties in the social order. Yesteryear, it might seem that this broader viewpoint should be reserved for the philosopher, or for the psychiatrist who had retired from the toil which is still the common lot of most of us. Today, the acceleration of social process has become so great that almost every psychiatrist has some occasion to realize that the first viewpoint is too narrow; that the level of general insecurity is rising, that the social order is in a sense itself gravely disturbed, and that psychiatry as a therapeutic art is confronted with new tasks that require a change of orientation and the perfection of new techniques.

I must necessarily confine myself, chiefly to that which we have learned in our efforts to participate helpfully in the lives of the mentally disordered. The broader aspects of therapy are scarcely ready for generalization. We can form some conceptions that are useful in dealing with relatively well-organized groups; for example, the armed forces, or the workers employed in the larger industries. We can formulate a number of principles that should be generally useful in the unhappy contingency of serious national emergency. But I, certainly, can offer nothing particularly inspiring for the general benefit of our people in their particular present state. I must say that I feel deeply disquieted by what I perceive to be the general attitude towards the course of world events. It seems as if our most remarkable development of education had failed to inculcate any deep sense of civic responsibility based on a clear understanding of the absolute dependence of personal welfare —of those of us who wish to continue our democracy—on the welfare of the nation as a whole and on the adequacy of its defensive personnel *and* matériel. This failure is manifest in the futile, the trivial and the positively harmful activities with which a great many of our people are responding to the increasing uncertainty, insecurity, and discouragement that is coming to be the common lot.

I make no apology for introducing this gloomy view as a preface to my consideration of benevolent psychiatric procedures. No other group of our citizens has a greater stake in the future of these United States than have the psychiatrists who are students of interpersonal relations. Our psychiatry emerged here in the peculiar setting of our national life; it has developed along lines of promise for reciprocal service in the evolution of ever-increasing human dignity, fraternity, and opportunity. It had looked forward with growing confidence to the time when the incidence of grave maladjustments of living would be greatly reduced by virtue of our increasing civilization. A crisis in world-events now imperils all this, and one may well wonder if the emergence of our psychiatry was not much too late in the era of realizing democratic ideals.

The therapeutic conceptions of modern psychiatry arise directly from the work of Freud, Meyer, and White. Were it not for Freud's formulations, we would probably still be frustrated by the obvious discontinuities in the stream of consciousness. Had it not been for Meyer's insistence that mental disorders are to be considered as dynamic patterns, as types of reaction to the demands of life, we might still be working in the laboratory on problems of neurophysiology and endocrinology. But it was White's ineffable zeal in teaching us to "determine what the patient is trying to do," his indomitable energy in training and in encouraging psychiatric investigators, and his vision and sagacity in the executive, administrative, and promotional aspects of psychiatry in the broader sense, that gave us most of our profit from Freud and from Meyer. Called early from a clinical career to the far more demanding application of his insight to the management of legislators, educators and physicians, Dr. White—convinced that psychiatry has to serve in order that it may study—found his 'patients' everywhere. His practice of psychiatry interpenetrated every aspect of his life. He came to be the very opposite of insular in his psychiatric formulations; he needed no special language and his appraisals of the work of others erred generally on the positive side.[59]

Early convinced of the lawful operation of the human mind, and of the usefulness of determinism as a premise for the study of human conduct, Dr. White received his first clinical orientation from Boris Sidis, and his first great research enthusiasm from Sigmund Freud. As Abraham A. Brill was shortly to become Freud's American protagonist, so Dr. White immediately became the champion of open-mindedness toward psychoanalysis among leaders of psychiatric thought. To him goes

[59] See, for his bibliography, *The Autobiography of a Purpose;* reference footnote 1, p. 1.

first honor for maintaining the healthy eclecticism that has characterized American psychiatry and that has carried it far beyond psychiatry elsewhere in the world. To his credit principally, and to that of Brill, Chapman, Meyer, Kirby and Oberndorf, is the fact that we regard psychoanalysis as one of the psychiatric techniques and require medical and psychiatric training as a preliminary to training for psychoanalytic practice. The foresight of these early students of Freud has greatly impressed me as I have observed the course of events in the period from my first personal experience with psychoanalysis in 1915 to the present.

I can scarcely avoid a tendency to be autobiographical at this point. My psychoanalytic reading began with Hart's *The Psychology of Insanity;* Jung's *The Psychology of Dementia Præcox,* and Freud's *Three Contributions to the Theory of Sex* followed; thereafter Jung's *Psychology of the Unconscious,* Ferenczi's *Contributions to Psychoanalysis,* Freud's *Traumdeutung,* and *The Psychopathology of Everyday Life.* There then came Kempf's *Psychopathology* with its case reports in importance second to none. It is my impression that, aside from Freud's discussion of the Schreiber case, and Groddeck's *Das Buch vom Es*—the ego is essentially passive; we are lived by unknown and uncontrollable forces—my subsequent reading of more purely psychoanalytic contributions has fallen under the law of diminishing returns.[60]

[60] Hart, Bernard, *The Psychology of Insanity;* Cambridge, Cambridge University Press, 1912 (ix and 176 pp.). Now in its 4 ed., N. Y., Macmillan, 1931 (ix and 191 pp.).

Jung, Carl G., *The Psychology of Dementia Præcox;* N. Y., Nervous and Mental Disease Publishing Co., 1909 (xx and 153 pp.).

Freud, Sigmund, *Drei Abhandlungen zur Sexual-theorie.* Tr. by A. A. Brill as *Three Contributions to the Theory of Sex* [3 ed.]; N. Y., Nervous and Mental Disease Publishing Co., 1930 (xiv and 104 pp.).

Jung, Carl G., *Die Psychologie der unbewussten Prozesse.* Tr. by Beatrice Hinkle as *The Psychology of The Unconscious;* N. Y., Moffatt Yard, 1916 (lv and 566 pp.).

Ferenczi, Sandor, *Contributions to Psychoanalysis* [Tr. by Ernest Jones]; Boston, Badger, 1919 (288 pp.).

Freud, Sigmund, *Traumdeutung;* Leipzig, Deuticke, 1900 (4, 371 and 4 pp.).

The focus of my interest from before medical school having been the schizophrenic states, a detail to duty at St. Elizabeths Hospital in 1921 finally brought opportunity for a variety of observations in an atmosphere of brilliant clinical psychiatry. This opportunity was greatly expanded by my transfer to the Sheppard and Enoch Pratt Hospital where nothing need interfere with the most intensive and prolonged study of informative patients. By 1925, I had convinced myself of the inadequacy of *any* extant formulation of the schizophrenic states, and offered a preliminary statement of the conservative as contrasted with the destructive aspects of these conditions: "the conservative aspects . . . . are to be identified as *attempts by regression* to genetically older thought processes . . . . *successfully to reintegrate masses of life experience* which had failed of structuralization into a functional unity and finally [had] led by that very lack of structuralization to multiple dissociations in the field of relationships of the individual not only to external reality, including the social milieu, but [also] to his personal reality." [61]

Tr. by A. A. Brill as *The Interpretation of Dreams* [3 ed.]; London, Allen and Unwin, 1927 (510 pp.). 9 ed. revised; New York, Macmillan, 1933 (600 pp.). New ed. revised; Macmillan, 1939 (600 pp.).

Freud, Sigmund, *Zur Psychopathologie des Alltagslebens;* Berlin, Karger, 1907 (132 pp.). Tr. by A. A. Brill as *The Psychopathology of Everyday Life;* London, T. Fisher Unwin, 1914 (vii and 342 pp.).

Kempf, Edward J., *Psychopathology;* St. Louis, Mosby, 1920 (xxiii and 762 pp.).

Freud, Sigmund, Psychoanalytische Bemerkungen über einen Autobiographisch Beschriebenen Fall von Paranoia (Dementia Paranoides). *Jahrbuch f. Psychoanalytische Forschungen* (1911) 3:9–68; and, Nachtrag zu dem Autobiographisch Beschriebenen Falle von Paranoia (Dementia Paranoides). *Jahrbuch f. Psychoanalytische Forschungen* (1911) 3:588–590; both published in *Gesammelte Schriften* and translated as Psychoanalytic Notes Upon an Autobiographical Account of a Case of Paranoia (Dementia Paranoides). *Collected Papers;* London, Hogarth (1925) 3:387–470.

Groddeck, Georg; *Das Buch vom Es;* Leipzig, Internationaler Psychoanalytischer Verlag, 1925 [2 ed. 1926]. Tr. by L. Pierce Clark as *The Book of the It;* N. Y., Nervous and Mental Disease Publishing Co., 1928 (244 pp.).

[61] The quotation is from Schizophrenia: Its Conservative and Malignant Features. *Amer. J. Psychiatry* (1924) 4:77–91. Muncie's *Psychobiology and Psychiatry*—reference footnote 10, p. 4—includes an "Historical Survey in Bibliography of Development of the Concepts Underlying the Principal Re-

Dr. White often remarked that an understanding of the schizophrenic states would also solve a great many other psychiatric problems. Some ten years spent in studying these conditions convinced me of the interpersonal nature of the psychiatric field. Another ten years in office practice with the closely related substitutive states, obsessional and other, has refined and consolidated the earlier insights. It is from this background that I bring what I can offer of therapeutic conceptions, including matters of differential diagnosis and prognostication.

Diagnosis and prognosis cannot be dissociated from therapeutic considerations. This comes about not so much because different therapeutic efforts are required for the various disorders. Rather, it follows because the information which one requires for making a diagnosis is most readily secured in a situation oriented to treatment. Let me develop this topic. For many years it has been the rule that psychiatrists shall conduct an initial more or less formally routine mental examination of their patients. This is all but invariable in many of the State Hospitals systems, where the manual edited by Kirby as Director of the New York State Psychiatric Institute has been widely adopted.[62] There are practical considerations that ren-

action Sets . . ." which shows that nothing of significance in the field of schizophrenia—excepting Cotton's focal infection theory and Lewis' primary cardiovascular aplasia theory—has happened in America since Meyer, Jelliffe, and Hoch gave their résumé of dynamic conceptions in 1911. Meyer's "Fundamental Conceptions of Dementia Præcox" appeared in *Brit. Med. J.* (1906): 757–760; and also in *J. N. & M. Disease* (1907) 34:331–336; Freud's "Analyse eines Falles von Chronischen Paranoia," in *Neurol. Centralbl.* (1896) 15:442–448.

[62] Kirby, George H., *Guides for History Taking and Clinical Examination of Psychiatric Cases;* Utica, N. Y., State Hospital Press, 1921 (83 pp.). The plan of the examination is basically that formulated by Meyer, who preceded him in the same post. A modification of this outline is given in Henderson, D. K., and Gillespie, R. D., *A Text Book of Psychiatry* [3 ed.]; London, Oxford University Press, 1932 (ix and 595 pp.). Most textbooks include advice as to the psychiatric examination. See, for example, White, William A.; *Outlines of Psychiatry* [14 ed.]; N. Y., Nervous and Mental Disease Publishing Co., 1935 (vii and 494 pp.) and Noyes, Arthur, *Modern Clinical Psychiatry* [2 ed.]; Phila., Saunders, 1940 (570 pp.).

der this procedure desirable. Most hospitals are understaffed and much of this work has to be delegated to relatively inexperienced medical officers. Expeditious achievement of some information in all the important fields of possible abnormality is facilitated by the use of a routine. The administrator of any hospital may be confronted by legal action amounting to a requirement that he show cause for the further detention of any recently admitted patient. If he fails, for want of information convincing to the judge or jury, an action to recover damages for alleged illegal detention of the patient may follow. However closely a hospital administration may come to Dr. White's dictum that in case of doubt the welfare of the patients shall determine policy, the legal responsibility and the enduring public attitudes to mental hospitals combine to require an early documentation of the patient's need for hospital care.

The differences of the interrogation for history taking and establishment of the "mental status," from the therapeutic interview are chiefly the results of lack of time, inadequate experience, and erroneous preconceptions on the part of the examining physician. The examination in either case is often conducted on the assumption that one person is obtaining information from the other. Our interpersonal viewpoint indicates that this is decidedly too naive a view. The interview situation is never so simply one-sided. It is never one who gives and one who takes. While it may be hard to see, in some cases, there is always a measure of exchange of information, and some consensual validation of expressed views. This touches on the greatest fault of the interrogation. There is so little of validation that neither the physician nor the patient are apt to be accurately informed as to the views of the other. The patient often receives misinformation which substantiates a body of his erroneous beliefs. The psychiatrist is often misled into formulating a history and a description of the present state of the patient that is a complex product of objectively valid fact and the preconceptions of doctor and patient. These unfortunate results of the formally routine examination have led some administrators to assign more experienced psychiatrists to the admitting services. These admitting medical officers make a brief but searching interrogation of each new patient, and incorporate their impressions in an Admission Note. In so far as the experienced psychiatrist deliberately or unwittingly gives the patient some valid insight into what is to be expected in the hospital, this is a distinct improvement. I think, however, that I might well illustrate, at this point, the evil effects that can be attendant on a hurried interview.

I worked at one time with a youth of 17 who manifested a severe and ominous schizophrenic state. We had some hour-long conferences, the first few of which amounted to very little, so far as communication was concerned. There came finally an hour in which the patient, as the end of the hour approached, mentioned the sexual performances in which he had been engaged by a boarder who had subsequently married the patient's mother, shortly before the psychosis occurred. I was then working in the room in which clinical conferences of the hospital staff were held. As the patient ended his communication, and I was attempting in haste to convey reassurance to him, the first group of the staff came in. I had to interrupt, continuing my remarks as I walked with the patient to the entrance of the hospital wards. On his way from that door to the door of his ward, he eluded the attendant who had joined him as we parted, rushed into a sun room, whipped off his belt, tightened it around his throat, and fought off an attendant and a nurse until he collapsed from asphyxiation. The subsequent course of his mental disorder was uninterruptedly unfortunate and he has resided for years in a State hospital. I have not since then permitted a patient to enter upon the communication of a gravely disturbing experience unless I have plenty of time in which to validate his reassurance as to the effect of the communication on our further relations.

Any interview presumes the existence of interlocking culture patterns, some approximate identities in acculturation of the people concerned. The most notable of these elements is generally the language. The risk here is the ease of assuming a full identity where there is only a superficial similarity. I could give such examples without number. Let me instead approach the subject from the standpoint of psychiatric discussion. It has for years been conventional among more psychoanalytically oriented psychiatrists to speak of some conditions as having resulted from "mother fixation." I have worked with a good many male patients from whom I came ultimately to understand the peculiar relationship in which each had stood with his mother. Far from becoming able to see an approximate identity in the significant features I learned from every patient new depths of meaning in the pattern of the mother-son relationship. Instead of learning the 'effects of the mother complex' so that I could use it as a sort of master symbol in thinking, I have learnt to avoid these generalizations. The significance in personality development of particular courses of events with others seems more generally to inhere in nuances than in the gross pattern more easily put into words.

I suggested early in the fourth of these lectures that the interview situation presumes a gradual evolution of awareness of the people actually concerned. The patient loses parataxic concomitants with which the physician is at first invested. The physician gradually refines his impressions as to what manner of person the patient may be. One of the more important factors involved in this growth of awareness is the purpose of the interview itself as the patient comes to see it. This purpose sometimes seems to be the humiliation of the patient. This is most diligently to be avoided, if one has any interest in therapeutic possibilities.

The processes that go on in the interview situation are determined by the whole body of integrating tendencies that the interpersonal situation calls into play. The perceptions of each person concerned and the actual verbal exchange are mediated by the respective self systems. Everything else goes on outside of awareness, and, unless the psychiatrist is both of wide experience in living and relatively very secure in the interview situation, a good deal is apt to escape his notice. The psychiatrist's formulation of historic development and present state of the patient is then apt to be relatively inconsequential if not quite irrelevant.

What is said in an interview is the part of the speaker's more or less cogent streams of revery process which is not suppressed by the self system concerned. Remembering that the self dynamism is a growing integration useful in dealing with others for obtaining satisfactions and avoiding insecurity; knowing that its growth is restricted by the function of anxiety which excludes from awareness all the data which would expand the self at the cost of insecurity; it must be evident that the patient cannot know enough to explain his present difficulties. What with the witting suppression of some considerable part of that which does appear in the patient's awareness, it must also be clear that far more than an interrogation is needed if one is to secure relevant and highly significant data about the sources of peculiarity in a patient's interpersonal relations.

An ideal psychiatrist with wholly unrestricted experience in living, whose self dynamism would be coterminous with his personality, if alert and intelligent, could observe in a sufficiently extended contact with any patient a great many of the actual peculiarities of the interpersonal relations in which the patient took part. Even this impossibly competent psychiatrist, however, could not infer with high probability the actual sequence of significant experience which lay behind the observed peculiarities. The most that he could infer with high probability is that certain events must have, and that certain other events could not have, occurred.

These inferences would be useful in guiding him in his further interviews with the patient, to the end that information rather than misinformation would be obtained, and no serious insecurities provoked as the patient became more fully acquainted with his own history—underwent an expansion of his self.

The principal problem of the therapeutic interview is that of facilitating the accession to awareness of information which will clarify for the patient the more troublesome aspects of his life. This requires that one circumvent the inhibiting processes which, on direct attack, would manifest themselves in severe anxiety, or anger and resentment, with disintegration of the therapeutic situation. This phase of the work is based on the fact that one has information about one's experience only to the extent that one has tended to communicate it to another—or thought about it in the manner of communicative speech. Much of that which is ordinarily said to be *repressed* is merely unformulated. The revery processes concerned with it are either non-verbal or of a highly autistic character. They do not recall the experience; in fact, their form is chiefly determined by a need to avoid recall. They often proceed in states of abstraction or inattentive preoccupation.[63] In other cases, they are actively preoccupying, making up the relatively meaningless recurrent ideation of a substitutive state. If so, their experiential subject-matter is sufficiently disguised so that nothing of it is recalled.

Before I leave the topic of the interview, let me anticipate something of that which I must say about therapeutic conceptions, and mention here the principal factors making for success and for failure in the interview. The successful conversation establishes various *consensi*. The physician is able to arrive with the patient at an agreement as to the time order of events, as to sequent and consequent, as to cause and effect.

[63] Revery processes have received very little attention compared to that given the processes of consensually validated, logical thought. See, in particular, the two books of the late Varendonck, J., *The Psychology of Day-dreams;* London, Allen and Unwin, 1921 (367 pp.); and, *The Evolution of the Conscious Faculties;* London, Allen and Unwin, 1923 (259 pp.).

The interview progressively *enfeebles restraint* on the free development in awareness of clear statements of unpleasant, embarrassing, or otherwise anxiety-laden experiences. The interchange *substitutes socially sanctioned* for anxiety enforced restraints or supervisions of behavior. The patient who uncovers and becomes clearly aware of an impulse the direct manifestation of which would probably be disastrous, sees the possibility of finding partial or symbolic satisfactions. It occurs to the patient who entertains impulses that would be acceptable to but few other people that he may *segregate his integrations* to suitable occasions and objects, and discharge the complicating resentments aroused by his individuation, perhaps in games.

These results come partly from the interpretation of clearly documented facts, the building of inferential bridges that carry one from particular concrete instances to a generalized formulation, and partly from considering alternative hypotheses for misleading formulations.

There are a great many misunderstandings about interpretation and inference. Some psychiatrists, particularly some psychoanalysts, are prone to much interpretation of the material expressed by their patients. I have worked subsequently with patients who have received this kind of treatment. Thus, one of them reported that her analyst had complimented her on the classical character of her "free associating." I was told of this gratifying circumstance because I had objected to the patient's uncommunicative verbalizations during our interviews, insisting that while they doubtless had purpose and meaning, they in no way informed the patient or me of anything concerned either in the patient's general difficulty in living, or in the present interpersonal situation. The analyst had on occasion been intrigued by the reveries provoked in him by the flow of language, and, with charming naïveté, assumed that what was going on in his awareness must have some validity for the patient. He, thus, expounded to the patient the meaning of the uninterpretable content—often to the patient's astonishment, sometimes to her perturbation; but by and large, to her final conviction. In other words, she came usually to accept the interpretations. It did not seem strange that some of her difficulties had not been remedied.

The supply of interpretations, like that of advice, greatly exceeds the need for them. Every patient has enough of his own misinterpretations and may well be spared the uncritical autistic reveries of his physician. At the same time, some interpretations are indispensable, if therapeutic results are to be achieved in a reasonable length of time. The first test for any interpretation should be as to its adequacy: does it cover the data to which it is applied? The second test should be as to its exclusiveness: are there other equally plausible hypotheses that cover the data? If so, the proposed interpretation justifies no presumption of its validity and, in general, it should not be offered.[64]

The psychiatrist must be resistant to precocious conclusions. In many patients, almost any inference is acceptable which *does not* clarify the problem in point. There is no particular anxiety connected with accepting the psychiatrist's mistake.

A great deal of the revery processes of many people are made up of what I have called *not-processes*. The patient thinks a great deal about what is not the case. This is greatly tributary

[64] Some people seem to have great difficulty in developing alternative hypotheses for any given set of facts. The first thing that comes to mind seems to them to be self-evident. Anything else is self-evidently erroneous. They can scarcely listen to a presentation of contradictory data; they may be polite and hear one out, only to renew the presentation of their previous view. These are mostly people who do not discriminate any more than they can help. They work preferably with conventional patterns of people and situations and are annoyed or puzzled by novelty. They show the all-black-or-white that I have associated with the manic-depressive psychosis. People interested in formulating 'types' of people call them *extraverted* or *cyclo-thymic*. The latter term refers to the swings of mood that often characterize them; they are either up or down, mildly elated and expansive or gloomy and 'blue.' Neither their moods nor their interpersonal relations have subtlety, and they are lacking in the capacity for *perseveration*—the carrying over of expression from an unsuitable to a subsequent occasion.

This sort of person and the one whose security depends on creating an impresson of omniscience are alike unsuited to the rôle of psychiatrist.

to security, for anything *is* but *one* thing, but *is not* an infinity of other things. One can proceed, therefore, by the not-processes to contemplate innumerable formulations, thereby easily avoiding the *one* formula that would be illuminating—and anxiety-laden. It is salutary, therefore, to see that all statements are finally offered in a positive rather than a negative form. Not the one of a possible infinity of statements as to what the patient does not think, did not do, or does not feel; but the single statement of what he thinks, did, or feels.

Even positive statements by the patient are usually misleading, unless they pertain to a concrete course of relatively impersonal events. The most forthright account of a conversation or other interpersonal event is apt to include a number of parataxic elements projected on the others concerned. Many patients include in their accounts long contexts about the other person's thoughts, motives, and intentions. The motives ascribed to the others are usually motives into which the patient has but rudimentary insight, in his own case. His interpretations, which he takes for granted and without any doubt, are therefore wholly unreliable. Whether they be correct, approximate, or entirely erroneous is simply beyond determination. Their relevance in therapy lies in their unquestioned acceptance by the patient. Their occurrence is a significant feature of his difficulties in interpersonal relations.

The pursuit of accuracy may be in itself a major handicap to communication. Some patients talk at great length 'to make something clear,' but qualify their various propositions so abundantly that the statement as a whole means simply nothing. As these vocalizations are often produced with much color of emotion and in good rhetorical form, it is easy for the bored or somnolent psychiatrist to pick out the part that interests him and to elaborate it into a conviction that the patient has told him something in particular. When he subsequently refers to this alleged communication, the patient may flatly contradict him. On the other hand, the patient may hasten to agree, but again embark on a course of qualifications which terminates the situation in a verbal fog.

"Agreement" is often a device for maintaining the illusion of one's omniscience. Patients suffering the substitutive disorders are often most ingenious at preventing the accurate formulation of the events which made up a situation. If, despite all the patient's efforts—parataxic interpretation, qualification, specious generalizations, and erroneous placing of events in time—the physician comes to grasp the actual facts and expresses them, one of a few processes is apt to follow. The patient may say, in essence, "Yes; but—." The proposition is then befogged. The patient, after a pause, may say, "Yes; that is quite true." The proposition then vanishes from active attention; the patient has asserted an omniscient control over the facts, which renders them unimportant. Or the patient may ask aid in understanding the implications, or ask some more or less relevant questions, and so lose the proposition in the pursuit of some details. It then appears that he has misunderstood the physician in all essential respects, and one is back where one started.

Even when a consensus is achieved in an interview, it may be short-lived. The factors which entered into it need not survive the interpersonal situation of its occurrence. Something apparently fatally contradictory to it may occur to the patient as soon as he has left the physician's company. Moreover, a disintegrating process may put in appearance near the close of the interview itself. There are some patients, for example, who show a marked change of attitude as they rise to go, and ask as if from a different position "Have we accomplished anything, today, Doctor?" This is a movement by virtue of which the significance of the interview is minimized and only the physician's opinion about it is given any importance. If this movement is not countered, the patient represses anything significant from the interview into a sort of dream-like vagueness, such that it is none of his business. This shift of attitude at the end of the interview is particularly conducive of the more autistic sorts of performances. The patient 'produces' a stream of unintelligible and uncommunicative revery processes, from which the physician is by some kind of a miracle supposed to achieve the patient's 'cure.'

Somewhat related to this interpersonally meaningless production is the patient's preoccupation with what one *ought* to do. A great deal of time and effort is wasted in discussion of will-power, choice, and decision. These three terms which refer to products of acculturation in the home, endure and are functionally very important because they are potent terms of rationalization in our culture. They are, in fact, embodied in various institutions of law and religion; and all too often are powerful factors in the work of the psychiatrist, himself.

The psychoanalyst, for example, may instruct his patient to say instantly every littlest thing that comes into his mind. The patient then charges off in autistic revery which gets nowhere, therapeutically. The analyst, if he is not entertained by parallel autisms, may interpret this as "narcissistic self-gratification" on the part of the patient. The patient may counter with the statement that he was told to say what comes to his mind and that is all he can do. There is no doubt that patients and others often have fun with their thoughts—and sometimes with gullible companions. The point is not this fact in itself. It is that there may be nothing else which could happen in the given situation. In any case, there is nothing else as powerfully motivated as that which is happening. The reason for this lies in the situation, not in the perversity of the patient, or his 'narcissism.' The physician, the patient, and the parataxic concomitants make up the situation. The punishing type of interpretation may obviate any necessity for the physician's seeing wherein the 'self-gratification' is the action which suits the integration. The situation is not necessarily integrated to the achievement of a therapeutic goal, and the physician, because of his relative freedom from personal handicap, is the one who can do most towards altering the integration in a desirable fashion. This is one of the more important uses of interpretation; in the case in point, the interpretation may be merely a statement to the effect that the physician does not see any connection between the expressed stream of thought and the current interpersonal situation.

All therapeutic conferences are made up of various patterns of some five types of process. There are processes which illuminate the immediate interpersonal relationship. These include the revelation of parataxic or "transference" phenomena. There are processes which clarify the action in some recent interpersonal situation, perhaps one in a relatively durable relationship with some person often discussed in the interviews. There are processes which revert from present and current situations to relevant situations in the patient's more remote past. There are processes which represent the pursuit into the future of aspects of current situations, by way of constructive revery. And there are processes called out by various crisis situations, in or outside of the therapeutic situation, many of which amount to acute maladjustive movements—one group of which is a preoccupation with current events of but trifling relevancy.

The patient's struggles to do the right thing, to overcome certain tendencies, or to stop certain manifest actions are all to be placed in the first and last categories of these processes. They are either parataxic adaptations to the psychiatrist as a moral censor, or preoccupations to avoid anxiety or conflict. I know of no evidence of a force or power that may be called a *will*, in contradistinction to the vector addition of integrating tendencies. Situations call out motivation; if there is conflict of motivation outside of awareness, a compromise or a temporary domination of behavior and suppression of the weaker motive occurs. If the conflict is within awareness, the self system is involved, with the corresponding element of insecurity. In these cases, more complex products result, but these too are vector additions, not interventions of some sort of personal will-power.

Decision, about which many patients have much trouble—their indecisiveness—is intimately connected with the illusion of choice, in turn entangled with dogmatic assertions of "freedom of the will," and of one's ability to choose between good and evil. Let me first settle the question of dogma, which is in this case both religious and legal. Dogmatic statements are necessary ingredients of any system of thought which cannot be deduced from generally demonstrable events. When I say that a burned child avoids the fire, I do not deny the possibility of some complex exceptions, but I do assert the prevalence of a type of behavior that could be inferred from almost any one's experience with being burned. When I assert that evil is any unwarranted interference with life, on the other hand, I am offering a complex formula that has arisen from my unique career among others. I do not know how to state a generally useful rule for assessing the warranty for particular interferences with, say, another person's life or living.

It will be a long time indeed before any group of people shall have come to a fully rational way of life, and in the meanwhile, man must have normative rules to govern his behavior with others, especially in the fields most modified by culture. Dependent on the particular course of culture evolution, these rules may carry social or transcendental sanction, or a blend of the two. This is of but indirect concern to the psychiatrist. He is concerned when the rules and the underlying and supporting culture-complex are so incongruent and so peculiarly contradictory that they give rise in some people at least to states of mental disorder—and probably in everyone to some measure of insecurity. As the rules of religious systems are relatively static, tend to be highly resistant of change; and as those of legal systems are susceptible to episodic modification only, these two fields of normative prescription are the least apt to keep closely in step with the developing culture-complex.

In the Western culture, into the second decade of this century, there was no devastating divergence of the religious rules from the main trends of the culture-complex. With the short-lived emergence of the Communist idealism and the still-spreading reversion to Totalitarianism as a doctrine of the state, the practical solidarity of the Western culture was destroyed.[65] There are now many significant differences in the culture-patterns which are impressed on children in home and school, and through the channels of mediate acculturation. A great deal that was unquestionable has now become controversial, if not obsolete. Whereas once one 'belonged' or was an outcast, the question now is rather *where* one belongs than *does* one. Each party, group, and clique has its own normative rules, its own orthodox attitude to the religious and even the legal systems. The differences in these respects between the most extreme groups are greater than any differences of belief that have previously influenced the peoples of the world. The ideologies (dogmata) that find devout believers even among our own people are strange indeed to survivors of a time when one's "conscience" could be one's guide.

Decision and choice are functions of memory and prospective revery—which often eventuates in foresight. They are, however, interpersonal processes; they do not occur in the vacuum of an isolated individuality, and they correspondingly

[65] I must not digress to contemplate the historic currents that prepared the way for these changes, nor shall I defend the statement that these two of a complex pattern of events are the most significant. In the first place, persons immersed in rapid culture change can seldom make valid judgments as to the relative significance of presenting signs and symptoms; in the second, I am not competent to discuss the economic factors which are doubtless of great importance. I will say that economics has developed with singularly little interest in the persons who manifest economic behavior, and economists do not interest themselves particularly in the personal effects of economic factors. I wish that the latter, at least, might not continue indefinitely to be the case, for economic factors cannot but be important elements in personal as well as in social security.

include the function of the self system. To that extent, they are influenced by all the factors involved in the pursuit of security or its maintenance. They may be, and often are, symptomatic of mental disorder and signatory of overcomplicated interpersonal situations. When they happen to be the decisions of a person who has come to subscribe to an ideology foreign to the culture-pattern of his childhood, they may be complex indeed. The person who believes that he *voluntarily* cut loose from his earlier moorings and *by choice* accepted new dogmata, in which he has diligently indoctrinated himself, is quite certain to be a person who has suffered great insecurity. He is often a person whose self-organization is derogatory and hateful. The new movement has given him group support for the expression of ancient personal hostilities that are now directed against the group from which he has come. The new ideology rationalizes destructive activity to such effect that it seems almost, if not quite, constructive. The new ideology is especially palliative of conflict in its promise of a better world that is to rise from the debris to which the present order must first be reduced. In this Utopia, he and his fellows will be good and kind—for there will be no more injustice, and so forth. If his is one of the more radical groups, the activity of more remote memory in the synthesis of decisions and choice may be suppressed almost completely, and the activity of prospective revery channelled rigidly in the dogmatic pattern. In this case, except for his dealings with his fellow radicals, the man may act as if he had acquired the psychopathic type of personality discussed in the third lecture. He shows no durable grasp of his own reality or that of others, and his actions are controlled by the most immediate opportunism, without consideration of the probable future.

The apparent psychopathy of persons entertaining more radical views arises chiefly from the institutionalization of their feelings of difference. If one is alone in this feeling, a paranoid state or a schizophrenic development is apt to ensue.

If, however, one finds not only a fellow, but a group who have a however feeble rationalization for active hostility to the 'in-group,' one is spared the more serious disorders. This comes about in part unwittingly by virtue of the group solidarity, and in part because of peculiarities in the verbal interchange in all militant minority groups. The more autistic thoughts of each person in such a none too secure group are rejected or modified by the others, while the more or less credible transfers of blame are elaborated into workable expressions of hostility and destructiveness. The group approaches a paranoid attitude to everyone outside it, but saves its members from deep regression under pressure of conflict. The aspects of the member's self which once might have conflicted with the destructive motivation are disintegrated by the revaluation of his past experience, or suppressed by the group norms. It is chiefly for these reasons that his dealings with people not of the group are so like those of a psychopathic personality.

The position of the person who *perforce* subscribes to an ideology foreign to his past is rather more simple, but by no means so comfortable. He is in essence a stranger in a strange land, but one who is surrounded by powerful people, not by infra-human creatures. The net result is that he has to take on a rôle of cautious subservience, and to live in a state of constant but obviously externally-conditioned insecurity. If his personality is one that permits the suppression of hostile impulses, all may go fairly well. If, however, he be of the incorrigible type, it is probable that some incompetent in the ruling clique will arrange his 'liquidation.' [66]

[66] Of more current interest to the American psychiatrist is the place of the *liberal*, the person who is not blind to the unsatisfactory state of things as they are, but who is not sufficiently disturbed in his interpersonal relations to yearn for a radical Utopian solution either on the far side of chaos *or* to be achieved by reversing the current of social evolution and regressing to the "good old days"—the equally morbid wish of the *reactionary* "conservative." The rational, liberal position exposes one to extreme vicissitudes of security from attacks by both the reactionaries and the radicals in our technically democratic society—some outstanding characteristics of which pertain less to the achieve-

Choice and decision are the products within awareness of the vector addition of motives called out by a situation, plus the constructive revery processes pertaining to them. The constructive revery, if its end stages are clearly within awareness, is said to constitute foresight. In many people, on many occasions, there is no clear foresight but rather a consciousness of determination that seems to be a thing in itself, a manifestation of the 'will.' These are simply cases in which the self system intervenes to suppress awareness of the forward-looking revery processes. Their unnoted presence is often indicated by disquiet experienced after the 'determined' action is started. This is a variety of anxiety; the foresight still tends to occur, and the self system is restricting awareness in the usual fashion.

A grasp on these processes is fundamental to the durable benefit of many patients. I shall, therefore, go to some trouble to illustrate what I mean. Let me take, as an illustration, the occasion of the lecture on explanatory conceptions, which was perhaps most unduly prolonged. This has a history. The topics of the individual lectures of the series were established some six months ago. The plan comtemplated an hour for each of the five topics. There seeming to be no possibility of foreseeing the real composition of the audience, I drafted the outline for the first lecture with an audience of psychiatrists and social scientists in mind. The audience as encountered included a signifi-

---

ment of human dignity, opportunity, and fraternity than to the safeguarding of special privilege at whatever cost to others.

I have no hesitancy in expressing these views for I am clearly of the privileged class, as are all of my intimate friends. I feel radical as to certain of the underprivileged, who would seem to have potentialities far greater than their socially-defined rôle permits them to manifest. I feel most reserved as to reactionary and radical groups—in part because I know intimately some of their leaders. I do not believe that the destruction of values is a necessary or even probable preliminary to their renaissance, and I know regression, professionally. I feel particularly hostile to all those among us who are incapable of appreciating our traditional almost accidental way of progress, who prefer instead to place confidence in the omniscience of a dictator. I do not believe that any one nurtured in the American culture-complex *can* have such sublime trust in another; I regard Totalitarianism as the political quintessence of personal despair.

cant proportion of people who belonged in neither category. The presentation would have to follow rather different lines of development than had been planned, *if* this series of lectures was to be of value to many of those who made up the audience. The change was foreseen to entail more than five hours for achieving any approximation to the initial purpose. The principal consideration encountered in my prospective revery seeming to be the very question of the scope of the psychiatric field—discussed at the start of the first lecture—to the broader definition of which I hold, my 'decision' was in favor of maximum usefulness to the audience as found rather than as anticipated.[67] The presentation of the first session was within the time as planned; each subsequent lecture—as the audience continued to be most encouragingly numerous—was more extended. The one which would require more than two hours, however, occasioned me some thought. I considered first the physical discomfort that each auditor might experience. How hard were the seats? Having never sat on one of them, I could only surmise that they might be unusually comfortable, in keeping with many other details of the auditorium. There then came the question of the durability of the auditors' attention. What motivation brought them? Noting that the occasion was an evening in a holiday week-end, I could assume that those who attended had a sufficiency of interest; could their attention-span extend over two hours? I had on one occasion approached a test of that very point, with a purely psychiatric audience. A 110-minute talk had succeeded. Psychiatrists were certainly no more apt to be interested in my views as to the relationship of clinical practice to psychiatric research; than the members of this audience, in my outlining explanatory

[67] It was also realized that the lectures as delivered would not approximate to written language; that the transcript would need revision before publication, in the course of which, adjustment for an even more varied audience would be desirable. I regret now that my judgment in this particular was not adhered to more rigidly, for the first two of these lectures are much too close to the transcript; the others have been entirely rewritten.

psychiatric conceptions. I foresaw then that a considerable part of the audience would stay to the end; I did not foresee how great a part would remain—after the opportunity for escape which I provided by way of a recess.

This inadequacy of foresight is a good example of the variations in constructive revery. My attitude towards interpersonal relations is rather pessimistic; a measure of personal success is, therefore, more frequent than is its anticipation. The attitude was fixed in the early years, not so much by a series of failures as by the continuing danger to my security which a failure due to over-optimism would have entailed.

Foresight is the product of constructive revery which often proceeds with great speed, so that one discards several possible courses of action as improbable of success, in a moment. The tracing through in this swift prevision of alternative courses of action of a way that will probably work results in an awareness of decision to follow that course.

The utility of the foresight must depend on the adequacy of one's insight into oneself and into the situation. To the extent that one's personal formulation includes complex abstractions, rationalizations—will-power, for example—foresight is misleading and one's 'decisions' are apt to get one into false positions and states of insecurity with others. To the extent that one is preoccupied with those power operations which are so striking in the substitutive states, one's foresight is useless, for insight in any given interpersonal situation is vestigial. One foresees trains of events in which all the people concerned are parataxic illusions, including the mighty magician, oneself. To the extent that powerful systems of motives exist in dissociation, foresight must be defective. In situations, multiply integrated by recognized and by dissociated impulses, there has to be a specific defect of insight, a so-called *scotoma* for the factors representative of the dissociated motives, although, as already indicated, prospective revery may still be efficient.

The effective, but unnoted revery processes that accompany many instances of inadequate foresight may be represented in awareness by a whole series of symptoms: dread, unreasonable doubt and 'indecision,' anxious 'uncertainty,' anxious 'certainty,' and perplexity. One may experience an apprehensive state on plunging into an action that will miscarry in the service of a powerful dissociated impulse; the 'decision' on which this action is based usually having been an emotional 'determination,' or else a blind impulse rising out of a painful state of 'blankness' of mind. When the self has not been quite so effective, the patient may express his discomfort by some such remark as "I am going to do so and so, but I dread it—or dread the consequences." The next step in the series is the one at which there is a 'decision,' but, no sooner is it reached, with all the trappings of foresight in the sense of clear probability of success, than there appear serious doubts as to the items in the chain of prospective revery. Again, the patient, seemingly clear on what to do, cannot begin. This may be because other revery processes reflect unfortunate possibilities—or sometimes present alternative, equally probable but significantly different courses of action. The patient may be uncertain, entertaining several courses of action with no index of relative probability of success, and with or without anxiety dependent on the degree of involvement of the self system and on the risk of becoming aware of something. Finally, there may be an equivalent in the field of foresight to the state of conflict. In fact, perplexity as to action often ushers in frank conflict. It implies an approximate balance of opposing motivation.

Clear as to the dynamic rôle of the self system, as to the power operations and the rationalizations by which insecurity is minimized, and as to the true rôle of constructive revery and foresight in determining action in a given situation, the psychiatrist is well equipped to project therapeutic action. He is clear as to the futility, often actual harmfulness, of requiring the patient to 'exercise self-control.' He knows that the 'controlled' adjustment of behavior to interpersonal demands can only arise from insight, from an expanded self which will include currently dissociated impulses, and information about situations towards which the patient must now be manifesting scotomata. He knows that 'self-control' is but one of a large number of alleged acts and abilities which a person cannot perform or manifest—except in the private theatre of his reveries—be he ever so firmly convinced of their possibility and desirability.

Just what can the psychiatrist reasonably expect the patient to do? In my opinion there are three groups of performances that are within human ability, although most people have to learn to do them well. The first is the *noticing of changes in one's body*—voice changes, molar movements, and increases and decreases of tension. Alertness in this field is necessary if the patient is to discover the unrecognized components of behavior, including the wholly unnoticed actions in the service of dissociated impulses. This is much more useful than is the learning of alertness for minor degrees of anxiety, because many patients experience but little anxiety. They are prompt and skillful in avoiding disturbing factors. They none the less undergo marked shifts in bodily tension, these being either themselves avoidance processes or occurring in lieu of anxiety at the start of the avoidance process. If these patients are not specifically interested in noting changes in somatic tension and movements, there will be very slow growth of insight. We hope that the patient will presently become alert not only to increases of tension—generically insecurity—but to its diminutions. These latter may mark the achievement of a new insight; but much more often indicate the miscarriage of a difficult constructive effort, of the occasion of which, otherwise, the patient may have no warning whatever.

The second collaborative effort for which the psychiatrist may reasonably ask is the *noticing of marginal thoughts*. This is an inadequate verbal reference to something in which everyone has some little experience. As, for example, I am now 'listening to myself talk,' somewhat the following is in progress. I am forming sentences, always at least a clause ahead of my speech. This is dominated by reference to an illusory auditor whom I shall call I_1—he is a rather unfriendly critic not very quick to understand—a particular aspect of my self. Mere talking organism and critic I_1 see to matters of formulation, vocabulary, grammar, rhetoric, and elocution. I am also hearing what is said, as it is spoken. This is dominated by reference to an illusory auditor whom I shall call I_2, a rather intelligent creature quick to see errors and incompleteness of exposition and some of the possibilities of misunderstanding. Insofar as it is true, it is my good fortune that I_2 really dominates the situation; requires reformulation and more lucid repetition, illustration, and the like. I say this because I_1 is, as it were, that which is going on in the center of awareness, while I_2 is only marginal, the fringe of awareness. If I were not rather secure in my ability to function with I_1, if I were "nervous" about my 'speech' or my speaking, most of the I_2 phenomena would receive no attention. I might now and then get a disagreeable surprise at the unconvincing sound of something that I had thought was quite clear; this awareness of an I_2 process would, however, have to be suppressed lest I be made too insecure to continue. Or, without becoming clearly aware of the 'weak' statements, I might then 'hem and haw,' or lose my place, and my viscera suffer increase of tension, if in fact some of my skeletal muscles did not tremble.

While my marginal processes of consensual validation aid in delivery of the lecture, in an insecure speaker they may seem to be a serious handicap. It must be obvious that this effect does not inhere in the consensual validation but in the insecurity and in the confusing efforts to suppress the I_2 processes. Let me now give another example of the same general situation. Let us suppose that the speaker is entirely oblivious to everything but the reading and uttering of a prepared speech, or the delivery of a memorized oration. Be he ever so unintelligible or utterly fatuous to his real audience, little will seem to have occurred in him except fatigue from the effort. His self system has obviated any feelings of insecurity by the simple expedient of complete preoccupation with the focal activity. Everything related to I_2 is transmuted into visceral tensions, outside of awareness. I believe these examples may have made clear the utility of the marginal processes. They may also have suggested the circumstances under which these marginal processes are in large part suppressed, and those under which there seem to be no marginal processes but only changes in bodily tension.

In practice, the patient often becomes intent on telling something to the psychiatrist. Either the account proceeds with difficulty, due to disturbing marginal processes, or it goes on with increasing smoothness, due to the security that comes from their complete exclusion. In either case, not the accounts but the marginal processes are the more useful for the growth of insight. This follows from the nature of the self system. To the extent that there is no disturbance of the self, to that extent nothing new is being learned by the patient about his living. We strive to teach the patient that the marginal processes, the interrupting thoughts, as it were, are very much the thing to be noticed.

The third possibility of collaboration is the *prompt statement of all that comes to mind*. The patient must learn to trust the situation to the extent of expressing the thoughts that it provokes. This is often a very difficult achievement, until insight into at least one of the parataxic processes has been achieved. After that, there are many recurrences of difficulty, but they are not very serious. Before this first great milestone of progress, however, the patient's 'mind' seems to be terribly troublesome. Waves of obscenities may flow in. Distressing recollections of most regrettable past performances may occur. Offensive thoughts about the psychiatrist may obsess the patient. False reports may press for utterance. Almost anything that is difficult to say, or any ideas that seem impossible to express, may be expected. It is for this reason that patients seek relief from the turmoil in a flow of autistic revery, a circumstantial account of some insignificant current event, or an extravagant report of the marvelous good results that have already, entirely mysteriously, been achieved by exposure to the psychiatrist.

The particular difficulties that stand in the way of achieving any and all of these three forms of collaboration are determined by the developmental patterning of the patient. The non-integrative or psychopathic person seldom seeks to enter a therapeutic relationship, and can scarcely achieve a beginning of any collaborative effort. The self-absorbed patient quickly makes an indoor sport of changes of tension, of marginal thoughts, and of astonishing communications. The pressure towards mental health is not lacking, but its manifestations have to be sought among the lush dramatics of hysteriod phenomena. One of these patients would go from my office to the home of another patient, long acquainted with her, and gush forth lurid accounts of the past, recollection of which had been provoked in our rather useless interview, concluding with the statement that I would give anything if she would only tell me about it. These patients make gratifying subjects for any spectacular form of treatment, although the effect on their difficulties in living seems usually to be a change of form rather than remedy. They 'just love' interpretations and can assimilate any number of them to the structure of their particular syndrome of mental disorder.

The therapy of mental disorders affecting incorrigible people is rough going. It is feasible only if one always knows what one is doing. The effort required in extreme instances, however, is not ordinarily available.[68]

The patient of negativistic developmental pattern presents no insuperable difficulties in the learning of collaboration. The

[68] See, for example, Aichhorn, August. *Wayward Youth;* New York, Viking, 1935 (xiii and 236 pp.).

more troublesome aspect of treating their mental disorders appears in connection with the use of interpretations. The negativistic patient resists all interpretations and often shows great ingenuity in delaying the occurrence of insight. This difficulty is mostly an initial handicap, however, and once past the first milestone of insight into a parataxic process, the resistance to interpretations passes gradually into a careful validating process that is useful.

At this point, I may well discuss the question of these initial insights which I regard as of fundamental significance in changing an allegedly therapeutic situation from a highly tentative and risky integration into a firm and reliable collaboration. I shall illustrate such an event by referring to a patient who consulted me because, she said, she had to divorce her husband. As people who are decided on securing a divorce have more need for an attorney than a psychiatrist, I inquired as to her expectation from consulting me. I found that she was well-acquainted with psychiatry, that, in fact, she had been under treatment for some time when she was in the throes of indecision about marrying this man. I then sought to discover the necessities calling for a divorce, and, to my growing astonishment, learned more and more of the husband's perfections. The only formula of the need for a divorce seemed to be a feeling that he interfered with the patient's self-realization. Wherein this interference was manifest, I could not elicit. This seemed to present a psychiatric problem, and I undertook to aid in discovering the facts underlying the situation.

In some three hundred interviews, I learned a great deal, but I could never be certain of the precise relationship of the information to what would have been observed by an ideally objective participant in the patient's career. In other words, no certainty had been achieved. A great deal was consistent and possible; it could all be complex misinterpretation and falsification. As an example, very early in our work I was told that the patient was puzzled because she had always heard that mental disorders arose from an unhappy childhood, whereas hers had been extraordinarily free from unpleasant incidents. There was much documenting of this early happiness, and the ultimate revelation that the patient's real childhood had been swamped in amnesia. As it finally came forth, it was appalling. The 'childhood' of which she had ready and elaborate recall was a serial story with which she had compensated herself in a desolately unsatisfactory home.

About the three hundredth hour, the patient came in with me from the waiting room in a peculiar state of agitation. She said that she was overwhelmed to discover that I looked quite different than she had hitherto seen me. She had known me as a fat old man with white hair. Disregarding the other characteristics, I can scarcely have had white hair. This is both an extreme and deceptively simple illustration of a parataxic distortion of the psychiatrist in the treatment situation. Gross illusions of physical attributes are not very common, and, needless to say, the fat old white-haired man was derived from a figure in the patient's past, and had been manifesting this other person's significant attributes, despite my efforts to avoid misinterpretations and to detect parataxic concomitants—at which I had been remarkably unsuccessful. When our grandfatherly figure had been located in his place in the patient's career; and when we had seen something of his rôle in the patient's development, as indicated in the now-accessible discrepancies between my performances and her misconceptions about them; the therapeutic situation then lost its tentative quality and became productive of durable results.

Until a patient has seen clearly and unmistakably a concrete example of the way in which unresolved situations from the distant past color the perception of present situations and overcomplicate action in them, there can be no material reorganization of personality, no therapeutically satisfactory expansion of the self, no significant insight into the complexities of one's performances or into the unexpected and often disconcerting behavior of others concerned. Up to this point, there is nothing significantly unique in the treatment situation; afterwards, however, the integration with the psychiatrist becomes a situation of unprecedented freedom from restraints on the manifestation of constructive impulses. This is the indirect result of the changes in the self system. The patient has finally learnt that more security may ensue from *abandoning* a complex security-seeking process than was ever achieved *by it*. This information is in itself an addition to security and a warrant for confronting other anxiety-provoking situations to discover the factors in them which are being experienced as a threat. The psychiatrist's reiterated statement as to the way by which one gains mental health now takes on something of the meaning which he has striven to communicate. The patient is beginning to understand what is sought, and its virtue. Up to now, the patient has been literally in Groddeck's words "lived by unknown and uncontrollable forces," however elaborately this fact was concealed from awareness.

Experience has taught me that it is useful to have clear and succinct statements with which to reply to the more general questions that are always, sooner or later, and again and again, asked by the patient. One may add new details to support the central formula, but it is unwise to vary from the central thought. This comes about because of the shifting relationship of perception to the underlying reality that is being perceived, due to parataxic concomitants representing activity of the self system. At best, we are none too certainly prompt in seizing even the more accessible meaning of a remark. When the remark pertains to some aspect of our living, our relations with others, even if there were nothing to conflict with any of its implications, the very act of perceiving it would have to include much related experience in the past, about which some contradictions and some definite misinformation may well be accessible to awareness. In the early phases of a treatment situation, many factors in the self conflict with the implications of any correct statement about the processes that are manifest in the mental disorder. Still more factors, practically the whole self system, conflict with *some* implications of a statement as to how the treatment situation is to do good.

One achieves mental health to the extent that one becomes aware of one's interpersonal relations; this is the general statement that is always expressed to the patient. Every one of my patients with whom I have had more than a consultative relationship has received this reply to many different questions, asked throughout the greater part of the work. This is the essential element in replying to the questions, "What ails me?," "How can I get better?," "What good will the treatment accomplish?," "Why can't I overcome this or that habit?," "What shall I do about my hatefulness—my hostility—my ugly disposition—my dependency—my domineering—my sensitivity—my suspiciousness—my uncertainty?" It is part of the framework that supports all explanations of what is going on, what might be going on, and what will presently be going on. It is one of the factual bases for interpreting unfortunate developments, unfavorable changes that are discouraging the patient. It is *the* necessary formula to which everything must be assimilable, if it is therapy.

This statement of the nature of curative change is for a long time a source of insecurity, and thus of anxiety or uncomfortable tension. It is prehended as an attack on the very core of the patient's personality. It denies the ultimate usefulness of the suppressive, the repressive, and the dissociating functions of the self system. For a long time, therefore, it is not understood in recognizable form. If the patient could seize even the most superficial of its implications, he would take it to mean that one could not make any progress without abandoning the hope of feeling secure in dealing with others. Even if one could exercise choice, one could not accept such a prospect. It would have to appear as the relinquishment of what little capability and comfort one had been able to maintain; as a grim preliminary to an incomprehensible next state. This might seem ever so desirable to the psychiatrist, but he is still a stranger of indefinite attitude to the patient.

Patients ask questions for various reasons; that is, as modes of behavior to resolve various aspects of the therapeutic situation. The physician is guided in his response by two considerations: the long-range probabilities about the situation, and the immediate phase of the treatment. The goal of the treatment, including the ultimate complete resolution of the patient-physician relationship, dictates the gradual evolution of valid insight. This calls out the succinct statements above mentioned. The momentary present state of what may be an extremely complex parataxic situation, on the other hand, can call for a great variety of actions. In general, if anything is to be said in reply to a question, both of these considerations should be subserved by it. In no case may the long-term aspect be ignored; if one relinquishes this orientation neither the physician nor the patient can long know what is going on.

I can now outline the more typical peculiarities that one encounters in treating the ambition-ridden sort of patient. I have spoken of patients' learning the three forms of collaboration. In the second lecture, I reserved the possibility of collaboration to persons who had entered or passed through preadolescence. Both of these views are relevant. The processes of psychiatric cure include the maturation of personality; that is, the evolution of capacity for adult interpersonal relations. Where the barriers to this achievement are practically insurmountable, or where other factors preclude the necessary procedures, the goal of cure is not to be sought, but only that of amelioration. I shall have more to offer in this connection, presently.

The ambition-ridden person comes to the psychiatrist to get what he can in the way of aid in his career. He may be willing to pay for this. He may be most determined in his efforts to achieve it. But he lives in a world of competitive violence and necessary compromise, and he will have none of the psychiatrist's skepticism about the finality of this formula. He cannot escape the competitive attitude, even in this regard, and all too frequently by dint of competing with the physician at every step, reduces the potentially therapeutic situation to a struggle about who is doctor and who is patient. If the psychiatrist remains detached in his attitude towards the incessant demands for recognition, the patient's insecurity is apt to disrupt the situation. The problem is chiefly one of following a course between a fraudulent acceptance of the juvenile motivation as satisfactory—in which case, the situation will proceed into a parataxic representation of an extremely important early situation *but* the psychiatrist will be too involved to assist in its clarification—and an emphatic insistence that even the patient's most satisfactory interpersonal relations are inadequate. Given the necessary interest, and tact and patience, one may come gradually to progress with one of these patients to a more mature relationship, whereupon the before-mentioned first milestone of progress can be reached, and the goal of cure posited. The long preliminaries are often interrupted before this achievement, often, I surmise, for the convenience of the physician.

Treatment situations integrated with patients of asocial development are chiefly characterized by the subtlety of distortion in the communicative processes. The structure of the self system of an asocial person is in one sense extraordinarily simple. Each tendency in this relatively simple organization extends, however, through innumerable nuances of experience back to childhood discouragement and to the sequential development of *detachment* from what I shall call representative participation with others. By this I mean that these patients even as children came to realize that their prehended reality was quite different from the illusions of them that the parents persistently entertained. The self of the asocial person is in this sense extraordinarily complex, for it is evolved on a duplex pattern of what *is* and what is expected. It is apt to be quite successful in avoiding insecurity, for the motivation manifested in any integration can shift from that relevant to the integration as perceived by the patient to that relevant to the prehended illusions of the others concerned. While we all show some ability in this regard, for more or less parallel reasons, the asocial person manifests it as a major characteristic, and often with relatively little parataxic distortion.

This does not mean that the asocial person always gracefully falls in with the other person's parataxes. He may have disintegrated most of his past interpersonal relations with anger and contemptuous disappointment. He may have left them with an increasing burden of inferiority as to his unsuitability to be a friend. He may come to the physician because he is intolerably lonely in an apparently close relationship which has endured for years. However all this may be, he will—if at least preadolescent—come fairly soon to learn the first two of my forms of collaboration, and will seem for the most part to have caught on to the third. Therapeutic processes will proceed rather smoothly for some time, but obscure difficulties will be encountered. Moreover, the patient will quite certainly become involved in powerfully-motivated integrations with one after another person outside of the treatment situation. Much that would be relevant in the treatment situation will then be discharged in these accessory situations.

In brief, these patients for a long time cannot entertain a durable conviction that the physician is what he purports to be. He cannot be so interested in the patient; he will 'let the patient down,' come to dislike or despise him. The patient protects himself with a parallel appraisal of the physician: he is not much good, he is of little importance to the patient, he is actually a rather shabby person who does psychiatry because he can't do anything else, the whole thing is probably a fraud, it is best to have somebody else to fall back on, and to help one keep one's skeptical perspective in the stress of the treatment situation. And none of this somewhat changing but essentially invariant content gets itself expressed by other than the most subtle indications. When it has finally come to its first clear expression, the treatment situation improves, but continues to be handicapped by the patient's feeling of remoteness and unlovability, convictions that will persist far past the first milestone as major problems of the treatment.

The inadequate person as a patient presents the great risk of developing a new phase of the self system in subordination to the physician. This device is a great handicap to treatment, for it cushions any attempts to reach the underlying frustration and humiliation, the dissociation of tendencies related to which is the principal factor in the maladjustment. These patients are for some time a boon to any domineering physician. They come usually to be rather like the albatross around the neck of the Ancient Mariner.

Of the treatment problems connected with handling patients of the homosexual developmental type, few require any special consideration. These people may be sufficiently evolved towards adulthood to enter readily into the therapeutic collaboration, in which case the physician's major problem is that of keeping the long-term goal always in sight. This goal must be the dissolving of the patient's barrier to full intimacy with persons of the other sex. The prevalent error is an effort to treat "homosexuality" as a problem in itself. This sometimes at least reflects the special interest of the therapist; it is always interesting, even if deeply disturbing, to the patient. As the homosexuality is an adaptive attitude in partial remedy of the real disorder, its successful 'treatment' in advance of remedy of the real problem could only precipitate a more grave maladjustment.

The special problems of treating the chronically adolescent are not very different from those just mentioned, and the greatest risk is of the same character; namely, the treating of an adjustive device as if it were the disorder, instead of attacking the underlying barrier to full interpersonal intimacy. Here, too, there is more than a possibility of impairing what mental health the patient brought to the treatment. With this, I shall leave the topic of special problems associated with the developmental syndromes and proceed to the question of general risks entailed in psychiatric treatment.

We have, thus far, discussed intensive and prolonged psychiatric treatment, the sort most often engaged in by physicians trained in the psychoanalytic technique. This constitutes but a small part of the work done by psychiatrists in an effort to benefit patients. I have presented it in some detail because it is the most revealing form of psychiatric treatment, both as to the actual possibilities of beneficial intervention, and as to the fortunate and unfortunate events that make up the cure, amelioration, or aggravation of mental disorder. There is a good deal of misinformation current in non-analytic psychiatric circles in this connection, and, as I see it, very little reliable information in the hands of the laity. This is in both cases the more regrettable because it shields the worst in alleged psychoanalytic practice from the valid criticism which it so richly deserves.[69] It also interferes with that reasonable con-

[69] It is perhaps even more regrettable because of its effects on the training of candidates to become psychoanalytic psychiatrists. The prerequisite psychiatric training is imperative. Undergoing a personal analysis is obviously necessary. Subsequent work under supervision is unquestionably wise. Didactic training in theory and seminar study of practical problems is excellent. But every step in education is in large measure a matter of interpersonal relations: the training psychiatrists and what the candidates learn from them; the 'training' analyst and what he cures, ameliorates, aggravates, and systematizes—which is what the candidate learns from him; and the supervising analysts and their particular interests and competence to remedy and refine what comes to them; all these and the lecturers and seminary leaders are people, in some parts people whose interpersonal relations are in measure decidedly immature and maladjusted. This could not but be the case, considering the recency of Freud's discoveries and their limited favorable reception. Were it not for a particular aspect of the situation, this need not distress us, as progressive improvement would occur automatically. The necessary remoteness of much of the practical performances from any competent criticism *is* troublesome. The possibility—all too often demonstrated fact—of continuing extraordinary influence over the performances of one's trainee, itself an evidence either of incompetent

sideration of probabilities to the advancement of which Dr. White devoted so much of his energy.

One hears again and again of the evils done by psychoanalysis and of the dangers attendant upon its use in this or that condition, notably in the case of those apt to undergo a schizophrenic episode. In psychoanalytic circles, one hears of subpsychotic, frankly dangerously disturbed periods in the course of the presumably adequate treatment of some patients. Some psychoanalysts seem to take this as a matter of necessary course. Plausible formulae are available to rationalize it, nay, even to rationalize the occasional suicide of a training or supervising psychoanalyst. A certain distrust of psychoanalytic practitioners, if not of psychoanalysis itself, comes thus to be quite understandable.

In psychiatric consulting practice one participates in many different kinds of interpersonal relations, to the end of recommending some course of action that will benefit the patient concerned. Among these situations is that of the young medical man, perhaps already somewhat trained in psychiatry, who seeks aid in furtherance of his training. He asks, for example, if psychoanalytic training, or a personal analysis at least, is an indispensable part of the technical equipment that he will need in order to be competent in practice. It would be easy to reply in the affirmative to this question. I cannot but recall, however, the case of a young man of extraordinary gifts to whom I gave an affirmative answer, some twenty years ago. I did not then know that this was but the beginning of discharge of my responsibility. He asked me whom I would recommend as a training analyst. We discussed several. He subsequently acted on some other advice and went to work with a psychoanalyst not of my personal acquaintance. After about eight-

therapy or of grossly unhygienic design, or both, coupled with manifestation of the prevalent ambition-ridden type of development in the person of the training analyst; this situation calls for more interest in psychoanalytic training institutions and the training of particular analysts than the general psychiatrist or the interested layman is now competent to show.

een months had passed, we met again, following the interruption of his analysis. He showed evidences of a transient paranoid state and a rather violent antagonism to psychoanalysis, root and branch. His career, so far as I can judge, has realized but a small part of his original promise. This story has been repeated, in my experience, on several occasions—with adoption of "psychoanalysis" as an important part of the paranoid systematization, which was *not* transient.

I learned finally that the necessity of psychoanalytic training for full psychiatric competence is not a technical but an intensely personal matter. The consultant on this problem is concerned with making a survey of the candidate's interpersonal relations, their successes and failures, and with formulating the probable outcome of treatment of the presenting disorders in terms of practically available facilities *and* personnel. He has discharged his responsibility to the candidate when he shall have communicated the following: an appraisal of the major assets and liabilities of the candidate's personality; an outline of the steps that seem necessary and feasible for achieving success in some field—one hopes, in psychiatry; and an outline of the factors that limit the candidate's probable achievements. The necessary and feasible steps include an assessment of many factors including available personnel known to be competent to deal with the person before one.

This optimum performance with patients is not always desirable. One encounters some situations in these consultations that forbid the frank expression of certain conclusions as to the mental disorder present. Quite aside from rationalizing his adequate performances, the psychiatrist realizes that it is futile, foolhardy, or actually viciously irresponsible to undermine any patient's security when one can offer nothing that will promptly be constructive.[70] Not psychoanalysis alone but

[70] In some instances, where I have found a complex of factors which seemed to me to preclude a successful career in psychiatry, among them some grievous disorder of personality, I have disadvised the pursuit of the career on the basis of my impression of its unsuitability to the person—but only *after* I had un-

modern psychiatry as a whole provides destructively motivated people with peculiarly effective tools for doing harm.

There is no valid question of danger in psychoanalytic treatment by a practitioner competent to handle the patient concerned. There are some patients who come to the consultant for the handling of whom no psychoanalytic psychiatrist of his acquaintance is certainly competent, and there are many patients for whom psychoanalytic treatment is wholly out of the question, by reason of economic, geographic, and other facts. As one whose practice has been chiefly among persons suffering schizophrenic and substitutive states, I have been able to observe the results of adequate psychoanalytic treatment in a variety of potentially and incipiently schizophrenic states. While treatment has not always been fully successful, I know that there is no danger of aggravating the mental disorder, and no necessity for phases of the work in which the patient is seriously disturbed. I have as a practitioner and as a supervising instructor followed rather minutely the processes making up the successful treatment, the cure, of potentially and of incipiently schizophrenic patients. The course of the work has been clear, often predictable as to developments days to weeks in the future. So much for what can be done; how often it works out this way is another matter.

It would be absurd indeed to recommend intensive treatment for all schizophrenic patients, or, for that matter, for all persons showing any pattern of mental disorder. A consideration of the collaborative performances on which cure depends should make this evident, without further discussion. The consultant sees many patients in the case of whom any direct interpersonal treatment is out of the question. These include some

---

covered some interest in an alternative course, *and* some of the experience that had eventuated in the 'choice' of psychiatry. By virtue of questioning the validity of the 'choice,' and recommending reconsideration, I have spared us both embarrassment about the actual personal problems. The tendency towards mental health does the rest, with no danger of serious disturbance to the candidate.

patients whose presenting condition is in all likelihood better than their probable future course. They include also some patients who are potentially of excellent outlook, but whose care entails their removal from mutually disturbing contact with any ordinary environment. These two groups, and those who fall between them, are in general the patients who require institutional care. I shall come to consider this, shortly. Besides all these, the consultant sees a number of people for whom, for a variety of reasons, he cannot recommend intensive treatment, but who would profit from further therapeutic contact with a psychiatrist.

Intensive psychiatric treatment, including psychoanalysis, proceeds by reintegrating dissociated motivational systems, and dissipating the continuing parataxic influences of unresolved historically past situations through which the patient has lived. This is a long-term procedure, often requiring many hundred hours of work for its adequate achievement. It is obviously of but very limited application to the great numbers of people who realize that something is the matter with their lives, that in some obscure way they defeat themselves in dealing with other people, that their children are not responding satisfactorily to the parental influence; in short, that they are unsatisfied and insecure. For most of these patients, the psychiatrist has to compromise with the ideal of cure and proceed along the line of amelioration.[71]

The office and the dispensary practice of ameliorative psychiatry is in some ways the most demanding form of treatment. The consultant sees the patient a few times, during which

[71] The notion of cure is, of course, a relative one. Very few patients who are rid of all marked handicaps in living will continue in intensive treatment to uncover trifling difficulties. Those who seem to be doing this are more probably moving towards the revelation of a serious difficulty that has not been noticed by the psychiatrist—if they are not in fact entangled with the psychiatrist in some mutually satisfactory, if unrecognized, durable relationship. This latter can scarcely be regarded as a successful outcome of treatment, as it represents a great shift in the rôle of the physician, and one contrary to the social sanctions which establish his relationship to his patient.

his activity must be therapeutic, but with as its main objective a wise recommendation as to the future, to be carried out elsewhere after his investigation is completed. The psychiatrist engaged in intensive treatment has to spend a great deal of time with each of his patients, has relatively little to say most of this time, and expects a good many erroneous statements, imperfect interpretations, and inadequate situations to work themselves out to no one's disadvantage. The average institutional psychiatrist works chiefly through mediate channels and in a field so complex that the outcome is not clearly within the scope of his psychiatric responsibility. The psychiatrist who receives a patient for non-intensive treatment has none of these advantages and is often vividly aware of the disastrous effects on his reputation of a suicide or anything else that might interest the sensational press. Under the circumstances, it is not strange that some of these practitioners do little more than play safe. For reasons that by now may be fairly evident, it is some of these 'cautious' practitioners—and the cruel-destructive ones—who have most of the misfortunes in their practice.

The responsible treatment of patients by way of occasional conferences is not often a brilliant success. I have for some years occupied myself in trying to determine if this must be the case. The history of many a patient shows a great and favorable change that allegedly followed a particular personal association, perhaps a brief contact. Some of these instances leave no doubt as to their authenticity. Moreover, ironically enough, marked improvements are sometimes obtained in the first few psychiatric interviews, only to fade out in those that follow. Part of the favorable change is to be credited to the mere act of finally seeking help, after months or years of struggling with the conviction that one ought to be man enough to handle one's own personal problems. The relief of asking help and finding that the psychiatrist does not regard one as a weakling is strongly reassuring. In this is included a large part of the trouble. The occasional psychiatric treatment is often addressed to improving the functional efficiency of the self, and not to the solution of the complications arising from the activity of the self. There is all too much of the attitude of which Frederick H. Allen gives a humorous summary: the patient is told to 'buck up' and if he doesn't buck up, one commits him to a mental hospital.

Efforts addressed solely to bolstering the self system are not ordinarily conducive of benefit to the patient. If the strivings towards mental health could manifest themselves, psychiatric aid would scarcely be needed. All that can obstruct them is the self, and increasing its efficiency is, therefore, tantamount to continuing the mental disorder. There are crisis situations to which these considerations are not cogent. I can illustrate this by referring to the case of a clergyman who sought treatment for a gastro-intestinal malady in a general hospital. A few nights after admission, awakening terrified, in a twilight state, he was so disturbed that he was transferred immediately to a mental hospital. The next morning, he was quite himself—nothing was the matter with him, there was no reason for his being in a mental hospital, he had no worries or problems. That night, too, he awakened in terror, hid under the bed, and was frantically combative. The next morning, he was in fairly good condition, but obviously unnerved. The third evening, he was anxious and unwilling to go to bed. He was given a powerful hypnotic, slept well, and was again quite himself. The next night, he was again disturbed, and shortly thereafter was definitely in a schizophrenic state. The use of the hypnotic was simply a support to the self. It interfered with the activity of the dissociated components and by protecting sleep reduced the fatigue which enfeebled the self function. It deferred the psychosis, a day or so. Such brief postponement of personal disaster may provide opportunity for truly remedial work—in this case, beyond my ability. The ephemeral calm that can thus be achieved sometimes enables a patient to regain perspective and to reach a wise decision about treatment, or in regard to some major change in his life situation that will be greatly beneficial in reducing conflict, anxiety, or tension. I know of few other indications for this sort of maneuver.

Direct enfeeblement of the self system is sometimes indicated, but, too, is apt to be devoid of lasting benefit. There are various ways of accomplishing this maneuver, of which one of the easiest is—as in the example of the clergyman—by chemical means. From the early days of the Egyptian culture, the use of beverages containing ethyl alcohol has persisted in the Western world. The pharmacodynamics of alcohol is most strikingly a relaxing of the inhibiting and dissociating power of the self.[72] Consideration of its remarkable power in this direction led me, some years ago, to use intoxication with alcohol as a means of obliterating conflict in schizophrenics whose exhaustion from chronic excitement or tension was dangerous to their survival. The gentleman of the imaginary stallion mentioned in the fourth lecture was the first patient so treated, and with complete success. A number of other patients in gravely disquieting condition were carried into freely communicative states by the same technique, with subsequent recovery or social restoration.

Under full doses of alcohol, the signs and symptoms of strong self function disappear. A patient, for example, in terror from the projection of cravings for perverse satisfactions—*craving* is the term by which we refer to the extremely unpleasant state which results when there is desire for the satisfaction of some zone of interaction so strong that it cannot be excluded from awareness, and at the same time so symbolized that it cannot be tolerated by the self; in other words, an abhorrent *yearning*—may be extremely excited, combative, and directly dangerous to himself and others. When thus intoxicated, his fear of people around him disappears, and with it, the excitement. After a

[72] One of the colleagues achieved a bon mot of the first water: the superego is the alcohol-soluble part of the personality.

More seriously, the findings about to be reported are well authenticated by repetition by other observers.

week or so of this alcoholically hazy existence—of which he retains memory and easy recall—*in a well managed environment* where nothing that will be regretted can occur, the patient has lost the necessity for terror and excitement. This is not solely due to the enfeeblement of the self function, but the weakening of the self system is prerequisite for the change.

The enfeeblement of the self by interpersonal processes is also possible. One works towards this in occasional treatment by calling in question some of the formulated inhibitory attitudes and normative prescriptions that the patient can express. In the intensive treatment, the patient works this out mostly for himself by recalling the situations from which the attitudes survive. The direct attack is not to be undertaken lightly; one must be quite clear as to both the direct and the more obscurely symbolized factors that are expressed in the accessible formula. It may, for example, be obvious that a patient is absurdly restrained about being what he calls 'forward.' We communicate this view to him with skill enough to make the point. He rapidly develops a distressing aggressiveness which makes him a nuisance to all his acquaintances. We have only succeeded in substituting a cruder for a more refined compromise; the underlying problems of the personality are not helped, in fact are aggravated.

In my consultative work with incipient schizophrenics, I seek often to enfeeble the self with respect to some restrictions of awareness. Thus a patient gradually unfolds a home situation both distressing and mystifying. Under methodic and persisting questioning, he becomes aware of a long-accumulating resentment about unreasonable restraints on his freedom that have been imposed by one of his parents—who has resisted the fact of his chronological maturity, and appropriate efforts to perfect his socialization. When this becomes clear, the mystery of his hostile acts disappears. He is more secure as a result of understanding the naturalness of a previously disconcerting series of events. He is less secure in knowing that he is hostile to the parent. It would not be wise to leave things in this state. One must go on to develop the natural inevitability of the negative feeling, and then to some interpretation of the parent's behavior that will provide the patient with a constructive technique for circumventing the situation without unnecessary exchanges of hostility.

The goal of occasional treatment being generally alleviation rather than radical cure, one sometimes has to interfere with the growth of awareness. This seeming paradox arises from several considerations. There are problems which, once clearly recognized, demand radical treatment if serious disturbance of the personality is to be avoided. I was once consulted by a patient 49 years of age who was sent to me because, in the face of a threat of chronic physical disability, he was entertaining well-formulated suicidal intentions. I learned that he suffered periods of insomnia connected with horrible dreams, that his enjoyment of social life was undergoing a marked recession, that while it had never included sexual intimacies with women, their company had until recently been delightful, but was now becoming repugnant to him. On the night before our fourth conference, he dreamt of something like a wrestling match in the course of which the two men engaged in some mutual sexual performance. The patient had reported one somewhat related boyhood experience. I provided this patient with no opportunity to concern himself with "homosexuality" as a part of the motives that expressed themselves in the horrible and disgusting dreams, and that were concerned in the change in tenor of his life.

The indications were chiefly for the remedy of his increasing loneliness, which was reducing the value of life. To this end, we made something of a detailed study of the women who had once been appreciated, and it gradually emerged that there were still a few who were attractive. From their characteristics, those of rather markedly differentiated women, it became reasonable to formulate a plan for specific avoidances instead of a blanket aversion to the sex. Some other matters were dealt with; my point is to show the way in which one of the less unfortunate compromises which one often encounters was utilized as a practical way out of a situation in which accumulating lust coupled with increasing social distance threatened to precipitate a very serious conflict.

At this point, in somewhat obscure apropos to the discussion of this patient, I shall comment on the utility of extra-verbal expression for the at least partial solution of mental disorders that for one reason or another cannot be treated intensively. Levy in his specific and general "release therapy" of problem children,[73] has worked out a technique of this kind. Moreno, in the "psychodrama" technique for older patients,[74] seems also to use this principle. The patient acts out under more or less controlled conditions a dramatization of personnel and performances connected with his conflicts. There is some encouragement of verbalization after the activity. Durably good results, however, seem to follow in some children and juveniles without their having had much to say about the meaningful play in which they were engaged.

My experience with intensive therapy in adolescents and adults leads me to think that verbalization is usually, if not always, necessary to insure permanent benefits. One of the problems of psychoanalysis is the *acting out* of troublesome motivation—in or outside of the therapy situation, and usually both—with little or no awareness of the meaning of the performances. Objectively, the activity may from the beginning be revealing, and it generally becomes progressively more obvious until the physician, at least, cannot overlook its significance. His interpretation then usually permits the suppression of the dramatization, and the production of verbalizations in its lieu. Let me repeat, in this connection, the statement that one has

[73] Levy, David M., 'Release Therapy' in Young Children. PSYCHIATRY (1938) 1:387–390.

[74] Moreno, J. L., Psychodramatic Treatment of Marriage Problems. *Sociometry* (1940) 3:1–23.

information only to the extent to which one has tended to communicate one's experience—through the medium of consensually valid verbal means. Theoretically, this last qualification gives somewhat undue importance to the use of words; by and large, it is a good principle to which to adhere in treatment work. Most patients have for years been acting out conflicts, substitutions, and compromises; the benefits of treatment come in large part from their learning to notice what they are doing, and this is greatly expedited by carefully validated verbal statements as to what seems to be going on.

A special case of this non-verbal expressive behavior to which people have recourse for the reduction of tension arising from unsatisfied tendency systems, or from conflict of motives, is made up of games and sports. It is often demonstrable that some activity of this sort has provided a symbolic discharge of motives that conflict with the self to a degree that makes the recreation an important factor in preserving relative mental health. Many a person has doubtless been able to preserve the peace, at home or in his community, in large measure by virtue of the symbolic satisfactions derived from hunting, trap shooting, or bowling. The rôle of card games in a prevailingly juvenile society can be far greater in importance than a relatively non-competitive person would guess. People who have but very limited ability for human intimacy can assuage loneliness through these instrumentalities, without any risk of troublesome interpersonal developments. Biological and other scientific avocations, and fishing, sailing, riding, golf, and swimming are activities that are in a special class, by virtue of the extensive contexts of integrating tendencies that may be involved. Various interpersonal stresses and dissatisfactions associated with one's necessary employment may be kept at an insignificant level by the elevation to prime personal significance of the intricate, long-span procedures, and highly personalized subject-matter, of, say, horticulture, the breeding of dogs or horses, or the study of ant-communities, as one's recreational avocation. Amateur astronomy and radio communication are two examples of the 'hobbies' which are scientifically and technologically absorbing, and associated with close but mediate relation with a well-organized group of co-workers. Riding, again often an attenuated participation in a group of like-minded people, is peculiarly significant because of symbolic investitures of the uniquely gifted sub-colleague, the horse. Golf is in most significant essence a consummately skillful performance that calls for remarkable development of perseveration, as well as for tonic and motor adjustments of almost all the skeletal muscles. It shares this with the game of billiards, with additional benefits connected with outdoor life. Fishing, sailing, and swimming have as a common element this outdoor life in its peculiar aspects that inhere in association with bodies of water. Swimming is rather in a class by itself, because it directly involves sub-cultural organismic factors that make for relaxation and repose, quite exterior to its often great symbolic rôle. I am sure that many an incipient schizophrenic has been able to reintegrate an approximation to mental health, by chief virtue of spending a summer in bathing suit at the seaside, away from any people highly significant to him. Camping expeditions to forests and mountains; mountain climbing; biological, anthropological, and archeological exploration; and activities which include moving at extraordinary velocity; these are some more of the forms of recreational behavior that have an extensive context of meaning in the non-verbal preservation of relative mental health.

Long the prescription of physicians as an adjuvant to or as the only treatment offered for a disturbed state of mind, activity as such has recently been made the basis of study as to its therapeutic possibilities. This came about somewhat indirectly, by way of a particular development in the institutional field, the *occupational therapy* with which Mrs. Slagel and William Rush Dunton were effective pioneers in psychiatry, and with the demonstration of general utility of which the treatment of those disabled in the World War—as by our Federal Board for Vocational Education, Rehabilitation Division—had much to do. In part because of the clearly demonstrable value of particular arts and crafts in rehabilitating disabled soldiers, sailors, and marines, and in part because of its leader's zeal for organizing, occupational therapy rather monopolized for some years the attention that should be accorded to activity-therapies in general. I believe that the part is now beginning to find its place in the whole, a change that I regard as decidedly constructive.

I shall turn now to the patients whose difficulties are treated in major part by a change of their cultural setting; more specifically, to those who are removed from their accustomed way of life to the peculiarly characterized culture-complex of the mental hospital. The fundamental principles of institutional treatment have had a long historical exemplification in the monastic orders and other religious and special communities—including such diverse institutions as the French Foreign Legion, the Chasseurs Alpines, and the Parisian Apaches. When life in the complex pattern of the times seems impossible, one may associate oneself—or forcibly be associated—with a group the social structure of which is less variously demanding in terms of fluid conformity.

The modern *custodial* mental hospital was brought into being largely through the almost incredible energy of Miss Dorothea Lynde Dix—1802 to 1887.[75] The *therapeutic* mental hospital began with the York Retreat established—as were several others, including the Sheppard and Enoch Pratt Hospital—by members of the Society of Friends. The work of the therapeutic institution has largely overshadowed the beneficial aspects of the merely custodial, although the great majority of those who have recovered from severe mental disorders have

[75] Tiffany, Francis, *Life of Dorothea Lynde Dix;* Boston, Houghton, Mifflin, 8 ed. 1892 (xiii and 392 pp.). Miss Dix in 1852 secured the passage by Congress of her District Hospital Bill as a result of which St. Elizabeths Hospital came into being as The Government Hospital for the Insane. She was thereafter Superintendent of Women Nurses, U.S.A., in the Civil War.

thus far been instances of so-called *spontaneous recovery*—the work of factors other than deliberate therapeutic intervention by the psychiatrist—that took place in custodial institutions.

In any society that permits a person to rise or fall in status as a more or less direct result of his own efforts, the possibility of favorable or unfavorable change in one's position in the hierarchy of personal valuation is apt to be important. Everyone knows that skill in dealing with important people is one of the effective ways to get ahead in our society of mobile vertical classes. Anything that handicaps the development or manifestation of this skill is, therefore, productive of keen insecurity. Any other source of insecurity is apt to act as just such a handicap, and thus to give rise to a 'vicious circle' of aggravating factors. It thus comes about rather generally that the severity of any mental disorder is to an important degree a result of insecurity about one's status. This part of the problem would be solved by removing the patient to a society in which vertical mobility is not possible. Just this, in effect, is achieved by his admission to the custodial institution.

The mental hospital is a sub-community strikingly different from the larger social system in which it is embedded. It exists communally with the larger society, but its organization is in a most significant way classless. It is primarily a social system made up of fixed *castes*, which does not permit any vertical mobility. Moreover, it is a social organization autocratically maintained in conformity to a relatively small number of simple, explicit, rules—in great contrast to the larger society with its however feebly democratic authority, coupled with complex, mostly implicit, often contradictory, demands that are variously and often inequably enforced by public opinion, group prejudice, the church, and the police powers of the community.[76]

[76] For two cogent sociological considerations, see Rowland, Howard, Interaction Processes in the State Mental Hospital. PSYCHIATRY (1938) 1:323–327, and Friendship Patterns in the State Mental Hospital. PSYCHIATRY (1939) 2:363–373.

For a sociological discussion of our social system and its effects on problems

Admission to the mental hospital is often the only way by which one can be separated from the particular people at home, in school, or at the place of employment, with whom one is integrated in an increasingly unfortunate situation, progressively aggravated as a result of fatigue, misdirected and misunderstood efforts, and the display of conflicting motives. As Dr. White used to say, the mental hospital is the only place where one can be "crazy" comfortably. It is used to these sorts of performances and, through its classification of patients, is more or less obviously able to deal with them intelligently. It has been unfortunate for mentally disordered persons that their voluntary admission to the mental hospital was until recently illegal or otherwise impractical. The practice was that of judicial commitment, perhaps after a brief residence on authority of a medical or other formal certification that the patient was a menace to himself or others. This had come about through legislative precaution called into being as a result of several factors; the bearing of severe mental disorder on property rights and various civil and criminal 'responsibilities,' coupled with some notorious XIX Century instances of the misuse of a custodial institution; many superstitions about "the insane" including vague to vivid convictions that mental disorders are in some fashion contagious; and a hatred of practices like the *lettres de cachet*. Many of the statutory safeguards showed no consideration of the welfare of the patient; until very recently patients in the District of Columbia had to appear before a jury and by them be found to be of 'unsound mind' before they could be retained beyond a brief period in St. Elizabeths Hospital.

Hospital classification of patients is in theory the segregation of patients on the basis of similarity of signs and symptoms. Hypomanic patients who are voluble, loud, and miscellaneously overactive, for example, would all be in the same ward

---

and current practices of preventive psychiatry, see Davis, Kingsley, Mental Hygiene and the Class Structure. PSYCHIATRY (1938) 1:55–65.

or group of wards, unmixed with patients who showed a different clinical picture. When one of them quiets down, he would be transferred to another ward, where he would find the other patients acting very much as he does.

The patient is transferred from one ward to another on the basis of his interpersonal performances, regardless of intentions, rationalizations, excuses, pleas, protests, "pull," or other of the thousand and one factors that make for inequality of opportunity in the larger world. Rumor and verbal tradition about the various wards may complicate the effects of patient classification, particularly in the hospital with restricted facilities for patient segregation. The basis of classification may also be inadequate or absurd. If, however, circumstances permit a reasonable approximation to the theory, the practice of classification is in itself of marked therapeutic significance.

A hateful manic patient in a ward that houses several catatonic patients is about as bad an example of non-therapeutic situations as one can find. Correspondingly, the disturbed wards of smaller hospitals are apt to be anything but areas of therapeutic segregation. Admission wards have to be the clearing area, from which patients are transferred to their appropriate group. They are the point at which effort may well be concentrated to inform the patient about hospital life, and about the non-punitive basis of classificatory transfers.

Systematic educational efforts to facilitate the adjustment of the patient in the mental hospital are not yet widely practiced. It is easy to see the difficulties that stand in the way. It is also easy to overlook the uncontrolled and often unfortunate educational influences that are bound to exist where acculturation to the hospital community is left to chance. Carefully formulated factual statements couched in relatively simple language might very well be made a part of the standard practice of all the hospital personnel who deal with newly-admitted patients. The barriers to communication with most of these patients may be great. This is all the more reason for being clear on just what one wishes to communicate. No one statement will serve with every patient, but good simple statements that are understood by the hospital personnel will usefully restrict the range of their improvisations in talking to patients, or among themselves, within hearing of patients.

In theory, the mental hospital is governed in accordance with an explicit policy calculated to achieve the practical maximum benefit of recognized principles of institutional psychiatric therapy. Its peculiar social structure requires an essentially rigid, if unusually simple, discipline of all the employees, and, along much more flexible lines, of all the patients.

The regimen of the hospital is in general mildly hygienic, sometimes markedly so. The rather rigidly enforced ordering of life by the clock is in the last analysis quite simple and understandable—probably, to many patients, a welcome relief from the irregularities to which they had felt driven. The variously encouraged participation in more or less intelligently prescribed and prosecuted activity therapy is often most helpful. If there is nothing more than work on wards, grounds, and hospital farm, it is much better than nothing.

In a few words, the aspects of the mental hospital community which are directly therapeutic are both numerous and of considerable positive value. The organization of people concerned into castes of the physicians, the technicians, the nurses, the attendants, and the patients, however undemocratic it may sound, is the product of centuries of evolution, and is therapeutically sound, irrespective of its effects on some of those who are not patients.

Besides the direct effect of the hospital community, benefit to the patient is obtained from some relatively generalized therapeutic procedures. Notable among these is *hydrotherapy*, the more or less scientific utilization of part of the historic "external hydropathy," wet packs, showers and sprays, and the continuous-flow tub. There are many complicated problems associated with the use of the wet pack, either for the patient alone in a room, or for a number of patients who receive packs in the same room. Besides the heat-transfer feature, there is that of a great degree of physical restraint. The beneficial effects of the pack in some phases of mental disorder seem to be fairly established. The benefits of the 'continuous tub' are unquestionable. Hydrotherapy, generally, and the use of showers and sprays in particular, often include, besides the hydrotherapeutic factor, a social influence. Patients moving among their fellows in *socially sanctioned* nudity, or approximations thereto, are in quite a different situation from that of the patient who insists on being nude in his room, or on the ward.

Something can be said in favor of the therapeutic use of seclusion and restraint. By seclusion is meant the separation of a patient from easy access to the company of others. By restraint is meant the use of some one of sundry devices to restrict the activity of the patient—from the sheet spread across the patient and wrapped around the sides of the bed, the unauthorized use of which may be overlooked by inexperienced physicians, to such devices as the camisole, wristlets, and anklets. As Dr. White has said, it has been fortunate for institutional psychiatry that the use of restraint was abolished; it made the psychiatrists use their minds. At the same time, if one could certainly obviate their abuse, restraint in some cases, and seclusion in many, are at times clearly indicated as positive therapeutic maneuvers. Seclusion can relieve the patient of the pressure of people and, as this effect is achieved, give him an opportunity to feel loneliness, the need for companionship.

The trouble with seclusion and restraint, as with the other instrumentalities of the hospital, is always the result of lack of intelligence, interest, and responsibility on the part of the physician who can prescribe—and, one hopes, supervise the use of—these restrictions. The psychiatrist, of all people, knows that rules and regulations, and principles useful in reaching conclusions, are all susceptible of gross misuse for rationalizing behavior in most blatant breach of their purpose. If re-education of those concerned is out of the question, he may well seek to abolish any and all practices that may be channels for inhumane indifference and cruelty.

To this briefest of glimpses into some of the useful factors in the more mediate treatment of seriously disordered patients, let me add a few words as to the psychiatrist's direct treatment of patients in the mental hospital. This may be intensive or occasional, continuing or only for the duration of some phases of the hospital residence. The hospital provides a setting for the active treatment of some patients, in the case of whom it would otherwise be contra-indicated because of the unpredictable or uncontrollable risk of suicidal misadventure, breach of the peace, or other serious concomitants. When therapy is the primary aim of the hospital, the beneficial factors inhering in the hospital situation can sometimes be so integrated that they facilitate the work of the physician to a degree almost beyond the possibility of any extramural setting. Unfortunately, however, the hospital setting is not generally useful for the entire course of an intensive treatment looking towards cure. The patient should ordinarily be paroled from the hospital some considerable time before treatment is concluded, if maximum benefits are to be secured—if, in fact, some disadvantageous factors are to be avoided. We are not yet clear as to how best to transfer a patient under intensive treatment from one psychiatrist to another, with but transient disturbance of progress. The treatment staff of the therapeutic mental hospital should, therefore, often carry on the treatment of patients after they have been paroled or discharged from hospital residence. As this is often impractical, the patients of therapeutic hospitals are apt to be discharged at the right stage of their reorganization but thereby separated from psychiatric collaboration, or retained in the hospital beyond the period of useful association with the hospital community, when their reassociation with ordinary life could much more profitably be under study.

For this reason, and because there are now many instances of hospitalization of young patients in episodes that might well be quickly remedied if so drastic a change of social situation as admission to the mental hospital were not experienced, I am greatly impressed with the desirability of an innovation in the shape of special communities in which some of the great advantages of the mental hospital could be made available, without incurring the necessary exposure to factors that now make for permanent institutional adaptation of many patients. Something at least remotely like what I have in mind has already been accomplished by the Civilian Conservation Corps, the various camps of which would be a rewarding field for study. It is desirable, during the developmental stage of a therapeutic camp or community, that it be in coöperative relationship with an accessible mental hospital with good facilities for classifying patients, and a therapeutic staff.

Even this addition to the institutional facilities of psychiatry would probably have little effect on one of the most embittering experiences to which the institutional therapist is constantly exposed. I refer here to the intervention of persons by blood or otherwise related to the patient. It is only natural that relatives should demonstrate some interest, real or assumed, in what is being done for the good of the patient. No hospital administrator would object to this. It is natural but not so unobjectionable that relatives should be firm in the conviction that their visits to the patient are wholly beneficial, while they are often precisely the opposite. The problem of the suspicious relative in this rôle can often be solved by restricting visits to some one person about whom the patient's history is encouraging, and to whose visits there seems to be a minimum of bad consequences. The peculiarly disheartening performance of relatives, however, is not a complicating but the most untimely *terminating* of a patient's treatment. They often remove the patient of otherwise excellent outlook in the midst of the most profitable phase of his work—often with consequences disastrous to the patient; but never, so far as I can recall, with subsequent self-recriminations—flatly against psychiatric advice.[77]

To conclude the matter of therapeutic conceptions, let me restate the steps by which the goals of psychiatric treatment are sought. Whether the work be intensive or occasional, institutional, extramural, consultative or informal; whether the end state of the patient has come to be the achievement of an extraordinary unfolding of hitherto potential capacities for living, the cure of a serious handicap, the amelioration of a difficult situation, or failure and adaptation to an institutional life, or even a grave dilapidation; in every case the events in the therapeutic effort will have been oriented in much the same way, the foresight of the psychiatrist will have sought ways to collaborate in much the same pattern of interpersonal relations. An analysis of this pattern into ultimate terms may now be useful.

The first effective step in the solution of any problem is the synthesis of perceptions and prehensions as to the problem-situation into a perception of that in which one is involved. This usually calls for the *release of one's alertness* from inhibiting influences which are manifestations of the self dynamism. There may be dissociated tendencies that are significant in explaining the integration of the problem-situation. There may be repressed, vaguely remembered, factors. There may be suppressive effects of the magnitude of a deletion or 'clouding' of consciousness, at some crucial phase of development of the problem-situation.

The history of the patient, secured retrospectively from the

[77] It is by no means mere spleen that leads the psychiatrist to conclude, in many instances, that the treatment was interrupted because the relative saw that the patient was becoming emancipated from a subordination to the relative which had pre-existed the psychosis; the, of course, unrecognized determination being that sick or well, the patient is not going to be free of the relative.

known presenting situation, will have revealed—or at least indicated as more or less probable—the more typical manifestations of complicated interpersonal relations in terms of the explanatory conceptions discussed in the fourth lecture. The elevation into awareness of the unnoticed influences that are giving rise to the problem aspect of the situation, is facilitated by training the patient to understand the pattern of maladjustive activity in terms of the appropriate explanatory conception—not in terms of its name, or the names of alleged dynamic entities, "complexes," which the patient might be said to be suffering.

Patients usually begin this learning from rather trifling instances, rather than from insight into deeply disturbing events. It seems as if this intrusion of apparently insignificant, 'accidental' events into the fabric of daily life, and remembered dreams of rather simple context, are the two chief ways by which the striving towards mental health ordinarily circumvents the general effect of the self system.

The psychiatrist often assists in this learning by simple interpretative behavior: he says something calculated to center attention on the momentary situation, recites in essential outline the course of the significant event as he has heard it, and perhaps asks if there can be something important which was omitted from the account, or if the action could have been meant to have such and such an effect, or if some detail can be recalled that would indicate that such and such an unrecognized end was being pursued. In another sort of this apparently insignificant event, he may intervene only to ask—with stress on the importance of the matter by preferably non-verbal, perhaps intonational means—as to how the patient could have been aware of the motivation of the other person concerned, or what the evidence may be that justifies the assumption that such and such is a durable characteristic of the other person. This latter sort of event and interpretative action is often called out by patients who show prevailingly substitutive processes.

As the release of the patient's alertness proceeds, there comes a time when it is possible to *identify* one of the *parataxic concomitants* that have been permanent complicating factors in the patient's perceptions of significant other people. Here again it will usually be an at first hearing quite insignificant, mildly irrelevant, remark that communicates the distortion of the patient's formulation of the psychiatrist.

Here also interpretation usually facilitates the learning. This, again, is often merely an interrupting, seriously expressed, question as to what the patient has just said; a repetition of the patient's statement in essential outline; and an inquiry as to its implication as to the psychiatrist, or as to the basis for the expressed belief.

The first awareness of a parataxically illusory personal characterization begins the therapeutic processes connected with it. In itself, the discovery is attended by a sharp fall in the patient's feeling of security; a disturbing 'mistake' has been made, a queer and disquieting 'misapprehension' has occurred. The patient feels that the psychiatrist is annoyed or disappointed, that his appraisal of the patient must be unfavorable. It is necessary that the essentially disintegrative, distance-producing security operations that are thus called out shall be handled in some conformity with the surmised pattern of the particular parataxis. It does not help if the physician offers reassurance in terms of his more real characteristics. This would but increase the insecurity of the patient because it asserts that there was a 'mistake' or 'misapprehension,' which the physician accepts as such.

The psychiatrist, having clarified the gross outlines of the expressed parataxic distortion, remarks to some such effect as "This impression that you have had about me must have a history, must be the recollection of some such a person who was once really important to you—perhaps you can recall someone. Let us listen to whatever comes to mind." Even if, as is frequently the case in the first instance of this kind, the patient silently 'searches his memory' and recalls no one, the interpretation will have communicated security *and* useful information about the sources of parataxic distortion.

It might be thought that, once the patient *has* recalled the historic, personal source of a particular parataxic distortion, that this parataxis would disappear. Nothing so spectacular is to be expected; if it seems to have occurred, the chances are greatly in favor of quite another explanation; namely, that the patient's insecurity was not resolved, and that there has developed an even more complex parataxic situation with the physician. The remarkable thing that has certainly happened—one trusts without the just mentioned unfortunate sequel—is insight into the actual fact of illusory, parataxic, distortions as a factor that complicates the patient's interpersonal relations. This constitutes the first therapeutic milestone, to which I have already referred.

Each recurrent recognition of a particular parataxic distortion of the physician brings with it more data as to the historic, personal source. The time comes when the patient recalls vividly a series of highly significant events that occurred in interpersonal relations with this person. This recall gradually expands into a more or less comprehensive insight; first, into the 'effects' of this earlier relationship on the subsequent course of the patient's dealings with others, on the formulation of ideals of conduct and relatively fixed valuational judgments of behavior. Besides this there comes insight into the less obviously interpersonal consequences of this former relationship; into direct symbolic associations made at that time, and into much more obscure resymbolizations, substitutions, and symptomatic and related actions that had their origin in, or in subsequent relation to, the significant relationship. As these complex remainders of previously unresolved motivational "sets" expand into easily understood meaning, the patient generally experiences a great deal of unpleasant emotion—to which may be added keen regrets for disastrous effects over the years, which are now seen to have stemmed from the early experience.

Progressively, in the course of identifying all the more important parataxically surviving, unresolved situations of the patient's past, and their consequent dissolutions, there goes an *expanding of the self* to such final effect that the patient as known to himself is much the same person as the patient behaving with others. This is *psychiatric* cure. There may remain a need for a great deal of experience and education before the psychiatric cure is a *social* cure, implying a more abundant life in the community. It may be impractical to achieve this more abundant life, the collaborative participation with others, in that particular community. A change of social setting may be mandatory but impractical, in which case adequate mediate relationships and clearly understood reformulations of some of one's interpersonal goals must fill the gaps. The possibility of achieving a social cure arises solely from the fact of psychiatric cure. The probability of its achievement is a matter of circumstances, limited chiefly by factors inhering in the culture-complex and selectively reflected in all the people available for interpersonal relations. Be social cure achieved or not, however, the person who knows himself has mental health. He is content with his utilization of the opportunities that come to him. He values himself as his conduct merits. He knows and mostly obtains the satisfactions that he needs, and he is greatly secure.

Sharply to be distinguished from the conception of social cure is the so-called 'social recovery' of the institutional psychiatrist. Patients are classified for discharge from mental hospitals as recovered, social recovery, improved, or unimproved. A person is socially recovered when he is both clear as to the fact that he was so mentally disordered that institutional care was required, and free from any manifest signs or symptoms of the disorder. Investigation sometimes reveals that the patient discharged as a social recovery still suffers marked mental disorder. He has learnt, however, to treat most people as if they had nothing to do with his troubles—of which, the less he has to say, the better. Many of these patients, like many of those somewhat benefited by other forms of non-intensive therapy, continue in a favorable course and require no further attention from the psychiatrist.

A Theory of Interpersonal Relations and the Evolution of Personality

BY PATRICK MULLAHY

THE FOLLOWING is an attempt to outline the group of central ideas and insights making up Harry Stack Sullivan's theory of personality and personality development. The impression that this useful body of theory has received less attention than it merits has led to this sometimes all too schematic review of the fundamental ideas in his published statements, supplemented by personal discussion.

Because of lack of space, several ideas can scarcely be more than mentioned in a paragraph or two. There are several concepts which, for sufficient clarity, would require a paper by themselves, but it is thought best to discuss them briefly.

What is psychiatry? Is it, as one might imagine, the study of the mentally ill? And what, precisely, does mental illness mean? What are the therapeutic conceptions of modern psychiatry? According to Sullivan, the therapeutic conceptions "arise directly from the work of Freud, Meyer, and White. Were it not for Freud's formulations, we would probably still be frustrated by the obvious discontinuities in the stream of consciousness. Had it not been for Meyer's insistence that mental disorders are to be considered as dynamic patterns, as types of reaction to the demands of life, we might still be working in the laboratory on problems of neurophysiology and endocrinology. But it was White's ineffable zeal in teaching us to 'determine what the patient is trying to do,' his indomitable energy in training and in encouraging psychiatric investigators, and his vision and sagacity in the executive, administrative and promotional aspects of psychiatry in the broader sense, that gave us most of our profit from Freud and from Meyer. . . ." [1]

The next step came with the realization that psychiatry is the study of interpersonal relations. "Psychiatry . . . is the study of processes that involve or go on between people. The field of psychiatry is the field of interpersonal relations, under any and all circumstances in which these relations exist. It was seen that *a personality* can never be isolated from the complex of interpersonal relations in which the person lives and has his being." [2] The full significance of these statements can only be progressively elucidated.

As a preliminary analysis, one may divide human behavior, interpersonal relations, into two closely related kinds or categories, characterized by the pursuit of satisfactions and the pursuit of security.[3] This does not mean, of course, that human behavior occurs marked, "For the pursuit of satisfactions," or, "For the pursuit of security." These are distinctions instituted by the psychiatric investigator in the course of inquiry, which help to make human behavior more intelligible. But these distinctions also are not "mental" or subjective. The attainment of satisfactions and security are seen to be the goals, *the end-states,* of human behavior, interpersonal processes. In popular language, they explain in general terms what one is after in any situation with other persons, real or fantastic, or a blend of both. From a slightly different point of view, they are "integrating tendencies." They explain why any situation in which two or more people are involved becomes an interpersonal situation. Furthermore, it is because of these needs

[1] See p. 177.
[2] See p. 10.
[3] See p. 12.

that one cannot live and be human except in communal existence with others. For preliminary analysis, they aid in clarifying interpersonal situations, and they lead to more illuminating and significant discoveries and interpretations.

The pursuit of satisfactions is a response to primarily biological needs. Food and drink, sleep and rest, the satisfaction of lust are all among them. "Throughout life," be it noted, "the pursuit of satisfactions is physiologically provoked by increased tone in some unstriped muscles, and the securing of the satisfactions is a relaxation of this tone, with a tendency towards the diminution of attention, alertness, and vigilance, and an approach to sleep." [4] In more popular language, the achievement of satisfactions causes a *decrease* of tension.

The other classification, the need for, and the pursuit of, security grows out of man's cultural equipment. The "cultural" is defined, anthropologically, as "all that which is man-made, which survives as monument to preexistent man." [5] It is, of course, imbedded in every person, the matrix of everything which he thinks and does. Without it, he would not be human, could not live. As Sullivan phrases it, "All those movements, actions, speech, thoughts, reveries, and so on, which pertain more to the culture which has been imbedded in a particular individual than to the organization of his tissues and glands, is apt to belong in this classification of the pursuit of security." [6]

How does the need for security arise? It arises from the fact that every person, through a long history, beginning at birth, becomes a social being. Through "empathy," a concept to be discussed later, every infant feels some effect of the culture by the attitudes of the significant person, mother or nurse, around him.[7] These attitudes of the significant person, or persons, are themselves socially conditioned. Long before the infant can

[4] See p. 88.
[5] See p. 13.
[6] See p. 13.
[7] See p. 17.

understand what is happening, he feels something of the attitudes of those who take care of him. After a while, the little one is deliberately trained and taught what is considered right and wrong. In other words, the impulses, the biological strivings, are socially conditioned, moulded according to the approved patterns of the culture. Unlike the attainment of satisfactions, the attainment of security requires the *maintenance* of some degree of muscle tonus, tension. It is said that some muscles are never completely relaxed, that most muscles are in a state of considerable tonus throughout the periods of deepest sleep. In fact changes in one's state of security are accompanied by spectacular change of tonus throughout the major muscular systems of the body. As will be seen subsequently, the attainment of satisfactions according to the socially approved patterns causes a profound feeling of well-being, of self-approval, of security. Not only does the person experience these felt needs but when, for certain reasons, they cannot be fulfilled according to the culturally approved patterns learned in early life, a feeling of intense uneasiness and discomfort, insecurity, *anxiety*, occurs.[8] This does not mean that the needs get converted into insecurity, anxiety, but that they are felt to imperil security; that is, they conflict with the necessity for achieving security.

An understanding of the power motive is fundamental, both psychologically and logically. For Sullivan, the power motive means much more than the usually restricted meaning of power in "power drive." A person is born with this power motive, or, in his cautious words, with "something" of the power motive.[9] This does *not* mean, however, that one is born with a "power drive." For Sullivan, power refers to the expansive biological striving of the infant and states characterized by the feeling of ability, applying, in a very wide sense, to all kinds of human activity. A "power drive," in the narrow sense, results from

[8] See p. 19.
[9] See p. 14.

the thwarting of the expansive biological striving, and the feeling of the lack of ability. In other words, a "power drive" is learned, resulting from the early frustration of the need to be, and to feel, capable, to have ability, to have power. A "power drive" develops as a compensation when there is a deep, gnawing, inner sense of powerlessness, because of early frustration of the expanding, developing latent potentialities of the organism. Later acculturation and experience may, and frequently does, add to the early frustration and sense of powerlessness. A person who has a feeling of ability or power does not need to gain, and will not seek, dominance or power *over* some one. A person who manifests a "power drive" does seek to dominate others. In the wide sense of the term, power is potential, and actual, accomplishment *along with* others. The accomplishment and the feeling of accomplishment are mutual. In fact, power refers to any activity where there is accomplishment, satisfaction of needs, mutual attainment of goals not distorted by unfortunate—that is, thwarting—experience. Power or ability "is ordinarily much more important in the human being than are the impulses resulting from a feeling of hunger, or thirst; and the fully developed feeling of lust comes so very late in biological maturation that it is scarcely a good source for conditioning." The power motive is more important because, in fact, it underlies them. They are expressions of biological needs. But biological needs are manifestations of the organism's efforts not merely to maintain itself in stable balance with and in its environment, but to expand, to 'reach out' to, and interact with, widening circles of the environment.

So important and fundamental is the power motive that the degree to which it is satisfied, fulfilled, and the manner in which it is satisfied and fulfilled mainly determine the growth and characteristics of personality. Stated negatively, the extent to which the power motive is frustrated, blocked, and the manner in which such frustration is accomplished, will mainly determine the development of personality. In Sullivan's words:

"The full development of personality along the lines of security is chiefly founded on the infant's discovery of his powerlessness to achieve certain desired end-states with the tools, the instrumentalities, which are at his disposal. From the disappointments in the very early stages of life outside the womb—in which all things are given—comes the beginning of this vast development of actions, thoughts, foresights, and so on, which are calculated to protect one from a feeling of insecurity and helplessness in the situation which confronts one. This accultural evolution begins thus, and when it succeeds, when one evolves successfully along this line, then one respects oneself, and as one respects oneself so one can respect others. . . . If there is a valid and real attitude toward the self, that attitude will manifest as valid and real towards others. It is not that as ye judge so shall ye be judged, *but as you judge yourself so shall you judge others. . . .*" [10]

To gain satisfactions and, particularly, security is to have power in interpersonal relations. So far as one cannot do so, that is to be power-less, helpless. As will be seen later, anxiety is an instrumentality of the self. But the self comes into being because it is necessary that one's interests be focused into certain fields that "work;" that is, attain satisfaction and security. And it is necessary that one's interests be focused into certain fields that work "in the modification of activity in the interest of power in interpersonal relations." [11]

It is perhaps advisable at this point to emphasize that the power motive, although given originally in the human organism, is not a fixed entity. It is manifested in activity, usually, although not always, in an interpersonal situation.

To be noted also is the fact that the energy of the infant, or rather its manifestations in the power motive, become quickly modified or transformed. But to modify or to transform is not to destroy. Sullivan's theories of interpersonal behavior are,

[10] See p. 15.
[11] See p. 20.

therefore, rooted in biology. But, if one may use a somewhat crude metaphor, the root is not the full-grown tree. On the other hand, the tree depends on its roots for its very life. The energy of a human being, however transformed as to its expression by acculturation, is still, obviously, biological. There is continuity between the biological and the cultural. A human being is an acculturated biological organism.

However, in the course of psychiatric inquiry, one discovers that it is not a person *as an isolated and self-contained entity* that one is studying, or can study, but a situation, an interpersonal situation, composed of two or more people. The locus of the study has shifted, and with it the reference frame of the investigator, or "participant observer." Furthermore, while one may *describe* an interpersonal situation which one has studied as though one had been a detached observer, in the actual study one becomes a constituent element or part of that situation. One becomes a participant observer. And to explain what occurred in the situation, of which one is a part, one must invent a new terminology in order to convey the new reference frame of the study.

According to Sullivan, to speak about impulses, drives, striving toward goals, is to use a figure of speech necessitated by the structure of the language.[12] One never observes such impulses and drives. What one does observe is a situation "integrated" by two or more people, and manifesting certain recurring kinds of action and behavior. How is one to explain what occurs? In common everyday language, it is said that "A is striving toward so and so from B." This mode of speech seems to imply that there are certain ready-made, isolated impulses or needs in A which B can satisfy, but which existed completely independent of any influence from B. The traditional psychology postulated and termed these apparently preëxisting and independent drives as "instincts." In an almost mechanical union or accidental association, a "response" was

[12] See pp. 50–51.

evoked which satisfied and fulfilled such drives. The goals of human behavior were thought to be rather rigidly fixed by the nature of such self-contained, independent, predetermined, instincts. Whatever reciprocal interplay, interaction, occurred between A and B was thought to be more mechanical than transformative. But, according to Sullivan, what one observes is action in a situation between two people. "Action in a situation between two people" can be a misleading phrase because the two people acting in a certain way together, reciprocally, make the situation. Their mode of reciprocal action, interaction, defines the situation. That is what an interpersonal situation is, a mode of interaction of two or more people. That is, he believes, what one should study. Preëxisting, fixed drives do not explain an interpersonal situation, because they are not observed. The action in an interpersonal situation *is* observed, and it is *this* that explains whatever there may be of preëxisting tendency to act. Extensive observation and study of human behavior has shown that such behavior, within certain limits, is almost infinitely varied. This is another way of saying that it is malleable, fluid, changeable to an almost incalculable degree. Furthermore, interpersonal behavior does not occur, obviously, in a mechanical, rigidly stereotyped manner. To some extent, at any rate, it is continually changing, and not haphazardly but with apparent purpose. Interpersonal acts make an intelligible pattern, a somewhat fluid, changing pattern. They are in process of becoming something. They *are* a process. They have beginning, direction, ending. Since they are reciprocal, they are transformative. The interaction brings about something different, new. Because these acts are in process of change, instead of being rigidly fixed and predetermined or haphazardly and willy-nilly occurring, they can to some extent be redirected. Goals can, therefore, be redefined, modified, changed. Within the human situation, there is a possibility of creativeness, of discovering and inventing new goals, new purposes. Human behavior is amenable to intelligence.

It is, then, a person-integrated-in-a-situation-with-another-person-or-persons, an interpersonal situation, which one studies. The interpersonal situation it is which manifests the determinate characteristics. "Many situations are integrated in which A wants deference from B, and B, mirabile dictu, wants deference from A. It looks as if there were something in A and something in B that happened to collide. But when one studies the situation in which A and B pursue, respectively, the aim of getting from the other person what he himself needs, we find that it is not as simple as it looks. The *situation* is still the valid object of study, or rather that which we can observe; namely, the action which indicates the situation and the character of its integration." [13] In other words, it is inaccurate, unscientific to speak of a person-in-isolation-manifesting-this-or-that-tendency-or-drive. What one observes is a situation, "integrated" by two or more people. The situation is an interaction, an integration, or rather an integrated interaction of two or more people. Because all but one of the people may be "illusory" personifications, or inhabitants of dreamland or the imagination, the problem is more complicated. A loving person is one who, generally, when circumstances permit, integrates situations having the traits categorized as love. A hateful person is one who, when the opportunity offers, integrates situations having the traits categorized as hate or hateful. To have an impulse or drive is to have or manifest a tendency to action in some kind of interpersonal situation. Impulses and drives cohere in "dynamisms," relatively enduring configurations of energy, which manifest themselves in numerous ways in human situations. The traits which characterize interpersonal situations in which one is integrated describe what one is. Because any person integrates interpersonal situations having many different traits, to determine whether a person may, in everyday language, be called loving or hateful, "neurotic," "psychotic," or "normal" is not an easy problem. The problem

[13] See p. 5.

is attacked more directly in his discussion of *self-dynamisms* and *dissociation.* Generally speaking, personality is, with a qualification to be noted later, a function of the kinds of interpersonal situations a person integrates with others, whether real persons or fantastic personifications.

The quotation about observing the action which indicates the situation and the character of its integration might easily be misleading. If it is taken to mean that all one has to do is *merely* to observe, in a passive manner, an interpersonal situation in order to find out what occurs, then it is misleading. Interpersonal processes, like all events, do not occur with their meaning written all over them. A situation in order to be understood has to be interpreted.[14] Because much of human behavior occurs according to stereotyped patterns, and because one has, more or less unconsciously, socially predetermined, ready-made standards and criteria for interpreting and judging such behavior, one is inclined to assume that all one does is *look at* such behavior, and that its meaning is quite independent of an observer. Actually, if, *per impossible*, one had no standards, no theories, to judge what happens, human behavior, or any configuration of events, would be an unintelligible, chaotic jumble. Every observer brings a vast and complex set of rules and standards, socially inherited, to understand events. Therefore, while it is true one never observes goals or tendencies, or impulses, in a situation, one must postulate them. A person is born with a substratum of biological needs and potentialities. Human behavior, one must assume, is purposive.[15] The participant observer has certain theories and insights about human behavior, which he has learned from experience, whether direct or mediated through the experience of others. Those in-

[14] Introspection is notoriously inadequate for understanding what one is about; nevertheless a skillful participant observer probably finds it indispensable in presenting clues and hints as to human behavior.

[15] To avoid confusion, one must make a distinction between logical and psychiatric interpretation, but it does not seem necessary to go into that phase of the subject here.

sights guide him in interpreting and understanding any given situation. At the same time he is trying out these insights, testing them, as to their explanatory value in illuminating and clarifying interpersonal situations. Mistakes as to what is significant and relevant are made, but a skillful observer learns to correct or at least take account of them. Psychiatric observation is progressive. It is also self-corrective, because the investigator learns that some "insights" are irrelevant, and have to be discarded for others which are more illuminating and which organize the data more satisfactorily. What is more illuminating for explaining and solving interpersonal problems is also progressively determined more precisely and accurately.

It is hoped that enough has been said to indicate that what is observed is not given ready at hand. The observer must interpret what he observes. His interpretations will be guided by his knowledge and skill. But his knowledge and skill will depend partly on his own automatic and spontaneous elaboration of his own experience and partly on subsequent elaboration from colleagues in the same and related fields. Finally, his own alertness on the occasion as to what rôle he is playing in the situation fixes the limits as to what he observes. And his alertness in the therapeutic situation, in which he participates—that is, integrates with the patient—will be determined by his own self-system.

However, according to Sullivan, one can do too much interpreting. He says: "The supply of interpretations, like that of advice, greatly exceeds the need for them. Every patient has enough of his own misinterpretations and may well be spared the uncritical autistic reveries of his physician. At the same time, some interpretations are indispensable, if therapeutic results are to be achieved in a reasonable length of time. The first test for any interpretation should be as to its adequacy: does it cover the data to which it is applied? The second test should be as to its exclusiveness: are there other equally plausible hypotheses that cover the data? If so, the proposed interpretation justifies no presumption of its validity and, in general, it should not be offered." [16]

Interpersonal situations are self-resolving processes. Otherwise, what is manifestly impossible would occur, a person would become transfixed in a situation. A change which is satisfaction-giving or tributary to security occurs. Since interpersonal situations are a system or configuration of processes, they are fluid, dynamic—they move on, so to speak. By appropriate action some "dynamic component" in each person is discharged or resolved. However as they pass into the history of the persons involved, they do not vanish without a trace. Their effects, to however small a degree, remain as a memory, whether conscious or not, and a potentiality for similar situations in the future.[17]

In passing it seems desirable to mention what will be discussed more fully in the exposition of the *self-system*, *selective inattention*, and *dissociation*. There may be, and frequently are, two or three kinds of dynamic component or impulse discharged in an interpersonal situation. One is the kind which occurs within the awareness of the person or persons; another occurs outside of awareness, unwittingly, "dissociated" or "selectively inattended." [18]

Before one can begin to understand Sullivan's theories of interpersonal relations, there are two or three concepts about the "epoch" of infancy which have to be grasped. These are *empathy*, the *parataxic*, and the *autistic*, which is a sub-species of the parataxic.

According to Ducasse, "empathy" is a word coined by Titchener to translate the German *einfühlung*.[19] For Sullivan, empathy refers to "the peculiar emotional linkage that subtends the relationship of the infant with the other significant

[16] See p. 187.
[17] See p. 51.
[18] See p. 52.
[19] Ducasse, Curt John, The Philosophy of Art; New York, Lincoln MacVeagh, Dial Press, 1929; (v and 314 pp.)—in particular p. 151.

people—the mother or the nurse." [20] It exists long before there is any understanding by the infant of emotional expression. Empathy is said to be an "emotional contagion or communion" between the infant and the significant adult. Sullivan assumes its greatest importance is perhaps from the age of six to twenty-seven months.[21] Because the attitudes and behavior of the mother or nurse are socially conditioned, the concept of empathy is very important for understanding acculturation. However, although the fact itself may be well-established, it is not explained. Two examples of this emotional contagion or communion are given.[22] One is of a mother who hates the pregnancy and looks with disfavor upon or deplores her offspring. When this happens there are great feeding difficulties. The other is of a mother who, although deeply attached to the infant, suffers a fright or gets worried about something around nursing time. On this occasion also there are feeding difficulties or the infant has indigestion. Whether or not this is a *post hoc ergo propter hoc* will have to be established by further study of infants. He seems to imply, however, that it is closely connected with, or related to, biological states. He says: "It is biological for the infant when nourished to show certain expressive movements which we call the satisfaction-response, and it is probably biological for the parent concerned to be delighted to see these things. Due to the empathic linkage, this, the reaction of the parent to the satisfaction-response of the infant, communicates good feeling to the infant and thus he learns that this response has power." [23] And this, he adds, may be considered the primitive root of human generosity, the satisfaction in giving satisfaction and pleasure. When *anxiety* and the *self-dynamism* or *self-system* are discussed it will be seen that empathy is a very important concept for understanding the theory of the self.

[20] See p. 17.
[21] See p. 17.
[22] See p. 16.
[23] See p. 17.

The concepts of the *prototaxic*, the *parataxic*, and the *autistic* are extraordinarily difficult to grasp and to formulate.[24] They are symbol activities. But as Sullivan uses the term, anything which stands for something else, or is a sign of something else, is a symbol. For example, in prototaxic symbol activities, a concept which will be discussed more fully at a more convenient place in the exposition, the mother's nipple represents, *in a vague way*, the Good Mother, as opposed to another representation, or "proto-concept" of the Bad Mother.[25] Prototaxic symbolization lacks formal distinctions. It lacks distinctions of time and space, of before and after, of here and there. Here a qualification is necessary. To say that the prototaxic lacks the distinction of before and after means that *no connection* is established. The infant vaguely feels or "prehends" earlier and later states without realizing any serial connection. Furthermore, prototaxic symbolization occurs without reference to an ego, to "I" or "me," because the infant has no, or only a rudimentary, self. As will be seen later, the prototaxic is chiefly related to the basis of memory, and can be described as instantaneous records of total situations.

Parataxic symbolization succeeds the first, the prototaxic. As the infant develops, he gradually learns to make some discrimination between himself and the rest of the world. He no longer reaches out from his nurse's arms to touch the full moon. Gradually he learns to shrink to life size. And he gradually learns to make elementary distinctions. His symbol activity now makes distinctions of a rudimentary sort.

"We learn in infancy," Sullivan says, "that objects which our distance receptors, our eyes and ears, for example, encounter, are of a quite different order of relationship from things which our tactile or our gustatory receptors encounter. That which one has in one's mouth so that one can taste it, while it

[24] The term "prototaxic" does not appear in Sullivan's published lectures. The concept of the parataxic as previously formulated is much narrower in range than the formulation conveyed orally to the writer.

[25] See pp. 78–79.

may be regurgitated to the distress of everyone is still in a very different relationship than is the full moon which one encounters through one's eye but can in no sense manage." [26]

With the development of the parataxic mode of symbol activity, the original undifferentiated wholeness, oneness, of experience is broken. But the "parts," the diverse aspects, the various kinds of experience are not related or connected in any logical fashion. Various experiences just happen together, or not, as the case may be. They are concomitant. The young one cannot yet relate his experiences to one another or make any logical distinctions among them. Expressed in another way, experiences which are related to one another are felt only as being concomitant. The young one can neither connect nor contrast his experiences. Of course, he feels no need of rigid distinctions. Later on he will learn them from the significant others in his environment. What is experienced is implicitly assumed, and certainly without reflection, to be the "natural" way of such occurrences, without question or comparison. As in the prototaxic, since no connections or relations are established, there is no movement of "thought." The symbolical activity is not a step-by-step process. Inferences cannot be made. Experience is undergone as momentary, unconnected organismic states.[27] The parataxic is that which is recurrent in the prototaxic.

Eyes and ears become increasingly important. Parataxic symbols are evoked mainly through visual and auditory channels.

As has already been mentioned, the autistic is a subspecies of the parataxic. The autistic is a verbal manifestation of the parataxic. It is explained thus: "The ability to make articulate noises and the ability to pick phonemal stations in vocal sound—that is, the peculiar ones of a continuum of sounds which are used in the forming of words, which varies, incidentally, from language to language—the ability, as I say, to learn phonemes, to

[26] See p. 34.

[27] Dreams are typical examples of parataxic thinking.

connect them into syllables and words, is inborn. That is given in the human organism. The original usage of these phonemal stations, syllables, words, however, is magical, as witness the 'ma' and as witness, for example, any of you who have a child who has been promised on a certain birthday a pony. As you listen to the child talk about the pony you realize perhaps sadly that twenty-five years from now when he talks about ponies, pony will not have a thousandth of the richness of personal meaning that pony has for him now. The word of the child is autistic, it has a highly individual meaning. And the process of learning language habits consists to a great extent, once one has got a vocabulary, in getting a meaning to each particular term which is useful in communication. None of us succeeds completely in this; some of us do not succeed noticeably."[28]

Read superficially, the passage seems inconsistent. He began by saying that the autistic belonged to the infant and ended by talking about the child. But this is how he distinguishes between what he calls the epoch of infancy and the epoch of childhood. When the infant learns the rudiments of language, he passes into the epoch of childhood.[29]

The symbol activity is arbitrary, highly personal, unchecked, untested, and necessarily so because of the child's limited equipment and experience with the symbol activity and experience of others. The capacity for verbal communication is only beginning to manifest itself and its tools are scarcely formed or realized. In Sullivan's language, consensual validation is lacking. In popular language, the imagination of the child runs riot, unchecked and undisciplined by "reality."

Another example will perhaps disclose the meaning and significance of the autistic more fully. Take the illustration of a child who has been presented with a picture book containing printed matter. There is, for example, a picture of a cat, below which there is written what the child later learns as c-a-t.

[28] See pp. 18–19.
[29] See p. 18.

The animal who runs around the house also is referred to by the same name as the colored or black and white pattern in the book. Sullivan goes on to discuss the significance of this:

"I am sure no child who can learn has not noticed an enormous discrepancy between this immobile representation in the book which, perhaps, resembles one of the momentary states that kitty has been in on some occasion. I am certain that every child knows that there is something very strange in this printed representation being so closely connected with the same word that seems to cover adequately the troublesome, amusing, and very active pet. Yet, because of unnumbered, sometimes subtle, sometimes crude experiences with the carrier of culture, the parent, the child finally comes to accept as valid and useful a reference to the picture as 'kitty' and to the creature as 'kitty.'

"The child thus learns some of the more complicated implications of a symbol in contradistinction to the actuality to which the symbol refers, which is its referent; in other words, the distinction between the symbol and that which is symbolized. This occurs, however, before verbal formulation is possible.

"From the picture book and the spoken word in this culture one progresses to the printed word and finally discovers that the combination of signs, c-a-t, includes 'kitty' in some miraculous fashion, and that it always works. There is nothing like consistent experience to impress one with the validity of an idea. So one comes to a point where printed words, with or without consensually valid meaning, come to be very important in one's growth or acquaintance with the world.

"There was first the visually and otherwise impressive pet, which was called 'kitty' (an associated vocalization); then came the picture of the kitten; now comes the generic c-a-t which includes kitty, picture of kitten, a kitten doll, and alley cats seen from the windows. And all this is learnt so easily that —since no one troubles to point it out—there is no lucid understanding of the sundry types of reality and reference that are being experienced. Familiarity breeds indifference, in this case. The possibilities for confusion in handling the various kinds of symbols, naturally, remain quite considerable." [30]

Consensually validated symbols carry a meaning which has been acquired from group activities, interpersonal activities, social experience.[31] They represent some degree of differentiation which can be consensually validated, and agreed upon by one's compeers. Autistic activity may use the socially inherited symbols, language, but it gives to them a unique and personal meaning. The meaning is determined by the personal experience of the child, *not* by the society which created them. The spontaneous feeling and imagination of the child invests the symbols, whether words or pictures, with a content that is determined by his own needs and experience, *not* by the requirements of the significant adults. But on the other hand, it is to meet with, and conform to, the requirements of the significant adults, for the purpose of gaining satisfactions and maintaining security, that the self is evolved.

Gradually, of course, the child learns something of the shared meaning of language. He must. But the autistic meaning is not thereby destroyed. Words, language, thus come to have a double meaning. In fact most people manifest a confused blend of both. This helps considerably for one to maintain a wide margin of misinformation and illusion. Autistic symbols, and, more generally, parataxic symbols are, among other things, peculiarly adopted for maintaining a type of activity later discussed under 'multiple me-you patterns." But, on the other hand, they are also well adapted for another type of activity, the creative.

Empathy, parataxic and autistic activity, and anxiety, a term whose meaning will become clear later, are fundamental to the origin and development of the self-dynamism. *Dynamism*

[30] See p. 35.

[31] Consensually validated symbol activity has more recently been called "syntaxic" thinking by Sullivan. It involves an appeal to principles which are accepted as true by the hearer.

has been defined as "*a relatively enduring configuration of energy which manifests itself in characterizable processes in interpersonal relations.* It is to be preferred to 'mental mechanism,' 'psychic system,' 'conative tendency,' and the like, because it implies only *relatively enduring capacity to bring about change*, and not some fanciful substantial engines, regional organizations, or peculiar more or less physiological apparatus about which our present knowledge is nil." [32] The self-dynamism is a process or a configuration—that is, a structure—of processes. *Self-dynamism, self-system*, and *self* are employed to express the same meaning. So the self is not a fixed entity, but a configuration of interpersonal processes. It seems well to emphasize that the self is always related to interpersonal relations.

Restraints on the child's freedom, necessary for his socialization, bring about the evolution of the self-dynamism. In this evolution there are also developed other, and no less important aspects of the personality, those which occur outside clear awareness, the *dissociated* and the *selectively inattended*. The *personality* includes all of them.

As previously noted, the infant—like certain animals—has a peculiar sensitivity to something which occurs in his immediate environment. This was called empathy. He could somehow feel the warm approval and delight of the mother in his expressive, expansive movements, called the satisfaction-response. Of course, this does not mean that he understood what happened, in the usual sense. He felt it. One might say that he felt the warm approval of the mother by means of the empathic linkage, but this does not add very much because no one seems to know anything much about this mode of communication. Nevertheless the good feeling, the warm, approving attitude of the mother was so communicated that his sense of well-being, his euphoria, was increased. At another

[32] Sullivan, Harry Stack, Psychiatry: Introduction to the Study of Interpersonal Relations. PSYCHIATRY (1938) 1:121–134; p. 123, footnote 3.

time, on the occasion of his crying, or not going to sleep, when the mother is perhaps irritated or tired, she manifests annoyance, displeasure, perhaps strong disapproval or anger. Again the mother's attitude is communicated. This time, of course, it is not warm approval. It is perhaps strong disapproval. And the infant feels the disapproval. Now his sense of well-being markedly decreases. The disapproval assures discomfort. The infant feels discomfort. To speak generally, expressions of approval from the mother or nurse increase the infant's state of well-being; expressions of disapproval, of dissatisfaction with the infant's performance, decrease his sense of well-being, arousing discomfort.[33] An important item to note here is that this occurs long before he can understand the meaning of what happens.

As the infant grows older, the mother begins deliberate training. For example, she trains him in the "proper" toilet habits, those considered proper by the culture she lives in. Not only that, but the time she begins to do so will probably be determined by what her culture considers the right time to begin training the young. Now training involves disapproval of some acts of the infant, and approval of others. Certain performances of the infant bring disapproval; others, approval. This is another way of saying certain performances result in a decrease of his good feeling, state of well-being; others, an increase. Gradually, the young one "catches on." He learns why, at first probably in a dim way, his sense of well-being, can decrease or increase. Sooner or later he learns that certain performances bring discomfort; other, a comforting state of well-being, good feeling. One might say that here he first dimly learns the relationship of cause and effect, although, no doubt, he is not yet much given to logical analysis. Of course, when the mother's, or the nurse's, attitudes are inconsistent, he has a bigger problem. And, it seems safe to say, no one's attitudes are always consistent. No one's behavior is rigidly

[33] See pp. 19–20.

consistent. In other words, the infant early learns, or at least feels, some of the inconsistencies of the significant people in his environment; that is, he early learns, or feels, some of the inconsistencies of the culture in which he will grow. It is an easy inference that the fewer inconsistencies, the more rapid will be his acculturation.

The first step presumably was somehow to note the referential relation of his acts, his behavior, to increase or diminution of his sense of well-being. As the infant becomes more educable, he is subjected to more numerous and more varied instances of approval and disapproval. Sooner or later, the young one perceives the disapproval or approval of the mother or nurse, while he previously only felt it. As his observation improves, his grasp on the patterns of action approved and disapproved becomes more refined. Gradually he has learned that when this kind of discomfort is present and something is done which brings approval and approbation, the discomfort is softened, assuaged, or banished.

The child learns to focus his attention not only on behavior which brings approval and approbation, but also on that which brings disapproval, so as to be better able to avoid it. He must, in order to achieve good feeling and avoid discomfort. Thus he learns to be alert to signs of approval and disapproval. His attention becomes concentrated on noticing signs of approval and disapproval. And out of this alertness to approval and disapproval, the self is first evolved. Thus, Sullivan says: "The self-dynamism is built up out of this experience of approbation and disapproval, of reward and punishment. The peculiarity of the self-dynamism is that as it grows it functions, in accordance with its state of development, right from the start. As it develops, it becomes more and more related to a microscope in its function. Since the approbation of the important person is very valuable, since disapprobation denies satisfaction and gives anxiety, the self becomes extremely important. It permits a minute focus on those performances of the child which are the cause of approbation and disapprobation, but, very much like a microscope, it interferes with noticing the rest of the world. When you are staring through your microscope, you don't see much except what comes through that channel. So with the self-dynamism. It has a tendency to focus attention on performances with the significant other person which get approbation or disfavor. And that peculiarity, closely connected with anxiety, persists thenceforth through life. It comes about that the self, that to which we refer when we say 'I,' is the only thing which has alertness, which notices what goes on, and, needless to say, notices what goes on in its own field. The rest of the personality gets along outside awareness. Its impulses, its performances are not noted." [34]

What is *anxiety?* In popular usage, it has various and obscure meanings. Anxiety has its origin in the discomfort felt by the infant at the empathized disapproval of the adult.[35] Stated in another way, the loss of euphoria—which is synonymous with a feeling of intense discomfort, due to the empathized disapproval—is, at a later stage, with the appearance of the self, called anxiety. Perhaps needless to say, when considerable hostility is felt, the infant undergoes acute suffering, without, of course, understanding what is happening to him. This capacity, under appropriate circumstances, to experience what is later called anxiety, endures without diminution throughout life. But as one grows older, one learns, if only in a dim way, how to avoid at least most situations which arouse anxiety. The avoidance of anxiety may, and usually does, occur outside clear awareness. Those who acquire facility in dealing with people learn that most situations are not threatening, or at least not to the extent which would evoke a degree of anxiety comparable to the discomfort felt in early life. In most people, to greater or lesser degree, knowledge triumphs over anxiety. But the capacity for experiencing a discomfort as intense as the original

[34] See pp. 20–21.
[35] See pp. 19–20.

remains. With the growth of the self, understanding also grows. There is some understanding of the relation of one's behavior to the feeling of acute discomfort, anxiety. At least some of the anxiety-provoking factors in the environment can be discriminated. The feeling of discomfort is now localized as in oneself. Nor is the whole environment threatening. There is refinement of meaning. The discomfort is no longer cosmic. A discrimination of oneself and the outside world has occurred, and with it, some discrimination about anxiety. Anxiety is an universal experience, although, of course, varying from person to person both as to intensity and the precise conditions for its occurrence.

The self limits and restricts awareness, and does it by means of anxiety.[36] There are two ways of interpreting anxiety. When something happens which is not welcome to the self, is not in harmony with the earlier experiences of approval and disapproval, anxiety occurs. The appearance of anxiety completely distracts attention so that one does not notice what occurs. Stated in another way, anxiety is the person's inner experience of the self-dynamism functioning so as to restrict or confuse one's awareness and prevent him from noticing and clearly understanding something which occurs. Usually the mere threat of anxiety, the mere possibility, the mere warning sign, of an occurrence not congenial to the self, is sufficient to bring about behavior calculated to avoid the experience, or prevent awareness of its significance. Anxiety restricts not only one's acts, but also one's conscious thoughts in the same way. One does not think, at least not clearly, of matters uncongenial to the self. And if a person is given to fantasy, it is certain that the fantasy will not be interpreted in a manner uncongenial to the self.

The learning of language greatly facilitates and enhances the development of the self. For the infant, the mode of communication from the outer world was empathy. The child at

[36] See p. 21.

first learns to use words, in a highly autistic way, of course, but they enable him gradually better to "catch on" to what occurs in his immediate environment. He has not yet lost the power of empathy,[37] but language is a better instrument for conveying what is expected of him, what is approved and disapproved. Thus language goes far to complete what empathy began, the person's acculturation.[38]

It is inherent in the nature of the self to facilitate and restrict its further growth in such a way as to maintain the direction and characteristics given to it in infancy and childhood. Experiences of approbation and disapprobation occur long before one can think, long before one has acquired the use of language and all that it implies for the purposes of socialization. To be unable to think, that is, logically or syntaxically, is to be unable to discriminate the meaning of what occurs. The earliest attitudes, therefore, which one learns, and also the most pervasive and "deep-seated," are acquired literally, unthinkingly. Besides the infant's biological helplessness, he is also spiritually or psychologically helpless. The young one must, therefore, accept the attitudes and codes of behavior of the significant others, not only because he depends on them for life itself but because he has no, or only incipient, ability to think, and no, or only rudimentary, social experience. The attitudes and codes of the significant others, therefore, are accepted, necessarily without criticism or discrimination. The question of their validity cannot readily occur to him. This is another way of saying they have for him a character of inevitability, unquestionability. He has not yet acquired the ability and experience to question and compare. What happens, therefore, is neither

[37] See p. 17: "We do not know much about the fate of empathy in the developmental history of people in general. There are indications that it endures throughout life, at least in some people. There are few unmistakable instances of its function in most of us, however, in our later years. . . ."

[38] The visual and auditory channels are also of considerable importance but as yet only obscurely understood. Facial expression, tone of voice, gestures are sometimes more effective than what is said.

right nor wrong, fitting nor unfitting; it just *is*. It happens.[39]

So it happens that the "facilitations and deprivations by the parents and significant others are the source of the material which is built into the self, because through the control of personal awareness the self itself from the beginning facilitates and restricts its further growth." The facilitations and deprivations in infancy and childhood are, usually, sufficiently consistent to give the self-dynamism a start in a certain direction. Although the parents or significant others are by no means always perfectly consistent in their behavior, their approval of some acts, and disapproval of others will tend to remain during a given period of development fairly constant. It is, therefore, the parents and significant others, brothers or sisters or nurse, who determine the nature of the self-dynamism. This is so because it is self-perpetuating, "tends very strongly to maintain the direction and characteristics given to it in infancy and childhood."[40]

In order to explain *dissociation*, it is necessary first to introduce the concept of *selective inattention*.[41] Selective inattention is a process whereby certain experiences and actions are not clearly noted or appraised, if they are noted at all. The person pays no attention to their character or significance. His attention has to be recalled before he is able to pay heed to them. Sullivan claims that selective inattention is the most frequent manifestation of the restriction of awareness. It is one of the ways by which the self dynamism hinders educative experience which is not in harmony with its current organization. In other words, when certain experiences and actions are tinged with anxiety, the person does not clearly note them, or their character and significance, because to do so would be to be confronted with the possibility or necessity of change. Sometimes in the course of an interview, when the therapist

[39] In other words, he is as yet limited to parataxic experience.

[40] See p. 21.

[41] The explicit formulation of *selective inattention* is not found in Sullivan's published lectures. It was communicated orally to the writer.

directly refers to something which is selectively inattended, one of two things may happen. Either a "security operation" is provoked—that is, something is provoked which functions so as to minimize anxiety—or severe anxiety results. And in the latter case, the therapist now has the problem of conserving the doctor-patient relationship. From one point of view, the difference between selective inattention and dissociation is one of degree as "measured" by the accessibility to conscious discriminated awareness of an experience or an overt action.

Dissociated dynamisms not only exist outside awareness but ordinarily are not accessible to the self.[42] Experiences and behavior which, because of selective inattention, are not discriminated—that is, occur outside awareness—when, for example, they are indicated by a friend, can be brought into awareness, accepted by the self. This cannot happen in the case of dissociation. If the friend were to point out, or call one's attention to, dissociated behavior no such expansion of awareness can easily occur. The result of the friend's efforts is very likely to arouse anxiety, followed by anger and heated denial.

The processes by which dissociation occurs are not formulated. All that one can say is the dissociated has been rejected by the self. In other words, those dynamisms to which the self refuses awareness and recognition, except under the impact of extraordinary influences, are dissociated. Processes existing outside awareness because of selective inattention can without great difficulty be reintegrated into the self because they do not imply any immediate considerable change as to basic direction and characteristics of the self. But dissociated dynamisms, once they are recognized by the self, involve an immediate and perhaps great alteration in the basic direction and characteristics of the self. In other words, the recognition and discrimination of previously dissociated dynamisms, imply a change, fre-

[42] See p. 22. The discussion of dissociation in *The Conceptions* is likely to be misleading because there is no differentiation of processes due to selective inattention.

quently a profound change, in the sorts of interpersonal relations in which one will be integrated. The pattern of future life is altered. By the reintegration of dissociated dynamisms, there is made necessary an extensive change in personality.[43]

With one exception, the self limits and restricts awareness. The exception is that of certain gifted people who can think within the field of awareness without consciousness of self, of "I," which is ordinarily the center of what goes on. A scientist can become absorbed in what he is doing, be clearly aware of some problem or activity, yet "forget" about himself, his "ego," and all the usual apparatus of self-consciousness.[44] Most people, however, are much too busy maintaining security and warding off anxiety to become aware of anything in an unself-conscious manner. Their waking hours are completely taken with activities which are strongly colored by a need for "success."

The result is that:

"Our awareness of our performances, and our awareness of the performances of others are permanently restricted to a part of all that goes on and the structure and character of that part is determined by our early training; its limitation is maintained year after year by our experiencing anxiety whenever we tend to overstep the margin.

"Needless to say, limitations and peculiarities of the self may interfere with the pursuit of biologically necessary satisfactions. When this happens, the person is to that extent mentally ill. Similarly, they may interfere with security, and to that extent also the person is mentally ill."

The peculiarity of the self is such that it may be said to be made up of *reflected appraisals*.[45] The child appraises himself as he is appraised by the significant adults. He lacks the expe-

[43] See pp. 142–143. At this point in the reference Sullivan is discussing the schizophrenic person, but the remarks about dissociation apply in some degree to everyone.

[44] This observation is also not found in Sullivan's published papers and was communicated orally to the writer.

[45] See p. 22.

rience and equipment necessary for a careful and dispassionate evaluation of himself. He has no guide except what he has learned from the significant adults. His evaluation of himself is, therefore, based on the appraisals of the significant adults. There may be no, or very little, conflicting data about his performances which would cause him to question the appraisals of those who take care of him. And in any case, he is far too helpless to question or revolt, because he depends on them for life itself. Therefore, he is not in a position to risk his security by doubting, challenging, questioning the treatment of others, even if he could doubt or question. He tends passively to accept the judgments, first conveyed empathically, and now by words, and gestures, and deeds, as to his worth. He "naturally," inevitably, feels his worth to be what the significant adults, conditioned by their own life-experience, find it to be. If an unwanted child meets with hostility and derogation from the significant adults, he appraises, he feels, his worth to be what they find it to be. He acquires a hostile and derogatory self. And as one respects or disrespects oneself, so one respects or disrespects others. The child from then on, in this case, will tend to be hostile and derogatory toward everyone. But since unremitting hostility toward others is dangerous to his security, it may have to be disguised, perhaps masked from himself and others by a great show of friendliness.[46] However, people who are good observers, or who are themselves secure in their relations with others, will not be long deceived, because such hostility will betray itself in unwitting behavior.

It must not be understood that the self-dynamism is synonymous with momentary self-awareness, of one's awareness of "I" at any given instant. The self-dynamism is not static; it is a configuration of processes. It has background and foreground, a before and after. Nor is it discontinuous with the rest of the personality. There are marginal processes which

[46] In another instance, the hostility may be dissociated.

merge the self with the dissociated. These marginal processes are frequently manifested just before one 'drops off' to sleep, or before one becomes clearly awake. For purposes of exposition, it seemed necessary sharply to distinguish the focal awareness of the self, but actually it fades imperceptibly into those marginal processes of awareness.

Anxiety tends strongly to preclude the experience of anything which might correct or modify the direction of growth of the self, whose organization represents the stabilizing influence of past experience. The self, by means of anxiety, controls and circumscribes awareness, thus inhibiting the learning of anything radically new and different. Even when the self is a derogatory and hateful system it will inhibit and misinterpret any dissociated feeling or experience of friendliness towards others; and it will misinterpret any gestures of friendliness from others. The direction and characteristics given to the self in infancy and childhood are maintained year after year, at an extraordinary cost, so that most people in this culture, and presumably in any other, because of inadequate and unfortunate experience in early life, become "inferior caricatures of what they might have been."[47] Not only the family, but various other cultural institutions less directly, all combine, more or less unwittingly, to produce this effect.

But the controlling, limiting function of the self is not absolute. As will be seen later, certain vital needs of the organism may, if thwarted by the self, prove too powerful even for the inhibitions of the self. And all people retain some capacity for change. Children, particularly, as they grow older, sometimes retain a considerable amount of plasticity, a certain capacity for acquiring new experience, even if not in harmony with the self. School can, in the early years, furnish some corrective experience. A kind and lovable teacher may undo, somewhat, the bad effects of a destructive parent. And *vice versa*, a de-

[47] See p. 56.

structive teacher can slow, or diminish the good effects of a kind and loving parent.[48]

There is a more or less precarious equilibrium maintained between the self and dissociated processes. Under extraordinary influences, some dissociated functions can be readmitted into the self, become integrated in the self. In fact, the self of "normal" people can exist and maintain its autonomy *only* by virtue of activities in sleep and unnoticed reverie, and waking behavior. In the schizophrenic state, the self-system, although unable to prevent the eruption into awareness of dissociated tendencies, cannot absorb them, cannot integrate them, and in general disowns them. These irresistible, formerly dissociated dynamisms, maintain an autonomy independent of the self. The result is that instead of anxiety there is fear and often terror. The conflict-provoking tendencies are accorded independent personality.[49]

It must not be thought that dissociation is necessarily a mark of very serious disorder of personality. In certain circumstances, tendencies in the self, which become unacceptable, are then gradually dissociated. Processes acceptable in infancy, for example, may at a later stage, be disapproved by the significant adults and become dissociated.[50] Phrased in another way, tendencies previously congenial to the self, now arouse anxiety and are blotted out of awareness. So the significant others determine not only the kind of self, but also the dissociated.

There is another point which is highly significant in a theory of the self. It is said that a "selecting and organizing factor determines what part of these observed judgments [51] of one's personal value, what of the information that one secures

[48] See pp. 39–40.

[49] See p. 142. At this point in the reference Sullivan is discussing the schizophrenic person, but the remarks about dissociation apply in some degree to everyone.

[50] See p. 46.

[51] . . . of praise and blame from parents, teachers, friends, and other significantly related people.

through secondary channels (*e.g.*, reading), and which of the deductions and inferences that occur in one's thinking, shall be incorporated into the self." [52] From this statement it might seem that there is a factor intrinsic to the self, maintaining its autonomy despite all the vicissitudes of experience. It is clear, however, that Sullivan does not mean that, because the self is made up of reflected appraisals, and tends very strongly to maintain the direction and characteristics given to it in infancy and childhood. To say that there is a selecting and organizing factor in the self is only another way of saying that the self-dynamism by means of anxiety selects and organizes the conditions for its further growth, both as to direction and characteristics, in order to maintain the direction and characteristics given to it in infancy and childhood. However, it will be seen later that there is an intrinsic biological tendency or "factor" in the organism, which is directed toward maintaining or achieving mental health.

The structure of the self-system is such that it is capable of manifesting many different "me-you patterns" in different interpersonal situations or even in the same situation.[53] Not only does the self-system generate, in an interpersonal context, of course, these "me-you patterns," but it limits them qualitatively to what is congenial to it.[54] Stated in a different way, the self-system is *the limit*, the containing manifold, the enveloping matrix of the "me-you patterns." Furthermore, the personality, the hypothetical entity postulated in order to make *all* one's behavior intelligible, is the limit of the self-system.

If a person exhibited multiple "me-you patterns" always only in different interpersonal situations, it might seem that they must be objectively justified. For example, if a person is hostile toward *A*, affectionate toward *B*, fearful toward *C*, one might assume that the person is objectively justified because *A*

[52] Reference footnote 32; p. 123.

[53] For the purposes of the paper, "same situation" may be considered as one where there is no change of real persons, or of place, or interruption of time.

[54] Reference footnote 32; pp. 122–132.

may be hostile, *B*, lovable, *C*, destructive. But when the person manifests different attitudes, hostility, affection, fear, indicative of the different "me-you patterns," in the same interpersonal situation, say, with *A*, the problem gets more complicated. Where now is the locus of the objective situation? And when *A*'s reactions are not "congruent"—that is, when, for example, *A* reacts with hostility toward the affectionate person—then the problem gets even more complicated.

To account for these varying or multiple "me-you patterns," Sullivan has formulated the concept of the parataxic.[55] Suppose a patient comes to a psychiatrist, having been recommended by the family physician. The psychiatrist is otherwise unknown to the patient. Furthermore, suppose the patient believes the psychiatrist is hostile or wishes to humiliate him. The psychiatrist, who, one may assume, is a kindly and affectionate person, knows that the situation does not justify such a reaction. In other words, he knows he is not hostile to the patient, who is a stranger to him. How can the patient's reaction be explained? People do not assume without cause that the other person, or persons, integrated in a situation are hostile. However "irrational" human behavior may seem, one can discover causes for it.

The actual situation, as understood and felt by the patient, is parataxic. The patient is reliving, or is integrated in, the situation in terms of an earlier situation. Here the rôle of parataxic symbol activity is obvious. Consensually validated symbols cannot be effectively employed because they are based on, and require, carefully formulated, discriminated, and validated distinctions. Multiple "me-you patterns" can occur only when carefully formulated, discriminated, validated distinctions are *not* made. Of course the patient believes, at least on a conscious level, that he is making valid distinctions, but that is no proof of anything. Actually he is forced, unwittingly, to

[55] See p. 92 and reference footnote 32; p. 126, footnote. This is an earlier formulation and much narrower in range, but it is quite consistent with the recent one. The former is an instance of the latter.

employ the earlier modes of symbol activity which lack clear-cut distinctions based on carefully formulated discriminations of experience. Great masses of early experiences can therefore be carried over and relived, or revoked, without fundamental alteration and expressed in subsequent interpersonal situations by means of prototaxic and parataxic symbols. Thus "new situations" can be lived parataxically. In this case the patient has carried over into the present situation a mode of interpersonal behavior justified by, or adequate to, an earlier situation, or situations, where the significant people were hostile and did ridicule him. The patient has a hostile and derogatory self—why? Because his experience, or a great part of it, with the significant people who took care of him in early life, taught him, convinced him, that he was a person to be ridiculed, ill-treated, abused. And since he consequently dislikes, or even hates himself, even though he may partially disguise it from himself and others, he must therefore dislike, or be hostile toward others. It is therefore quite natural, inevitable, for him to expect hostility in the new situation, one which is for him closely on the model of earlier situations.

Now most people are not so unfortunate as to meet with unalloyed hostility from the significant adults who cared for them in early life. Usually children experience a mixture of attitudes, affection, indifference, as well as hostility, although one kind of experience may, and usually does, predominate. Their experiences are varied and contradictory. Hence they are raised with contradictory, or at least inconsistent, attitudes about themselves, and therefore about others. It is not surprising, therefore, that their interpersonal behavior is erratic, is inconsistent. It is not surprising, on the contrary it is inevitable, that a person's behavior may be at one time lovable, at another, hostile, and still again, indifferent toward another. By means of selective inattention, attitudes and occurrences not favorable to the prevailing "me-you pattern" are not discriminated.[56]

[56] It seems reasonable to assume that parataxic symbols are an instrumentality of selective inattention.

This accounts for the multiple "me-you patterns" in an interpersonal situation.

When one kind of experience, say love, predominates, the person has generally, when circumstances permit, a loving attitude toward himself and others. A "me-you pattern" characterized by love will predominate in his relations with others. This is another way of saying that he will tend to integrate loving interpersonal relationships. The "me-you patterns" characterized by hostility or indifference will occur less frequently because hostility or indifference is less powerfully imbedded in the self system and in the whole personality. The person is less inclined to act with hostility or indifference. His self, in order to maintain the basic direction and characteristics given to it in infancy and childhood, is, in the main, conditioned toward integrating loving relationships. When a loving person becomes integrated in hostile or derogatory relationships, the basic direction and characteristics of his self, which is a loving one, become threatened. Anxiety may intervene and disintegrate such relationships. In everyday language, a loving person does not want, as a general rule, to get involved with prevailingly hostile or prevailingly destructive people, that is, those who cannot love. The loving person, one who has respect for himself and others, one for whom the satisfaction and security of his friend, the loved one, are equally important, or nearly so, as are his own, knows that love, the genuine solicitude for the other fellow's well-being and happiness, is by far the best way, the only adequate way, to obtain, or maintain, his own satisfactions and security.

Personality is the hypothetical entity postulated "to account for the doings of people, one with another, and with more or less personified objects." [57] It "is made manifest in interpersonal situations, and not otherwise." [58] It is the most inclusive category of interpersonal behavior, including not only the self

[57] Reference footnote 32; p. 121.
[58] Reference footnote 32; p. 121.

system, with its multiple "me-you pattern," but also what exists outside awareness because of selective inattention or dissociation. As analysis will reveal, it is the reservoir of creative activity and original thought. From the personality, the self system can, under appropriate circumstances, obtain enrichment for a deeper and wider awareness. In an ideal psychiatrist the self would be coterminous with personality.[59] Needless to say there are no ideal persons because there are no ideal cultures.

It might seem that the personality compensates for the limitations of the self by accepting and maintaining dissociated tendency systems. And this is so, with a qualification. Since by definition dissociated tendencies exist outside awareness, they cannot be deliberately noted, formulated, appraised and evaluated. They are beyond the easy reach of logical thought and elaboration. It is possible for them to exist, however incompatible, inconsistent and disharmonious they may be. Since they cannot be thoughtfully, that is, logically appraised within awareness, they escape rational criticism, their status may be blind, impulsive, irrational. On the other hand some dissociated tendencies may be superior—in terms of love, freshness of feeling, freshness of insight, for example—to any tendency systems in the self. So when the self system is impoverished by toxic experience, the whole personality tends also to be impoverished. When loving tendencies have to be dissociated, the person may save, in this furtive fashion, a precious part of life experience, but such tendencies, so long as they exist in dissociation, are denied a fair chance to be deepened, expanded, fructified by conscious elaboration and experience. Such tendencies are likely to remain relatively undeveloped, immature, struggling along, so to speak, in a makeshift fashion, as best they can. When they are expressed, it is unwittingly, or in dreams, or in fantasies.

But, someone may object, what about the person who goes to bed with a mathematical problem he cannot solve and wakes

[59] See p. 184.

up in the morning with the solution? Clearly there are, or seem to be, mental processes which go on outside awareness and yet are highly fruitful. The answer is, according to Sullivan's theories, that this is *not* an example of a dissociated dynamism. Not all psychological processes going on outside awareness are dissociated dynamisms. There are two other modes of symbol activity besides the consensually or socially validated symbol activity of the self.

There are, first, "prototaxic symbols." [60] Prototaxic symbols are, as one might expect, indicative of the rudimentary state of development of the infant. All that the infant "knows" are momentary states. He has not yet developed, or learned, the forms of time and space, of before and after, of here and there. His ability to discriminate, if any, is quite rudimentary. He has no ego, because the self has not yet developed. Therefore he has no understanding of himself as a separate object from the outer world. His experiences are all of a piece, undifferentiated, undefined, not delimited; in other words, they are "cosmic." Everything belongs to the infant's own "cosmic entity." [61]

Long before the infant can utter words, or learn them, he perceives, or rather "prehends" the *mothering* one. Her nipple "provides the first of all vividly meaningful symbols—a vaguely demarcated 'complex-image' or proto-concept with very wide reference." [62] Gradually the mothering one gets distinguished as not being a part of oneself. The mothering one who contributes to the increase of euphoria, feeling of well-being, of the infant becomes characterized as the Good Mother. Since she will at times, for one reason or another, also cause a decrease of euphoria, another "complexus of impressions" becomes the Bad Mother.[63] To the infant, the two are vaguely limited but distinct people. The nipple becomes an attribute of the Good

[60] Prototaxic symbol, complex-image, and protoconcept are used synonymously.

[61] See p. 33.

[62] See p. 33.

[63] See p. 79.

Mother. It "stands for" or represents the Good Mother, in a vague way. The nipple is a pre-concept or proto-concept. Some people throughout life show evidence of this original bifurcation of interpersonal experience. Gradually, as the infant develops, this kind of symbol activity fades from waking life.

There is said to be a close resemblance between this kind of psychological activity and certain schizophrenic states where the person, for reasons too complex to be mentioned here, has regress to a very early state of development.[64] An ordinary bench can become the footstool of God. The schizophrenic is surrounded by cosmic forces.

In prototaxic symbolization, there is no movement of "thought." For the infant, experience is unconnected, discrete. The symbolization expresses momentary experiences. These momentary experiences form the basis of memory. Sullivan says that "living beings *fix*, somewhere and somehow, meaningful traces of everything they live through, not as 'perceptions' or 'states of excitation of the cortex' or the life, but rather as the pattern of how the organism-and-significant-environment existed at the moment." [65] It is on these momentary organismic states that subsequent experience is built. Subsequent experiences are "colored" by these earlier ones. In other words, subsequent experience is undergone in terms of the original felt experiences of early life. In a sense, later experiences are, on the subject side, pyramidal. So the experiences of infancy and childhood are enormously important for later experience. This does not mean that later experiences are undergone so as to repeat the earlier one. But it does mean that subsequent experiences do not make a fresh start. They are conditioned by previous experiences which perhaps, to some degree, extend to the prenatal.

The next stage of development begins with the appearance of the parataxic. Its verbal manifestation is the autistic. How-

[64] See pp. 150–152.
[65] See p. 105.

ever, the requirements of the developing self-system, which is another way of saying the requirements of the significant people, require that the use of words, the verbal symbol activity, be more refined and "consensually validated." Words then take on a more precise, a more scientific reference. The overt autistic behavior tends also to fade from waking life. In order to 'get on' with the significant people, in order to gain satisfactions and maintain security, the child has to conform, more or less, to *their* ideas, modes of behavior, and *their* use of language, *their* reference-frames.

But in deep sleep one can still carry on these earlier forms of symbol activity. In dreams one does not have to conform to the ideas of the significant adults. To a considerable extent, this is also true of fantasy—a kind of waking dream.

It is clear, then, that these earlier modes of mental activity persist. In a waking state, the needs of the self, the requirements of society, oblige one to be more or less "rational," to be "logical," to be consciously aware of what one is about. Meanings have to be relatively precise; that is, thought must have relatively precise reference frames. Furthermore, thinking tends to be more of a step-by-step activity. Of course, the thinking may not actually follow the rules of inference very carefully, but one must, the self must, at least make a pretense of doing this, in order to impress oneself and others for the purpose of maintaining prestige. People who do not at least make a pretense of logical thought are branded "queer" or "crazy." This means their chances of gaining satisfactions and maintaining security are endangered. And seriously to endanger these, may endanger one's very life.[66]

To be noted is the fact that the necessary refinement and precision of symbol activity carried on in healthy interpersonal relations is both a great gain and a great loss. In order to be

[66] These observations are not explicit in Sullivan's published writings. They were communicated orally to the writer.

understood with any degree of accuracy one has to use words with some referential precision. At least, words must have a shared and recognizable meaning. Science, in its more refined branches, strives for rigorous definition of terms and meanings. But, from another point of view, there is great loss. Imagination, except in rare instances, and feeling are checked. Mathematics is the outstanding example, where a special language is invented, whose symbols are devoid of all specific content and have no direct reference to anything outside the system. It is true that for a very few gifted people mathematics has a charm of its own, not to mention the great practical benefits which can be attained with its application in other fields. But traditionally people regard mathematics as dry, uninteresting, tedious, a bore. And in a modern industrial society, with the aid of the newspaper, the radio, the movies, words become hackneyed, stereotyped. Having become insipid and banal, they certainly do not stir the imagination and feelings.

The result of all this is that everyone, to some extent, and some people to a large extent, have to fall back on earlier modes of mental activity. In fact, one can distinguish three reasons for falling back to the earlier modes of symbol activity. The first is that dissociated dynamisms have to be discharged somehow, if one is to maintain a tolerable degree of mental health. They usually are discharged in sleep, in dreams, or, to a lesser extent, in undiscriminated fantasies whose meaning is not clearly understood, as well as in more overt activities. The second reason is that there is not time to do everything in a deliberately logical fashion. Nor is it necessary. If one were to think out step by step everything that one does getting up in the morning, one would never get to the office. The third reason is that these two earlier symbol processes can have a richness of emotional content which everyday experiences and activities lack. Those who can use their imagination freely know that the world of fantasy can sometimes have a richness, an intensity, a variety, and a quality which one rarely experiences, unless one is unusually fortunate, in the everyday world. Indeed, one might say that the world of art has for one of its functions, at least, to compensate for the lacks of this everyday world of humdrum activity.[67]

So the pre-conceptual, or prototaxic, mode of symbol activity characteristic of early infancy, and the parataxic and autistic characteristic of childhood, continue to be primary forms of creative thinking and spontaneous feeling. Here one is free to ignore, for the time being, in dreams and fantasy, the demands of "normal life," of "reality," the common and shared everyday world. Of course, all meaning which is to be shared by others must be expressed in symbols understood by others, and by one's own self. Feeling, also, if it is to be understood and shared by others, must employ conventional expression. But the reshaping and transformation of the earlier symbols into conventional expression comes after, just as in one's life history.[68]

In order to avoid confusion, it must be indicated that, while dissociated dynamisms are also frequently discharged in dreams and fantasy which employ the earlier modes of symbol activity, it does not follow that all mental activity, other than rational, conscious thinking, is an instance of dissociation. Just how much non-rational mental activity represents dissociated tendencies depends on the course of the self-dynamisms. A self-respecting person will probably manifest far fewer dissociated tendencies than a self-derogatory person. But it does not follow that a self-respecting person, a loving person, will manifest less of the earlier kind of thinking and feeling. The contrary may be the case.[69]

[67] It is not meant that this is, or should be, the primary function of art. Ideally, at any rate, art is an enrichment of life, not an escape from life.

[68] These observations are not explicit in Sullivan's published writings. They were communicated orally to the writer.

[69] These observations are not explicit in Sullivan's published writings. They were communicated orally to the writer.

The self dynamism "uses," or functions by means of, rational thinking but it obviously is not synonymous with rational thought.[70] The dissociated dynamism "uses" parataxic—with its sub-species, the autistic—symbol processes but is also not synonymous with them.[71] In the first case, rational thinking frequently is an instrumentality of the self. For the discharge of dissociated tendencies, the earlier modes of symbol activity are frequently employed, but they certainly did not originate for that purpose, and they exist, that is, function, independently. In other words, they have a status of their own.

One can say that the dissociated tendencies are analogous to the self, because they definitely involve the existence of others. Dissociated tendencies are discharged in actual interpersonal situations unwittingly, or in dreams or fantasies. Powerful impulses, desires, and needs are thus discharged. In an actual interpersonal situation, dissociated tendencies are "communicated" in a disguised fashion, outside the awareness of the person manifesting them. If the other person, or persons, are skillful observers, they will recognize such manifestations. In any case, they will have to take account of them.

Rational thinking can also occur as a spontaneous activity, within conscious awareness, but without reference to the self. But it occurs thus in relatively few people and under very restricted circumstances. By its very nature, rational thinking tends to be limited not only by the needs of the self, but by the constitution of things as they are, or are implicitly maintained to be by the culture one lives in. Except for a relatively few gifted people, rational thought is not the vehicle of imagination. And even in the case of great scientific discoveries, there is considerable evidence that new ideas frequently "come in a flash" and are only later elaborated according to logical procedure.[72] The earlier modes of symbol activity are not limited either by things as they are, "reality," or what one's culture

[70] It also functions in the parataxic mode.

[71] The dissociated can also use rational thought.

[72] However, one must not underestimate the importance of logical analysis.

says they are. They are free to express any fantasies, ideas, creations of the mind, subject only to the imaginative and creative power of one's mind. One can experiment with them. They give the imagination free play. And if one is sufficiently talented, one can with their aid achieve artistic creation or new scientific theories.

Sullivan has said that the "personality tends towards the state that we call mental health or interpersonal adjustive success, handicaps by way of acculturation notwithstanding. The basic direction of the organism is forward." [73] Here is ascribed an intrinsic tendency of the personality toward mental health. It implies that one is not a completely passive and helpless victim of unfortunate experience. Otherwise the prescriptive rôle of the self dynamism would entirely succeed in preventing or thwarting the effects of corrective experience, or any experience not acceptable and congenial to it; that is, in harmony with its basic direction and characteristics. Some people, at least, *do* learn better. The self-dynamism does expand somewhat, despite great resistance as manifested in anxiety. And some elements of the personality, like the need for companionship, or lust, when dissociated, are so powerful that they may force their way into awareness, even despite great suffering. Under certain circumstances dissociated elements can be re-integrated, become a part of the self.

Nevertheless, the resistance to change is very great. And for most people in this culture, and probably any other culture now existing, only a small percentage of their potentialities is ever realized. "It inheres in the nature of being human that one will relinquish, so to speak, a relative security and undergo anew a previously intolerable conflict within awareness *only* if one perceives a probability of speedy relief." [74] In the more

Among other things, it reveals implications in a system or concept which would otherwise be missed.

[73] See p. 97.

[74] See p. 130.

severe mental disorders, the problem of change is enormous —why? "To 'accept a dissociated tendency system into the self' is tantamount to undergoing an extensive change in personality, implying a marked change in the sorts of interpersonal situations in which one will have one's being. Not only is there this element of great change, but also there is no possibility of foresight as to the direction and extent of the change. Finally, one could not foretell that this change will be tolerable; there is every prospect of its including serious conflict, for the self dynamism includes powerful tendency systems which are responsible for the character of the present life course. The metamorphosis is scarcely an attractive prospect, even theoretically. Practically, there is no such prospect; there is only the stable course of life in contrast with terrors and anxieties, easily referrable to the unknown." [75]

If one speaks of an objective situation in interpersonal relations, what can be validly meant by such a statement? Is there such a thing; and if so, can it be understood? Are the constituents of an interpersonal situation so determinate that they can be appraised with accuracy? Or are the guiding principles sufficiently well established and reliable to make possible a reasonably correct analysis? Since the psychiatrist participates in the situation he is studying, can he at the same time remain sufficiently detached so that his own peculiarities will not seriously interfere with understanding? Can he participate in the situation and yet remain objective?

Yes, Sullivan would say, one can achieve a relative objectivity. "The psychiatrist," he states, "in developing his skill in interrogating informants, learns to integrate situations the configurations of which provoke the elaboration of information that was previously potential. He thus obtains more data from the informant than the latter has clearly perceived. The informant, so to speak, tells more than he knows. The data are

[75] See pp. 142–143.

more significant to the psychiatrist because he has more experience and more freedom in formulating interpersonal processes. He is alert to implications; his alertness is oriented to understanding interpersonal processes; and he has many fewer specific inhibitions of alertness in the interpersonal configurations in which he participates. From the relative accessibility of his own past, and from intimate contact with the developmental history of a number of people, he has a considerable grasp on the actual dynamics of interpersonal relations. He knows more about the processes that can occur in these configurations; in particular, he knows that certain alleged processes are highly improbable. Reports of these alleged events are, therefore, most probably rationalizations, and he is able, from experience or by inquiry, to secure clues to the unwitting motivations that underlie these conventional statements.

"Certainty about interpersonal processes is an ideal that should seldom concern one. Information about any situation should be considered as a formulation of probability. . . .

"When one has regard for the multiple me-you patterns that complicate interpersonal relations, for the possible differences in individual prehension of events, and for the peculiarities of language behavior which characterize each of us . . . the practical impossibility of one-to-one correspondence of mental states of the observer and the observed person should be evident. We never know all about another, we are fortunate when we achieve an approximate consensus and can carry on meaningful communication about relatively simple contexts of experience. Most of us spend the greater part of our social life in much less adequate contact with our interlocutors, with whom we manifest considerable skill at avoiding frank misunderstanding, with whom in fact we agree and disagree quite often with very little consensus as to subject of discussion. The psychiatrist of all people knows the relative character of his formulation of the other person, even if he has gained such skill that he is often quite correct." [76]

The objection is sometimes made that one cannot derive valid conclusions about "normal" people merely, or perhaps at all, from people who are mentally ill. To this Sullivan would probably reply after the following fashion:

"At this point, I wish to say that if this series of lectures is to be reasonably successful, it will finally have demonstrated that there is nothing unique in the phenomena of the gravest functional illness. The most peculiar behavior of the acutely schizophrenic patient, I hope to demonstrate, is made up of interpersonal processes with which each one of us is or historically has been familiar. Far the greater part of the performances, the interpersonal processes, of the psychiatric patient are exactly of a piece with processes which we manifest some time every twenty-four hours. . . . In most general terms, we are all much more simply human than otherwise, be we happy and successful, contented and detached, miserable and mentally disordered, or whatever." [77]

In another place he says:

" 'Mental disorder' as a term refers to interpersonal processes either inadequate to the situation in which the persons are integrated, or excessively complex because of illusory persons also integrated in the situation. It implies some—sometimes a great—ineffectiveness of the behavior by which the person is conceived to be pursuing the satisfactions that he requires. It is not, however, to be envisaged as an equivalent of *psychosis*, 'insanity,' or the like. The failure to remember the name of an acquaintance at the opportune moment is just as truly an instance of mental disorder as is a fixed delusion that one is Napoleon I." [78]

[76] Reference footnote 32; pp. 132–134.
[77] See pp. 15–16.
[78] Reference footnote 32; p. 122, footnote.

How does a patient get well? And what does "getting well" mean? Nothing miraculous is accomplished, but only an indication of the process can be given here. The patient, because of the relative freedom of the therapeutic situation, and because of skillful interpretation and guidance at opportune moments, is enabled to understand better the significance of his past and the rôle it plays in his present behavior and his outlook on life. The possibility of a different and more satisfactory mode of interpersonal relations and a new outlook on life gradually dawns upon the patient. Thus:

"Until a patient has seen clearly and unmistakably a concrete example of the way in which unresolved situations from the distant past color the perception of present situations and over-complicate action in them, there can be no material reorganization of personality, no therapeutically satisfactory expansion of the self, no significant insight into the complexities of one's performances or into the unexpected and often disconcerting behavior of others concerned. Up to this point, there is nothing significantly unique in the treatment situation; afterwards, however, the integration with the psychiatrist becomes a situation of unprecedented freedom from restraints on the manifestation of constructive impulses. This is the indirect result of the changes in the self system. The patient has finally learnt that more security may ensue from *abandoning* a complex security-seeking process than was ever achieved *by it.* This information is in itself an addition to security and a warrant for confronting other anxiety-provoking situations to discover the factors in them which are being experienced as a threat. . . ." [79]

The patient eventually grasps the significance of the statement, "One achieves mental health to the extent that one becomes aware of one's interpersonal relations. . . ." [80] He learns to understand what he is doing. "Most patients have for years been acting out conflicts, substitutions, and compromises; the

[79] See pp. 205–206.
[80] See p. 207.

benefits of treatment come in large part from their learning to notice what they are doing, and this is greatly expedited by carefully validated verbal statements as to what seems to be going on." [81] There is "*an expanding of the self* to such final effect that the patient as known to himself is much the same person as the patient behaving with others." [82] But it takes a good deal of education and experience effectively to grasp the meaning and significance of uncomplicated interpersonal relations, to realize the full benefits of a more abundant life. Increasing knowledge and insight make possible a less complicated, richer experience. New experience in turn makes possible still greater insight. This process does not stop with the end of treatment. Theoretically, at any rate, it continues throughout life.

Personality development is divided into epochs or periods of growth. These epochs are not rigidly fixed, since, he says, they vary, at least in the later stages, from culture to culture. Nevertheless, he seems to think that, although subject to variation, they are universal. One can attempt merely an outline of them here. They can be fully understood only in the light of all of Sullivan's fundamental theories of interpersonal relations. On the other hand these epochs, or rather his theories about them, are an intrinsic part of a theory of interpersonal relations. Despite some repetition it seems best to recapitulate the various epochs. One may not be able to explain interpersonal behavior solely in terms of a person's past history, but one cannot adequately explain or understand such behavior without a knowledge of the past. No one's acts are always free of parataxic elements. The several epochs are: infancy, childhood, the juvenile period, preadolescence, adolescence, and mature adulthood.

He describes the course of existence of what is later to be a human being from fecundation of the ovum as "parasitic, new-born (animal), then infantile (human)." [83] Since the new-born

[81] See p. 223.
[82] See p. 237.
[83] See p. 33.

is completely helpless, if unaided by people, he is "modified by this personal element" from the earliest stages of life outside the womb.[84] But "the long stretch of postnatal life required by the human young for the attainment of independent competence to live" is one of the factors which make civilization possible.[85] The "*mothering one*" becomes the infant's first vivid perception. Here the fact of empathy assumes primary importance. By this yet unclear mode of communication, the affection, loving care, good feeling, or their opposites, of the mothering one are perceived or felt by the infant. The nipple becomes the first vividly meaningful symbol, vaguely demarcated. Gradually by attending to outer objects which do not directly satisfy physico-chemical needs, the infant begins to mark off the limits of his own private world.

He begins to explore the possibilities and limits of his own body, and certain outer subjects. He "experiments." Summarily, infancy is "the period of maturation, of experimentation, of empathic 'observation,' and of autistic invention in the realm of power." [86]

As previously noted, the transition from infancy to childhood occurs when the rudiments of language are learned. It is during this period that the folkways of the culture begin to be deliberately taught. The development of the self-system, which, at least in a very rudimentary form, begins in infancy, proceeds rapidly with deliberate acculturation.

"Childhood includes a rapid acculturation, but not alone in the basic acquisition of language, which is itself an enormous cultural entity. By this I mean that in childhood the peculiar mindlessness of the infant which seems to be assumed by most parents passes off and they begin to regard the little one as in need of training, as being justifiably an object of education;

[84] See p. 33.
[85] See p. 33.
[86] See p. 16. *Parataxic* should probably be substituted for *autistic*, since the latter term is now confined in Sullivan's formulation mainly to verbal manifestation of the *parataxic*.

and what they train the child in consists of select excerpts from the cultural heritage, from that surviving of past people, incorporated in the personality of the parent. This includes such things as habits of cleanliness—which are of extremely good repute in the Western culture—and a great many other things. And along with all this acculturation, toilet habits, eating habits, and so on and so forth, there proceeds the learning of language as a tool for communication." [87]

During childhood, as already seen, autistic activity, the unchecked and undisciplined use of words, is pronounced. Also during this period the manifestation of anxiety, as an instrumentality of the self, begins to be discriminated.

"The era of childhood ends with the maturation of a need for compeers. The child manifests a shift from contentment in an environment of authoritarian adults and the more or less personalized pets, toys and other objects, towards an environment of persons significantly *like* him. If playmates are available, his integrations with them show new meaningfulness. If there are no playmates, the child's revery processes create imaginary playmates. In brief, the child proceeds into the *juvenile era* of personality development by virtue of a new tendency towards coöperation, to doing things in accommodation to the personality of others. Along with this budding ability to play with other children, there goes a learning of those performances which we call competition and compromise." [88]

For the young in this culture, schooling begins in the juvenile era, an experience which in itself is fraught with great consequences.

Preadolescence is said to begin between the ages of eight-and-one-half and twelve years.[89] In this period the capacity to love is developed. According to Sullivan, love exists when, and only when, the satisfactions and security of the loved one are

[87] See p. 18.
[88] See p. 38.
[89] See p. 41.

as significant to one as one's own satisfactions and security.

"This state of affectional rapport—generically love—ordinarily occurs under restricted circumstances. In the beginning many factors must be present. Some of these may be called obvious likeness, parallel impulse, parallel physical development. These make for situations in which boys feel at ease with boys rather than with girls. This feeling of species identity or identification influences the feeling involved in the preadolescent change. The appearance of the capacity to love ordinarily first involves a member of one's own sex. The boy finds a chum who is a boy, the girl finds a chum who is a girl. When this has happened, there follows in its wake a great increase in the consensual validation of symbols, of symbol operations, and of information, data about life and the world." [90]

He goes on to say that, with the appearance of love, when another, the chum, matters as much as oneself, "the great controlling power of the cultural, social, forces is finally inescapably written into the human personality."

The concluding remarks of this chapter are significant for the present state of cultural development. The author believes, "for a great majority of our people, preadolescence is the nearest that they come to untroubled human life—that from then on the stresses of life distort them to inferior caricatures of what they might have been." [91]

The stages of personality development, he says, previous to adolescence are closely, though obscurely, related to somatic maturation. "Adolescence begins with the most spectacular maturation of all, the puberty change, with its swift alteration of physiological processes to the completion of bodily development." [92] This period is characterized by maturation of "the genital lust dynamism." It is subdivided into three eras: "early adolescence, from the first evidences of puberty to the com-

[90] See p. 43.
[91] See p. 56.
[92] See p. 57.

pletion of voice change; mid-adolescence, to the patterning of genital behavior; and late adolescence, to the establishment of durable situations of intimacy such that all the major integrating tendencies are freely manifested within awareness in the series of one's interpersonal relations." [93]

Sullivan emphasizes the rôle of experience in determining sexual, or genital, behavior and the emotion of lust. "I have to add a word of caution, here," he says, "for there are those among us psychiatrists who make of sex a nuclear explanatory concept of personality, or at least of personality disorder. This is an error from insufficiency of the data. The highly civilized Chinese of the pre-Christian era were not bowled over by sex. A number of the primitive peoples who have been studied by anthropologists are found to take sex rather in their stride. Even the American Negro crashes through adolescence with relative impunity—if he is of the lower classes.

"The lurid twilight which invests sex in our culture is primarily a function of two factors. We still try to discourage pre-marital sexual performances; hold that abstinence is the moral course before marriage. And we discourage early marriage; in fact progressively widen the gap between the adolescent awakening of lust and the proper circumstances for marriage. These two factors work through many cultural conventions to make us the most sex-ridden people of whom I have any knowledge." [94]

Lust cannot easily be dissociated, or in the traditional language, be "repressed." He says:

"What happens when the sexual impulses, the impulses to genital behavior, collide with the self system . . . ? Under certain circumstances, the self is able to dissociate lust and the impulses to genital behavior. This can be achieved only by the development of new and elaborate 'apparatus' in living. . . .

[93] See pp. 57–58. Sullivan now divides the adolescent era into early and late adolescence, the former ending with the patterning of genital behavior.

[94] See pp. 58–59.

The point I wish to emphasize now is that, late as it is in maturing, the genital lust dynamism is something that can be dissociated only at grave risk to effective living, and that in most people it cannot be dissociated at all. It will again and again, at whatever great expense to security, whatever suffering from anxiety, manifest itself."[95]

What about "sublimation," or as Sullivan would phrase it, the sublimatory reformulations of interpersonal relations? Sublimation is defined thus: "a motive which is involved in painful conflict is combined with a social (culturally provided) technique of life which disguises its most conflict-provoking aspect and usually provides some representation for the opposing motive in the conflict."[96] Sublimation as he uses the term has a much wider range than the usual denotation and can refer to any tendency system or drive. A disguised and partially fulfilled satisfaction is combined with the achievement of personal security. Sublimatory reformulations sometimes work, and "work beautifully;" but they do not always work.[97]

Mature adulthood, the "fully human estate," is obviously not synonymous with chronological adulthood. The characteristics of a mature adult are only briefly mentioned. If one has had fortunate experience in living and has successfully reached and passed through adolescence, he emerges, so to speak, inevitably as a mature person. Once adolescence is "successfully negotiated, the person comes forth with self-respect adequate to almost any situation, with the respect for others that this competent self-respect entails, with the dignity that befits the high achievement of competent personality, and with the freedom of personal initiative that represents a comfortable adaptation of one's personal situation to the circumstances that characterize the social order of which one is a part."[98] In other

[95] See p. 63.
[96] See p. 126.
[97] See pp. 126–141.
[98] See p. 57.

words, adequate self-respect, respect for others, personal dignity, personal initiative adequate for one's station in life are necessary conditions for the achievement of mature personality.

Sullivan's language has been a considerable barrier to understanding. The result has been that his theory of the self, among other theories, has been misunderstood. For example, it has been thought that he believed acculturation necessarily limits the self or the personality, two concepts which in the minds of some people have been confused. What he does believe is that adequate and inconsistent acculturation limits the self and impoverishes the whole personality. The self is a product of acculturation. Without acculturation there could be no self.

The concept of psychiatric cure has also been misinterpreted. He says that along with psychiatric cure "there goes an *expanding of the self* to such final effect that the patient as known to himself is much the same person as is the patient behaving with others." It is worth noting that he does *not* say the patient as known to himself is much the same person *as he is known to others*. The practical consequences may not seem great. But there is an important theoretical difference. The patient as known to others may be, and very likely is, accompanied by parataxic distortions, because others are by no means likely to be free of limitations resulting from their own life history. If the patient knows himself as he is known to others, very likely he has an inadequate idea of himself. Ideally, the patient knows himself as he is behaving with others, free of all illusory "me-you patterns." This certainly does not mean that he will integrate situations having the same traits with everyone. A loving person, however free of self-distortion, cannot love a hateful person, because the latter is incapable of responding in a loving way. A situation having the qualities categorized as love cannot be integrated because opposites do not unite. There can only be conflict or withdrawal. In the latter case, the situation is disintegrated. If an interpersonal integration occurs and persists, it can only be on the basis of hostility, because a hateful person cannot love, but a loving person, under appropriate circumstances, can be hostile, if only for his own defence.

Individuality, as applied to a person, is a term Sullivan finds objectionable. In a somewhat obscure passage he has declared, "The unique individuality of the other fellow need never concern us as scientists." [99] Here he seems to be emphasizing the fact that a person is not an isolated entity, that personality is revealed and has its being in interpersonal relations, and is observable only in such interpersonal relations. Elsewhere this meaning is explicit.[100] He says that the personality which can be studied by scientific method cannot be observed directly, and that unique individuality would not be any concern of the psychiatrist. There seems to be some confusion on this point. In the first place, scientific method is not limited to a study of only that which can be observed directly. Furthermore, it is an open question whether any psychiatrist uses the term "individuality" when applied to a person in the same sense as when applied to an electron.[101] The criticism seems to be misdirected.[102]

It seems to be based on a confusion of two different concepts of individuality. The first is analogous to the traditional concept of "soul." Traditionally, the soul is a unique spiritual entity or substance, which can subsist independently. Some people talk about individuality as if it were literally a spiritual essence.

But there is a quite different concept of individuality. A sense of personal worth and dignity, and a recognition of solidarity or oneness with others in interpersonal relations, crea-

[99] See p. 12.

[100] Reference footnote 32; p. 121.

[101] Reference footnote 32; p. 121.

[102] Compare Welldon, Jr., J. E. C., *The Nicomachean Ethics of Aristotle;* London, Macmillan, 1930 (lxvii and 352 pp.); p. 14. "But when we speak of self-sufficiency, we do not mean that a person leads a solitary life all by himself, but that he has parents, children, wife, and friends, and fellow-citizens in general, as man is naturally a social being."

tive ability, love as self-affirmation and the affirmation of others —these express this second concept of individuality. There is nothing in the ideas which have been discussed repugnant to such a concept. Prototaxic, parataxic and in some cases rational symbol activity are all indicative of the creative potentialities of people. Self-respect, respect for others, the dignity of competent personality, freedom of personal initiative are said to be marks of adult maturity. Love is said to exist when and only when the satisfactions and security of another are equally important with one's own. So there seems to be no need to reject individuality on the ground that it implies "a self-limited unit that alternates between a state of insular detachment and varying degrees of contact with other people and with cultural entities." [103] In rejecting the notion of individuality, Sullivan exposes himself to the superficial misunderstanding that he believes personality is a passive instrument of acculturation or the equally dubious notion of cultural relativism.

The view that is argued for here is that every situation is individual, is unique. It has an immediately pervasive quality. Psychologically the situation as a qualitative whole is immediately sensed or felt. "Distinctions and relations are instituted *within* a situation; *they* are recurrent and repeatable in different situations." [104] One must, therefore, be careful to distinguish between psychological, that is *felt*, uniqueness, individuality, and the distinctions and relations instituted by discourse in investigating the situation. These distinctions and relations are necessary instruments for determining interpersonal involvements or interactions. The distinctions and relations are recurrent in studying different interpersonal situations.

When the psychiatrist is studying an interpersonal situation, he institutes distinctions and relations. Terms like *parataxic*, *dissociated*, *schizophrenic*, are terms in discourse, meanings, in order to determine or indicate how people sometimes become

[103] Reference footnote 32; p. 121.

[104] Dewey, John, *Logic, The Theory of Inquiry;* New York, Henry Holt, 1938 (v and 546 pages); p. 68.

involved with one another. These terms refer to recurring modes of interpersonal behavior. So far as these recurring modes of behavior are modeled on past experiences, are, in other words, parataxic, they prevent, or tend to prevent, radical newness in an interpersonal situation. The problem for psychiatry would seem to be *not* the supposed scientific inaccessibility of individuality, but, in dealing with people who are mentally ill, their lack of ability to experience the uniqueness of new situations. In other words, the mentally ill are not sufficiently able to feel and sense and understand the uniqueness and differences of interpersonal situations. For them the situation is, erroneously, of course, felt to be not unique but modeled on, or paradigmatic of old situations.

There would still be, of course, recurring distinctions and relations, but the problem for the psychiatrist and the patient would seem to be to learn what ones are valid and what are not valid.

If the understanding of living in order that it may be facilitated is the purpose of psychiatry, it leads one eventually to seek an understanding of the social order in which people live. The ultimate causes of mental disorder, it would seem, have to be sought in the social order itself. Expressed in another way, the study of interpersonal relations leads pretty directly to a study of the social order which is their matrix. It is now rather obvious that the inadequacies and the contradictions which the culture manifests is a fertile breeding ground for the mentally sick and the mentally handicapped. The psychiatrist, if he is to function with social effectiveness, can no longer stand aloof. He must, while maintaining his own specialty, join hands with other social scientists. This broader point of view requires a new orientation and the perfection of new techniques.[105]

NEW YORK, N. Y., *May*, 1945

[105] See p. 175.

Index

HARRY STACK SULLIVAN, M.D.

THE Psychiatric Interview

Edited by

HELEN SWICK PERRY *and* MARY LADD GAWEL

With an Introduction by OTTO ALLEN WILL, M.D.

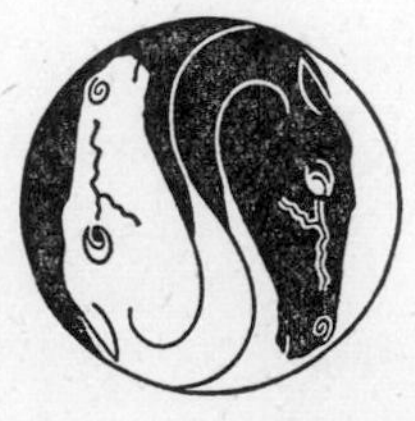

W · W · NORTON & COMPANY · INC · *New York*

Prepared under the auspices of
THE WILLIAM ALANSON WHITE PSYCHIATRIC FOUNDATION
COMMITTEE ON PUBLICATION OF SULLIVAN'S WRITINGS
Mabel Blake Cohen, M.D. Dexter M. Bullard, M.D.
David McK. Rioch, M.D. Janet MacK. Rioch, M.D.
Clara Thompson, M.D.
Helen Swick Perry, *Editorial Consultant*

PRINTED IN THE UNITED STATES OF AMERICA

Contents

Editors' Preface

This is the second of the posthumous books of Harry Stack Sullivan prepared under the auspices of the William Alanson White Psychiatric Foundation, Sullivan's literary executor. This book is based on two lecture series which Sullivan gave, in 1944 and again in 1945, under the title of *The Psychiatric Interview*. These lectures were given in the Washington School of Psychiatry, which is the training institution of the Foundation. While the lectures were directed primarily toward psychiatrists, Sullivan also meant them for all those who engage in dynamic interviewing. The lectures were recorded, and this book is based both on these recordings and on two Notebooks, one for each year, which Sullivan used as a guide in presenting his lectures. In general, Sullivan's own scheme of organization of the material, as he refined it in the second year, has been followed, and the best material from each year has been selected to cover the various topics. This has been supplemented by material drawn from three lectures on psychiatric interviewing which Sullivan included in a more general and theoretical lecture series in 1946–47. Thus this book endeavors to present all of the best of Sullivan on this topic and at the same time not to depart radically from Sullivan's organization of an approach to this topic.

Insofar as possible, Sullivan's language has been left intact. However, repetitions and digressions more appropriate to the lecture room than to the printed page have been omitted or footnoted, and obscurities have been clarified by reference to Sullivan's Notebooks, to what he said on the same points at other times, and by listening to the recordings themselves for the emphasis and meaning of sentences as spoken. The headings and subheadings in the book are mainly derived from the headings in Sullivan's Notebooks, a procedure which proved useful in the preparation of the first of these books.

Much of the material in the first two chapters of this book appeared first in the journal *Psychiatry* [(1951) 14:361–373 and (1952) 15:127–141]. In organizing this into book form, it has been necessary to shift some of the material and to make other minor modifications incident to the making of a book.

In presenting this book to the public, the Foundation wishes to make special mention of the contribution of Otto Allen Will, M.D., to the work on the clinical papers in general and this book in particular. Shortly after Sullivan's death, Dr. Will became interested in the possibility of organizing all of the various clinical lecture series into books. He began to put some of the various clinical lectures into readable form so that the richness of the material could be more easily recognized. His voluntary assumption of this role has played no small part in the Foundation's program for publishing this series of books. The selection and the preliminary assessment of the material in this book was done by Dr. Will, and he has acted as medical consultant in all phases.

In the preparation of this book we are particularly indebted to Philip A. Holman, a staff member of the journal *Psychiatry*, who has helped extensively in the editing and at various stages of the preparation of the book. For the typing of the final manuscript and the proofreading we wish to express our gratitude to Marguerite A. Martinelli.

Finally, we would like to pay tribute to the friends of the Foundation—students and colleagues of Sullivan's, for the most part—who continue to give financial support and encouragement to the whole project.

HELEN SWICK PERRY
MARY LADD GAWEL

Introduction

In this book psychiatry is defined as the field of the study of interpersonal relations, emphasis being placed on the interaction of the participants in a social situation, rather than being centered exclusively on the supposedly private economy of either one of those participants. The psychiatric interview is a special instance of interpersonal relations, and the term, as used here, does not refer exclusively to the meeting of a psychiatrist and his patient. The interview is characterized by the coming together of two people, one recognized as an expert in interpersonal relations, the other known as the client, interviewee, or patient, who expects to derive some benefit from a serious discussion of his needs with this expert. The situation is designed to make clear certain characteristic patterns of the client's living with the prospect that such elucidation will prove useful to him.

The term psychiatric as used here simply indicates that the interview is considered to be an interpersonal phenomenon, and that the data for its study and comprehension are to be derived from the observation of what goes on between the participants—or, to phrase it in another way, from an observation of the field of their interaction. Also implied in the term is the concept that patterns of living are to be clarified and that in that process benefit may accrue to the client. Interview situations in which the goal is the obtaining of factual data from the interviewee—as in the presenting of a questionnaire —and in which subsequent benefit to the interviewee is of little or no importance, are not by this definition "psychiatric."

Thus the term psychiatric interview, as used in this book, has broad implications, and the discussion of it presented here is practically related not only to the psychiatrist and his patient, but to the interviewer and interviewee in a wide variety of situations. The term interview does not apply to a certain fixed period of time, but rather to a course of interpersonal events which may be encompassed to some degree in a single conference of sixty or ninety minutes' duration, or developed to a greater extent during the course of several meetings, or elaborated in the many sessions of intensive psychotherapy. Contained in a single psychiatric interview are the essential characteristics and movements of the more prolonged therapy. So it is that much of what is discussed here in terms of the interview has application to the entire course of a psychotherapeutic endeavor.

We often speak of the "art" of this or that—the art of salesmanship, of medicine, of living, of interviewing. Used in this way the term art may indicate that an important part of the profession or task is an interpersonal relationship, the skillful handling of which plays a large part in the success or failure of the enterprise. The word also suggests that the particulars of the relationship are not subject to observation and description; they are "intuitive," "subjective," or "personal," and likely to be damaged in some way by close scrutiny, or they are "insignificant" and "unscientific," and unsuited for objective study. Thus, to speak of the art of interviewing may imply that the processes in that interaction are not observable, and that for reasons not entirely clear, the situation might best flourish in an atmosphere of privacy.

Sullivan thought that the scientific method could be applied to study of the interpersonal field, and that patterns of action in the interview could be identified, observed, and defined in a manner that would move the entire process to some extent away from the obscurity of an art and toward the clarity of a science. He made some progress in this direction by paying considerable attention to the nonverbal components of the situation—tone of voice, patterning of speech, facial expression, bodily gesture, and so on—the ways by which so much of meaning is transmitted between people, and the observation of which is often indiscriminately labeled by some such term as intuition. Sullivan also observed that the processes in the interview are kept obscure by the mutual anxiety of the participants. Thus it is easier for the patient to think of his relationship to the therapist as puzzling, irritating, frustrating, unsatisfactory, or even wonderful, than to recognize the anxiety which has led to his puzzlement, irritation, wonderment, and so on. The therapist, likewise, may find it more comforting and less disturbing—although hardly more profitable—to consider his role in the interview as an artistic performance not subject to observation, thus avoiding a study of the interactions with his patient in which his own anxiety plays a significant part.

In the lectures from which this book originated, Sullivan was formulating his thinking concerning a theory of interpersonal relationships as applied to the special instance of the interview. A portion of the lecture time was spent in group discussion, the approach being one of inquiry, of formulating questions, and of suggesting approaches to the study of human behavior, rather than one of attempting to discover definite "answers" to alleged "problems." In later years this process or operational approach was further developed by Sullivan in a series of seminars concerned with interviewing. These were lively meetings in which students presented case material, discussion was encouraged, and the business of psychiatry as demonstrated in the group interaction was seen to be very much a matter of interpersonal relatedness. Except for notes made by students, there are no records of these seminars, and they are not reflected in this book.

Although the coming together of two people for the purpose of developing a meaningful exchange of ideas directed toward their mutual enlightenment is a fundamental characteristic of the interview, such a meeting is complicated by the disjunctive force of the anxiety experienced by both participants. The psychiatrist and the patient—the interviewer and the interviewee—are motivated to meet with each other by certain obvious considerations. The psychiatrist looks upon the meeting as a way of practicing his profession, and of earning his living. The patient comes in order to learn more of certain characteristics of his behavior which he finds to be in some ways a handicap, with the prospect of altering these to his greater satisfaction. Despite such motivations, which would seem to favor the rapid progress of communication, an outstanding feature of interviews is the fact that the patient will not find it simple to present his case, will frequently engage in evasions, the subtleties of which he may be unaware of, and may wish to withdraw from the situation before much benefit has been obtained. The psychiatrist may find his work interfered with by his own anger, boredom, inattention, and other responses which are seemingly inappropriate to the expert in this specialty. Thus both psychiatrist and patient, while strongly motivated to meet, are also driven by anxiety to withdraw from each other. This interplay of movements—multiple variations of advance and retreat—is characteristic of the field of the interview. These operations on the part of both psychiatrist and patient are inevitable accompaniments of an interview and therefore cannot reasonably be looked upon as cause for rejoicing or lamentation. Because of their display the patient need not be labeled as difficult or uncooperative, nor the psychiatrist as incompetent. Although the psychiatrist is expected to be alert to these subtle interactions, it is not likely that he will immediately identify all of them. The goal of interviewing is not to do away with these movements, but to recognize them, explore their origins, and come to an understanding of their significance in the current situation. It is with such relationships of forces in a social field that the present book is concerned.

There is nothing extraordinary in the concept that the participants in an interview may experience emotions which promote their mutual withdrawal. Although the experience of anxiety is always unpleasant, there is little likelihood in our world that we can avoid it at all times, despite our great capacities for developing remarkably effective patterns of behavior as forms of defense. If early acquaintance with anxiety has been markedly painful, he who has endured this will be cautious in his dealings with people, and loath to expose himself to relationships which may threaten his feeling of security. Such a one may not welcome becoming either a psychiatrist or a patient—the personal contacts which are an ingredient of either role may seem too painful to risk. Nevertheless, without the experience of anxiety one would not become a patient; and without such experience it is not likely that one would be so preoccupied with the subtleties of human performance as to become a psychiatrist.

For the psychiatrist his experience of anxiety can be put to good use in his dealings with his patients, as well as with others. For such experiences to be forged into a useful therapeutic tool they must be identified, brought into awareness, their origins and modes of expression understood, and their reality accepted as part of life without fear or shame. All this is simply a part of the business of being a competent psychiatrist and interviewer as these terms are used here.

Sullivan spent some time at St. Elizabeths Hospital in Washington, D. C., where he worked in association with William Alanson White, and had the opportunity of observing large numbers of patients diagnosed as schizophrenic. He then moved to Sheppard and Enoch Pratt Hospital in Maryland, where he passed several years in investigating the difficulties of acutely disturbed schizophrenic patients in a small hospital unit. During this period, Sullivan was studying the difficulties that people have in "making sense" with each other, in finding out what the other fellow "means." In doing this he came to an observing of the interaction of forces in a social field, and began to develop a method of thinking increasingly congenial with the concepts of the modern physical sciences, and with the trend of the social sciences. He was moving in the direction of the so-called operational approach to the study of communication.

In his work with schizophrenic patients Sullivan observed that they often used language more as a means of defense than of communication; their speech served to keep people at a distance, thus protecting an already low self-esteem. One who has experienced a great deal of anxiety in contacts with others tends to withdraw from those others. He may do this by physical avoidance, by "keeping his thoughts to himself," or by speaking in such a fashion that his listeners are bored, irritated, puzzled, call him "crazy," and in turn withdraw from him. All of this is not "conscious" or planned, but is a complicated response to anxiety; and the end result is very successful avoidance of people.

Following the period at Sheppard, Sullivan spent some time in working with those who are known as obsessional. Although their behavior was more conventional and socially acceptable than that of many schizophrenic people, the obsessional use of language could be comprehended as another elaborate defense against the decrease of self-esteem at the hands of another person, and the accompanying experience of anxiety. Certain aspects of human living in our culture were becoming increasingly clear. It was evident that anxiety was a common experience, that it had its origins in the relationships of people with one another, and that in response to it, defensive patterns, or security operations, were developed which served to isolate people and keep them at some distance from each other. In certain exaggerated form these patterns were known as symptoms and indicators of "mental disease." Psychiatric patients were being understood as essentially no different from other humans, and as but striking examples of the common human experience—namely, that from people can come not only great good—but also great harm. This most children learn early in their lives; they learn that they cannot exist without human contact, and they also learn that some of that contact is dangerous in its arousal of anxiety—as well as in other ways. Experience that leads one to emphasize the dangerous aspects of human contact, and to erect great barriers against these, is the background of those recognized as mentally disordered and of many another whose difficulties may be concealed by a conventional façade.

As he came to a greater understanding of the general destructive effects of the experience of anxiety, its commonness in everyday life, and the intimate relationship between what is called normal and abnormal living, Sullivan shifted his interests to teaching and to the furthering of the collaborative efforts of workers in the various fields of human relations. If the psychiatric patient was not a peculiar form of human mutation, or other expression of biological disaster, but was to a large extent a reflection of group living which directed the patterning of his behavior, just as it directed that of successful and normal people, then the role of the psychiatrist must change. Biological wreckage might be isolated and supervised in institutions, and scatterings of human deviants be treated by clinicians of a medical specialty. But as the interest of the psychiatrist widened, keeping pace with the newer concept of his patient as at least a partial expression of the social group, it became increasingly evident that psychiatric problems were hardly to be solved by the creation of large numbers of practitioners, however skilled, to minister to those who might conceivably benefit from their efforts.

It was a realization of something like this that led Sullivan to turn his attention from the details of dealing with anxiety in individual therapy to the problems concerned with the diminishing of anxiety—or tension—as it appeared in groups. From what he had learned in his study of the person in terms of the social setting, he came to a greater recognition of the importance of the social structure in relation to mental health and mental disorder. In 1948, the year before his death, he was active in forming the World Federation for Mental Health, and in serving as a participant in the UNESCO Tensions Project, established by the United Nations to study tensions affecting international understanding. In developing greater comprehension of the intimate relationship existing between the socially productive person and the emotionally disordered and less productive one, Sullivan came to look upon anxiety as a destructive commonplace in human living, as the motor of much group tension, and as a force of such significance in its effects that it should be dealt with by group and public-health measures. Preventive psychiatry and the application of psychiatric knowledge to other fields of study seemed to him of greater urgency than an exclusive preoccupation with individual therapy. In this thinking he was in the medical tradition. Few practitioners would relish treating tubercular patients without the backing of the public-health measures which are so effective in reducing the incidence of that disorder. If it is once clearly understood that a goodly number of the emotionally disordered are a reflection of their life experiences, and if it is also understood that few people even remotely approach any full realization of their potentialities, and that such wastage of human potential is practically expensive and destructive to the larger social group, serious attention might be paid to efforts directed at the prevention of such loss. For the psychiatrist the task is, at least, the increased clarification of the difficulties as he sees them in his patients, and the relating of those difficulties to the broader social scene, with an accompanying promotion of a wider recognition of those relationships.

Throughout his career Sullivan was concerned with problems of communication as these were demonstrated in a variety of situations—in numbers of patients in large hospital wards, in the obscure behavior of schizophrenic patients observed in close personal contact, in the more conventional life of the obsessional person, and in the interaction of groups, large and small. This book on the interview, based on lectures given in 1944 and 1945, is concerned with the phenomena that interfere with the freedom of communication, as they are revealed in the special instance of two people sitting down together for a supposedly common purpose—improving the living of one of them. No patient—and few people under any classification—come into the presence of another without considerable caution and some expectation of rebuff. The understanding of such blocks to communication, reflecting underlying anxiety and anticipation of hurt from another human, is a major goal of the interview. The interview itself may be looked upon as a miniature of all communicative processes, containing within it the essential qualities of all human relationships, and much data relevant to the getting along of people in any social setting.

It should be clear that this book does not present a definite schematization of just what the interviewer should do in conducting the interview. It is not intended as an outline guide for action, but rather as a provocative succession of ideas which may prove stimulating to the thinking of anyone who conducts an interview. Many of us, doctors, nurses, and others, have been brought up in the tradition of identifying problems and then doing something about them; as practical people we want to deal with a clear statement of a difficulty and a prescription for action. We want to see a beginning, a solution, and an end to a situation. If we could only be told that a patient's trouble arises at point A, that it can be defined as disease B, and that it can be relieved by the application of remedy C, through the use of technique D, we would feel as if we were getting somewhere. This book does not give such answers.

Sullivan was trying to make some formulation of a process, by which I mean an always progressing, never stable movement of interactions taking place between people. This dynamic interplay of forces in a social field is in constant motion even though the outward behavior of the participants suggests that an equilibrium exists. Such an equilibrium is dynamic in character, the relationship being maintained by the ever-shifting patterns of behavior of the parties involved in the field. The psychotherapeutic process—and the psychiatric interview seen as a segment of that process—may be looked upon in this operational manner, in which the person observed can be comprehended only in terms of his relationship to others who influence him in his "life space," or field of living, and in terms of the behavior of the observer—the therapist or interviewer—who is, of necessity, a part of that field. In this sense the study of the interview becomes a study of the process or the interaction which results from the presence of the participants in that field. From this study certain rather accurate inferences may be drawn as to the past experience of those participants as reflected in the current action. Questions and answers about such a field must then be what is often referred to as "open-ended"—that is, they cannot be conclusive, final, and in all ways precise. They *can* be suggestive, provocative, and useful in guiding further inquiry as one participates in and moves along with the process under study. The attempt to deal in fixed quantities—raising questions as to 'Just what do I say here?', 'Just what does the patient mean when he says that?'—presents a static and somewhat unreal picture of the interview. 'What I say' and 'what the patient means' can be determined only in terms of the total context, and that context itself is not static. Thus in his consideration of the interview Sullivan reflects a movement in his own thinking toward an operational, field approach to the study of psychiatry, and his writing can be understood best when this developing point of view is kept in mind.

In working with schizophrenic patients, Sullivan found that the technique of so-called free association did not always yield great profit. The mute patient did not respond, the paranoid patient tended to repeat his paranoid stereotypes, and the patient who was near panic often came nearer to panic, engaging in great displays of "crazy" behavior which frequently effectively interrupted the relationship. The hebephrenic patient was usually not responsive to any suggestion to speak freely and easily. The obsessional person might speak at great length, but often with little apparent relevance to anything that might seriously constitute a problem in his living. The manic patient associated with all too great a show of freedom, and the depressed person withdrew even more when asked to relax and talk freely.

In this book Sullivan is not speaking "in favor of" an interview which is entirely directed by the therapist, and he is not speaking "against" the uncensored expression of the free flow of ideas. He is, however, opposed to the casual prescription of courses of action without there being some idea of how such action is to be effected. I recall that some years ago, when engaged in the more general practice of medicine, I advised a certain patient with high blood pressure to "take it easy." This gentleman was very polite, thanked me for my advice, and departed. Later, at my leisure, I was able to ponder on how this man, who supported a wife and three children by his labors in driving a dump truck, might apply my prescription. I decided that the prescription was not suited to the case, or that I should have devoted more attention to discovering how practical use might be made of it.

So for Sullivan and the matter of free association. He thought that the concept was excellent, but saw that the reasons for the difficulties of its application are intimately related to communication in the interview. To speak freely and without censorship implies a very low level of anxiety, a condition which rarely exists in the interview situation, unless the anxiety is covered by defensive maneuvers which in themselves are not useful expressions of free association. The questions raised by Sullivan are simply, 'How do you get people to associate freely?', and 'If there is trouble doing this, what is the nature of the trouble, and what can be done about it?' The very raising of such questions may be productive in improving the communication.

In these lectures Sullivan does not discuss countertransference as such, but he does place great emphasis on the role of the physician or interviewer. An important aspect of this role is the fact that one's observations of another may be considerably influenced by unrecognized anxieties arising from previous relationships with people. Such distortions we call transference or countertransference, depending on their reference to the patient or to the therapist. In Sullivan's thinking there is no situation in which the interviewer is a "neutral" figure in the therapeutic field; he is inevitably a participant, and the field of social action is altered by his presence. Thus the therapist can never observe his patient *acting-as-if-I-weren't-here-and-he'd-never-met-me*, but can see him only *acting-in-terms-of-his-past-and-including-me-also*. With this in mind it is evident that the removing of transference distortions does not do away with the fact that the social field is composed of the participants as real people plus the ways in which each experiences this current "reality" as a reflection of his previous experiences in living.

Sullivan had no great confidence in the accuracy of anyone's recall in reproducing either the content of an interview or its vocal and gestural accompaniments. Yet he thought that the taking of notes during an interview interfered with the exchange of ideas, and for a time was of the opinion that recording machines might unfavorably disturb the field. However, he was very much interested in the making of detailed observations of the nonverbal aspects of communication, and in the later years of his life he used a recording machine during some of his hours of therapy, listening back to such recordings in an attempt to learn more clearly "what had gone on." He also listened to recordings of colleagues' work with their patients and hoped that in this way he would be able to increase his effectiveness as a consultant.

In 1948 Sullivan was instrumental in getting under way a project in which the entire course of therapy with three patients (each with a different therapist) was recorded, and subjected to careful review by the therapists and consultants. In this way there was a movement in the direction of subjecting the work of the therapist to detailed scrutiny, thus getting a closer look at what is so casually spoken of as the "therapeutic operation."

At present the recording of interviews and their study are increasingly commonplace. The next step—which has already been taken by some, and was proposed by Sullivan [1] in the late 1920's—is the photographing of interview sessions, with the goal of obtaining a good look at the nonverbal gestural components of communication. In doing this we may come to a greater understanding of many things which in this book are but suggested, implied, or not as yet clearly formulated.

These lectures on the interview present some clues regarding the not-always-easy business of getting to "know" another person, as we put it, and give some examples of the ways in which the experience of anxiety gives rise to protective patterns of behavior which invariably complicate this. In any interview a certain characteristic of speech becomes quite clear, namely that speech is used not only for the transmission of ideas but for keeping matters obscure, for the maintenance of distance from another, and for the protection by rather magical means of one's self-esteem.

One of the truly remarkable characteristics of man is his development of speech, which is so extraordinarily suited to his purposes. When one observes a child, he sees a person who is interested in all that goes on about him, who is curious, who asks all manner of questions, and who uses speech as a wonderful means of getting acquainted with the world which opens out before him. Then comes the experience of anxiety in rela-

[1] "Affective Experience in Early Schizophrenia," *American Journal of Psychiatry* (1927) 6:467–483.

tionship with others—which is not to discount the influence of anxiety in the preverbal years—and the child discovers that certain magical qualities of speech may somehow save him from these painful decreases in his self-esteem. He learns that certain phrases such as "Excuse me," "I'm sorry," and other elaborations of words may win some semblance of approval. Thus a remarkable process occurs. At the very time when the child is expanding his knowledge of the universe and the people in it, and is beginning to acquire skill with the marvelous tool of speech—which, when joined on to his lively curiosity, will hasten that expansion—he undergoes a change which is marked by withdrawal and constriction. His curiosity is curbed, his interest in people is dulled, and he may become more concerned with the protection of his self-esteem, and with the use of language for this purpose, than with much else. This process apparently occurs to some extent in all people in our culture—and in any other of which I have any knowledge. There is almost a race between the circumstances which favor the use of language for the communication of ideas, and the circumstances favoring its use for their concealment and distortion. Should the experience of anxiety be so intense that the concealment value of language is of primary importance, there is a considerable reduction in the person's curiosity and in the possibilities of his experiencing anything like a marked realization of his potentialities. Such are those whom the psychiatrist sees as patients—and many others who never come his way. It is this remarkable intermingling of the communicative and defensive aspects of speech which characterizes every interview. This, and the background of anxiety which gives rise to it, is the central theme of these lectures.

This book stresses a certain important ingredient of successful interviewing which is frequently more adequately conveyed by gesture and tone of voice than by words. This quality or ingredient is shown by the interviewer's being keenly responsive to the needs of the interviewee, and doing nothing to lower that one's self-esteem. The skilled interviewer knows that those who come to his office have no great excess of security, and he does not become involved in heroic attempts to increase it by some magical means. That is, he does not attempt the impossible by engaging in unproductive reassuring gestures. What he does do is to demonstrate a very simple and serious respect for the other person in the interview. Now it is very impressive that such a display of honest, undecorated respect for another person brings out, in response from that other, not only reciprocal feelings of respect for the interviewer, but, most wonderfully, some feelings of increased respect for himself, the interviewee. That is exactly what one would expect to occur in a social field. When it happens in an interview, the prospects for some benefits to all concerned are excellent.

OTTO ALLEN WILL, M.D.

The Psychiatric Interview

CHAPTER

I

Basic Concepts in the Psychiatric Interview

SINCE THE field of psychiatry has been defined as the study of interpersonal relations, and since it has been alleged that this is a perfectly valid area for the application of scientific method, we have come to the conclusion that the data of psychiatry arise only in participant observation. In other words, the psychiatrist cannot stand off to one side and apply his sense organs, however they may be refined by the use of apparatus, to noticing what someone else does, without becoming personally implicated in the operation. His principal instrument of observation is his self—his personality, *him* as a person. The processes and the changes in processes that make up the data which can be subjected to scientific study occur, not in the subject person nor in the observer, but in the situation which is created between the observer and his subject.

We say that the data of psychiatry arise in participant observation of social interaction, if we are inclined toward the social-psychological approach, or of interpersonal relations, if we are inclined toward the psychiatric approach, the two terms meaning, so far as I know, precisely the same thing. There are no purely objective data in psychiatry, and there are no valid subjective data, because the material becomes scientifically usable only in the shape of a complex resultant—*inference*. The vicissitudes of inference is one of the major problems in the study of psychiatry and in the development of practical psychiatric interviews.

I am not going to discuss anything like the theory of psychiatry or attempt to investigate the reasons why a good many of the things that I say seem to me to be of practical importance. In considering the subject of a serious conference with another person, I shall discuss only that which seems capable of being formulated about the steps most likely to lead to the desired end. These comments will apply whether the other person is a patient in the sense of someone seeking help for what he calls his personal idiosyncrasies, or peculiarities, or other people's strange treatment of him; whether he is someone looking for a job; or whether he has been sent by his employer to discover why he fails to make good. Any interviews calculated to meet certain criteria, which I will shortly outline, may use the same techniques as those used by the psychiatrist in attempting to discover how he can serve the professional needs of his patient. In referring to the interviewee or client, I shall sometimes speak of him as the patient, but I imply no restriction of the relevance of what I say to the medical field, believing that, for the most part, it will apply equally well to the fields of social work or personnel management, for example.

A Definition of the Psychiatric Interview

As a point of reference for comments often somewhat rambling, it may be useful to attempt a definition of what I have in mind when I speak of the psychiatric interview. As I see it, such an interview is a situation of primarily *vocal* communication in a *two-group*, more or less *voluntarily integrated*, on a progressively unfolding *expert-client* basis for the purpose of elucidating *characteristic patterns of living* of the subject person, the patient or client, which patterns he experiences as particularly troublesome or especially valuable, and in the revealing of which he expects to derive *benefit*. Of course, any person has many contacts with other people which are calculated to obtain information—if only the directions for how to get where he wants to go; but these are not properly regarded as instances of the psychiatric, or serious, highly technical inquiry.

The Vocal Nature of the Communication

The beginning of my definition of the psychiatric interview states that such an interview is a situation of primarily vocal communication—not verbal communication alone. If one assumed that everyone who came to a psychiatrist or other interviewer had to be pinned down, as one too often hears in psychiatry, or cross-examined to determine what was fact and what was fiction, then interviews would have to go on for many, many hours in order to make any sense of the other person. But if consideration is given to the nonverbal but nonetheless primarily vocal aspects of the exchange, it is actually feasible to make some sort of a crude formulation of many people in from an hour and a half to, let us say, six hours of serious discourse (I might add, not six consecutive hours, though I've even done that). Much attention may profitably be paid to the telltale aspects of intonation, rate of speech, difficulty in enunciation, and so on—factors which are conspicuous to any student of vocal communication. It is by alertness to the importance of these things as signs or indicators of meaning, rather than by preoccupation only with the words spoken, that the psychiatric interview becomes practical in a reasonable section of one's lifetime.

The experience that gives me a peculiar, if not an important, slant on this whole matter is that I was initially intensely interested in schizophrenic patients. Schizophrenics are very shy people, low in self-esteem and subject to the suspicion that they are not particularly appreciated or respected by strangers. Like many other people, they are rather sensitive to scrutiny, to inspection, and to being "looked in the eye." Perhaps in all too many cases they are full of ancient traditional hokum from the culture about the eyes being the windows of the soul, and things being seen in them that might not otherwise be revealed —which seems to be one of the most misguided ideas I've ever known. In brief, schizophrenics are embarrassed by being stared at.

As I wished to learn as much as I could about schizophrenics (and with good fortune, perhaps about other humans as well), I very early in my psychiatric research work abandoned the idea of watching people while they talked with me. For years, seven and a half at least, I sat at an angle of ninety degrees from the people whom I interviewed, and usually gazed at something quite definitely in front of me—very clearly not at them. Since the field of vision is so great that one can observe motor movement in another person over an extraordinarily wide range, I think I missed few of my patients' starts, sudden changes of posture, and one thing and another, but certainly I could not see the fine movements of their faces.[1]

In order to become somewhat at ease about what was going on, I necessarily developed further an already considerable auditory acuity so that I could hear the kind of things which, perhaps, most people are inclined to deceive themselves into thinking that they can only see. I do believe that the majority of clues to what people actually mean reach us via the ears. Tonal variations in the voice—and by "tonal variations" I mean, very broadly and generically, changes in all the complex group of things that make up speech—are frequently wonderfully dependable clues to shifts in the communicative

[1] A visual study to determine what there is about other people's faces that gives away falsehoods and so on immediately demonstrates the gross absurdity of thinking that their eyes provide us with any clues. Even in the lower part of the face, which is distinctly more expressive and closely related to the mental state of the person concerned, the tensions are not by any means so labile that they keep up with the changing mixture of truth, best appearances, untruth, and frank falsehood that make up a great deal of communication.

situation. For example, if somebody is attempting to describe his work as a journeyman electrician, things may go on quite well until he is on the verge of saying something about the job which pertains to a field in which he has been guilty of gross disloyalty to his union, at which time his voice will sound altered. He may still give the facts about what a journeyman electrician should be and do, but he will sound different in the telling.

In the psychiatric interview a great part of the experience which one slowly gains manifests itself in a show of mild interest in the point at which there is a tonal difference. Thus the interviewer would perhaps say, "Oh, yes, and the payment of exactly 2½ per cent of one's income to this fund for the sick and wounded is almost never neglected by good union members, I gather"; to which the other might reply, again sounding quite different from the way he had earlier, "Exactly! It's a very important part of membership." And then, if the interviewer feels sure of the situation, he might say, "And one, of course, which you have never violated." Whereupon the other person sounds very different indeed, perhaps quite indignant, and says, "Of course not!" If the interviewer is extremely sure of the way things are going, he might even say, "Well, of course you understand I have no suspicion about you, but your voice sounded odd when you mentioned it, and I couldn't help but wonder if it was preying on your mind." At this the other person may sound still more different, and say, "Well, as a matter of fact, early in my journeymanship I actually did pocket a little of the percentage, and it has been on my conscience ever since."

Thus the psychiatric interview is primarily a matter of vocal communication, and it would be a quite serious error to presume that the communication is primarily verbal. The sound-accompaniments suggest what is to be made of the verbal propositions stated. Of course, a great many of these verbal propositions may be taken as simply matters of routine data, subject to the ordinary probabilities and to such further inquiries as will make clear what the person means.

I do not believe that I have had an interview with anybody in twenty-five years in which the person to whom I was talking was not annoyed during the early part of the interview by my asking stupid questions—I am certain that I usually correctly read the patient's mind in this respect. A patient tells me the obvious and I wonder what he means, and ask further questions. But after the first half-hour or so, he begins to see that there is a reasonable uncertainty as to what he meant, and that statements which seem obvious to him may be remarkably uncommunicative to the other person. They may be far worse than uncommunicative, for they may permit the inexperienced interviewer to assume that he knows something that is not the case. Only belatedly does he discover that he has been galloping off on a little path of private fantasy which clearly could not be what the patient was talking about, because now the patient is talking about something so obviously irrelevant to it. Thus part of the skill in interviewing comes from a sort of quiet observation all along: "Does this sentence, this statement, have an unquestionable meaning? Is there any certainty as to what this person means?"

For example, during an interview one may learn that a person is married, and if one is feeling very mildly satirical, one can say, "And doubtless happily?" If the answer is "Yes," that "Yes" can have anything in the way of implication from a dirge to a paean of supreme joy. It may indicate that the "Yes" means "No," or anything in between. The logical question, I suppose, after learning how happily the person is married, might be, "Was it your first love?" The answer may be "Yes," at which one may say, "Is that so? That's most unusual." Now, nobody cares whether it's most unusual or not. In fact, it is *fairly* unusual, but it isn't *most* unusual. The "most unusual" makes it an issue, with the result that the informant feels that it requires a little explanation; he is not quite sure whether or not it is something to be proud of. And at this point the interviewer may begin to hear a little about the interviewee's history of interpersonal intimacy with the other sex. Frequently, for example, in cases of marriage to the first love, there is a very open question of whether love has ever entered the patient's life, and one discovers that the marriage is nothing very delightful.

The Two-Group

To return to my definition of the interview, the next point is that this communication is in a two-group, and in that suggestion there certainly is a faint measure of irony. While it is practically impossible to explore most of the significant areas of personality with a third person present, it is also true that even though only two people are actually in the room, the number of more or less imaginary people that get themselves involved in this two-group is sometimes really hair-raising. In fact, two or three times in the course of an hour, or more, whole new sets of these imaginary others may also be present in the field. Of that, more later when I discuss what I call parataxic distortion.

Voluntary Integration of the Participants

The next point I would like to make concerns the patient's more or less voluntary entrance into this therapeutic situation on an expert-client basis. Psychiatrists are accustomed to dealing with people of all degrees of willingness, all the way from those who are extremely unwilling to see them but are required to do so by process of law, to those who are seriously interested in getting the benefits of modern psychiatry. I think that these startling extremes only accentuate the fact that probably most people go into any interview with quite mixed motivations; they wish that they could talk things over frankly with somebody, but they also carry with them, practically from childhood, ingrained determinations which block free discussion. As a result, people often expect that the psychiatrist will be either a great genius or a perfect ass.

Now, the other side of the picture: There are some more or less voluntary elements in the psychiatrist's attitude. He may vary from enthusiasm for what he is about to discover, to a bored indifference about the patient—and these attitudes unhappily may be determined very early in the interview. The attitudes of the interviewee are data. But any striking emotion on the part of the interviewer is an unhappy artifact which amounts to a psychiatric problem. For example, any intense curiosity about the details of another person's life, particularly his sexual life or drinking habits, or something like that, is a very unfortunate ingredient in a psychiatric interview. On the other hand, a more or less disdainful indifference to what the patient may have to offer amounts to a quite serious evidence of morbidity on the part of an interviewer.

As I shall presently suggest, there is no fun in psychiatry. If you try to get fun out of it, you pay a considerable price for your unjustifiable optimism. If you do not feel equal to the headaches that psychiatry induces, you are in the wrong business. It is work—work the like of which I do not know. True, it ordinarily does not require vast physical exertion, but it does require a high degree of alertness to a sometimes very rapidly shifting field of signs which are remarkably complex in themselves and in their relations. And the necessity for promptness of response to what happens proves in the course of a long day to be very tiring indeed. It is curious, but there are data that suggest that the more complicated the field to which one must attend, the more rapidly fatigue sets in. For example, in dealing with a serious problem in a very competent person, the psychiatrist will find that grasping the nuances of what is reserved, and what is distorted, and what is unknown by the communicant but very relevant to the work at hand, is not easy. So an enthusiasm about psychiatry is preposterous—it shows one just hasn't grown up; but at the same time, for the psychiatrist to be indifferent toward his work is fatal. The more dependable attitude of the psychiatrist in a psychiatric interview is probably simply to have a very serious realization that he is earning his living, and that he must work for it.

Whether the patient thinks at the beginning that he is very eager to see the psychiatrist or the interviewer, or whether he thinks he is bitterly opposed to it all, is less important. This does make some slight difference at the start, because one tries to accommodate, insofar as one readily can, to the mood of the patient. In other words, if a person comes to you quite angrily, it is not particularly helpful to beam on him and say, "Why, my dear fellow, you seem upset. Do tell me what's troubling you!" That is probably too reminiscent of the worst of his past experience with maiden aunts and so on. When people approach you angrily, you take them very seriously, and, if you're like me, with the faint suggestion that you can be angry too, and that you would like to know what the shooting is about.

Thus the initial attitude—be it willingness or unwillingness, hesitancy or reservation—of the client determines somewhat the attitude, and perhaps the pattern, of the interviewer's initial inquiries. But the client's attitude is not in itself to be taken very seriously; many very resistant people prove to be remarkably communicative as soon as they discover that the interrogator makes some sense and that he is not simply distributing praise, blame, and so on.

The Expert-Client Relationship

The expert-client relationship, which I have mentioned, implies a good deal. As defined in this culture, the expert is one who derives his income and status, one or both, from the use of unusually exact or adequate information about his particular field, in the service of others. This "use in the service of" is fixed in our industrial-commercial social order. The expert does not trade in the implements or impedimenta of his field; he is not a 'merchant,' a 'collector,' a 'connoisseur,' or a 'fancier,' for these use their skill primarily in their own interest.

The psychiatric expert is expected to have an unusual grasp on the field of interpersonal relations, and, since this problem-area is peculiarly the field of participant observation, the psychiatrist is expected to manifest extraordinary skill in the relationship with his subject-person or patient. Insofar as all those who come to him must be by definition relatively insecure, the psychiatrist is peculiarly estopped from seeking personal satisfactions or prestige at their expense. He seeks only the data needed to benefit the patient, and expects to be paid for this service.

By and large, any expert who traffics in the commodities about which he is supposed to be an expert runs the risk of being called a fancier, or a connoisseur, or a sharper, or something of that kind. This is because people are at a peculiar disadvantage in dealing with the expert who has an extraordinary grasp on a field; and if he traffics in the commodities concerned, as well as in the skill, people are afraid and suspicious of him. By cultural definition, they expect him to be a purveyor of exact information and skill, and to have no connection with the commercial-industrial world other than to be paid for such services. This is poignantly the case with psychiatrists, who work in a field the complexity of which is so intimidating that very few of them maintain for long the conceit that they are great experts at psychiatry. It is very striking to consider the cultural definition of the expert as it applies to the psychiatrist: he is an *expert* having *expert* knowledge of interpersonal relations, personality problems, and so on; he has no traffic in the satisfactions which may come from interpersonal relations, and he does not pursue prestige or standing in the eyes of his clients, or at the expense of his clients. In accordance with this definition, the psychiatrist is quite obviously uninterested in what the patient might have to offer, temporarily or permanently, as a companion, and quite resistant to any support by the patient for his prestige, importance, and so on.

It is only if the psychiatrist is very clearly aware of this taboo, as it were, on trafficking in the ordinary commodities of interpersonal relations, that many suspicious people discover that they can deal with him and can actually communicate to him their problems with other people. Thus the psychiatrist must be keenly aware of this particular aspect of the expert's role—that he deals primarily in information, in correct, unusually adequate information, and that he is estopped by the cultural attitude from using his expert knowledge to get himself personal satisfaction, or to obviously enhance his prestige or reputation at the expense of the patient. Only if he is keenly aware of this can the expert-client relationship in this field be consolidated rapidly and with reasonable ease.

The Patient's Characteristic Patterns of Living

To return again to my definition of the psychiatric interview, I said that it is for the purpose of elucidating characteristic patterns of living. Personality very strikingly demonstrates in every instance, in every situation, the perduring effects of the past; and the effects of a particular past event are not only perhaps fortunate or unfortunate, but also extensively intertwined with the effects of a great many other past events. Thus there is no such thing as learning what *ails* a person's living, in the sense that you will come to know anything definite, without getting a pretty good idea of who it is that's doing the living, and with whom. In other words, in every case, whether you know it or not, if you are to correctly understand your patient's problems, you must understand him in the major characteristics of his dealing with people. Now, this relationship of difficulty in living to all the rest of the important characteristics of a personality is a thing which I must stress, because we are such capable creatures, we humans, that we do not always know anywhere near what we have experienced. Psychiatrists know a great deal about their patients that they don't know they know. For example, caught off guard by the offhand question of a friendly colleague—"Yes, but damn his difficulties in living! What sort of *person* is this patient of yours?"—the psychiatrist may rattle off a description that would do him honor if he only knew it.

And do you think that this is restricted to psychiatrists? What you know about the people whom you know at all well is truly amazing, even though you have never formulated it. It may never have been very important for you to formulate it; it hasn't been worth anything to you, you might say. All that it's worth, of course, is that it makes for better understanding; but, if your interest lies in what the person does and not in understanding him, you probably don't know how much you know about him.

In the psychiatric interview, it is a very good idea to know as much as possible about the patient. It is very much easier to do therapy if the patient has caught on to the fact that you are interested in understanding something of what he thinks ails him, and also what sort of person his more admiring friends regard him to be, and so on. Thus the purpose of the interview is to elucidate the characteristic patterns of living, some of which make trouble for the patient.

Many people who consult psychiatrists regard themselves as the victims of disease, or hereditary defect, or God knows what in the way of some sort of evil, fateful entity that is tied to them or built into them. They don't think of their troubles, as they call them, as important, but not especially distinguished, parts of their general performance of living in a civilized world with other people. Many problems are so thoroughly removed from any connection with other people—when they are reported by the patient—that the young psychiatrist would, I think, feel rather timid about suggesting to the patient that perhaps he did not experience these problems in his relations with everybody, but only with some particular people; and I think that even the very experienced psychiatrist would scarcely wish to expose the patient to such unnecessary stress. But one can always ask *when* the trouble occurs—in what setting it is most likely to be seen. Remarkably often one of these patients who has an "organic" or "hereditary" neurosis that has nothing to do with other people can produce instances of his neurosis in which five or six different people have been involved—and for the life of him can't think of any other settings in which it has been demonstrated. It is only when he has come to this point that the psychiatrist can say, "In other words, you don't have this difficulty, so far as you know, with your wife and her maiden sister, and so on and so forth?" The patient stops, and thinks, and quite honestly says, "No, I don't believe I ever do." Only then is he on the verge of realizing that perhaps the other fellow *does* have something to do with the difficulty; only after being led around to making that discovery from his own data can he begin to realize that it is the interpersonal context that calls out many troubles.

I am not attempting to say here that there is nothing that makes living difficult except other people and one's inadequate preparation for dealing with them. There are a vast number of things, such as blindness in one or both eyes, and harelip, and poor education, which make difficulties in living. But the psychiatric interview is primarily designed to discover *obscure* difficulties in living which the patient does not clearly understand: in other words, that which for cultural reasons—reasons of his particular education for life—he is foggy about, chronically misleads himself about, or misleads others about. Such difficulties stand out more clearly and more meaningfully as one grasps what sort of a person he is, and what that person does, and why.

To sum up, a patient's patterns of difficulty arise in his past experience and variously interpenetrate all aspects of his current interpersonal relationships. Without data reflecting many important aspects of the patient's personality, the patient's statement of symptoms and the psychiatrist's observation of signs of difficulty are unintelligible.

The Patient's Expectation of Benefit

This brings me to the final portion of my definition—that the patient has at least some expectation of improvement or other personal gain from the interview. This statement may not sound particularly impressive; yet I have participated in long interviews that have been very unpleasant to the patient but which have come to some end useful to him and satisfactory to me only because he caught on to the fact that there was something in it for him. The *quid pro quo* which keeps people going in this necessarily disturbing business of trying to be foursquare and straightforward about one's most lamentable failures and one's most chagrining mistakes is that one is learning something that promises to be useful. Insofar as the patient's participation in the interview situation inspires in the patient a conviction that the psychiatrist is learning not only *how* the patient has trouble, but *who* the patient is and *with whom* he has trouble, the implied expectation of benefit is in process of realization.

I wish to put a good deal of emphasis on this, because there are interview situations in which there is no attention paid whatever to what the interrogee—the victim, one might say—gets out of it. Instead, it is a wholly one-sided interrogation. Questions are asked and the answers are received by a person who pays no attention at all to the anxiety or the feeling of insecurity of the informant, and who gives no clue to the meaning of the information elicited. These one-sided interrogations are all right for certain very limited and crudely defined purposes. For example, if you want to accumulate in fifteen minutes some clues as to whether or not a person will probably survive two years in the Army under any circumstances that are apt to transpire in two years in the Army, then you can use this type of interrogation. But, out of a large number of people interviewed in this way, the percentage of error in your judgment will be high. How high this percentage is, nobody has yet very adequately determined, for even the people who set out to use one-sided interrogation undoubtedly interpret a good deal that goes on besides the answering itself.

One can, in a rather brief interview, reach certain limited objectives. For example, an interviewer can determine that a person should not be given a job as a telephone operator by discovering that he has no capacity for righting himself after a misunderstanding, or that he is unnerved by someone's being unpleasant to him. But for purposes anything like those of the psychiatric interview, in which one is actually attempting to assess a person's assets and liabilities in terms of his future living, some time is required, and a simple question-answer technique will not work.

The interviewer must be sure that the other person is getting something out of it, that his expectation of improving himself (as he may put it), of getting a better job, or of attaining whatever has motivated him in undergoing the interview, gets encouragement. As long as this personal objective receives support, the communicative situation improves, and the interviewer comes finally to have data on which he can make a formulation of some value to himself as an expert, and to the other person concerned.

To sum up, the psychiatric interview, as considered here, is primarily a two-group in which there is an expert-client relationship, the expert being defined by the culture. Insofar as there is such an expert-client relationship, the interviewee expects the person who sits behind the desk to show a really expert grasp on the intricacies of interpersonal relations; he expects the interviewer to show skill in conducting the interview. The greater this skill, other things being equal, the more easily will the purpose of the interview be achieved. The interviewer must discover who the client is—that is, he must review what course of events the client has come through to be who he is, what he has in the way of background and experience. And, on the basis of who the person is, the interviewer must learn what this person conceives of in his living as problematic, and what he feels to be difficult. This is true whether one is interviewing with the primary idea of finding the person a doctor, of curing him of a so-called mental disorder, of getting him a job, of placing him in a factory, of separating him from some type of service, or of deciding whether he can be trusted in a certain position. In finding out in what areas the interviewee has his trouble in functioning, the interviewer would do well to remember that no matter how vastly superior a person may be, there is enough in the culture to justify his having some trouble. I have rarely experienced the embarrassment, or the privilege, of being consulted by a person who had no troubles, and I may say that when this did appear to be the case, it rapidly proved to be an artifact. Thus we may assume that everybody has some trouble in living; I think it is ordained by our social order itself that none of us can find and maintain a way of life with perfect contentment, proper self-respect, and so on.

The interviewer's learning wherein his client encounters headaches in dealing with his fellow man and achieving the purposes of his life, which is of the essence of the psychiatric interview, implies that the other fellow must get something in exchange for what he gives. The *quid pro quo* which leads to the best psychiatric interview—as well as the best interview for employment or for other purposes—is that the person being interviewed realizes, quite early, that he is going to learn something useful about the way he lives. In such circumstances, he may very well become communicative; otherwise, he will show as much caution as his intellect and background permit, giving no information that he conceives might in any way do him harm. To repeat, that the person will leave with some measure of increased clarity about himself and his living with other people is an essential goal of the psychiatric interview.

The Psychiatrist as a Participant Observer

As I said at the beginning, psychiatry is peculiarly the field of participant observation. The fact is that we cannot make any sense of, for example, the motor movements of another person except on the basis of behavior that is meaningful to us—that is, on the basis of what we have experienced, done ourselves, or seen done under circumstances in which its purpose, its motivation, or at least the intentions behind it were communicated to us. Without this past background, the observer cannot deduce, by sheer intellectual operations, the meaning of the staggering array of human acts. As an example of this, almost all the things pertaining to communication form such highly conventionalized patterns and are so fixed within the culture that if my pronunciation of a word deviates from yours, you may wonder what in the world I am talking about. Things having to do with your own past experience and with proscriptions of the culture and so on that were common in your home; activities which are attached to you as the person concerned in their doing, and activities to which you respond as if you were the person primarily, directly, and simply concerned in them—all these are the data of psychiatry. Therefore, the psychiatrist has an inescapable, inextricable involvement in all that goes on in the interview; and to the extent that he is unconscious or unwitting of his participation in the interview, to that extent he does not know what is happening. This is another argument in favor of the position that the psychiatrist has a hard enough job to do without any pursuit of his own pleasure or prestige. He can legitimately expect only the satisfaction of feeling that he did what he was paid for—that will be enough, and probably more than he can do well.

The psychiatrist should never lose track of the fact that all the processes of the patient are more or less exactly addressed at him, and that all that he offers—his experience—is more or less accurately aimed at the patient, with a resulting wonderful interplay. For example, one realizes that statements are not things that can be rigidly fixed as to meaning by Webster's or the Oxford Dictionary, but that they are only approximations, sometimes remote approximations, of what is meant. But that is just the beginning of the complexities of the participant character of the psychiatric interview—for that matter, of all attempts at communication between people, of which the psychiatric interview is an especially characterized example.

That does not mean, as some of our experts in semantics might lead us to suppose, that before a psychiatrist starts talking with his patient he should give him a list of words that are not to be used. It simply means, as I said earlier, that the psychiatrist listens to all statements with a certain critical interest, asking, "Could that mean anything except what first occurs to me?" He questions (at least to himself) much of what he hears, not on the assumption that the patient is a liar, or doesn't know how to express himself, or anything like that, but always with the simple query in mind, "Now, could this mean something that would not immediately occur to me? Do I know what he means by that?" Every now and then this leads to the interviewer's asking questions aloud, but it certainly does not imply the vocal questioning of every statement. So if the patient says, "The milkman dropped a can of milk last night and it woke me up," I am usually willing to presume that it is simply so.

On the other hand, a patient may say, "Well, he's my dearest friend! He hasn't a hostile impulse toward me!" I then assume that this is to explain in some curious fashion that this other person has done him an extreme disservice, such as running away with his wife—or perhaps it was a great service; I have yet to discover, from the interview, which it was. And I say, "Is that so? It sounds amazing." Now when I say a thing sounds amazing, the patient feels very much on the spot; he feels that he must prove something, and he tells me more about how wonderful his friend's motivation is. Having heard still more, I am able to say, "Well, is it possible that you can think of nothing he ever did that was at least unfortunate in its effect?" At this the poor fellow will no doubt remember the elopement of his wife. And thus we gradually come to discover why it is necessary for him to consider this other person to be such a perfect friend—quite often a very illuminating field to explore. God knows, it may be the nearest approach to a good friend this man has ever had, and he feels exceedingly the need of a friend.

The more conventional a person's statements are, of course, the more doubtful it is that you have any idea of what he really means. For example, there are people who have been trained to cultivate virtue (and the cultural motives that provided this training were horrible) to such an extent that they are truly almost incapable of saying any evil of anybody.

The psychiatrist, the interviewer, plays a very active role in introducing interrogations, not to show that he is smart or that he is skeptical, but literally to make sure that he knows what he is being told. Few things do the patient more good in the way of getting toward his more or less clearly formulated desire to benefit from the investigation than this very care on the part of the interviewer to discover exactly what is meant. Almost every time one asks, "Well, do you mean so and so?" the patient is a little clearer on what he does mean. And what a relief it is to him to discover that his true meaning is anything but what he at first says, and that he is at long last uncovering some conventional self-deception that he has been pulling on himself for years.

Let me illustrate this last by telling you of a young man who had been clearly sinking into a schizophrenic illness for several months and who was referred to me by a colleague. Among the amazing things I extracted from this poor citizen was that, to his amazement and chagrin, he spent a good deal of his time in the kitchen with his mother making dirty cracks at her, saying either obscure or actually bitter and critical things to her. He thought he must be crazy, because he was the only child and his mother, so he said, was perfect. As a matter of fact, he had two perfect parents. They had done everything short of carrying him around on a pillow. And now he had broken down just because he was engaged in a couple of full-time courses at one of our best universities. In other words, he was a bright boy, and had very healthy ambitions which represented the realization of the very fine training that he had been given by these excellent parents. I undertook to discover what was so surprising to him about this business of his hostile remarks to his mother, and he made it quite clear that the surprising thing was that she had never done him any harm, and had actually enfolded him in every kind of good. To all this I thought, "Oh yeah? It doesn't sound so to me. It doesn't make sense. Maybe you have overlooked something."

By that time I was actually able to say something like this: "I have a vague feeling that some people might doubt the utility to you of the care with which your parents, and particularly your mother, saw to it that you didn't learn how to dance, or play games, or otherwise engage in the frivolous social life of people of your age." And I was delighted to see the schizophrenic young man give me a sharp look. Although he was seated where I didn't have to look directly at him, I could see that. And I said, "Or was that an unmitigated blessing?" There was a long pause, and then he opined that when he was young he might have been sore about it.

I guessed that that wasn't the whole story—that he was still sore about it, and with very good reason. Then I inquired if he had felt any disadvantage in college from the lack of these social skills with which his colleagues whiled away their evenings, and so on. He recalled that he had often noticed his defects in that field, and that he regretted them. With this improvement in intelligence, we were able to glean more of what the mother had actually done and said to discourage his impulse to develop social techniques. At the end of an hour and a half devoted more or less entirely to this subject, I was able to say, "Well, now, is it really so curious that you're being unpleasant to your mother?" And he thought that perhaps it wasn't.

A couple of days later the family telephoned to say that he was greatly benefited by his interview with me. As a matter of fact, he unquestionably was. But the benefit—and this is perhaps part of why I tell the story—arose from the discovery that a performance of his, which was deeply distressing to him because it seemed irrational and entirely unjust, became reasonably justified by a change in his awareness of his past and of his relationship with the present victim of his behavior. Thus the feeling was erased that he was crazy, that only a madman would be doing this—and, believe me, it is no help to anybody's peace of mind to feel that he is mad. His peace of mind was enhanced to the extent that it was no longer necessary for him to feel chagrin, contempt for himself, and all sorts of dim religious impiety; but on the other hand he could feel, as I attempted to suggest in our initial interview, that there wasn't anything different in his behavior from practically anybody else's except the accents in the patterns of its manifestation. As he was able to comprehend that the repulsive, queer, strange, mystifying, chagrining, horrifying aspects of his experience reflected defects in his memory and understanding concerning its origins, the necessity to manifest the behavior appeared to diminish, which actually meant that competing processes were free to appear, and that the partitioning of his life was to some degree broken down. The outwardly meaningless, psychotic attacks on his mother did not give him the satisfaction that came from asking her more directly why in the devil she had never let him learn to play bridge. With the substitution of the possibility of a more direct approach, the psychotic material disappeared and he was better.

Thus whenever the psychiatrist's attempt to discover what the patient is talking about leads the patient to be somewhat more clear on what he is thinking about or attempting to communicate or conceal, his grasp on life is to some extent enhanced. And no one has grave difficulties in living if he has a very good grasp on what is happening to him.

Everything in that sentence depends on what I mean by "grave," and let me say that here I am referring to those difficulties unquestionably requiring the intervention of an expert. It is my opinion that man is rather staggeringly endowed with adaptive capacities, and I am quite certain that when a person is clear on the situation in which he finds himself, he does one of three things: he decides it is too much for him and leaves it, he handles it satisfactorily, or he calls in adequate help to handle it. And that's all there is to it.

When people find themselves recurrently in obscure situations which they feel they should understand and actually don't, and in which they feel that their prestige requires them to take adequate action (a somewhat hypothetical entity, since they do not know what the situation is), they are clearly in need of psychiatric assistance. That assistance is by way of the participant observation of the psychiatrist and the patient, in which the psychiatrist attempts to discover what is happening to the patient. A great many questions may be asked and answered in the psychiatric interview before the patient sees much of what the psychiatrist is exploring; but, in the process, the patient will have experienced many beginning clarifications of matters which will subsequently take on considerable personal significance.

As an example of such an obscure situation which seemed to demand action, I would like to mention a patient whom I saw for a brief interview a number of years ago in New York. She was a young lady of forty-three or so who presented, as her trouble in life, the fact that at night her breasts were frightfully tampered with by her sister who lived in Oklahoma. Now, such a statement is a reasonable sign of something being a little the matter with the mind. It also developed that the pastor of one of the more important New York churches gave the only help that she had ever been able to obtain in this cursed nuisance perpetrated by her sister. Since I always appreciate any help that anybody can get, particularly from somebody besides me, I was pleased to learn this and wondered why she had sought me out.

At this I learned that there were other difficulties. She was coming to suspect that a woman who worked in her office had been employed by her sister to spy on her—this nice psychotic lady, like many others, was earning a living. I said, "Aha! Now we are getting somewhere! Tell me all about that." Whereupon she bridled, realizing that it was risky to admit psychotic content to a psychiatrist. It developed that she had been controlling increasing rage against this woman in her office for weeks, and that she had been consulting her pastor with increasing frequency about the problem. I didn't ask what he did. But I did happen to look at the clock at that point and discovered that I had been keeping another patient waiting twenty minutes. So I said to the young lady, "Well, look here. I don't believe it would be practicable for me to attempt to substitute for the friendly adviser who is considerable comfort and support to you. But I do want to say one thing, which I have to say both as a psychiatrist and as a member of society: If you feel impelled to do something physical to square yourself with this persecutor in your office, then, madam, before you do it, go to the psychopathic pavilion at Bellevue and apply for voluntary admission for two or three days. In the end that will be much better." And she said, "Oh, you're like all the other psychiatrists!" With which the interview was over. I am quite certain that she derived considerable benefit from the finish of that interview.

The Concept of Parataxic Distortion

Now let us notice a feature of all interpersonal relations which is especially striking in the intimate type of inquiry which the psychiatric interview can be, and which is, in fact, strangely illustrated in the case I have just mentioned. This is the parataxic, as I call it, concomitant in life. By this I mean that not only are there quite tangible people involved (in this case the patient's sister living in Oklahoma and a fellow employee in the patient's office), but also somewhat fantastic constructs of those people are involved, such as the sister tinkering with the patient's breasts in her Manhattan room at night, and the fellow employee acting as an emissary or agent of her sister. These psychotic elaborations of imaginary people and imaginary personal performances are spectacular and seem very strange. But the fact is that in a great many relationships of the most commonplace kind—with neighbors, enemies, acquaintances, and even such statistically determined people as the collector and the mailman—variants of such distortions often exist. The characteristics of a person that would be agreed to by a large number of competent observers may not appear to you to be the characteristics of the person toward whom you are making adjustive or maladjustive movements. The *real* characteristics of the other fellow at that time may be of negligible importance to the interpersonal situation. This we call *parataxic distortion.*

Parataxic distortion as a term may sound quite unusual; actually the phenomena it describes are anything but unusual. The great complexity of the psychiatric interview is brought about by the interviewee's substituting for the psychiatrist a person or persons strikingly different in most significant respects from the psychiatrist. The interviewee addresses his behavior toward this fictitious person who is temporarily in the ascendancy over the reality of the psychiatrist, and he interprets the psychiatrist's remarks and behavior on the basis of this same fictitious person. There are often clues to the occurrence of these phenomena. Such phenomena are the basis for the really astonishing misunderstandings and misconceptions which characterize all human relations, and certain special precautions must be taken against them in the psychiatric interview after it is well under way. Parataxic distortion is also one way that the personality displays before another some of its gravest problems. In other words, parataxic distortion may actually be an obscure attempt to communicate something that really needs to be grasped by the therapist, and perhaps finally to be grasped by the patient. Needless to say, if such distortions go unnoted, if they are not expected, if the possibility of their existence is ignored, some of the most important things about the psychiatric interview may go by default.

CHAPTER II

The Structuring of the Interview Situation

The Cultural Role of the Psychiatrist as an Expert

I HAVE ALREADY stressed the cultural definition of an expert. I now want to discuss further the peculiar aspects of that definition as it applies to the psychiatrist, or to anyone who functions in the general field of the psychiatrist—that is, to a serious student of, shall I say, practical aspects of human personality and living.

I think that what society teaches one to expect is important. The person who comes to the interview expecting a certain pattern of events which does not materialize will probably not return; he will not say nice things about the interviewer if the latter, feeling that the things expected by his client are irrelevant or immaterial, ignores these expectations and presents the client with something much "better." In other words, what a client is taught to expect is the thing that he should get—or, at least, any variation should very clearly depart from it in a rather carefully arranged way. To illustrate, a person comes to you expecting the satisfaction, let us say, of a thirst for contentment. You may feel, in contrast, that it would be a great thing for him to learn how to make a living. But, before you expect success in offering him help in making a living, please pay attention to the fact that he is there to gain contentment, and that you will have to take what he expects into consideration if you wish to wean him from his interest in contentment and induce him to follow you in developing an interest in making a living. The social or cultural definition is very important indeed in the earlier stages of an interpersonal relation; in fact, it is finally important if one of the people concerned overlooks it, since this means that the relationship will not be developed in any meaningful sense. Something will happen, but the person who has overlooked the cultural definition of the situation will not know what has happened, and the course of events thereafter will not particularly suit him. The psychiatric expert, or anyone who sees a stranger on the assumption that he will find out about him and possibly be useful to him, may well pay considerable attention to what is traditionally, in informed society, accepted as the function of one in his particular expert role.

Let me mention now some of the ways in which the psychiatrist, in his work, illustrates this social definition. The psychiatric expert is expected to have an unusual grasp on the field of interpersonal relations, one which is very extensive, or very wonderfully detailed, or both. He is supposed to be at least somewhat familiar with practically everything that people do one with another, and to know more than his client does about the interpersonal relations in any field of interest that may be discussed. He is supposed to have such an unusual grasp on the technique of participant observation that when he talks with another person, he learns more than could be expected of any reasonably intelligent ordinary mortal. He catches on to more; he is more informed about what goes on in his relations with others than are even really talented, but not expertly trained, people. And he is expected to show his expertness in the management of his relation with the patient—an expectation in which many patients are woefully disappointed now and then. In other words, since the psychiatrist is an expert in interpersonal relations, it is not at all strange that the patient comes to the physician expecting him to handle things so that the patient's purpose will be served: namely, that his assets and liabilities in living will be correctly appraised, and that his difficulties will be tracked down to meaningful and remediable elements in his past—or that he will be advised, for instance, to divorce his wife in case she is really his trouble instead of his past. The psychiatric expert is presumed, from the cultural definition of an expert, and from the general rumors and beliefs about psychiatry, to be quite able to handle a psychiatric interview.

Now this statement implies that the demonstration of expertness in the psychiatric interview takes place, as Adolf Meyer once said, in the "here and now" of that interview. It does not take place somewhere else—for example, in the office of the physician who says, "You ought to see a psychiatrist, and I think so-and-so is a marvelous psychiatrist." That is all right; it may get the patient into the subway, or over the bus system, on his way to the psychiatrist's office, but it does nothing to establish the expert-client relationship which is the underlying factor in the possibilities of success of the psychiatric interview. The psychiatrist must demonstrate to the patient, in terms of the rumors and beliefs prevalent in the particular stratum of society from which the patient comes, that the psychiatrist is at least something of the person he is expected to be.

The psychiatrist demonstrates that he fulfills the expected role—insofar as these expectations make any sense and have any significance at all—if the patient experiences, in the course of the interview, something that impresses him as a really expert capacity for handling him, the patient. If you will pause to consider the people whom you look upon as "understanding"—that is, able to handle you expertly—you will notice that they demonstrate a very considerable respect for you.

Meeting such a person can be a really significant event; it is almost a privilege to have him around. This respect for you, which is so impressive when experienced, not only takes the general form of endorsing your worth as a companion in the same room, but is also shown by a certain warning of any severe jolts that you might receive in the discussion, and by a certain tendency to come to your rescue at those junctures at which you would feel better if you had some information that you don't happen to have, and so on and so forth. In other words, you are well managed, first, when you are treated as worth the trouble, and second, when the other person is keenly aware of, and sensitive to, disturbances in your feeling of personal worth, in your security, while in his presence.

Thus when a certain question is going to touch on a topic or field regarding which the patient feels insecure or anxious, the psychiatrist makes a little preliminary movement which indicates that he is quite aware of the unpleasantness that will attend this question, but also that it is obviously necessary that he should know the information; in other words, he gives the patient a little warning to brace himself. Now and then he may recognize that the patient is anxious about something which to the psychiatrist seems to be among the most natural things on earth; at that point he may say, "Well, do you feel that that's unusual?" The patient may say, "Well, yes, I'm afraid I do"; and the psychiatrist replies, "Dear me! Why, I never heard anybody talk honestly who didn't mention that." Thus respect for the other person, and awareness of the other person's feeling of security, is the first element of the expertness in interpersonal relations which any client will look for in an interviewer who is engaged in a psychiatric or quasi-psychiatric task. And if the client does not find it, no amount of propaganda by the family physician is going to make it look to him like a good situation, or make the results of the interview very deeply illuminating.

RELEVANT AND IRRELEVANT DATA

Both the culture and the social order—what is taught from the cradle onward—may support the psychiatrist in saying that as an expert he is "entitled to" or has a "right to" certain relevant and significant data about the person who consults him. In other words, such data are necessary on the basic assumption that the psychiatrist must understand who the client is and how things happened in his life. Anyone's being "entitled to" or having a "right to" anything is, of course, a very obscure reference to something very complicated. But so prevalent is this notion that there are inherent and indwelling rights connected with you, your family, your job, and so on, ad infinitum, that the client usually accepts it. The social order is such that no sooner do you as a psychiatrist indicate this assumption than the overwhelming movement in the client's personality is toward the conclusion: "Why, of course, the doctor is entitled to it. He must have it to make any sense of this problem of mine." And thus the psychiatrist engages in no arguments concerning the "right" or "wrong" of his being given data, or in debates relating to the "propriety" of his hearing this or that, or the "necessity" for the patient to reveal thus and so. He simply assumes that data must be given in order to make any sense at all of the always much too obscure processes of living; he avoids extended discussions with his patient about the origins of or the reasons for the assumption, presenting it as a sort of dogma, to be accepted of necessity if the work is to go forward and make any sense at all. Of course, if the patient does not accept this assumption, and wants to know what in the world I'm talking about, I tell him, but without amusement, because it requires so very many words.

Thus the expert insists on getting what he must know, emphasizing the fact that without the information it is impossible for him to guess what sort of person his client is, or to know what ails him. This applies, with certain changes in phrase, to interviews for the purpose of deciding whether a person should or should not be employed, should or should not be fired, can or cannot perform this or that, and so on. The expert is entitled to the relevant and significant data, and he therefore sets out to get it. If there is any great difficulty, he explains how necessary it is to have the information, and when that is made fairly clear, then he inquires why in the world he can't get it.

Sometimes difficulties in living are illuminated at that very point. For example, in paranoid states there is the utmost secrecy about all sorts of things which, so far as I know, are of no interest to anybody but the patient. The psychiatrist, in trying to get at various things that he needs to know, may bump into these areas of secrecy; in such circumstances he may say, for example, "Am I to understand the difficulty that you have with this troublesome neighbor of yours without any information at all about it?" At this the patient may glare for a while, being in somewhat of a dilemma, because, as far as he is concerned, the psychiatrist really should be able to do just that; yet it *does* sound rather peculiar when put that way. If then the psychiatrist says, "Or is it some secret that you don't want to confess?" he may draw himself up, really indignant at this point, and say, "Well, I think that these things are not at all improved by discussion." Now that helps to make it very clear that the psychiatrist cannot be useful to him, and so the psychiatrist simply comments on that. Thus it becomes fairly evident that there are some very remarkable secrets in this person's life, secret even from him.

The interviewer is also entitled to exercise his skill in discouraging trivia, irrelevancies, graceful gestures for his amusement, and repetitions of things he has heard. It is perhaps harder for the younger interviewer to demonstrate his expertness in this respect than it is for him to insist on the data he must have. But if you are an expert in interpersonal relations, you are likely, for good reason, to doubt that you have too much lifetime ahead of you, and therefore you want to utilize it as well as you can. It is also profoundly impressive to people, in the lucid interval after they leave you, to realize that you have kept them to something that made sense, and that when they started telling you a thing all over again, you said, "Yes, yes. Now we want to inquire into so-and-so." In other words, the expert does not permit people to tell him things so beside the point that only God could guess how they happened to get into the account. And so from his first meeting with the patient until the end or interruption of an interview or series of interviews, the psychiatrist handles himself like an expert in interpersonal relations who is genuinely interested in the problems of the patient. He is careful to get all the details necessary to avoid misunderstanding and to clarify erroneous impressions unintentionally given by the patient, yet he is chary of encouragement toward any repetitive, circumstantial, or inconsequential detail in the report and comment of the patient. There is no time to spare in a psychiatric interview. If he sees that the patient is repeating himself, going into circumstances which are in no sense illuminating, or wandering into inconsequentialities about some fourth, fifth, or sixth removed person, he may, without unkindness, discourage such moves, tolerating only a minimum of wasted time, since he knows that there is plenty to do. Actually this is a kindness to the patient, for it communicates to him that the psychiatrist seems to know what he is doing, and with such hope in mind he will put up very nicely with what the psychiatrist does.

The psychiatrist also foregoes the satisfaction of any curiosity about matters into which there is no technical reason to inquire. He foregoes this in a *passive* fashion, in that he does not ask, for example, what particular fore-pleasures the person has learned in intercourse with his wife or sweetheart, when that is of no moment; moreover, he foregoes it very *actively*, by cutting off accounts when he has heard what is important, even though it would be thrilling to hear the rest. Again, the patient greatly appreciates this. First, he is spared the perhaps marked embarrassment of going into harrowing detail. Second, he realizes, even if only after he leaves the office, that "This doctor was trying to find out what *ailed* me. He wasn't trying to amuse himself." Such a discovery goes a long way in making for the durable benefit which I wish to come from a psychiatric interview. Patients are really immensely pleased to learn that the doctor can end matters when he gets what he wants to know, and that he can then turn his curiosity off and apply it to something else that really matters.

PSYCHIATRIC BANALITIES

Still another thing that the interviewer should eschew is all meaningless comment and clouding of issues. At the same time, he avoids giving tacit consent, by absence of comment, to delusion or grievous errors expressed by the patient—a point which I shall discuss later. We often fail to realize just how meaningless many comments are. A lot of bromides from the culture and psychiatric banalities are handed out with the utmost facility, but I defy anyone to determine what most of them mean. For example, people refer to a "mother-fixation"—and when this is done by a psychiatrist in the course of a psychiatric interview, I think it deserves nothing short of a spanking. I grew up in the psychoanalytic school, and in studying schizophrenics—males only, after I found that I couldn't study female schizophrenics without getting more puzzled than they were—I discovered many mother-fixations. That is, I listened to a number of accounts of people's relationships with their mothers, but these were in every case accompanied by a wealth of detail which made of the relationship something which could never be appropriately and meaningfully condensed under the rubric, "mother-fixation." Nor could such a term be meaningful to any of these patients, who experienced their mothers in a great many ways, both devastating and wonderful. In other words, "mother-fixation" may be a beautiful abstract idea, useful for the psychiatrist's private ruminations; but to the person who suffers the "mother-fixation," the term is as nearly devoid of meaning, as near to being claptrap, as anything I can think of. Thus the psychiatrist tries to avoid meaningless comments and psychiatric banalities that prevent both his and the patient's learning anything, and merely give the patient a vague feeling that, "My God, I must have been terribly stupid; of course, that must be so, but why didn't I think of it?" In such a situation, there was nothing simply and usefully clear in what the psychiatrist said; he merely clouded the issue.

Thus, insofar as it is possible—and all of us fail now and then when one of our private interests is touched upon—the psychiatrist remembers that his role is that of an expert. He tries to keep to this role, no matter what attractive cul-de-sacs the patient may open up to him; if he does take an interest in the interview other than that of a person who is very hard at work in the most difficult of all labors—namely, understanding who somebody else is, what ails him, and what one can do that will be wise and durable in its results—he recognizes it and regrets it. From beginning to end, to the best of his ability, the psychiatrist tries to avoid being involved as a person—even as a dear and wonderful person—and keeps to the business of being an *expert;* that is, he remains one who, theoretically and in fact, deals with his patients only because he (the psychiatrist) has had the advantage of certain unique training and experience which make him able to help them.

In all this, the psychiatrist eschews with the greatest care all procedure which is calculated chiefly to impress the patient, to show that the psychiatrist is clairvoyant, or that he is possessed of omniscience. A psychiatrist, or any other expert interviewer, should have developed a certain humility, so that he may not be too inclined to act as if he knew all and his mind penetrated all, at a glance. He may feel that interviewing is hard work, as I recommend everyone should. It is, beyond perchance, very hard work.

Cultural Handicaps to the Work of the Psychiatrist

In the expert-client relationship with the patient, some of the extraordinary difficulties which the psychiatrist encounters in being expert arise from what may be called "antipsychiatric" elements in the culture itself—that is, elements in the culture which make the performance of psychiatric expertness far more difficult than is the demonstration of expertness in a great many other fields. Under this topic I could discuss a great many cultural attitudes that have been conspicuous throughout historic time, but I shall attempt to generalize only a few of those that constantly harass the psychiatric expert, just as they have always harassed people of Western European culture. First, in attempting to be psychiatric experts, we are very much afflicted by the fact that all people are taught that they *ought not* to need help, so that they are ashamed of needing it or feel that they are foolish to seek it or to expect it. And along with this, they come for psychiatric assistance with curious expectations as to what they are going to get, perhaps partly because this is so necessary to prop up self-esteem.

Second—and this is very widespread in the cultural heritage, so that people are taught it quite generally—is the belief that they should "know themselves," know what a fixed something-or-other called "human nature" is, know "right from wrong," and "good from bad," and be able to see through others in respect to all these important matters.

And third, people are more or less taught that they should be governed by "logic," or have "good sense"; or if they can't claim particularly good sense, then at least they should have "good natural insincts" and "good intuition," which ought to govern them in choosing the "right" way to act and to think about themselves and others.

Another idea which is very generally ingrained in personality is that one should be ashamed if one has not risen above and overcome the limitations of one's past, one's misfortunes, and one's mistakes; or if one hasn't, then one should occupy oneself with producing a very rich crop of verbalisms to show why, in spite of one's fineness and so on, these misfortunes were too much to be risen above and overcome.

Finally, as a sort of generalization of all of these, or in some people as yet another and separate antipsychiatric view: one should be independent. One should have no need for anyone else to tell one what to do or how to live. It was the culturally endorsed notion of independence which made the story of Robinson Crusoe so attractive in our unhappy youth—and a more recent demonstration of this notion appeared in a book which set up as the ideal of human maturity that one should be dependent only when sick, which I hope I have made clear is a somewhat dubious idea.

The Use of Methodic Procedure for Overcoming Personal Handicaps

The psychiatrist encounters extraordinary difficulties in being expert, not only because of these very widely spread antipsychiatric attitudes in the culture, but also because of inadequacies of his technical information. At the present stage of psychiatric knowledge, that is inevitable, because we do not yet grasp enough of the processes making up interpersonal relations to be adequate to all of the problems that arise in the course of our attempting to be psychiatrists. In addition, there is in all cases some measure of handicap arising from the psychiatrist's ignorance of interpersonal factors, which interferes with or precludes his participating as an expert in certain phases of the doctor-patient relationship. Now this may be a recurrent handicap in every one of his doctor-patient relationships, or practically every one—in which case one strongly surmises that the ignorance of interpersonal factors pertains primarily to the psychiatrist's grasp on himself. Or the handicap may vary from one of his doctor-patient relationships to another—in which case the handicap primarily pertains to characteristics of particular patients which the psychiatrist, because of his particular background and training, is unable to note, to observe.

None of us, with reasonable humility about the incompleteness of psychiatry and of our personal orientation, can expect to escape such handicaps. Therefore, in order to reduce the chances of serious difficulties arising from our ignoring or overlooking interpersonal processes in the psychiatric doctor-patient relationship, it is wise to make use, practically to the point of habituation, of a more or less methodic procedure for developing these relations with patients. While I cannot tell other psychiatrists just what procedure will be ideally suited to them, still there are some gross outlines which probably would be useful to practically anyone who does interviewing. Therefore I want to discuss a sort of diagram of method—or a diagram of the way in which one can develop methods for handling psychiatric interviews. By unobtrusively following such a method of procedure, the psychiatrist both saves time and demonstrates skill.

The psychiatric interview may be considered as made up of a series of stages which, while really hypothetical, fictional, abstract, and artificial, can be very useful for the psychiatrist to have in mind in arranging his time with the patient. More important, I believe that they are quite necessary for the achievement of the purpose of an intensive relationship of this kind. These stages are: first, the formal inception; second, the reconnaissance; third, the detailed inquiry; and fourth, the termination.

I shall discuss these stages in considerable detail later on, and for the moment shall outline only very briefly what I mean by them. The *inception* includes the formal reception of the person who comes to be interviewed and an inquiry about, or reference to, the circumstances of his coming. It should also include a brief, but considered, reference by the psychiatrist to any information already at his disposal; this is important not only to promote a feeling of confidence on the part of the patient, in the interviewer's straightforwardness, but also to provide an opportunity for the patient to amend the presumptive data which the psychiatrist may have received from another source, if necessary. Finally, an adequate reason for the conference must be established; that is, the psychiatrist should obtain adequate justification for the use of his skill.

Throughout this stage of the interview, the psychiatrist must remember that the person who consults him is a stranger—even though in other circumstances he may be an old friend. Thus the psychiatrist cannot know what impression anything that he says or does may make on this stranger, for he knows nothing of his background and nothing of the parataxic elements which may be very powerful in influencing his impressions. The psychiatrist must, therefore, be very alert to learn something of the impression that he and certain of his performances give, and at the same time very alert to learn how he himself is affected by certain things that the stranger may do and say. The interviewer should proceed in such a way that no complicating situation develops in this stage, for the inception of the interview may either greatly accelerate the achievement of the result desired or make that result practically unattainable.

The second step in procedure, the *reconnaissance*, which should be initiated as "naturally" as possible, consists in obtaining a rough outline of the social or personal history of the patient. In this stage, the interviewer is concerned with trying to get some notion of the person's identity—who he is and how he happened to get to be the person who has come to the office. Thus the interviewer asks conventional questions about age, order of siblings, date of marriage, and so on; he does not try to develop a psychiatric history, but tries to orient himself as to certain basic probabilities. The skill of the interviewer in obtaining and interpreting this history may often largely determine the ease or difficulty of the succeeding detailed inquiry. Moreover, the time to be spent in achieving the purpose of the interview or series of interviews may depend on the concise accuracy with which this history is obtained.

The next stage, the *detailed inquiry*, depends considerably, although not exclusively, on the ostensible purpose of the interview—a topic which I shall discuss shortly. The larger part of these lectures will deal with the principles and techniques of the detailed inquiry—that is, with some of the particulars that make up the almost unlimited variety of subtleties and complexities of this long stretch of inquiry into another person's life and problems. For the moment, I will say only that while the interviewer is governed in this inquiry by the ostensible purpose of the interview, he never carries out a good interview if he forgets what it is really for—namely, to permit an expert in human relations to contribute something to another person's success in living.

The fourth step of the interview, in this particular abstract scheme, is either the *termination* or the *interruption* of the psychiatric interview. By termination, I mean that the interviewer does not expect to see the person again; he is through. And by interruption, I mean that the interviewer has seen his client as long as he is going to on that particular day, and will see him again on the next day, or at some future date. If the interview is interrupted, the psychiatrist should give the patient a prescription for the interval, as a setting for the next session—for example, he may suggest something that the patient might try to recall. If the interview is terminated, the interviewer should make a final statement. In general, the main purpose to be attained, either in terminating an interview or in interrupting it for any length of time, is the consolidation of what has been achieved in terms of some durable benefit for the interviewee.

CHAPTER III

Some General Technical Considerations in Interviewing

Types of Psychiatric Interviews

BEFORE I DISCUSS the stages of the psychiatric interview in detail, I would like to mention several considerations which affect the course of the interview as a whole, and which affect the detailed inquiry in particular. One is the ostensible purpose of the interview. If the interview is for the purpose of finding out whether there is an adequate reason for firing a person whom somebody wants fired, naturally the interviewer does not cover all of the same topics that he would cover if he were attempting to discover, for example, why the person has precocious ejaculation in all of his attempts to establish his heterosexual prowess. Thus the interviewer is governed by the ostensible purpose of the interview; yet the assumptions I have named are not changed, and the attempt of the interviewer to be of some use to the person cannot be yielded, for this is the reason why the person does reveal what the interviewer needs to know.

To give some idea of the formal spread of ostensible purposes in psychiatric interviews, let me mention, first, the consultation carried out for purposes of diagnosis with a view to advising and perhaps facilitating the securing of competent treatment elsewhere. That is, the psychiatrist tries to determine the nature of the interviewee's personal difficulties in living, and to advise him with whom, and in what way, treatment or benefit may be obtained. Even though the interviewer in this case does not himself contemplate undertaking intensive treatment of the patient, he still must accomplish a good deal therapeutically, in the broad sense that I have spoken of; the patient may not be able even to reveal many of his greatest difficulties in living unless it becomes evident that this doctor will be useful in encouraging him to survive them for the time being, at least.

Then there is the interview which is, in fact, the initial conference in either brief psychotherapy or a potential continued-treatment situation; that is, the interviewer undertakes both diagnosis and the establishment of a professional acquaintance with a view to carrying on treatment himself.

These two are very different matters. In the former type of psychiatric consultation, it is a foregone conclusion that unless the patient proves to be charming beyond his wildest dreams, this particular doctor will simply tell him where to get treatment. I think that that is a distinctly easier job than the interview in which the psychiatrist not only finds out, it is hoped, some of the major ailments of the patient, but also communicates to him the conviction, which the psychiatrist himself shares, that he can aid the patient in getting rid of them. The element of the future relationship so strongly colors some interviews of the latter type that I have known psychiatrists to overlook what ailed the patient in the process of arranging to treat him, as a result of which the treatment was somewhat difficult. On the other hand, when it is a foregone conclusion that this particular interviewer will perform no miracles, but will just tell the patient where to go and why, getting the necessary data is greatly facilitated.

The next type of interview I wish to mention is held again for the purpose of diagnosing a difficulty in living, but with an emphasis on influencing the environment rather than the patient. For example, wives sometimes come to discuss treatment for their husbands, or ladies their sweethearts, or vice versa, with the idea that this might take some kinks out of the relationship. For all I know, it sometimes does. Schoolteachers sometimes come to discuss getting treatment for difficult children, with the idea that this might make it easier to live and teach in the same room with them. And clergymen have been known to feel that they needed a little technical knowledge about their relations with communicants. Parents, custodians of jails, judges, and very intelligent members of law firms sometimes wonder if a little technical advice about the mental health and probable needs of their clients might not be an aid in helping them. In such cases, the psychiatrist is supposed to produce the benefit, so far as the given situation is concerned, by some effect through other people, or institutions, or something of that kind. That does not suspend the necessity for also helping the person who comes to the interview, if the interviewer is really to get the data he needs; it does not forbid that something should be done for this person to help him to live.

There is also an increasing field of interviewing in connection with industrial or commercial personnel management. Thus the psychiatrist may be asked to interview a prospective promotee or transferee for some organization which has an enlightened official who thinks that there is something to be gained from the study of personality. Or if a person repeatedly fails to show up for work because of ill-health, he may be advised to see the psychiatrist; such procedures are becoming accepted in the growing field of industrial medicine. Incidentally, there seem to be an increasing number of major generals in the British, American, and doubtless the Russian armies, who have already discovered that the company commander who gets somewhat acquainted with his troops—the one who might say, "You look sort of down-in-the-mouth today, Joe. What's the trouble? Bad news from home?" and hears in return something like, "Well, I think my girl has fallen for somebody else," and then talks to him a little—is the commander whose company has very few absences without leave, and a strikingly small proportion of acute psychoneurotic disturbances under fire, and so on. In other words, it is beginning to be clear in many places that a great deal of the seeming difficulty in the productiveness of people is related to obscure problems away from the job—in the home, in the community, in the church, or elsewhere—and that it can be very useful to have someone around who is not too free with advice but who can be fairly skillful at finding out what the person is really worrying about, so that he can say, "Well, isn't this or that probable, and can't you brace yourself for one or the other of them?" Such an apparently simple thing as that has an immensely useful effect on these apparent difficulties in management–labor relations, commissioned officer–enlisted man relations, and various other types of elaborately organized interpersonal cooperation.

As I have said, the ostensible purpose of the interview has a good deal to do with the exact procedure, but nevertheless it is fundamental that the interviewer convey to the interviewee more feeling of capacity, of adequacy to go on living, and of doing perhaps better as a result of the conference—even, for example, in a case where the interviewee may get fired as a consequence of his and the interviewer's finding that he is really greatly handicapped for dealing with the particular organization in which he happens to be. It is not enough that the interviewer should find out something and give a really convincing demonstration of it. The interviewee must also get something out of it.

The Use of Transitions in Interviewing

The topic of transitions is of such peculiar significance in connection with the whole procedure of the interview that I want to discuss it before proceeding any further. Although the making of transitions is strikingly important in the detailed inquiry, it is a necesary part of the technique of interviewing at every stage. And it is so peculiarly an abstraction of technique that it has nothing to do with the ostensible purpose, but is worth while for the interviewer to have organized in his mind no matter on what basis he interviews another person.

When I talk about how to make transitions, I simply mean how to move about in the interview. It is imperative, if you want to know where you are with another person, that you proceed along a path that he can at least dimly follow, so that he doesn't get lost completely as to what you are driving at. When he gets lost, very often you do too, and one or the other of you may not know it. The law of diminishing returns then begins to operate with great vigor without the patient's quite realizing it—and often without the psychiatrist's quite realizing it. It is ideal, if you can, to go step by step, with sufficient waving of signal flags and so on, so that there is always something approaching a consensus as to what is being discussed. Unfortunately, with many people that would mean that you would have to live several months with them; and so, when you are conducting a psychiatric interview, you may need to vary from this idea of always proceeding toward a goal which is unknown but can nonetheless be designated so that the patient can see what you are driving at. Actually, the interviewer must change directions quite frequently. He chokes off topics which, although they interest the patient, he identifies as improbably useful—that is, as taking vastly more time than any probable utility will justify. He must ask about some things which the patient is very skillful at eluding, and, as a result, the interview must sometimes move from one obscure situation to another, with the interviewer not always being certain that the patient knows just what he is asking about or certain that he understands exactly what the patient is trying to say.

I look upon transitions in interviews as one of the very important technical details that ought always to get considerable attention, requiring a sort of quiet, continuing alertness in all your work in dealing with strangers in a serious and intimate fashion. Notice that when you speak of changing the subject—

that's one way of putting it—it doesn't tell the whole story. There are people who, I believe, have never stayed on the same subject for two consecutive remarks. And there are interviewers who seem to do little better. It is very easy to move from what you were discussing to something else that has popped into your mind; and if you do that without noticing what you have done, it is quite possible that you may obtain the most fantastic ideas of your interviewee. Thus it is always well to notice—with the same ease with which people can notice such a world of things that are going on without losing their place—when you change the subject. The changing of the subject can very well be treated in one of at least three ways, which are important and are by no means artificial abstractions.

The first of these we may call the *smooth transition.* When the interviewer wishes to change the subject, he can make the transition by a more or less adequate, and at least superficially truthful, statement which definitely says, in effect, "Well, now, that brings up the topic of so-and-so. Eh?" The patient might wear himself out trying to guess how it brought it up, but at least the interviewer has taken him by the hand and led him to the new topic. There are a good many times when the interviewer may use some little comment such as, "Oh, yes, well, sometimes that's due to so-and-so. I wonder if by any chance you've had experience of that kind?" In other words, he moves from one thing to another quite smoothly, so that the other person feels that this is really a very clear, collaborative inquiry. Now, an interviewer is not apt to do that if he does not realize that he is going to change the subject. And if he doesn't realize such things, he may lose his client.

In the *accentuated* or *accented transition* you do not use one of these polite ways of moving yourself and the patient hand in hand from one topic to another, but you rustle your feathers, as it were, and somehow indicate that, "Well, the world is about to undergo some mild change." In my case I usually begin to growl, rather like a ball bearing with some sand in it, just to indicate that something is about to happen. I want to drop what is going on, emphatically; not in such a way that it is forgotten forever, but with such emphasis as to disturb the set, as the old experimental psychologists might call it. I want that which has been discussed not to influence that which is now to be discussed. Suppose the person has just been showing me what an unutterably lovely soul he has. I will then sort of growl a bit as a preliminary to saying something like, "With what sort of person do you find yourself really hateful?" As a matter of fact, I probably wouldn't do anything quite that crude. But the point is that as long as he is full of the idea of convincing me of his beautiful soul, it would really be uncouth for me to proceed smoothly to attempt to find out how the devil he is a nuisance. But with the accented change, he may forget what he was talking about. People are apt to get a little insecure, you know, when it is suggested that the weather is going to change, and the predictions aren't dependable. In any case it causes a little pause, a sort of empty pause, which is not being smoothly, socially conversational. And then, without commotion—without startling the patient—I introduce the new topic. In this way the later data is not poisoned by the exploration that was in progress before, as it might be with a smooth transition.

Then there is the *abrupt transition*, at which, I am sorry to say, many interviewers seem to be past masters—and I should not wish to encourage them to improve their art. Nevertheless, it has its uses. I am not, however, suggesting a transition so abrupt that the patient is suddenly so startled that he can't guess what on earth the interviewer has said. I mean, rather, that a new topic is introduced which has relevance, but which is introduced at what would be described as a socially awkward point, and without warning. This sort of thing may be done to avoid, or to provoke, anxiety. I may say here that many an interview passes from the informative to the nebulous because the patient has become acutely anxious; but, on the other hand, some interviews would never get to be psychiatric interviews if the patient were not made anxious. The question relates to the way in which the patient is made anxious. It is properly done when the patient is taken through an upsetting period to definitely reassuring material, or from something that was going on with greatly increasing risk to the situation to something which is remarkably reassuring.

To sum up, the smooth transition is used to move gently to a new topic; the accented transition saves time and clarifies the situation; and the abrupt transition is ordinarily used either to avoid dangerous anxiety or to provoke anxiety where you can't get anywhere otherwise.

The Taking of Notes During the Interview

I am often asked my opinion about the making of written notes during the course of the interview, considered from the point of view of its effect on the psychiatrist and on the patient. There is a great variation among people in the degree to which certain behavior is automatic; and so there may be people so expert at shorthand that they can jot down rather automatically a great deal of what they are listening to and still leave the field of awareness free to participate in the work of the interview, and there may even be people who can make longhand notes which are useful to them later without particularly occupying their attention during the actual session. The only times that I have ever made notes during an interview with the feeling that it did not seriously interfere with the work that I had to do was when I dealt with people whose production rate was very low—certain puzzled schizophrenics, and one patient with a serious disorder in the region between schizophrenia and the obsessional illnesses. Schizophrenic patients have great difficulty in completing their sentences, often losing their place before they are through with a sentence, and they speak relatively infrequently, spending a good deal of time in starting and stopping. Since I was greatly interested theoretically in what the disorder of thought and speech was, I did take down quite completely a great many of my hours with a few puzzled schizophrenics. In fact, I had one patient who talked so slowly and had such a theoretically very important condition that I wrote down verbatim what he said. Unhappily, I fear that this record will not become available to posterity, because I can't translate my writing without taking two or three times as much time as it took to conduct the interviews. That, in its way, tells a story: the fact that I was not paying enough attention to write legibly suggests that I was busy with something else. And the obverse of that is more or less my opinion about taking notes: if enough attention is paid to them so they are legible, this is very apt indeed to interfere with things of much greater importance to the patient, if not to the psychiatrist.

The psychiatric interviewer is supposed to be doing three things: considering what the patient could mean by what he says; considering how he himself can best phrase what he wishes to communicate to the patient; and, at the same time, observing the general pattern of the events being communicated or discussed. In addition to that, to make notes which will be of more than evocative value, or come anywhere near being a verbatim record of what is said, in my opinion is beyond the capacity of most human beings.

Even if the interviewer were able to do all this, when he deals with patients who are quite suspicious, even paranoid, in their attitudes, the making of notes will probably guarantee that the interviewer hears an exceedingly studied group of communications, in which all the nuances which he might otherwise catch on to are missing. Nevertheless, there are occasions—for example, when I am getting the gross social data about a person—when I do feel that I should have a few notes. On such occasions I tell the patient that I have really a gift for forgetting things that might be handy, and therefore, if he doesn't mind, I shall make a few notes as to the number of siblings and one thing and another. At other times, however, when I have felt that something of great importance could be obtained from an interview, I have taken considerable pains to see that the recording of the interview was entirely exterior to the patient's awareness.

In the interrogation of patients before staff conferences, the patient is not only in the presence of a shorthand reporter, but also of a large number of psychiatrists. Many psychiatrists consider this a relatively barbarous practice, but since I found it in existence at several places where I worked, I put it to such use as I could. I think that the fact that a record is being made is initially quite distressing to many of the patients, but there are so many other things that are distressing about the interrogation that most of the patients, I think, forget that a record is being made before the session is over. Nevertheless, the reporting does not facilitate communication.

To put the whole thing succinctly, I think that most psychiatrists, if they are really engaged in conducting and understanding a psychiatric interview, are too busy to have much time to make written notes, even if making notes did not have a distinctly estopping effect on the patient. I think that patients, like the rest of us, can usually talk with relative freedom if only their own and the other fellow's memories are later to be consulted as to what was said. All of us become considerably more cautious if there is to be a written record of it. I myself can, through long experience, talk in the presence of a recording machine; I am able to be more interested in whether or not I have gotten across what I am trying to present than preoccupied with the inhibiting effect of the recording machinery. Yet if I knew that a stranger was going to take over the record before I had a chance to look at it, I might feel differently about it—in spite of the fact that I have considerable faith in saying what I mean, aside from minor accidents in speaking, and fatigue that sometimes prevents me from finding the words I am looking for. These are advantages rarely possessed by a person undergoing a psychiatric interview; even if in his better moments he feels quite able to speak the language, the psychiatric interview is a situation of considerable stress, in which he is likely to feel at a disadvantage, and the idea that a record is being made increases his disadvantage still more.

A verbatim record of an interview, until it has been heavily annotated, is almost invariably remarkably misleading. I have had some recordings of interviews which I have regarded as astonishingly good teaching material, but when I have sprung these on intelligent colleagues, I have often found them barking up trees that I hadn't seen—if, indeed, such trees were ever there, and I came to realize that they weren't. In other words, the complete meaning of a conversation is not to be found in the verbatim verbal context of the communication, but is reflected in all sorts of subtle interplay. For example, very slight changes of tone suggesting the faintest hint of irritation on the part of the psychiatrist often switch the patient from an attempt at concealment to a very reasonable compromise between what he thinks it is safe to tell and what the facts may have been. Such things do not appear in the most perfect verbal record. Thus, to give a third person a notion of all that happened in an interview, one would have to annotate the written record by adding the impressions that went with different statements, explaining why things were put as they were, and so on; only in this way could the richness of the interchange in a two-centered unitary situation begin to be apparent.

The Interpersonal Integration of the Interviewer and Interviewee

I would now like to review some of the things that I have said from a somewhat different standpoint. What I have said about the course of the interview through its various stages and the transition during the interview from topic to topic may be seen to imply the beginning, course, and termination of an interpersonal situation. Psychiatry studies interpersonal relations, which occur only in interpersonal situations; such situations imply something more than the presence of two people somewhere; they concern two people who are *involved* with each other—and that we call *integration*. Further, an interpersonal situation, of which the interview situation is a particular instance, is integrated by—brought into being by, held together by, and the course of its events, to a certain extent, determined by—something in the two people concerned which is *reciprocal*, and the manifestations of which coincide approximately in time. Thus one may say that the interview situation, or series of situations, is *integrated by coincident reciprocal motivation* of interviewee and interviewer.

A great deal about the psychiatric interview can be learned if we consider it from the standpoint of the reasons for its occurrence—that is, if we examine the reciprocal motivation that coincides in a particular interview. From what we know about the integration of interpersonal situations I derive the statement which I have already emphasized so much: an interview must promise to be of some use to the interviewee; he feels entitled to, and should have, some gain from it. If his expectation is in no way met, the interviewer will not have much of an idea of what is going on. Thus, no matter how apparently inferior, or unfortunate, or needy, or what not, another human being may be, the interviewer must realize that his profit from the interview must be more than imaginary. He must have a sufficient motive for going on with it; otherwise, even though he may sound as if he were really answering the interviewer's questions, he will actually be doing something different.

As an expert in the participant observation of interpersonal situations, the interviewer has the task of so influencing the interview situation that the closely observed course of his participation will reveal the major handicaps and major advantages in living which are relatively durable characteristics of the interviewee. Now, that is a very big requirement, and my experience suggests to me that many of us, having discovered a *few* of the patient's handicaps, may use a very lively imagination to provide us with something like a comprehensive picture of him as a person. The need to do that is understandable, but the practice yields distorted data. Of course, the inconspicuous intervention of the psychiatrist will not serve to reveal all of the patient's reasonably probable handicaps and assets fully, and will not result in their being documented or proved; some of them will be indicated only. But they should not be entirely overlooked or left to the interviewer's imagination in retrospect when he is writing his report.

It is the interpersonal events and the pattern of their course which generate the data of the interview; that is, the interviewer experiences the ways in which the interpersonal events follow each other, what seeming relationships they have to one another, what striking inconsistencies occur, and so on. Thus the data of the interview may come, not so much from the answers to questions, but from the timing and stress of what was said, the slight misunderstandings here and there, the occasions when the interviewee got off the subject, perhaps volunteering very important facts which had not been asked for, and so on. And so as an interviewer grows more skillful, he realizes with increasing clarity that what he must do is to watch the course of events and observe how they, as a pattern of progression, give rise to a very wide field of data about the other person with whom he is concerned. His use of this data, and his skill in drawing inferences from it, will grow with experience. Yet, until he has the information to be gained from this kind of participant observation, he has nothing with which to begin; and it cannot be obtained by the charmingly simple procedure of sitting at a desk and, with a feeling of utterly detached isolation from the person out in front, shooting questions at him, and perhaps checking his answers on a form.

The all but inevitable extreme obscurity of the events early in the interview, and the continuing complexity of so many of those events making up its course, make it useful to be unobtrusively methodical, as well as constantly alert. In other words, the interviewer is quite clearly aware of the type of significant data that he may reasonably expect in different phases of the interview; he takes steps to secure these data; he validates, or marks for subsequent validation, anything which seems needlessly indefinite or improbable; and he notes most carefully any occasion when material reasonably to be expected *has not* come forth. All this implies what I have already stressed—the advisability of very methodically, although unobtrusively, including in each interview the four phases which I have mentioned, and of accomplishing in the formal initiation of the interview certain very definite steps. Because of the sometimes impossible complexity of relations with a comparatively unknown other person, it is wise for the interviewer to ingrain in himself an outline of the ways in which these steps can be taken, developing patterns of action which will work so effectively and so unnoticed that he will not have to take time out to consider what the next step is to be.

But since no outline can possibly anticipate the variations that may occur in a personal relationship with a stranger, it is not enough that the interviewer knows just what he expects to do; he must also be alert for any suggestion that something has happened which is unexpected, because the *novelties* which occur in an inconspicuously methodical investigation are the things that distinguish its results. For example, among the most significant characteristics in the course of events making up an interview are the absences of those events which all or most of the interviewer's previous experience leads him to expect. A person may build up a course of historic data which, in the interviewer's experience, has always meant that certain events would follow. When this sequence does not appear in a particular patient's account, the interviewer does not necessarily get excited about it, but he does not overlook the omission. The fact that the data reasonably to be expected from a certain movement in an interview have not appeared *may* be highly revealing, and, in any case, is far too promising a matter to be overlooked or forgotten.

Somewhat similarly, the psychiatrist notices any points at which the patient seems to have no grasp on things which the psychiatrist regards as necessary or important in life, or in the patient's work. At such points, instead of concluding that he is dealing with someone stupid, the psychiatrist offers some hints as to what the information might be, to determine if it actually is lacking. If it is, he may offer some comment which is as simple, unassuming, and clear as he can make it, to see what happens, because there are a good many people who require only a hint to catch on to long streams of implications, and it is very useful to discover that.

Or, as another example, the psychiatrist may be puzzled by something the patient says. This does not always justify the interviewer in immediately jumping into the situation and asking about it; there are times when it is very wise to wait to resolve any puzzle or doubts. However, if events have not been made clear at some particular point, the interviewer should *know* that such is the case, so that when there seems to be an opportunity for a perfectly good transition, or when nothing in particular seems to be going on and the patient is waiting for questions, he can bring this point up again and indicate that he is in doubt as to the precise meaning. People very quickly come to understand that what they have said may not communicate perfectly to the listener, and they are quite reasonable about illustrating the various conclusions that they have stated.

Now, observing all these things is a function of the interviewer's *alertness*. No matter how smoothly things are going, he must be alert for something new or unexpected. Alertness is a function that is in a sense intimately related to that type of activity which people call "thought," but which is actually vastly more extensive than that which we know as "thought." For more precise purposes we may apply to this activity the term "covert process"—something that cannot be observed, but only inferred—which is in contrast to the other type of referential operations, the *overt*, which can be observed, although sometimes only by the initiate. Some may say that covert processes can be observed by introspection. Doubtless some covert processes could be observed this way, were it not that the process of introspection is apt to destroy the clarity of the covert process. In any case, the field of covert processes concerned in human behavior is vastly wider than anything that anyone has ever discovered by introspection.

Since one's alertness is a *function of covert processes*, it is useful in training for interviewing to have in mind the genera of data to be expected from phase to phase in the interview. That can be put, if you please, as "knowing what you are looking for"; however, I hesitate to describe it that way, for anyone who thinks in such terms is in very serious danger of believing that he looks from an isolated observing standpoint on performances to which he is related solely as an observer, and this the interviewer cannot do. There are no psychiatric data that can be observed from a detached position by a person in no way involved in the operation. All psychiatric data arise from participation in the situation that is observed—in other words, by participant observation. Thus, instead of "knowing what one is looking for," one wants to be *alert to the possibilities of the immediate future of the relationship in which one is involved*. This is why I cannot say, "Here are seventeen tables of events that can characterize interviews; now, you memorize all these and then you will always know just what to expect." No such thing is possible.

Alertness can never be brought about in a useful fashion solely in response to things that can be precisely communicated in words, unless the communication is of a peculiarly extraordinary character. Of course, if without warning I look wildly toward the door and shout, "Fire!" I do use a word, and the hearer's alertness would be very powerfully influenced by that communication. But that is most exceptional, and even so, it is scarcely *verbal* communication. It is a queer kind of warning of great danger, very little different from the ringing of a very large gong. Thus I cannot teach anyone *what* to expect—what to be alert to so that he will not overlook important events. Instead I am attempting to encourage the organization of thought in a fashion that will include, in this very broad sense, the functions of the covert processes, a great many of which cannot be formulated accurately.

But, when I say that the psychiatrist must be greatly alert, I do not suggest that he uses this alertness simply in observing the *patient*, the *patient's* behavior, what the *patient* says, and so on. Instead, he is at all times conscious of the fact that this is a performance of *two* people, in which the patient's behavior and what he says are adjusted, to the best of the patient's information and ability, to what he guesses about the psychiatrist. Correspondingly, the psychiatrist's comments, questions, remarks, innuendoes, and so on are effective to the extent that he is aware of the patient's attitude toward him, and is aware of all that he has thus far learned of the patient's background, his experience, and what sort of a person he is. Thus the psychiatrist, insofar as it is possible, concentrates his attention on the processes going on between himself and the other person, or involving himself and the other person, and not on something as remote as, "What is this patient of mine doing and saying?" If, however, he should add, "with me and to me," then he begins to make sense.

CHAPTER

IV

The Early Stages of the Interview

The Formal Inception

I WISH NOW to discuss rather fully, within the frame of reference I have tried to set up, the first of the four phases which I have mentioned: the *formal inception* of the interview, including the reception of the interviewee and the overt establishment of the type of interpersonal situation that is expected to ensue.

First, let us consider the actual "physical" encounter with the interviewee. He may be an utter stranger found unexpectedly sitting in one's waiting room, or he may be an old friend who disconcertingly converts himself, in the course of a commonplace conversation, into a client seeking expert advice. Or, of course, he may be someone who has made an appointment by telephone to see the psychiatrist. The way in which the interviewee is received can greatly accelerate the achievement of the result desired, or it can make the result practically unattainable. From the moment that the interviewer and interviewee first see each other, very important aspects of the psychiatric interview are in progress. And from this moment, the interviewer must realize that his own convenience, his own past malfeasances, and so on, are not anywhere near as important as the assumption that here is someone to be treated with respectful seriousness because he wants to be benefited, or at least can be benefited.

That means that the interviewer does not greet his patient—who may be both penetrating and hostile—with a lot of social hokum that might be all right in meeting aged maternal relatives. I think that the social manner of some doctors has antagonized a larger proportion of their really life-size patients than have their failures in skill and their obvious stupidities of judgment. Any person who notices what is going on is not amused at being treated simply as another statistical instance of a patient who must be made to feel comfortable, a procedure which some interviewers suppose they accomplish by treating the patient like an animated art object, or an imbecile, or something of the kind. Formal statements are perhaps not the ideal way to start psychiatric interviews; habitual utterances—especially those accompanied by the kind of handshake which reminds one who is sensitive of a curious relationship between what he has in his hand and a dead fish—are not conducive to establishing the claims to interpersonal expertness to which I have referred. And per contra, astonishing greetings such as, "Oh, *hello*, come in!" which might be all right with a person recently returned from London, are not useful substitutes.

May I suggest that a stranger is fully as bothered about meeting the interviewer as the interviewer would be in a similar situation. Thus while I don't try to show a great welcome to the patient, I do try to act as if he were expected—that is, I try to know the name of a person who makes an appointment to see me for the first time, and to greet him with it, relieving him of any morbid anxiety as to whether he came on the wrong day, and so on. And I suggest that he come in, which is a form of hospitality that extends to many branches of civilization, and is, in fact, I suppose, indispensable wherever there is a doctrine that a man's house, or office, is his castle. I take a good look at him while he is at the door, and after that I do not stare at him. Once he is in, I indicate where he should sit. I think most of us have experienced the relief, in a difficult situation, of having someone indicate where we may sit; it relieves us of all the wondering about where the other person intends to sit, where it is proper to sit, and so on. One experience of mine impressed this on me: A great man, who had invited me to confer with him about a paper, courteously asked me in, and then sat down and looked at me for a long time without asking me to be seated. I decided that that was a poor way to treat a stranger.

Next I tell the patient what I have learned so far as to why he is there. If he telephoned me to make the appointment, I may say, "I gathered from our conversation over the telephone that you have a problem of such-and-such a nature," putting a little question mark at the end. If I am aware that he is there because someone else sent him, I may say, "Doctor So-and-so," or the chief of the division, or what not, "sent you, I understand, for such-and-such reasons," again with a question mark. In other words, I show that I have paid attention to what little data have been presented to me—I have, for example, taken the trouble to notice what was said to me over the telephone. And I am straightforward to the extent of my data —and even though in certain special circumstances that is not true, at least I try to give the client something of my impression of why he is there. These first data are probably irrelevant; for instance, what he told me over the telephone may well have been merely an excuse for seeing me, or the boss' reason for sending the client may have represented a complete misapprehension on the boss' part. But by laying my cards on the table—insofar as is practicable—I give him, at the very beginning of things, a magnificent opportunity to correct the situation, to revise the information I so far have. Thus when I give him my impression of the story that I have either from him or from somebody else, he can react with anything from, "Yes, that's right, Doctor, and it's a great problem," all the way to, "What? Why I never dreamed of it. How is it possible for you to have such a misunderstanding?" In the latter case, I certainly don't say, "Well, that's the case." Instead, I say something like, "Well, now tell me what really *is* the case." And he begins to tell me. Thus the interviewer operates so that no complicating situation develops in this first meeting with the stranger.

In this way, it is easier for the patient to get started if he doesn't happen to be the person the interviewer thinks he is—and he usually isn't. He begins to feel, "Well, we've begun." And as a matter of fact, we have begun; something has gone on with the fewest possible words, and with the least vacant utterance and gesture. The end of this first stage comes when he has made some statement that I can assume gives him the feeling that he has transmitted to me some idea of his problem and of himself. But I don't try to *find out* at this stage what ails him, for, as I have already said, no one can understand what ails a person without knowing that person. But I try to let him feel that I do know something—that he has, at least, explained his presence. By that time we are ready for the second stage.

Since I have touched on the psychiatrist's use of collateral data—that is, information obtained from some source other than the patient himself—perhaps I should go into this further at this point. A question is sometimes raised as to whether the psychiatrist should receive such data. The problem, as I see it, is not so much one of whether he receives such data, but of what he does with it.

When very grave issues are concerned—for example, if the patient is seriously disordered, or fairly obviously in danger of serious mental disorder, and is confronted with the making of decisions that vastly transcend his ability, so that other people are badly worried about his having to make them—I would regard it as simply quixotic devotion to some curious doctrine for the psychiatrist not to avail himself of any information he can get that will bear on the problem concerned. But what he *does* with that information is often a very delicate problem of technique.

Whether the interviewer has sought out information from sources other than the patient, or whether it has been thrust upon him in the shape of a document that precedes the interviewee, or something of that kind, I have gradually come to feel that it is very important indeed to conduct the interview on the basis of that which is given *in the interview*. However, on some occasions I may use collateral data in unobtrusively directing the course of the interview.

For example, I may be asked to see a man who is applying for a certain government job because the chief of the bureau that is about to employ him feels very uncomfortable about him. From the bureau chief, I hear all sorts of things, including the fact that this man was once a patient in a mental hospital for two years, allegedly with a very serious mental disorder. In the course of the interview, I am able to inquire several times whether something that was being discussed ever got serious enough to be genuinely incapacitating. The answer in each case is, "Oh no! No indeed!" There is no suggestion that this man has ever had anything remotely like a mental disorder; the possibility is denied categorically, from every approach. Toward the close of the interview, I take counsel with myself and discover that I am not quite clear on his chronology of employment. I then say, "Now let's track down, year after year, just what you were doing and where." When he comes to the fatal years there is a pause, and things don't go so well. I say, "Well, you continued in your former employment through that year?" "No. No, I didn't." I wait for about thirty seconds, and then I say, "Well?" And he says, "As a matter of fact, I had some difficulty with my wife at that time, and had to take some time off from my employment. I was actually so upset by this business that I stopped work for a year and a half and took a trip." I say, "Well, well. Where did you go?" The man tells about the start of a trip, and then suddenly says, "Did you know that I was in a mental hospital?" To this I say, "For God's sake! Tell me about it." And he does.

I am pleased with that, because I would not have asked him about this. In this relationship, I have not told him in the beginning what I know, while he has become highly informative about many things that are both good and bad, from his standpoint—excepting that he has reserved something from me; I think he would go away feeling that he had been in the hands of a crook if I were to reveal in the end that I knew all about that something. The very thing that I insist is of vital importance in the psychiatric interview—namely, that the patient get something from it—would be endangered by his discovering that the cards had been stacked against him all the time. But, as a matter of fact, I don't know that very many people who reserve something from the doctor really feel, on sober second thought, that they have pulled the wool over the doctor's eyes. Many people who never overcome the inhibitions they set on themselves before coming to the interview wonder, in the two or three hours after they leave, whether they haven't been fools for not revealing the data which they suppressed. During the interview, they carefully protected this omission, this gap in the data, but because I have given them so many chances to fill it in, they can hardly help but notice in retrospect that it has appeared as a gap. It may then occur to the patient that such success in concealment has in it elements of personal failure.

This is an exception to what I have already stated: that in general, when a person meets me for the first time by order of, or recommendation of, someone else, I establish the situation as best I can by giving him, with as much frankness as I can, a very condensed outline of the highly significant things that I have been told or asked to determine, or what not. But in telling him this, I am chary with any rich detail, any possibly misleading emphasis, and so on, which the informant may have conveyed. I refrain from communicating any of the innuendo which is almost always present in a third person's talking about a second person, and I literally disadvise any interviewer's being very much influenced by such innuendo. It is not that those who send people to the interviewer intend to deceive him in advance; they simply don't know any better. Most people in referring somebody to a psychiatrist try to show that they know something about psychiatry—an innocent conceit, but one which is unfortunate if the psychiatrist enters into it.

Thus I tell the interviewee any presumably incontrovertible facts which have been laid before me, entirely minus any elements of interpretation by the person who communicated them to me. Telling the patient the gross facts as they have been given to me often saves a good deal of time. If what has been told me is not true, I want to hear the correction immediately.

In general, there is no reason in the world, so far as I know, for not letting the patient in on the facts as the psychiatrist was told them, *unless* some of them may be very disturbing. There is no reason to pronounce the patient insane as a preliminary to helping him regain his sanity. For example, the psychiatrist may be told so many disturbing things about a person that it seems practically a foregone conclusion that he has a serious mental disorder. But there is no sense in engaging in a prolonged psychiatric examination if the psychiatrist accepts all this as fact. In a great many years, I have rarely found the facts given to be literally facts. Even when the patient was fully as sick as had been indicated to me, the picture that I obtained in four, five, or six hours of inquiry was quite different from the picture I had been given in advance, and implied possibilities of treatment in the future which had not been implied by the information transmitted to me.

In general, collateral information should not be refused without good reason. However, when somebody very obscurely related to or probably hostile to the patient volunteers information, certainly one should discover the reason for this very "helpful" intervention before accepting it. For example, a husband may consult me because his wife is threatening divorce. In a couple of days the wife calls me, and wants to talk with me. It is a good idea to inquire what the lady has in mind: Does she feel the need of a psychiatrist for her own troubles, or what? No, she doesn't; she wants to tell me all about her husband. My general attitude in such cases is rather forbidding. For instance, I may say, "I should like very much to get the facts, but since I'm just beginning to understand your husband's difficulties, I do think we ought to wait a little while. I don't want to be unduly confused by too many facts all at once." Thus, when the interest of the informant is definitely hostile to the person with whom the interviewer is dealing, it pays to maintain a very judicious detachment in receiving this information and in venturing any comments on it; the interviewer is entitled to notice that the motivation for the action may not be constructive. That doesn't necessarily make the data bad, but it should inspire caution in the use of the data. And since it is very often greatly to the interest of an enemy to know what the psychiatrist thinks of his patient, ordinary caution would suggest that the psychiatrist speak in such a manner that it would be very difficult to put together what he says into any very definite reflection of his opinion.

This is a matter of the confidential relation of the expert and his client, which is deeply ingrained in our culture, and which we can't easily suspend. If we do choose to suspend it for cause, then I trust we will be very skillful indeed in avoiding the evil consequences which may flow from carrying out a role contrary to the expectations defined by the culture. A person who consults anyone with the idea of establishing a frank relationship with him has already overcome some pretty heavy inhibitions laid down by the culture. If the interviewer then chooses to violate the confidential relation, he must be very skillful in doing it, and quite sure that he has adequate cause for so doing—and I would define "adequate cause" as something closely related to movements designed to further the patient's progress toward finding more satisfactory ways of living.

Throughout the inception of the interview, the psychiatrist certainly, and any interviewer in some measure, should "know how he acts"—that is, he should have learned from experience the *usual* impression obtained of him in the particular circumstances of encountering the sort of stranger that the interviewee at first glance *seems* to be. In other words, the psychiatrist should have some idea of how he affects the stranger and how he facilitates or retards certain things that the stranger may have thought of doing. The psychiatrist should also have learned what sorts of immediate impressions he himself obtains from the appearance and initial movements and vocal behavior of another, noting that in such a relationship what one hears first from the other person, no matter how free and easy, or how conventional, represents that person's repertoire of operations to be addressed to a complete stranger. The psychiatrist, who is, in this situation, such a stranger, has the peculiar necessity of having some idea of how these operations affect him; otherwise he is as bad off as is the man on the street, who will perhaps waste hours of one's time arguing about the excellence of his first impressions.

It is useful for the therapist to review these details with great care at the start of his career, gradually catching on to what phenomena have made what impression on him; correspondingly, by observing the larger context of what the other person has done after the formal beginning of the interview, he can begin to develop dependable impressions of how he himself must have affected that person. For example, he may observe that, if a person says, "Hello, Doc," when he answers the door, he usually gives that person an impression of being very reserved and forbidding. He may, of course, find that the next person who greets him with "Hello, Doc," immediately thinks that he is a very fine fellow indeed. Nevertheless, he should note that this kind of rash friendliness—"Hello, Doc"—leads him to frown forbiddingly, which in turn leads many people to think that he is not a very pleasant person. Why should they think otherwise, when from the very first act with the psychiatrist, he registers this mood on his face? Thus it is useful to keep in mind what the *usual* reaction is, even if no one can swear that it will recur tomorrow.

If it has not occurred to the psychiatrist to sort out what his own particular classification of strangers is, and what effect these immediate impressions of his have on his own expression and other behavior—which in turn affect the interviewee's impression of him—he will not learn a great deal and will not improve very much. If he does look at his initial reactions from this really very simple sort of standpoint, then he will begin to make interesting observations. For instance, a great deal that we show on our faces does not ordinarily come into clear awareness, but "just happens," as it were, without our being "conscious" of it. Needless to say, becoming aware of such things is a particular aspect of alertness which requires some cultivation. Thus we can come to discover certain telltale things that we do "without thinking" which have a powerful effect in handicapping the favorable development of an interview situation. Then, after the general fashion of the exceedingly capable creature called man, once we have learned what the trouble is, it tends to disappear; we don't go on doing it.

To what does this "knowing," this "having learned," actually refer? Does it, for instance, mean that a really skillful psychiatrist "knows just what role to take," "just how to behave," in order to impress the patient in the way that the patient should be impressed? Yes; *but with very great qualifications.* It is much more accurate to say that the experience of the psychiatrist is synthesized into *an aptitude to do nothing exterior to his awareness* which will greatly handicap the development of the interview situation, or which will direct its development in an unnecessarily obscure way.

For example, many inexperienced interviewers, quite exterior to their awareness, communicate to their interviewees a distaste for certain types of data; and their records of interviews are conspicuous for the fact that the people they see don't seem to have lived in the particular areas contaminated by that distaste. Until such interviewers realize that they are rather unwittingly prohibiting, or forbidding, or shooing the interviewee away from a particular type of data, they continue not to encounter it. Thus, "learning how to act" is largely a matter of being aware of what one does, and aware of it in terms of how it affects the setting of the interview. As an interviewer does this, he stops doing those things which interfere with the fuller development of the interview.

As another aspect of "learning how to act"—or perhaps as a special instance of this awareness of one's actions which I have been discussing—the interviewer should learn to avoid any deliberate attempts to give an impression which it is *impossible* or *impracticably difficult* to sustain under the circumstances. A remarkable number of actions by psychiatrists to impress the patient have come to my attention. Not infrequently the impression that was to be conveyed to the client by certain more or less elaborate and studied behavior was quite out of keeping with the picture of the psychiatrist as seen by others. Thus all that could possibly come from this pomp and circumstance was a distinct feeling of puzzlement on the part of the interviewee. I doubt that an initial feeling of being puzzled by one's expert is an indication of his skill, and I scarcely need stress the inadvisability of acts which are calculated to produce impossibly good impressions, for these come too close to home in all of us.

While I have suggested that the psychiatrist must be alert to learn, insofar as possible, the immediate impression of him which is created in a stranger, I should at the same time emphasize that this is something which he cannot *know*. He can at best have a useful surmise of *alternative probabilities*, based on experience with other clients, and including the information he has picked up in the initial observation of the behavior demonstrated by this particular client. Now, why do I say surmises of at least *two* probabilities? I don't mind if the interviewer has a dozen, although it is very difficult to keep track of that many probabilities. But if he doesn't have more than one, he is operating on faith, which is the method of performance characteristic of people who never pause to doubt their heaven-sent ability to know all about another person by talking with him for five minutes. For such people, their *one* surmise of probability amounts to a certainty. But if the interviewer has *alternative* probabilities in mind, he is moved to explore further, whereupon the probability of one increases and that of the other diminishes; and by this simple device he moves toward reasonable accuracy. The best that a psychiatrist can have in the very early phases of his contact with a stranger is a surmise of perhaps two possible impressions that he may have created with that stranger. Such a conjecture is useful; it is the beginning of coming to know, rather roughly, how he impresses such people. The only way that he ever learns such things is by being careful to avoid closing his mind the moment he has a hunch. Closing his mind prematurely is likely to be very gratifying or very distressing, depending upon his needs at the moment, but it will have very little effect in helping him to do better in later interviews.

An aphorism credited to ex-President Mary E. Woolley of Mount Holyoke comes to my mind as being well worth attention at this point. On one occasion this great lady said this, the truth of which rendered me all but speechless for hours after I first heard it: "It is often very important to distinguish between the merely very difficult and the actually impossible." The recognition that some things are impossible, and not just difficult, is a great economizer in any field involving very complex operations—and the psychiatric interview is probably a very complex operation. It is therefore useful, very early in one's contact with strangers, to have a lively realization that there are a great many things which would be wonderful if they were possible, but which, since they are *not* possible, it is well not to spend time on. For example, if you recall your personal observations in meeting people, you will realize that there are limits to how much it is possible to accomplish in the formal reception of a stranger. You may go to the door and call him in, or look up and say, "Oh, you are Mr. Jones," and follow this by getting the newcomer seated and so on. Such simple and conventional operations are about all that is possible at this stage with any conceivably understood result—and everything in the psychiatric interview should be sharply focused on *quite easily understood results*. When I say "understood," I refer to data that fairly readily fall into alternative hypotheses as to their probable meaning, which alternative hypotheses can then be tracked down, so that one hypothesis gains in meaning and the other fades into unimportance.

I would now like to sum up much of what I have been saying, in another aphorism which may be credited to me: *The interviewer should be alert to, so that he can correctly recall, all that he has said and done in the formal inception of each interview, so that he can learn to do better*. It is only when an interviewer can recall a course of events correctly, both as to movement and pattern of movement—that is, the timing of movement, what preceded what, what followed what—that he has the material from which to make a useful analysis of the processes which were involved, from which, in turn, he can synthesize an improving grasp of the particular aspect of living concerned. Since the interviewer is trying to be an expert at assessing the movements of another so as to get a useful view of this other person, his training may well start with the idea that he must be intensely alert to just what he himself says and does.

Sometimes a patient mentions some incredible error which the psychiatrist made long past. If the psychiatrist has a vivid recall of what he said or did, the discovery that this was an incredible error might be a big step forward. Very often, however, the psychiatrist does not have any precise idea of what he did. The patient tells him something that sounds very much like what he vaguely recalls, but he doesn't know the facts clearly enough to be sure, for he was not alert enough at the time. He only knows that some serious misinterpretation has occurred of something which went on between him and the patient, which is regrettable; but so far as I know, regrets don't do people much good.

Thus one learns to devote an immense amount of alertness to the work at hand—a sort of watchful clarity as to what happens. That doesn't mean that the interviewer acts as if he were afraid that the stranger will blow up in his face, or anything like that. People can be so alert as to have a microscopically correct record of small events and yet engage congenially in all sorts of things that don't require any particular attention. And the interviewer learns that there is communication from the first visual encounter with the stranger—not only communication by speech, but communication by gesture, broadly conceived, an interchange by expressive movement other than speech.[1] That which is communicated starts the growth by inference of working hypotheses about the other person.

The Reconnaissance

As I have already suggested, by the end of the first stage the patient should have come to feel, "Well, now the doctor knows why I'm here." The psychiatrist can then say, in effect, "Well, who are you?" In other words, he sets out in this second stage to obtain a rough social sketch of the patient, which is to be

[1] A notion of the extent of this interchange can be obtained from the "Tentative Classification of Expressive Movements," pp. 24–35, in Gordon W. Allport and Philip E. Vernon, *Studies in Expressive Movement;* New York, Macmillan, 1933.

brief, and not an extended life history. This is the stage to which I refer as the reconnaissance.

I customarily begin this stage by saying, "Now, tell me, how old are you? Where were you born? Are your mother and father living?" And if one or both of them are dead, "When did they die and of what?" If the patient doesn't know what his father died of, for example, this may lead to the discovery that the father hasn't lived in the home for the past twenty years, and that while the patient is pretty sure his father is dead, he doesn't know any of the circumstances. Here are some interesting data. Next I inquire as to the number of siblings, including any who died. If a sibling died during the memory span of the patient, that may be quite significant, but it is also important to note those siblings who died before he can remember, because they might have been of particular significance to his parents and thus have a considerable effect on him. I ask about his place in the time-order of siblings, and I try to get it right. Then I ask who, besides the parents, was chronically or frequently in the home in his first seven years. For example, if grandma—or a maiden aunt, or even the sheriff—was very frequently in the home during those years, this may leave a quite permanent effect; it is wise to be warned as early as possible of this, because otherwise one may make great mistakes in induction. Sorting out such data is truly impressive to a great many people. They may have actually forgotten that grandma was the one bright spot in the home in their first seven years, and are glad to be reminded of it.

I then ask what the father, or the mother, or whoever earned the money, did for a living. I probably by now have derived a notion of the family's economic circumstances—if I haven't, I ask specifically. I then ask if there was any sharp change in the economic circumstances at any time. (All this was, of course, impressed on me because I went into private practice just as the Great Depression arrived.) Marked economic disturbances usually have either general or special reasons, and have very marked effects on the course of personality development. Parents almost always aim their children at something, which the children either seek or avoid at all costs, but big economic change may lead to tragic revision of the parental ambitions with corresponding effects on the children's goals and so on, and may leave permanent marks. If there were changes, I try to notice how old the patient was when they occurred. If they occurred very early, before the patient was eight, they may have greatly influenced the parental utterances and efforts to direct the life of the child. If the changes occurred when the patient was around twenty, they may have affected his getting a university education—or if he was headed for medicine or the law, they may have affected his educational goal even though he was older. If the changes occurred after he completed his education, they have probably not made very much difference except insofar as they have made other people dependent on him.

And when I have all this information—and note that I am proceeding in what has gradually been ingrained in me as a system of values that seems natural to Americans—I become curious, sometimes to the patient's amazement, as to what sort of a person his father was. People are anything from extremely vocal to helpless in the face of such a question, and if a patient's helplessness seems to be a real lack of verbal formulation, I say, "Well, how was he regarded in the community?" If he still cannot formulate this, I may mention the pastor of the church, and the family doctor, and the druggist with whom he had an account, and the grocer, and so on, asking, "What would they have said of him, offhand?"

A slight haste in the face of obscurity does no harm here, because brevity about these things is not solely for the physician's convenience; it also has a certain relevance in the matter of what the patient is there for. You see, he really isn't there to give me an adequate biography of himself; and so, if I seem a little hurried in getting what I want of his biography, his grievance is minimal. When I have obtained some idea of what sort of person the father was, I become curious to learn whether it was a happy family. Were the parents happily married? Then I want to know about the mother. And for reasons that I would never try to put into words, while I ask *what sort of a person* the father was, I ask the patient to *describe* his mother. When we have developed this point somewhat—the patient usually has an exceedingly vague idea of the lady—I then remember any other stray people who were mentioned earlier as being around the house a great deal in the very early years and ask what sort of people they were. This is usually such a relief to the patient after trying to describe his mother that I often get quite an account of the third, the semiparent; and that semiparent may prove to be illuminating, if only in understanding the role that I may play later on in the relationship.

At this point, I usually sigh—for sufficient reason—and ask the patient to tell me something about his education; and when we have gone through that as rapidly as possible, I want to know his occupational history. In the educational history, I don't believe I'd waste a minute with most people to find out whether or not they were held back in a grade in grammar school, unless I felt that they were probably feeble-minded. Education is, so far as I am concerned, a clear index of the combination of foresight and blind ambition on the part of parents, wealthy relatives, and the patient. The educational history can be quite, quite brief, such as, "Well, I went from high school to such-and-such a prep school, and then to such-and-such a college, and I finally got a Ph.D. from such-and-such a place." That is enough; it merely tells me that he is lucky, as the average person goes.

The occupational history, while it still includes big factors of the general economic situation, the particular geographical opportunities, and so on, is much more illuminating as to the patient's ability to get on with people and to get somewhere in life. Therefore, I now want to know what he has done ever since leaving school, and I am rather curious about this. The sicker people are, the more they omit from their occupational history. And so here, for the first time, I quite generally do something which is a very important part of the psychiatric interview: I tell the patient what I have heard, and then inquire whether that is the whole story, by saying something like, "Well, aside from these two jobs you have had no other occupation?" Whereupon many people reveal that, oh, yes, they have had twenty-five other jobs, but they haven't held them long. This is much more important information than that about the two jobs mentioned first. Thus one should discover whether or not there is more occupational history than the interviewee at first reports. However, I watch the clock as I do it. That is, I don't want to know how bad the foreman was; all I want to know is what jobs, how long, and where—thus getting an idea of whether the person was advancing in his work; whether he was so driven by a need for money that he held a job only long enough to get one that paid more; whether he held each job long enough to know what the work was about and then took another one, in a curiously thorough but superficially morbid pattern of learning something about life; whether he quarreled with everybody that he ever tried to work with; and all that sort of thing. I don't want details, but I do want a sketch of the facts.

At this point I become curious as to whether the person is married, and if so, how long he has been married. I ask somewhat casually, "Quite happily?" And if it isn't a happy marriage, the patient usually takes a moment to say "Yes." Sometimes I look at him then, and ask if there are any children; and I may ask if it is the first marriage. Quite often a person will say, "No, no, I was married before," sounding as if I should have known this, when everything he has said so far was not in any sense calculated to suggest such a thing. Then I want to know about the early marriage. The great thing is: Was it the first love?—and if there is a little hesitancy there, then comes, of course, the inquiry, "Why did you marry?" Sometimes it was just because the family thought it was a great idea. I receive all this information without surprise, for an expert is not surprised at getting what he wants.

With that I'm through. Of the labels which the patient's neighbors and casual acquaintances attach to him, I have tried to pick up those that have some measure of probable significance for understanding what he does. He feels that I know a great deal about him—in part because a good deal of these data are ordinarily not discussed in his relations with strangers. In a vague way, I do know a good deal, because from now on I just watch which of the customary indices prove to be correct in his case, and wherein he is an exception to the probabilities which are implied in the semistatistical data of his past, his family position, and so on.

For example, there is some probability that the fifth and last child in a family, who is the only male child, and who is born ten years after his nearest sibling, will be dreadfully spoiled. On discovering that a person occupies that position in the family, I immediately think, "Hah! The probability is that this fellow has gotten away with murder since his early years." And so I notice this, I begin with it, but I hope that I recognize any very striking exceptions that I encounter. That is what the brief sketch is for. The interviewer utilizes as much as he can of the dubious, but still respectable, generalizations that he has picked up in all his previous life and study, remembering, however, that those generalizations are statements of probability; they are never statements to the effect that "under these circumstances so-and-so is inevitably the case." We don't have that sort of absolute knowledge about human living, and, therefore, we shall remain eternally young. If it turns out that *nothing* about the patient fits with any of the interviewer's past experience, he will really have a grand and difficult task in being useful to this patient.

Some psychiatrists, having discovered that someone is the

youngest child and the only male, born many years after the nearest sibling, consider it a certainty, rather than a probability, that he is dreadfully spoiled. Those folks ought to go into the natural sciences, rather than deal with human living. The exceptions to the probabilities which arise from this type of crude data about people are very striking. They may not approximate 50 per cent, but they are still a very significant group of exceptions; and since the interviewer is supposed to show some expertness in dealing with people, it is well for him not to close his mind to them. But insofar as the probabilities that he has come to accept hold true in a given case, those data are easy to keep track of from then on. And when he encounters exceptions, simply because everyone is respectful of exceptions from their very nature of being somewhat against the rule, he finds them a little easier to recall than if he had blundered into them somewhat blindly while listening to a long life history and perhaps getting all wrapped up in Aunt Hattie's peculiar attacks that came on at the menopause, which are relevant only if one is curious as to whether there is lunacy in the family, which can be a dreadful waste of time.

Thus the second step is a very hurried picking up of the kind of clues which ordinarily can be rather useful in considering anybody's personality and habits. But notice that I haven't asked anything about the person's personality; I have simply tried to find out how he comes to be here—in the sense of time and space—to find out what the grossest landmarks are that have characterized his course up to now. Nevertheless, by the time these gross social data have been completed, the psychiatrist will have been impressed with many characteristics of the person with whom he is dealing. Because of the great number of topics covered in the social outline, and because of their real importance and yet apparent lack of relationship, the patient is much more apt to show meaningful signs, without perhaps quite knowing it, than would be the case if he were conversing freely about something in which he more or less had control of the topics. Later on, in the detailed inquiry, unless for some reason the psychiatrist really must resort to cross-examination, it is to a large extent necessary to leave the patient more or less in control of the topics; things have to flow, for otherwise they are apt to be so disconnected that the interviewer does not quite know what he has learned.

But in the reconnaissance, in which the interviewee is more or less answering an organized stream of questions, the interviewer has an opportunity, by alert listening and some seeing, to pick up a great many clues for further exploration. For example, the interviewer notes in this stage the relative ease or difficulty of the relationship, which reflects the degree of the interviewee's concentration on the procedure; his sensitivity to the other person—in this instance, the interviewer; and his "attitudes," as one commonly describes them in such terms as reserved, guarded, suspicious, hostile, defensive, conciliatory, apologetically inferior, superior, supercilious, mutually respecting. The interviewer may also observe the interviewee's attitude toward his own memory—whether he seems to trust it or not; his attitude about "answering questions"—whether this makes him feel at a disadvantage or not; the apparent extent of his need for reassurance; and so on. Later on, when I discuss the interview as a process, I will discuss in more detail the kinds of gross impressions which the interviewer can gather during this stage of the interview, and the ways in which he evaluates these impressions and tests their validity.

The Reconnaissance in Intensive Psychotherapy [2]

The reconnaissance may take about twenty minutes, in a case where I never expect to see the person again, or it may take from seven and a half to fifteen hours, which I think is about the average when time is not of the essence, or it may

[2] [*Editors' note:* The remainder of this chapter is taken from a series of lectures on *Conceptions of Modern Psychiatry*, which Sullivan gave in the Washington School of Psychiatry in 1946–47, and in which he discussed some aspects of psychiatric interviewing.]

take even longer. Once in my actual experience, literally a little over three months was spent in this phase which I call the reconnaissance; the person concerned was a candidate in training who had done a great deal of thinking about his personal history, and therefore the personal history itself was rather rich in data, and already pretty well organized.

The skill which an interviewer can manifest in obtaining and interpreting this outline history has a great deal to do with the ease or difficulty of the subsequent detailed inquiry—which, if the interviewer is a psychiatrist undertaking treatment of a patient, ordinarily means the long stretch of intensive psychotherapy. Depending on the concise accuracy of the outstanding points in this reconnaissance sketch of the personality, the detailed inquiry may be reduced, I suppose, as much as 90 per cent.[3] I am quite sure that the reason for the unending spans of lifetime spent in supposed intensive psychotherapy of patients is in some instances simply the fact that the psychiatrist had no particular hints of how the particular patient had got

[3] [*Editors' note:* In a question-and-answer session at the end of the 1944 series of lectures, Sullivan made the following remarks in response to a question about brief psychotherapy:

"I have long held that 'brief' psychotherapy was to be achieved by improving the utilization of the psychotherapeutic minute. If one is governed by no principles, but only by some vague beliefs—as in something like 'free association'—I think brief psychotherapy is very likely to be measured in terms of decades. But if one is interested in a precisely defined, recurrent difficulty that people have in significant relations to others, it is quite possible that a good deal can be done in a rather short time. If a good deal *is* to be done in a short time, neither the patient nor the doctor can permit long sustained digressions about their mutual admirability, or about interesting shows in the theater, or something of the sort. In fact, the psychiatrist must follow events closely enough so that whenever a digression seems to be in progress, or some subordinate problem seems to be in the center of things, he can inquire whether such is truly the case, or whether the topic actually does fit in with the business before them. In those circumstances, the patient may come to see that the psychiatrist knows what he is doing, and that there is good reason to collaborate in doing it. Incidentally, I think that the frequency of interview is important only from the standpoint of the limitations of the psychiatrist; and that is a matter of his ability to recall. It usually takes me a little while, in each interview, to recall what has been going on; usually the patient says something which brings up the right recognition, and we are then off to where we were at the time of the previous session."]

to be the person who had come to the office; instead, the psychiatrist depended on what is called free association to find all that out. Since association can be extremely free indeed, by the time that the psychiatrist had some notion of the life history of the patient I'm afraid he had the wrong notion. Thus the ideal time to make this sort of inquiry—to try to find out "How come this patient?" in terms of his rudimentary life history—is right after the thing has begun, as soon as a potential doctor-patient relationship has been established. If the doctor does that, then he is in a position to have views which are not transcendental. And even if half the facts told him then are wrong, they will be corrected fairly soon.

Suppose, on the other hand, that a person comes to the psychiatrist and says, "I've been diagnosed as an obsessional neurotic and told I need psychoanalysis. Can you take me?" and the psychiatrist says, "Yes, let us begin." What is assumed there? First, that a competent diagnosis has been made; and second, that the psychiatrist is a godlike person who is bound to be successful—or that he is an unprincipled scoundrel who will take money without any thought of what the patient is going to get for it. I suggest that a psychiatrist find out something about a person before he makes or implies expansive promises about what he will do, or what ought to be done, and particularly before he begins to do something which may or may not have any earthly constructive influence on the patient. I insist that the psychiatrist should in the beginning try to find out something about the patient, not in the sense of developing a psychiatric history according to this or that outline which he may find in the mental hospital library, but from the standpoint of orienting himself as to certain basic probabilities according to the developmental scheme of things.

I do not mean to imply that all of the reconnaissance is always rather sharply separated from all of the detailed inquiry. In actual fact, there are matters that come up in such a way in the course of developing this social outline that it is obviously highly advantageous to pursue the topic immediately in detail. It is very much better to go into the details when it is opportune than to be in any sense obsessional about following the rest of the social outline before getting anything to hang on it. Unless something is deferred smoothly and in a fashion which the interviewee experiences as natural, it is not apt to be the same thing when it comes up again. For example, in inquiring about the mother, the interviewer may have learned that she was a wonderful woman, except that she had a violent temper and at times really seemed a little bit out of her mind from anger. If, after he has heard a statement like that, he then shifts to an inquiry about someone else, the patient is apt to suffer over the baldness of his original statement. As a result, when the interviewer gets around to asking about the mother again, he may hear a stream of apologies about what was first said, the patient having by then convinced himself that it is necessary to be much less frank in his statements. By this time the interviewer cannot be nearly so sure of what he is getting. But if, when the original statement is made, the interviewer invites a few examples—what sort of thing was apt to precipitate the mother's violent anger, and so on—before going on with other matters, then the topic is opened wide, and eventually the details may be gone into with much less distress.

THE USE OF FREE ASSOCIATION

During the reconnaissance, the interviewer may hear of some situation at some time in the patient's past which seems significant, but which is unclear; when the interviewer asks supplementary questions, he may get to a point where something he would like to know is not accessible to the patient. The patient is unable to recall it; to use the old slang, the material has been "repressed." Here is an opportunity to do something very educative. The interviewer may say, "Well, I really wonder what might have been the case; tell me, what comes to your mind?" Partly because of the pressure, partly because of the objectivity of the inquiry, and partly because the patient really is trying to get something out of his contact with psychiatry, he often has a very surprising experience indeed in discovering what comes to his mind. In other words, by attacking blind spots in the patient's recollection in this very simple way, the interviewer is actually giving him a hint as to the nature of free association that might be terribly hard to give otherwise.

As a matter of fact, trying to tell patients what is meant by free association, and trying to get them to do it, can be quite a problem. I used to collect prescriptions given to patients by analysts about how to go to work. Of course, the first instruction in the old days was, "Lie down on the couch and relax completely." One of unnumbered variants of this prescription went on, "Feel as much at peace as possible, and say every littlest thing that comes to your mind." Trying to relax completely always stymied the patient, so the psychiatrist didn't have to worry about anything else for a while; some patients could spend the next six months trying to relax completely, without one success. If the psychiatrist tells patients to do things that they can't do, they very rarely have the good sense to say, "Yes, Doctor, how do you do it?" Instead, they just presume that the psychiatrist knows what he's talking about, and try. If the prescription doesn't work, such patients then have proof that they can't get any benefit from psychiatry.

None of these prescriptions ever got anywhere in my hands. I finally concluded that the only way to get a patient to doing free association that is of any good to him or to me is to impress upon him the faculty of his personality to present unknown data by more or less free flow of thought. And I also concluded that the way to impress this on him was not by talking about it, but by having a few demonstrations of it. The ideal circumstance for this is when a valid question arises and the patient has nothing in the way of an answer. Thus, when we take up some problem that has emerged in the reconnaissance, and run into blind areas concerning it—that is, areas where the self-system is at work—I try to get the patient to talk more or less at random as things come to his mind; and then, as often as not, the patient gives a very convincing demonstration of moving toward useful information. In other words, when the patient has no answer for a question which is obviously of real importance to him, the functioning of the personality is such that the following process is likely to ensue: as the patient begins to talk about the things that come to his mind, his thoughts will begin to circle, in the most curious fashion, toward the answering of the question. It may be, of course, that the process will start and stop many a time before a very significant question is answered.

Only after the patient has had a few examples of the fact that free association makes sense can the psychiatrist lay down injunctions about it—even useful injunctions as to the inadvisability of his selecting what to report. When the patient has actually accomplished something by a more or less free report of his covert processes, he will begin to understand that the leaving out of ideas because they seem irrelevant or immaterial may cause the therapeutic process to miscarry. I have often heard people start out on what seemed to be a simple evasion of an anxiety-fraught position—that is, they seemed to be talking about something irrelevant; but if they were really faithfully reporting what went on in their minds, it wasn't irrelevant very long, for the mind usually does not spend much time on irrelevant and unimportant details. Of course, when a person keeps on talking about the bees and the flowers, and so on, I may say quite sardonically, "This seems to be *really* free association, but I wonder what on earth it pertains to."

Thus my way of getting this very valuable aspect of personality to work is to induct the patient into the reporting of relatively free-flowing thought before giving him any hint that that is a very important method. One might think that everybody by now knows all about free association, and cannot be entrapped into doing it by such a simple technique. But if you are doing a fairly good job of the reconnaissance, patients are much too interested and busy to be thinking about the latest psychoanalytic movie they have seen, for they are really at work on something of importance to them. So the psychiatrist should try to get something to *happen*, that he can then refer to as having happened, instead of telling the patient to say every littlest thing that comes to his mind, or something of the sort.

SUMMARIZING THE RECONNAISSANCE

In my proxy [4] experience of the last three years, I have found it useful to recommend that the psychiatrist—particularly in a series of interviews with one patient—conclude the preliminary reconnaissance with a summary statement. Thus the summary statement would be made at the end of, say, seven to fifteen hours of interviews, and it would precede the detailed efforts of psychotherapy. In this summary statement, the psychiatrist tells the patient what he has heard and what he sees as a problem that seems well within the field of psychiatric competence. In my experience, such a statement has without exception proved extremely useful to the patient and gratifying to the therapist. In fact, even in cases where a patient who was being seen for a single interview was enraged by the summary, and apparently closed the door to all psychiatric help, I have sometimes found out later through collateral information that the patient was benefited. In a long series of interviews, it is important to establish the justifiability of the patient's seeing the psychiatrist; the relationship should not be left tacit as to its basic nature for very long. The psychiatric situation is formally established when there is a consensus—even if unwilling—that the patient and the psychiatrist might well talk further about the problem which has emerged from the reconnaissance.

4 [*Editors' note:* Sullivan is referring here to his supervisory and consultative work with psychotherapists in the Washington area.]

The summary at the end of the reconnaissance should be presented with as much economy of time as possible, short of rudeness; if the psychiatrist is prolix at this time the patient is likely to become vastly more prolix in the course of the detailed inquiry. In presenting the summary, the psychiatrist should explain that he now wishes to tell the patient what has impressed him in the reconnaissance, and that he would like the patient to bear with him until he is through, so that he will be relatively uninterrupted; at the same time, the psychiatrist should tell the patient that at the end of the summary the patient will be asked to amend and correct those things which the psychiatrist has misunderstood, and to point out any important things which the psychiatrist has missed.

Many therapists on first attempting to use this method have encountered remarkable impulses in themselves to procrastinate about summarizing, and have felt profoundly uncertain as to what to put in the summary, and so on; in fact, they usually have had to make an extraordinarily firm resolve before actually getting around to summarizing. I have great sympathy with the psychiatrist's reluctance to tell the patient what he has learned about him. As psychiatrists, we can all advance the perfectly reasonable argument that psychiatry is a very complex field and that, at a given time in therapy with a patient, we haven't had enough time to verify the facts. Many psychiatrists who have not had the experience of using the summary statement have a gloomy feeling which might be verbalized somewhat as follows: "If I were to tell the patient how little I've caught on to of what he has told me, he'd be completely discouraged." But the brute fact is that in all of my experience by proxy with this procedure, this gloomy anticipation of how badly the psychiatrist will show himself up with the patient has never been realized once; in each instance, the summary has resulted in the patient's showing a very marked respect for the psychiatrist. The psychiatrist, you see, is peculiarly qualified—by virtue of his psychiatric education—to sort out the relevant details of another person's life and throw them into meaningful patterns, as compared with any of the infinite number of voluntary advisers that the patient, like everybody else, has been dealing with previously.

One of the reasons for the psychiatrist's initial hesitancy in revealing by means of a summary how at sea he feels in the interview situation is that the sort of things that he summarizes is determined by his own experience and his own grasp on living. That is what is behind the feeling of helplessness that we all have at times in undertaking a summary. But the psychiatrist's own limitations of experience and lack of grasp on living are handicaps in working with the patient, particularly in the detailed inquiry, whether or not the psychiatrist is aware of them. In addition, sometimes it is actually beneficial for the patient to realize that the psychiatrist, because of his own experience, is somewhat insensitive to certain areas of living. The most crushing outcome of such a revelation would be that the patient would find another psychiatrist, which in some cases might be of real usefulness for the first psychiatrist if he were able to learn something from it.

When the psychiatrist seriously attempts to summarize what has happened at the end of the reconnaissance, the patient will have an experience which in some ways is quite startling. Things that the patient has known all of his life and which he has told the psychiatrist in the interviews will be reflected back to him in the summary in a newly meaningful fashion—in spite of what the psychiatrist thinks of as his own stupidities and forgetfulnesses. Thus to the extent that the summary represents a somewhat expert view of the data that the patient had accessible in his awareness and was moved to report in the interview, it will be a very uplifting experience to the patient—a very definite step in the patient's education as to how psychiatry works. And quite often the summary shows the patient some of his conventional evasions and distortions.

In presenting the summary, the psychiatrist has to use some

judgment in determining when he has an outline of reasonably significant things; and he will never know how good his judgment is in that respect until he has tried it. After the psychiatrist has summarized the situation and given a sort of recommendation of what he feels might well be more or less the point of immediate attack, he should, as I have said, encourage the patient to amend and correct the statement. Real amendment and correction on the part of the patient are important, for, in this way, the psychiatrist can learn a lot more about what he has on his hands than he could find out in the same time by any other means. In fact, this is an immensely good way of getting things started on something like a consensually valid basis. Of course, if the psychiatrist sees that the patient is merely amending in an obsessional way—just gilding the lily—he should interrupt the patient and say, "Yes, yes. Well, I gather that you're in approximate agreement with my view. Of course, I can't cover all the details that you've covered."

Actually most of the patient's amending at the end of the summary has consisted, in my own experience, of reminding me that I have dropped out some important figure. In those cases in which two or three people had much the same influence on the patient's difficulties in living, I quite often forget all but one of these people. And the patient at the end will think, "But where was Aunt Agatha?" and mention the fact that I have forgotten the importance of this figure. He is unable at that juncture to generalize about these figures; but he is quite content when I say, "Oh, yes, Aunt Agatha was also like such-and-such a person." He then sees that I am aware of the important experience, even if I don't recall all the significant figures. In the single interview of an hour and a half, I have often used a ten-minute summary at the end of an hour and fifteen minutes to try to tell the patient what I thought was quite important in what I had heard. The patient may sputter around for the last five minutes about what I have left out of the summary, but quite often he ends the interview by indicating that he will follow my suggestion about what to do next, in this way indicating that my summary has been of use to him. Despite the fact that the psychiatrist will leave many gaps in this brief summary, he should be able to give the patient a clear notion of what he considers an important problem.

Somewhat tangentially, I would like to mention that it is useful in a series of interviews to have the patient prepare a chronology of his life. This is quite helpful for a psychiatrist like myself who has great difficulty in getting abstract names attached to concrete people. In addition, it saves time in dealing with patients who are particularly productive of names and who mention, in the course of the work, everybody with whom they have had any dealings. I suggest that the patient prepare a record, showing in one column the date or the year and his age, beginning with his birth and coming up to the present, and in another column, opposite this time scale, brief statements of where he lived, who was living in the household at the given time, and any very significant events, including those that he has been telling me about. I explain that such a record might help him to recall certain things that had not shown up in the early reconnaissance and that it would be very valuable to me in keeping track of the various people and when their influence was felt by the patient. I point out that this will save a good deal of time for both of us, and that it will help me to avoid misunderstandings. Very frequently, indeed, the patient adopts this suggestion and both of us profit from this procedure.

The question of what to include in the summary, in terms of the patient's problem as the psychiatrist sees it, is a very real one. To be simply frank in psychiatric work would often result in a situation in which the psychiatrist was as cruel and destructive as possible. When we later consider the development of the self-system, it will become somewhat clearer that a great many people are easily exposed to extremely severe anxiety unless they can maintain certain conventional defensive operations which represent the anti-anxiety manifestations of the self. The psychiatrist therefore always has the responsibility of presenting a problem in the patient's living in such a way that it does something more than precipitate intense anxiety. At the end of the reconnaissance it is possible for the psychiatrist to present problems in such a way that the patient won't become too anxious to continue to work with that psychiatrist. In some instances, I have given a patient a rather grim statement at the end of, say, seven hours that would have terminated treatment had I tossed it out as a conclusion at the end of the first hour. But in the period of the reconnaissance the patient has had hints that the encounter makes sense and that the psychiatrist did not put things as brutally, unfeelingly, contemptuously, and superiorly as possible; and these earlier hints have made it possible for the patient to rally from the effect of the rather grim summary.

Perhaps an example might illustrate the sort of summary that can be useful without being too anxiety-provoking. In commenting on a patient's particular pattern of disparagement of others, I might say, "Well, it seems to me that this pattern of giving lip service and then undermining the other person, which you were forced to develop with Aunt Agatha, has stayed with you ever since." If said in another way, this might be extremely offensive to the patient and intensely provocative of insecurity. But such a pattern of behavior, when placed in its historic setting, does not seem quite as horrible as when it is placed in a more immediate context. Once the patient is able to recall what I'm talking about in that setting, then I can say, "Well, this pattern seems to have gone on, huh?" In a vague way, there's a sort of transfer of blame to Aunt Agatha in this approach. More important, I have indicated that I am interested in how things began, and that I am not surprised that some of them go on still, even though the patient has not recognized this pattern up to now and, having recognized it, is not particularly happy about it.

Sometimes the problems in living which the psychiatrist encounters in the reconnaissance are so grave, so close to the structure of the most serious mental disorders, that it would be simply disastrous to toss them in the patient's face. The psychiatrist cannot expect a patient who is deeply disturbed to give up his shadowy vestiges of security by agreeing with the psychiatrist that he is psychotic. Even in those cases, however, I believe that the patient should be presented with something. If the psychiatrist omits all emphasis on what in the patient's behavior actually demonstrates psychosis, he can sometimes refer to what are in essence the patient's psychotic difficulties with others, without actually communicating the idea to the patient that these difficulties constitute a particular very severe mental disorder. Under those circumstances, it is by no means uncommon for the patient to be quite clear on the fact that in a rather objective and undisturbing fashion, the psychiatrist has said, in essence, that he is psychotic; and this is established without any serious movement of anxiety, and with the patient's feeling that it might be possible to get somewhere with the psychiatrist.

Perhaps a case which I happen to remember at the moment will illustrate some of the points that I have been making about the summary. Some time ago, I had occasion to see a patient who revealed in the first interview that he had a homosexual problem. The upshot of the reconnaissance was that I told him that I had no psychiatric time available—and I didn't know anybody else who had—for his interest in homosexual problems. If, on the other hand, he wanted to find out why he could never hold any one job for more than six months—despite an initial curiously ascending progress at amazing speed—and was always in ever-increasing, terrific danger of being completely discredited and expelled by the organization he worked for, then I thought I could find him a psychiatrist. Believe it or not, the patient was quite content to go to work on the problem of why, in the space of six months or so, each one of his bosses came into such open collision with him that he left. The curious thing about this story is that in the process of studying his difficulties with bosses, the great homosexual problem sort of caved in. This kind of success story doesn't happen very often; in general, homosexual problems or any other problems don't just cave in. The important part of this story is that, as a result of a brief reconnaissance, I declined entirely to have anything to do with what the patient considered his problem. Instead I indicated a problem that needed very urgent treatment and that I thought psychiatry could help him with. The patient agreed, and we went to work on this second problem—that is, we began the detailed inquiry.

Thus in my summary of the reconnaissance, I strive always to outline for a patient what I see as a major difficulty of his living which seems well within the field of psychiatry. In doing this I imply that if we work together I hope that we can get somewhere on this problem. Although I call this a major problem, I have no prestige whatever involved in its being *the* major problem of the patient's life, or the one that we will spend many months on in a long series of interviews. As a matter of fact, many people cannot bring into the open the major problem of their living until they have found themselves in an almost impossibly secure interpersonal situation. In such cases, it may well be long after the reconnaissance that *the* great major problem of living will become clear.

If by the end of the reconnaissance, the interviewer is not able to clearly define any major problem of the patient, he should not be at all hesitant to indicate something quite minor that ails the patient. Perhaps the patient may think, "Oh, yes, but that's just a trifle; the doctor just doesn't know what really ails me." But the patient also knows that the reason the doctor is unclear about the more important problems is that the patient couldn't show them to the doctor. And if the doctor has stated a problem, however minor, in an adequate fashion, this statement has not foreclosed all sorts of discoveries in the future; he has merely indicated that, so far as he is concerned, this problem is worth working on. The important thing is that the doctor and patient now have something to work on.

Without this statement of a problem in living, treatment situations are apt to be quite defeating. They are painfully reminiscent of the steel plant where I once worked; after a sleet storm, the little narrow-gauge locomotives with their loads of ingots would struggle along the icy tracks and progress would apparently be made, when suddenly everything would slide back to just where it had been before. In the psychiatric interview, this business of much ado, no achievement, and a sort of aching void, in which the doctor must try to whip up excitement again, can all be remedied by the simple expedient of establishing something to work on at the end of the reconnaissance. The doctor then goes to work on that particular problem. If the patient seems to drift away from that problem to no purpose, the doctor investigates what has happened. But if the patient moves from this problem to something which seems to be much more important, then the doctor can rest. The point is that the psychiatrist tries to have something to work on, and he continues to work on it until something more worthy of his attention comes along. And in some ways that's the whole story of intensive psychotherapy.

CHAPTER

V

The Detailed Inquiry: The Theoretical Setting

During the early stages of the interview, the interviewer will have received a good many impressions of the sort of person whom he is participantly observing. These impressions derived from the two initial phases of an interview should stand him in very good stead in quickly putting into effect the procedures which make up the long haul of actual detailed inquiry. Most unhappily, these impressions will be in need of a great deal of revision as a series of interviews proceed, or even during one long interview. Again I say that impressions are, in their purer sense, hypotheses, and like every other hypothesis they should be tested. Thus the impressions that one gains during the first two stages are tested in the prolonged detailed inquiry.

From my years of experience with the interview I would say that there are enough merits in one's early impressions of a stranger to justify some conceit. But this fact can become a very great handicap to any distinguished success in interviewing, since there are enough instances of singularly incorrect impressions to justify a very thorough realization that one must constantly test alternatives and try to keep an open mind as to the essential correctness of his impressions. It is foolish to assume that one's first impression is any good except in a very general sense. There is no magic by which even the most experienced human being can assess in a relatively simple series of relationships the dependable patterns of another personality. Nor can the psychiatrist determine after a few interviews the durable characteristics of a patient so accurately that predictions can be made of the patient's performance in any given situation. I know no evidence whatsoever that any such magic can be performed. If the interviewer finds that his impressions at the start of an interview situation have been rather close to his impressions at the end of an interview, then he can feel immensely encouraged; it is another of the unnumbered manifestations of the extraordinarily gifted character of the human being. But if the interviewer begins to rest on his laurels by assuming that an early impression of a stranger has more than purely experimental importance, then he is not yet ready to do interviewing.

The stage of detailed inquiry in the psychiatric interview is a matter of improving on earlier approximations of understanding, in which process a really revolutionary change in one's impressions may occur. A good many times I have had to make really phenomenal revisions of early impressions of a patient, on the basis of data in the detailed inquiry. Often the statements that misled me would have misled anyone who was paying attention only to what these statements *presumably* meant. For example, patients may tell a psychiatrist things which have so little to do with their durable characteristics that he finally realizes that one of the great difficulties in the interview is the patient's effort to suit him, to impress him. Although this is not a matter of deliberate malice or of stupidity on the patient's part, it does subtly color the way things are presented. Thus the patient is completely unaware of any intention of deceiving the psychiatrist or defeating him in his efforts to find out what is going on; and things which are actually grossly misleading get themselves said as simply as if they were absolute truths.

This element of unreliability in making responses to questions is not uniquely a part of the psychiatric interview. In any life situation, when a person is asked a question his reply varies greatly in its appropriateness, significance, communicativeness, and so on, according to what area of contact with reality the question seems to pertain to. I can ask you, for example, how to get from your house to the nearest streetcar stop, with a high probability that I will get a communicative response. Questions of geometric or geographical orientation addressed to a hundred persons in series would bring something like forty responses which would be incomplete and very much off the point. However, more than fifteen out of a hundred answers would be responsive to the question, and prove to be fairly adequate reflections of what might be described as fixed aspects of reality.

In this realm of alleged spatial relationships which have no particular significance except their immediate utility to the person involved, one can expect some degree of adequacy in the response. In the next category of relationships—those which refer to time—there seems to be an increase in the fringe of irrelevance, uncertainty, misinformation, and so on. If I were to ask a group of sightseers, "Did you go to this place or that place first?" I would discover from the answers that there is not nearly as high a probability that the honest, solemnly helpful answer has any useful relationship to the facts, as those facts would be perceived by a third person, or revealed in a crude statistical analysis of the actual data.

We could proceed to study, through gradation after gradation, the probability of a particular request for information calling out something usefully related to a significant course of events. When in this long series of gradations, which I shall not attempt to outline now, we would finally come to questions about one's belief about how one should act under a given situation—such as asking several people, "How do you believe that you *should* behave about so and so?"—amazingly enough we would find that the responses contained practically no uncertainty; suddenly each answer would be very close to the so-called norm of conduct in that particular. Now if we were to alter the question a little and ask, "How *did* you act under such-and-such circumstances?" referring now to a real event, the answers would be really amazing; the fringe of irrelevancy in the replies, the immateriality of them, and so on, would closely approximate 100 per cent. In other words, a person can't tell you accurately how he acted in an important situation unless by almost sheer chance the way he *did* act happened to coincide with his idea of how he *should* have acted—a rather uncommon coincidence in which the answer is just as good as a geographical direction. In other words, everyone knows in a particular cultural situation just how he ought to act. If his behavior coincides with what he thinks he ought to have done, he can report the matter accurately. If, as is very much more frequently the case, there is no such coincidence between the act and the ideal, one finds that there is a truly astonishing decrease in the likelihood of the response being valid.

Thus it seems to be almost impossible for any of us, in dealing with strangers at least, to say anything which will perfectly succinctly demonstrate that we are inferior to our demands on our own behavior. We all know when we are "at fault" about what we did—an idea which is first learned in childhood from the authority figures. When we start to report something that doesn't come up to our standard of behavior, we know that it doesn't come up to this standard. That goes on in covert processes very quickly. What we then produce, however, is no simple statement. It is a stream of words aimed at what we trust is the unskeptical ear that is listening.

The work of an interviewer is largely concerned with evaluating such statements—apologies for failure, extravagant exaggeration of successes, and studious minimization of errors. Thus the detailed part of the psychiatric interview, in order to be significant, has to be exceedingly far from a conversation made up of simple, correct answers to clear questions. The uncertainties of this part of the interview arise from the interviewee's feeling that what occurs to him isn't "good enough." The real facts of the interview situation might be expressed: "If I tell the doctor the truth, he won't think well of me." Or, "Well, I must put a good face on that; otherwise I might make a bad impression." Or again, "My God! If I do things like that, of course he won't authorize my employment." All of these covert operations show an attempt on the part of the interviewee to read the interviewer's mind. A great many of them form defects in the process of communication, for all of them spring from a dreadfully troublesome and significant question in the mind of the interviewee: "What will he think?" The complex products which the interviewer gets from the interviewee arise from the latter's attempt to avoid even the faintest sign of an unfavorable answer to that question in his mind. There isn't the remotest chance that any person in this social order, and probably in any other extant in the world today, will not try to put his best foot forward, which means that each of us in talking about any of our past performances will try to guess what we can say that will minimize the unfavorable aspects of such performances. This is such a universal phenomenon that it would be utterly absurd for an interviewer to be annoyed by all the complex answers—this walking around the obvious—that he gets from questions which he poses to the interviewee.

If we translate this phenomenon into the psychiatric situation, we find that from the psychiatrist's standpoint all of his contacts with any patient are marked by *the patient's strange dependence for some kind of comfort on what the patient believes the psychiatrist thinks of what is being discussed.* It is hardly necessary to say that the patient's idea of what the therapist is thinking about the patient's remarks is often far from accurate. When it occurs to a patient that he does not have a fair idea as to what the therapist is thinking, his distress is often pathetic. The hesitancy—the attempt to cover two horns of a dilemma with one foot—is poignant, and is really distressing to the patient. It may be much more comfortable for the patient to hold the opinion that he "knows" what the psychiatrist is driving at, that he has some idea of what the "right" answer is, and that he can with some accuracy estimate how his prestige stands with the psychiatrist, than it is to have any reasonable appreciation of the simple fact that the psychiatrist is giving forth with no signs whatsoever on which to base any reliable interpretation of the psychiatrist's attitude. When the conservation of time is quite important, it is very convenient for the psychiatrist to develop a way of behavior that gives no clear index as to his favorable or unfavorable response to what he has heard. Under those circumstances the patient usually operates under the assumption that he can accurately guess whether he is making a good impression on the psychiatrist and will get somewhere, or whether he is making a bad impression and won't. The patient feels much more comfortable if he is completely deluded in his impressions of the psychiatrist's impressions, whether or not he is working on an important aspect of his personality. Although all this seems to be an impractical way to handle the business of living, it is, I assure you, quite understandable once you have some reasonable grasp on what I shall now discuss.

The Concept of Anxiety

The concept of anxiety is central to this whole system of approach. In other words, one might say that anxiety is the general explanatory concept for the interviewee's trying to create a favorable impression. More important, it is this concept which gives the psychiatrist the most general grasp possible on those movements of the patient which mislead him, whether those movements are found in the statements of the informant or in the psychiatrist's interpretation of what he hears. The use of abrupt and accented transitions in the interview becomes understandable in terms of this same concept, for the transitions make it possible for the psychiatrist to alter communicative sets, or to restrain or increase the development of anxiety in the interviewee. And this concept of anxiety can be understood in terms of what everyone of us has known most intimately and continuously from the beginning of our available memory.

An important part of a reasonable grasp on the concept of anxiety might be stated quite simply as: *The presence of anxiety is much worse than its absence*—which is in essence what I have said previously at great length. Under no conceivable circumstance that has ever occurred to me has anyone sought and valued as desirable the experience of anxiety. No series of "useful" attacks of anxiety in therapy will make it something to be sought after. This is, in a good many ways, rather startling, particularly when one compares anxiety with fear. While fear has many of the same characteristics, it may actually be sought out as an experience occasionally, particularly if the fear is expected or anticipated. For instance, people who ride on roller coasters pay money for being afraid. But no one will ever pay money for anxiety in its own right. No one wants to experience it. Only one other experience—that of loneliness—is in this special class of being totally unwanted.

Not only does no one want anxiety, but if it is present, the lessening of it is always desirable, except under the most extraordinary circumstances. Anxiety is to an incredible degree a sign that something ought to be different at once. As the interviewer studies the circumstances of his contact in the interview situation with any stranger, he will observe that those times when the stranger is clearly at a loss to know what the interviewer thinks of him are occasions on which the stranger is suffering considerable anxiety. And anxiety is such a distressing condition to be in that it is often easier for the interviewee to think privately that he is reading the interviewer's mind than to evaluate a situation more realistically. If the interviewer is to have any skill at the work of interrogating, he must realize that he doesn't know what the other fellow is thinking. Yet it is so much more comfortable, even for a psychiatrist, to be carried away by the hope that one does know, that sometimes one acts just as if he did. The only conceivable explanation of this singular travesty of human ability is that it is better than feeling more anxious.

How in the world does it come to be that anxiety exerts such a powerful influence in interpersonal relations? Why does it have this ubiquitous effect of making people act, you might say, like asses? People act so in the exceedingly dubious hope of not being uncomfortable. They may still be terribly uncomfortable when the events are finished, but they haven't suffered as much anxiety as they might have without the use of the defensive behavior. Quite often in the therapy situation, if the patient suffered more anxiety, the returns might be highly desirable. He might not need to experience further anxiety about that particular problem. But that fact makes little difference to the patient. Anxiety rules.

The Development of the Self-System in Personality

It is so extremely important for all of us to maintain any level of euphoria that we are experiencing that we develop a vast system of processes, states of alertness, symbols, and signs of warning, in order to protect what sense of well-being we do have. Although this has its beginning in the relation of the infant and the mothering one, it is first clearly evident in the child as he develops general skills to avoid forbidding gestures; and in the last half of childhood, these skills become elaborated into a great many verbal techniques for putting a somewhat better face on difficult situations. This vast system of operations, precautions, alertnesses, and so on could perfectly properly be called the *self-system*—that part of personality which is born entirely out of the influences of significant others upon one's feeling of well-being. This organization of an enormous number of complex operations comes into existence solely for the purpose of avoiding drops in euphoria which are related to the significant other person with whom the child is integrated. Since these drops in euphoria are, in fact, the same thing as the experience of anxiety, the psychiatrist must realize that every patient carries with him experiences from extraordinarily early in life which make him somewhat cautious about too ready an expression of himself to another by word or gesture. In infancy, we would say that the self-system seeks to protect one's feeling of well-being, of relative euphoria, from a drop in level; and any drop in the sense of well-being is experienced by the infant as anxiety. When we think of the more adult years of existence, it is more informative, more illuminating, to consider the operation of the self-system in terms of operations calculated to protect one's self-esteem; and any lowering of self-esteem is experienced as anxiety. While the formulation is different, we are, in fact, talking about the same thing.

Whether we are talking about infancy or the more adult years of existence, we will speak of these operations for the protection of the self-system as *security operations*. In other words, all anti-anxiety operations are security operations; all efforts to protect one's self-esteem are security operations. It is somewhat easier to see the security element in the processes by which all of us in an adult world practically read into the people around us the movements of our own self-esteem. But I also use the term security operations to refer to the operations of the self-system in the infant, for the adult security operations have their beginnings in the infant's protection of his relative state of euphoria or well-being. One of the great profits that we derive from experience that is well assimilated is better foresight in avoiding unpleasant experience and in gaining good experience. This rather obvious notion about human living can be applied generally to the avoiding of anxiety. Since the other fellow from the beginning to the end has been capable of injuring one's self-esteem, of lowering one's euphoria, it is logical that the self-system should develop into a singularly subtle apparatus for watching for signs of approval and disapproval in the other fellow. But one must remember that the signs that one sees in the other fellow don't necessarily mean too much about him. There is no such thing as "objective" observation; it is participant observation in which you may be the significant factor in the participation.

Thus everybody who comes to the interviewer is very busy interpreting the interviewer while the interviewer is interpreting him. There is some small chance that the interviewer will interpret correctly, but there is little chance that the interviewee will interpret correctly, for the interviewer is not engaged in being anything like a well-rounded person whose durable characteristics would be pertinent to the interview. He is engaged in being an expert at determining what the durable characteristics of the interviewee are. The interviewer's durable characteristics may interfere to some extent with the manifestations of his expert skill in getting a fairly dependable idea of the interviewee. To that extent the interviewer is getting in his own way.

I do not mean to suggest that the perfect interviewer is opaque and free from meaningful gestures and so on. Were any one of us to be interviewed about a significant aspect of our living by a person who gave us no clues as to what he thought and how we were doing, I think we would be reduced to mutism within a matter of minutes. Our uncertainty would be frightful, and we would simply be too acutely anxious to go on. In short, none of us feel that safe, and we won't feel that safe until the social order has greatly improved in its utility for living. The interviewer actually gives signs by tonal gestures, by physical gestures, and by verbal statements, which can be, and are, interpreted and misinterpreted by the interviewee. The skill in interviewing lies in not doing this in the wrong way. These gestures and signs of the interviewer may not be greatly revealing of his ideas regarding the discussion currently in progress, but they do serve to indicate to the interviewee that the interviewer is a human being, and that is sufficiently reassuring, makes the interviewee sufficiently comfortable, so that he is able to go on without getting completely tied up in his uncertainty and anxiety.

Frequently the patient thinks that he has learned just what impression he is making on the therapist, and gets quite enthusiastic about what he thinks he is conveying to the therapist. The patient will probably continue to be enthusiastic until a simple and commonplace question by the therapist shows him that his concept of the impression he was making was all a mistake. At this point the patient will experience considerable anxiety. No matter how painful the experience, the patient often does not seem to learn anything from it. Having recovered, he may immediately start the cycle over again, building up in his mind another version of the therapist's impression of him, until it is interrupted by the therapist and the patient again experiences anxiety.

In other words, the one thing the therapist can always depend on in psychiatric interviews is that the patient's self-system will be very active indeed. Unless the interviewee is revealing data bearing on his aptitudes for living, on his successes, or on his unusual abilities as a human being, the operations of the self-system are always in opposition to achieving the purpose of the interview. That is, it always opposes the clear revelation of what the interviewee regards as handicaps, deficiencies, defects, and what not, and it does not facilitate communication except in the realms where that which is communicated clearly enhances his sense of well-being, his feeling of making a favorable impression. It is well for the interviewer to calmly assume that this is the way the world is. This is a perduring aspect of reality; it is no cause for lamentation, for contempt of the other fellow, or for irritation at how hard the interviewer has to work for a living. He will then understand that, in his role of participant observer, a very great part of the work of the detailed inquiry is his use of skill to avoid arousing unnecessary anxiety, and at the same time to obtain dependable indices of what the interviewee considers to be significant misfortunes about him, unfortunate incidents in his past, handicaps that he has in dealing with people, and so on. But I trust that I am making it amply clear that the successful psychiatric interview is *not* largely a matter of "showing up" the interviewee.

As I have said, one of the remarkable aspects of the self-system is that after suffering defeat it immediately pulls itself together and goes to work again. This fact has some practical implications for the interviewer's handling of those actions, remarks, processes, and events which are chiefly purposed to protect the self-system of the interviewee. Thus if the interviewer is unduly impressed by the fact that anxiety can be an absolute barrier to interpersonal processes, he may become too "considerate" of the feelings of the interviewee. In that case he will obtain a great deal of data on the manifestations of the interviewee's self-system, but the data won't be of any particular use, for it will do no more than clearly demonstrate that, like all other human beings, the interviewee tries to make a good impression. That discovery will not be enough to solve any problems.

On the other hand, the interviewer may have nothing to do with the interviewee's movements toward reassuring himself, toward putting his best foot forward, but may immediately consign them to oblivion; thus the interviewer precipitates anxiety every time the interviewee tries to avoid it, and the interview becomes unproductive. If the interviewee is a patient, it is perfectly certain he won't return. If he is a candidate for a job, or something of the sort, it is perfectly certain that he will not give the interviewer any adequate basis for forming an opinion.

Now how does one get the data one needs despite the interviewee's anxiety? In the early part of this discourse I laid great stress on the orientation of every interview situation to the achievement of some useful, beneficial effect for the interviewee. I did this with the following in mind: There is a great deal of fairly subtle data to support the notion that every human being, if he has not been tediously demoralized by a long series of disasters, comes fairly readily to manifest processes which tend to improve his efficiency as a human being, his satisfactions, and his success in living—a tendency which I somewhat loosely call *the drive toward mental health*. If one's operations with another person begin to connect with an anticipation on his part of favorable outcome of the experience, then, however unpleasant the details may be, he will begin to be not so immediately deflected by anxiety. If, for example, as a result of very sustained and well-directed efforts on the part of the psychiatrist during three months of intensive therapy, the patient finally sees that the procedure might work, then he will be able to go on despite some increasing anxiety. In fact, if this conviction of favorable change becomes quite strong, the patient will at opportune moments be able to undergo rather rapidly increasing anxiety, even though it may reach a point where his conventional skills are seriously impaired—for example, his speech may be disturbed.

Thus the interviewer, whether he is a psychiatrist or a personnel manager, must learn to facilitate this movement in the interview situation which renders the interviewee's anxiety less immediately deflective—remembering that no intervention, no matter how skillful, can ever render anxiety desirable. When the interviewee's 'tolerance' for anxiety has increased, he can even discuss things that he is quite sure will harm the interviewer's esteem of him.

Remember this, however: The psychiatrist can—if he is both skillful and stupid enough—precipitate intense anxiety and "smash," as some people put it, the patient's defenses; he can "pin him down to the facts," as some have a damnable habit of saying; but he will not get useful information in this way. He will be presented with a great many "phenomena," but there will be no way that he can guess what they are all about. For example, the doctor may feel quite conceited at having brought a patient to the state of practically generalized bodily tremor, whereupon the patient says something like, "Well, Doctor, it really wasn't so. What I actually did was to hit him with an ax." He may have hit somebody with an ax, but when the patient is at that level of anxiety the psychiatrist cannot be sure of anything that he hears. Once in while the beautiful account of the blow with the ax is only a wild guess by the patient as to what the therapist is insisting he must say, and has no particular reference to any other aspects of the patient's past. Anxiety of that intensity puts a terrible strain on the prospects of further results, and gives the psychiatrist data which are useless to him.

But the interviewer does have to deal with anxiety almost eternally. This dealing with anxiety in relations with others is a work of exquisite refinement and crucial importance, at least until the other person sees a high probability that something useful is going to come of it. After that has happened—and the interviewer must be judicious in judging *when* it happens—he may not have to worry quite so much about doing the wrong thing. If he provokes a little anxiety when he doesn't need to, it can usually be assuaged by some sort of mildly reassuring gesture. But until the interviewee becomes convinced that some good will come out of the interview or series of interviews, the psychiatrist must avoid any carelessness about provoking anxiety, or any insensitivity to its manifestations. And he cannot afford to object to the existence of anxiety and its manifestations. To fail in any of these respects is to promote disaster.

Anyone who proceeds without consideration for the disjunctive power of anxiety in human relationships will never learn interviewing. When there is no regard for anxiety, a true interview situation does not exist; instead, there may be just a person (the patient) trying to defend himself frantically from some kind of a devil (the therapist) who seems determined (as the patient experiences it) to prove that the person (the patient) is a double-dyed blankety-blank. This can be a spectacular human performance, but it does not yield psychiatric data relevant to therapeutic progress.

What I have been saying about anxiety and security operations will become more meaningful if you will make a careful study of the next awkward situation that you get into with your boss, your husband or wife, or what not. Needless to say you will only be able to study this awkward situation retrospectively. Although these situations often include various complexities, they are always characterized by anxiety and they always manifest almost simon-pure security operations. That means, of course, that you won't just think about what bright answer you could have made, or something of that kind, but you will actually study all that you can recall of how the situation grew, how you felt, what you did, and so on. Any one of these awkward situations—which, unhappily, most of us have at least one time a day—shows, in microcosm, practically all that anyone needs to really understand about security operations in order to become fairly skillful at provoking them or by-passing them in dealing with other people. When you study particular awkward situations, you may eventually be able to discover that, for instance, a particular remark in a particular tone was what made you feel uncomfortable. This feeling of acute, sort of diffused discomfort is anxiety—however it is experienced, whatever guises and whatever language you attach to it in order to make it feel less unpleasant. The first few times you attempt it—even though you try hard to analyze clearly in your recollection just what went on, one event after another, dealings, thoughts, this and that—you are apt to find that you didn't have any particular discomfort. The other person made you angry, he humiliated you and you were annoyed, you humiliated him—all that sort of thing. But you are then missing completely the thing I am striving to describe—namely, the anxieties that started the fireworks. Until you are able to discover that the first experience in this sequence of events is acute discomfort, you won't make much sense of what I am talking about.

This comes about because anger is much more pleasant to experience than anxiety. The brute facts are that it is much more comfortable to feel angry than anxious. Admitting that neither is too delightful, there is everything in favor of anger. Anger often leaves one sort of worn out, and one thing and another, very often makes things worse in the long run, but there is a curious feeling of power when one is angry. In other words, the expressive pattern of anger tends to drive things away. Not only is anxiety thus avoided, but the initial index of its presence fades from observation, and you are left with no clear idea of how this all came about. In somewhere around 94 per cent of all occasions on which you are anxious, the security operations called out by that anxiety are the things you are perfectly clear on, whereas the precipitating anxiety is obscured.

Discomfort, tense discomfort, a definite sudden transition from fair to worse, a feeling of general ill-being, all of these are of a single genus—they indicate anxiety. It is anxiety which starts you off on the manifestation of these security operations, shown by protesting your rightness, and so on. There are an infinity of ways in which these protective devices, security operations, are displayed. In suggesting that you attempt to notice the movements of premonitory anxiety in yourselves, I am well aware that it will be difficult, if not impossible, to capture the experience of anxiety, since it moves so swiftly into these security operations. But you may be able to discover that in addition to the immediate activation of the security operation, there has been a covert operation which gives you some notion of what in the other person angered you, and so on. You will find that immediately after whatever causes you anxiety you develop an unfavorable estimation of the other person and that you react in response to this. In addition you may discover that the character of your action gives a clear index to the character of your unfavorable appraisal of the person who injured you.

So it is that in interviewing, the interviewer must learn to recognize the anxiety that underlies the security operations in the interviewee. Otherwise he doesn't make very much sense in trying to develop the fairly subtle sensitivity which makes it possible to operate in the field of recurring anxiety with steadily increasing useful results in communication. He studies, by such skills as he can acquire, the indices by which the interviewee indicates his supposition about what the interviewer is thinking. This supposition is the formulated part of what the interviewee thinks he is doing with the interviewer. The interviewer, as he studies these indices, permits the security operations to go on long enough so that he can develop reasonable certainty regarding the sensitivities that called out these security operations—that is, by observing the security operations, he seeks for clues to the location of the underlying anxiety. And when the interviewer has developed a good hunch as to what the insecurity is about, he then tests that hunch by the use of some question designed to suddenly destroy the patient's illusion that he is doing fine in making a good impression. The successive movements in the situation may indicate whether or not the patient is experiencing anxiety, and thus whether the interviewer's hunch was reasonably probable or quite beside the point.

To refer again to your study of your own experience of an awkward situation, you may be able to discover that an acute feeling of ill-being is followed by what looks like two streams of processes. One of these is that you are engaged in some sort of action, often angry action, toward the other person with whom you are involved. The other process, which goes along with the first, is that you are analyzing the situation as one in which this other person has injured you, belittled you, or done something to you which is decidedly unpleasant. If the psychiatrist keeps these processes in mind as he observes his patient, he may notice that the ways in which the patient responds, his angry remarks, and so on, are rather strikingly a revelation of, a communication about, the interpretation that he has made of a particular situation. In other words, if the patient defines a situation as being injurious or anxiety-provoking, what he does shows it. But if the psychiatrist does not recognize that anxiety lies behind the whole performance, he will look in the wrong place for an explanation of the behavior.

Thus the interviewer sees both attempts to make good impressions and angry behavior as security operations which occur under somewhat different circumstances. He observes the pattern of these security operations; he gets some idea about what sort of theory about him, and about the situation, is behind this pattern of activity. He formulates this idea as a hypothesis which must be tested in order to become useful. If he has two hypotheses, all the better, as I have said earlier. In order to test his hypothesis, the interviewer does something designed to disturb the field of operation, and what follows may confirm his hypothesis about where the patient's sensitivity lies. Now, if the hypothesis is correct, none of this is pleasant for the patient, for he ends up with some felt anxiety, unprotected for the moment by his security operation. It is quite important that this should not happen exterior to the interviewer's clear awareness and thus to no useful end. The interviewer must not go through this performance of listening to the interviewee's somewhat rosy account of something, for instance, and then perforate it without trying to learn something from what he is doing. Otherwise the interviewer is manifesting utter disregard and disrespect for the other person concerned, or he is showing an obtuseness, or a deep preoccupation with something else—all of which violates the whole basic notion of the essentially therapeutic or helpful relationship.

It is inevitable that from time to time the interviewer punctures—often very clumsily—the self-esteem of the interviewee.

That is all right if the interviewer knows what he is doing, and learns something from it. But if he does it because he is insecure or absent-minded, the detailed inquiry will not develop very satisfactorily. Instead, the interviewer will gather a quite fictitious collection of data about some quite fictitious creature, innocently believed by the interviewer to be the person he is interviewing.

CHAPTER

VI

The Interview as a Process

A GREAT DEAL of our discussion of the interview has suggested that it is a process, or a system of processes—and the word *process* of course implies change. I wish now to present a generalization of this change—that is, a way of looking at it—which will help the interviewer to keep track of what is going on. One kind of change which may go on in the interview situation is *a change in the interviewee's attitude*. A change in the attitude of the other person is fairly easy for anyone to notice in any conversational dealing. But noticing another, equally important group of changes which may occur in an interpersonal situation requires more training, more centered interest. In the interview situation, these somewhat more recondite changes are *changes in the interviewer's attitude, as reflected by the interviewee*. In other words, the interviewer must ask himself: What attitude of mine is being reflected by the interviewee? What does he seem to be experiencing about my attitude? What does he think I am doing? How does he think I feel toward him? A great many useful clues to the complex processes making up the interview first appear when the interviewer begins to think in such terms. Part of his development of skill comes from observing, more or less automatically, what is *probably* the case with respect to the interviewee's feelings about the interviewer's attitude. The interviewee's impression may, of course, be very far from what the interviewer would call "accurate." In other words, even though the interviewer is being highly objective and entirely, respectfully impersonal, it may seem to the interviewee that the interviewer is engaged in showing him up to be no good. The interviewee's operations give clues to what he is experiencing, and in many cases these point toward the type of difficulty that he will have with anyone who impresses him as superior in capability or in position.

Thus it is is quite important to realize that there are two groups of processes directed to the interviewer: one is the *direct attitude* of the interviewee toward him; and the other is that part of the interviewee's performances which are faithfully related to the *supposed attitude* of the interviewer.

Gross Impressions of the Interview Situation

In order to observe change, it is necessary to have some point of departure; and for the detailed inquiry, that point of departure is those gross impressions obtained in the stages of the formal inception and the reconnaissance. The changes from these initial gross impressions which are observed during the later course of the interview are useful as data.

The first rudimentary, gross impression that any interviewer has of a particular interview is in terms of its efficiency: perhaps the interview is "hard going"—that is, the interviewer feels that he really earns his money to get any information at all out of his client; or perhaps the interview is rather "run-of-the-mill," and not in any way unusual; or it may be remarkably productive. It is not difficult to obtain such gross impressions; the interviewer can scarcely avoid noticing it if he must make unusual effort to obtain results, or if, on the other hand, he is required to do very little to gather relevant information. Having obtained this grossest of impressions, he begins to analyze it from several different points of view—and here I will use some popular expressions that point in the direction of what I mean. First he considers the interviewee in terms of his *general alertness*—that is, how keen he is, and in how many areas, and how clearly the implications evoked in his mind of the other person's remarks and questions are related to what might reasonably be expected. In other words, the interviewee's *attention* to what is going on may vary greatly. Some people are *intent* on everything the interviewer says, and are very careful about everything they produce, but at the same time are not guarded; they are simply determined to get something out of the interview. There are others who are *distracted;* noises outside, or things that are going on in their own minds, get in the way of their following closely the questions, comments, and suggestions of the interviewer. Occasionally a person's attention in the interview situation may be appropriately called *vague*. Such people seem to have only the most casual and foggy contact with what the interviewer is trying to get at, and the responses that they produce seem to have at best a tenuous or nebulous relationship to what the other person has said.

Along with all this, the interviewer develops an impression of the "*intelligence*" of the interviewee. First impressions of the intelligence of another person can be quite misleading. For example, every now and then in employment interviewing one encounters a person who literally doesn't seem to know the language. Inquiry into his employment history, however, may show that he has made extremely rapid progress in handling complex machinery in an industrial job, and the interviewer realizes that to have done this he must have very high general intelligence. Thus one must always realize that intelligence, in the sense of something which is useful as an aid in living, is by no means necessarily measurable by verbal dexterity. Verbal dexterity is closely related to intelligence only if there has been opportunity for the development of verbal skills.

Finally, in this group of very general characteristics, the interviewer may notice the *responsiveness* of the interviewee. People who are quite responsive—a very broad term in the sense that I use it here—are apt to be commended by their friends as having a peculiarly "sensitive understanding"; that is, they are likely to be sufficiently sensitive to such things as minor tonal indices so that they are able with a minimum of awkward questions to catch on to those things which are embarrassing for other people to communicate. Responsiveness includes a group of complex elements in the personality which, other things being equal, make for ease in living, and which in their very highest manifestation, perhaps, add up to what is ordinarily called "tact." In the interview situation, the responsiveness of the interviewee can vary from *understanding cooperation*, in which he almost knows what the next question will be, and provides a succinct and illuminating answer as soon as it is asked, to an *obtuseness* such that he gets completely lost trying to guess what the interviewer is driving at, apparently deriving very little from those indications that would suffice for an "understanding" person. Sometimes obtuseness seems to border on something that is probably hostile; in other words, there are people whose dumbness is all but deliberate. Sometimes there is a certain *unwillingness to be led*, so that it is singularly difficult to get the interviewee to deal with the topics that one presents, although he may be very productive about something quite irrelevant, or about something that is important but tangential at the moment. Occasionally there are interviewees—sometimes court cases, sometimes difficult children—who are, the interviewer is apt to think, *deliberately obstructive*. It clearly seems that such an interviewee is engaged in trying to prevent the interviewer's getting his points across, and is attempting to keep anything of interest from the interviewer.

These are only hints of the kinds of gross impressions that the interviewer has gathered by the time he begins the detailed inquiry; such gross impressions, which may, of course, be wrong, form the point of departure from which he observes change.[1]

[1] [*Editors' note:* This chapter is taken from the 1945 series of lectures. In his 1944 lecture on the same topic, Sullivan mentioned two other gross impressions which the interviewer may obtain, which he described as "related to the elaboration of observation rather than to observation itself":

"It is useful to note the patient's *habitual attitude toward his recall or*

He realizes, of course, that at the same time that he is picking up these gross impressions of the interviewee, the interviewee is picking up gross impressions of him. Thus it is quite rewarding for the interviewer to be curious about those signs in the remarks and performances of the interviewee which reflect to the interviewer the sort of person that the interviewee surmises him to be.

I would now like to mention some of the more specific terms which are used quite frequently by the interviewer to describe the interviewee, and which provide a somewhat more refined

---

memory. Recall is a function of motivation, and the person's attitude toward his own recall—be it assurance, vague uncertainty, or emphatic pessimism—may be quite revealing. By an attitude of assurance, I do not mean that anyone knows that his memory will always work, for nobody's memory always works. I, for example, find it extremely difficult to recall ordinal data—names of telephone exchanges, names of people, and so on and so forth—but I usually recall anything which I need badly, and so my attitude toward my recall function is rather trusting. I expect it to work if there is a reasonable cause for it to do so; however, I don't expect to be able to remember poetry, for instance, since, so far as I know, it will never be useful to me. In contrast, there are people who almost always wonder if what they recall from the year before last is right or wrong. They don't seem to have any particular optimism as to their success at recalling anything; they simply don't trust their recollection. I think that most of these people don't mention this distrust; it is something they don't brag about. On the other hand, when you encounter someone who talks about how rotten his memory is, the chances are that he *does* trust it—and that you can't trust his statements. Thus the interviewer can make some estimate of the patient's recall. Is what he has lived through handy to him, available to him when he needs it? Or are many matters of the past to be looked upon as lost, strayed, or stolen? It is not that recall is important in itself, but that the person's *attitude* toward recall gives a valuable clue to the simplicity of his motivation. If his recall is relatively useful to him, he has probably been proceeding toward more or less clearly foreseen goals for a long time, and having some success at getting nearer them; and his motivational system is relatively simple. In trying to trace some unhappy people's motivational history, one may get into quagmires which take hours to wallow through, whereas one could have found a useful and immediate clue to much the same thing by noticing to what extent they could depend on their memories.

"An inference can also be made in regard to the patient's *habitual feeling about answering questions*. Some people are at an atrocious disadvantage with almost anybody if they are put in the position of answering questions; and no matter how suavely one handles the interview, such people will soon discover that they are being required to answer a lot of questions, and will feel this very keenly. This attitude reflects certain things about the interview-

impression of the processes that go on to make up the interview. The following sets of attitudes suggest patterns which the interviewer will use as starting points in observing change in his relation with the interviewee. While these are words of common speech, I also hope to have them carry some fairly specific meaning. In the early stages of the interview, the interviewee may seem to be, for example, *reserved*, *guarded*, *suspicious*, *hostile*, or *contemptuous*. A quite different set of five terms may also characterize the same interviewee from a somewhat different standpoint: his manner toward the interviewer may be *supercilious*, *superior*, *conciliatory*, *deferential*, or *apologetically inferior*. There are two situations which may be presented by the interviewee in the early stages of his work which are of peculiar difficulty, and for that reason it is very important for an interviewer to consider carefully how to deal with them. One is presented by the *insolent informant;* in certain types of interview work the informant may be thoroughly insolent—and it is nice indeed when this changes. Something which is much more common in psychiatric work, and also quite common in all other forms of interviewing, is the situation presented by the *evasive informant*.

---

ee's past, but it also gives the interviewer a fairly important hunch as to how much faster things will proceed if he can only get this person to talking about things, so that the interviewer can be quiet and listen, only coming in now and then with a conversational remark. Of course, if time is very limited and the problem is very complex, one can scarcely have recourse to this. Under such circumstances, when somebody goes into a mild upset because a question is flung at him, one can sometimes, believe it or not, diminish the evil effects by saying, 'Do you feel I'm questioning you?' At that, any completely sane person would say quite angrily, 'I *know* you are questioning me!' But people who are upset are so glad to have anything that looks like a straw thrown to them that they don't notice the preposterous character of such an inquiry, and actually feel better about what the interviewer is doing, having somehow slipped away from the anxiety connected with being questioned."]

The Observation of Changes in the Interview Situation

The interviewer's interest is in observing the *changes* that appear in such sets of attitudes—in observing what in the situation is improving or what is deteriorating. Sometimes, of course, it is the impression of the interviewer that there is little or no change. Perhaps during the inception of the interview and the reconnaissance the interviewer has, as nearly as he can judge, developed impressions of the interviewee which are fairly accurate. Perhaps the interviewee began as a somewhat supercilious person. As the interviews progress, he still sounds as if he thought the interviewer were one of the very great headaches that it had been his misfortune to encounter; there isn't a bit of change. These situations in which there seems to be no particular alteration in the attitude of the informant in the course of a well-conducted interview are highly significant, for reasons which I trust I shall be able to make clear a little later. Sometimes, of course, the psychiatrist sees a *mutually respecting* person—one who shows such obvious self-respect, and therefore respect for the other person, that the interviewer has the feeling, "Well, bless us! What on earth does this man need of a psychiatrist?" Sometimes the answer is that these people are not seeking cures, but are seeking jobs or something else, for the interview is used for many purposes besides finding cures. A fairly clearly self-respecting attitude, with respect also shown for the other person—the one does not exist without the other—is not likely to undergo very much change during an interview or series of interviews unless the interviewer very seriously disappoints the person who possesses it.

Besides noting change, and having some idea of what that change is, in terms of what is improved, what is deteriorated, or what has shown no change at all, the interviewer tries to pick up, more or less automatically, impressions of what in his own performance has had some bearing on the change. If the situation is bad—the interview is hard going for some reason or other—it is well for the interviewer to have some idea as to what operations of his are responsible for the failure to produce any change, even though he may have thought they were well adjusted to improving the situation. If he knows what he was trying to do, and if he is able to study—in the interstices of other things, as it were—how well he did it, how flatly it failed, or how dramatically it succeeded, then he will have important data related to the motivational system which characterizes the interviewee.

As I have already suggested, the interviewer will have a gross impression of the informant's changing impression of the interviewer, as shown by the informant's attitude. There are in this field three areas, if you please, of major importance. First, the interviewer may ask himself: Is the patient being impressed with the therapist's *expertness in interpersonal relations?* Second: Is the patient coming more and more to appreciate the therapist as an *understanding person?* That is, whether the therapist is friendly or austere, does he show an interest in sparing the informant's "feelings"—or, more accurately, does he pay as much respect as possible to the informant's need to feel self-esteem? As an indication of what I mean by "understanding," consider a situation in which a therapist, for some reason or other, is interviewing a seventeen-year-old about the details of his sex life. Some interviewers would ask blunt questions, which might serve the purpose of giving the adolescent some new ideas about possible sexual ventures which had not occurred to him before, but would usually have the main result of producing such anxiety that the adolescent would not even be able to stutter, and nothing useful would go on, either visibly or audibly. Other interviewers in such a situation would be so careful that unhappily they would not get any useful information either; even though they thought they did, further inquiry would show that they did not. Thus the really understanding person is not so tender to the interviewee that he prevents his doing what he is there for, but he does not make it any more distressing than he can help, even though he may seem very cold and remote. The third major question about the patient's impression of the interviewer is this: Does he seem to feel a *simplicity of motivation* in the therapist—that the therapist is solely interested in doing a competent job? In other words, to what extent does the patient seem to consider that the therapist is concerned primarily with getting valid data from which to reach valid conclusions about him and his troubles; and to what extent does he seem to think that the therapist is activated by ulterior motives?

Assessing changes in these areas is important. Insofar as the patient seems to be more and more impressed by the doctor's expert skill, and more and more relieved by his understanding way of doing things, and perfectly convinced that the doctor has no objective except finding out who the patient is, and what ails him—to that extent the serious work of the interview is being vastly expedited, and the difficulties in the patient's personality will be increasingly presented with a minimum of wear and tear on the doctor. When these impressions are not so favorable, the data are presented in such a way as to make their interpretation more difficult, since there is less freedom of movement in the interpersonal field—that is, the patient's ability to express himself is more restricted.

Impressions as Hypotheses To Be Tested

These gross impressions that I am talking about are, in fact, rough hypotheses, and, like all hypotheses in interpersonal work, they should be subjected to continuous, or recurrent, test and correction. Sometimes the interviewer is able, almost as automatically as a calculating machine, to add up negative and positive evidence of this and that so that he simply knows, without any particularly laborious thinking, that the patient is, let us say, improving. In such a case, the interviewer has so continuously and automatically tested his hypotheses that he knows the answer without bothering to do anything about it very consciously or deliberately.

But more frequently the interviewer obtains impressions which on scrutiny may or may not be justifiable. More or less specific testing operations should be applied to those impressions with the idea of getting them more nearly correct. One way these impressions are tested is by more or less *unnoted inference*. However, the testing of hypotheses cannot safely be left wholly to relatively unformulated referential operations. Instead it is well for the interviewer now and then to think about the impressions that he has obtained. The very act of beginning to formulate them throws them into two rough groups: *those about which one has no reasonable doubt* and *those which, when noted, are open to question*. The latter, of course, need further testing. A so-called "highly intuitive" interviewer who does not formulate his impressions, but relies solely on his unnoted inference, is likely to find that after an interview is over some most pregnant questions arise in his mind —and he has failed to secure any clues whatever to the answers. That is the danger if one depends on the machinery outside of awareness to do all the work, instead of attempting now and then to take stock of one's impressions. The other way of testing hypotheses is by *clearly purposed exploratory activity* of some kind. The interviewer asks critical questions—that is, questions so designed that the response will indicate whether the hypothesis is reasonably correct or quite definitely not adequate.

The Situation of Improving Communication

Let us consider now the general case in which the interview situation shows, more or less continuously, or at least from period to period, definitely improving communication. This is the situation in which everything is going well. For the inexperienced interviewer, that can be a great misfortune, for he may fail to notice carefully and as completely as possible all of the context—the operations, the remarks, and their patterns—which lead to distinct improvements in the situation. If the interviewer knows how the situation came to be going so well, in the sense that he knows at which points of his operations the patient's communicability increased, he has quite valuable indices to the informant's covert security operations—that is, his security operations which are only inferentially evident. In other words, the interviewer can find, in the context that led to distinct improvements in the interviewee's freedom of communication, fairly clear grounds for inferring what sort of thing led him to suffer anxiety; improvement in the patient's communication at a particular time implies that the patient at that time experienced relief from the feeling that he would make a bad impression, give away something disastrous, or something of the sort. Looking back a little further, the interviewer can then begin to see the general pattern of the interviewee's precautions, the security operations by which he was guarding some particular area until the interviewer did something that made it seem safe to go ahead.

Thus, unless the interviewer pays close attention to the more or less episodic improvements in the interview that goes "wonderfully," he may miss a great deal of the data that might show what the interviewee would be like in a more difficult situation that didn't go so smoothly. The same things are to be found out about the interviewee in the interviews that go well as in the interviews that go badly, but in the first instance they are revealed only if the interviewer notices each favorable change, and thinks of it in terms of what the patient was doing earlier, which has now been made unnecessary.

The Situation of Deteriorating Communication

Now let us consider the special case in which deterioration of the communicative attitude is occurring: the patient is getting less communicative and acts as though he thought that the interviewer were anything but an expert. When things seem to be going from bad to worse, I should counsel any therapist to control his anxiety for the moment, if possible, and to try to study the deterioration in the relationship by retrospective survey, for a great deal may be gained in this way. (I trust that it is becoming clear why I emphasize that it is well for the interviewer to have some recall of what has gone on—which is unlikely if he simply shoots out questions as fast as he can, ignoring the answers.) The interviewer may begin this study by trying to sort out the time when deterioration first seemed to characterize the relationship. Sometimes a psychiatric interview goes badly from the inception, from the time the interviewer uttered his first remarks to the stranger. More often, the bad going begins during the reconnaissance. Perhaps the interviewer, by his way of getting the gross social history of the patient, has fallen over some security apparatus of the patient—and if this is so, it is a very good thing to know. Or in retrospect the interviewer may realize that the inception of the interview was characterized by a certain willingness and mutual regard on the part of both, that they got through the reconnaissance or outline of social history quite well, and that actually for some time in the detailed inquiry everything seemed to be quite all right—until at a certain point the interviewer asked something, the patient replied, and events seemed to go sour thereafter. Such a discovery is very useful indeed, both as a basis for rectifying the deteriorating situation and, much more important, as data for achieving the purpose of the interview. Things don't have to be lovely for an interview to succeed; some quite unpleasant interviews may give the interviewer a pretty good impression of what ails the other fellow. I might add that the longer the interviewer has been working with a particular person, the more possible it is to be reasonably certain of what did happen. Early in a relationship, the interviewer may know what *he* said, and he may know what *the patient* said; but nevertheless it was as if two strangers were talking to themselves. Later interviews often progress to what amounts to singularly subtle communications of fact. The longer the relationship has gone on, the greater is the possibility of the interviewer's being reasonably certain of just when things went wrong, and what was probably the situation at the time deterioration appeared.

In considering this question of timing, the interviewer should note whether the situation began going from bad to worse insidiously or relatively abruptly. If its appearance was relatively abrupt, careful review in the interviewer's own mind of the apparent circumstances will give him a hunch as to what was the matter, and this hunch can then be tested in various ways. If in retrospect the interviewer cannot determine any particular time at which things seemed to get worse, but feels that matters have been getting worse insidiously from the beginning, he has something on his hands which may be quite intricate. In this case, *first*, he may well *review the factual basis for his earlier more favorable appraisal of the situation.* Sometimes he may discover in retrospect that his own enthusiasm, rather than that of the patient, was responsible for his feeling that things had been better in the beginning. In other words, in some supposedly insidiously deteriorating situations, matters have been very bad from the beginning, and the patient has been more and more driven to impress upon the interviewer how bad things are, until the interviewer finally catches on. But that is not deterioration. When the interviewer grasps the fact that the situation is bad, that is, if anything, a slightly favorable change, since communication has improved. Thus it is well to look back to see whether there was any valid reason for thinking that things were once going better and now are going worse.

Second, and this is very important in the situation which really is deteriorating, the interviewer should review what has happened as best he can to *learn whether anything discouraging as to the outcome of the interview has occurred.* Has the interviewer said or seemed to imply something, or encouraged the patient to say something (which the interviewer has not neutralized) which discourages the patient's hope of a useful outcome of the interview? When a person loses heart about an interpersonal relation, things begin to be dull, and the person tends to think about how to get out of it politely. Most psychiatrists have had this unpleasant retrospective realization that they have said, or have permitted the patient to say without rejoinder, something which is seriously discouraging. After that things may go much worse. In some instances, the patient is so far ahead of the psychiatrist that he soon realizes that things are not going to work with this particular psychiatrist, and so, practically from the start, he is thinking about how he can escape and try it with someone else.

Third, it is well for the interviewer who is looking for the facts about a deteriorating interview situation to *observe what relation the current situation has to his own attitude toward this interviewee*. He should consider what his attitude has been from the start, or what it has been since some particular event—for example, perhaps the interviewee said something which displeased the interviewer, or which caused a sudden concentration of the interviewer's interest. Sometimes the young doctor finds data about mother, and father, and maiden aunts, and so on, rather boring and uninspiring, but gets greatly interested in some "problem" such as masturbation—and sometimes interview situations deteriorate lamentably after such a sudden evincing of unexpected interest on the part of the doctor. Thus when things are deteriorating rather insidiously, it is well for the interviewer to check up on whether he took a dislike to this patient when he came in; whether the patient offended the interviewer in some way; or whether, unfortunately, the interviewer showed undue interest in some aspects of the data in such a way that the intelligent patient could interpret it as meaning that the interviewer was very little interested in him, but was interested in some aspect of life of which he happened to be the present entertaining example.

I now want to mention several further attitudes which may

appear as changes in the interview, either on the part of the interviewer or the interviewee. Let us consider particularly the situations in which the informant becomes *bored*, is definitely *amused* at an inquiry by the interviewer, is clearly *irritated*, or is frankly *angry*. Changes in the interview situation represented by the appearance of any of these attitudes on the part of the patient are none too cheering. These same attitudes may, of course, appear in the interviewer; on occasion some of them may be deliberately assumed by the interviewer. There are times when it is well for the interviewer to express boredom, mild amusement, or even irritation; however, if the interviewer is genuinely angry, I would say that this is probably tantamount to a serious defect in his equipment for interviewing. Then there are patients who are from the beginning, or become at some later stage in the work, *frivolous*, *flippant*, *arrogant*, *insolent*, *sarcastic*, or *ironic*. On the part of the interviewer, there are occasionally circumstances, if the interviewer is sufficiently expert, in which it may be useful for him to express any except the first two and the last of these attitudes. So far as I know, a frivolous attitude is never under any circumstances useful on the part of an interviewer. I also very firmly disadvise the least flippancy under any circumstances—and that applies with all the greater force to dealings with the patient who begins interview situations flippantly. Patterning one's activities after the informant in that case leads to distinctly less than nothing. And an ironic attitude by the interviewer is often wasted and may cause a lot of trouble; for irony, if at all subtle, may easily be misleading and may get one into rather inextricable situations. Thus I warn the interviewer against being ironic.

Informants at times show rather abrupt changes by becoming decidedly more evasive than they have been up to that time. Occasionally they become quite *actively obstructive;* they insist emphatically on talking beside the point, so that the interviewer can scarcely overlook the definite unwillingness to follow him and to deal with what he considers to be urgent. Especially in the psychiatric field, the interviewer encounters every now and then a patient who grows, the interviewer feels quite sure, *obscurely suspicious.*

These attitudes which I have now named are all rather important indices to change in the interview situation. I shall try to be a little more informative later on, but at present I am trying to build a sort of very rough fence on which we may or may not be able to grow a few vines later. Let me now present a rule which the interviewer might well engrave somewhere on his interior: *All through the interview process, even in the terminating phases, it is important for the interviewer to covertly verify his observations; he must not merely automatically, perhaps unwittingly, "react" to the patient's expressed attitudes, whether by tone, by gesture, or by words.* All of us are very prone to the automatic response—in fact, life is so exceedingly complex that we need a great many ways of handling things on the spur of the moment—but this has very little place in the intensely complex and therefore rather extraordinarily uncertain work of the psychiatric interview. While the appearance of spontaneity is desirable in the interviewer's responses to affective movements and changes in the patient, these responses should never be automatic in the way they might be with his wife, or his child, or the bus driver, for in the very act of the automatic response, selective inattention probably eliminates about half of the useful data. No interviewer can afford this.

The Theorem of Reciprocal Emotion

Now let me shift to a somewhat more theoretical consideration of the matters which I have been discussing. As I have already indicated, the interview is a system, or a series of systems, of *interpersonal processes*, arising from participant observation in which the interviewer derives certain conclusions about the interviewee. Under these circumstances, interview situations fall under a general principle which I have organized as the *theorem of reciprocal emotion.* That theorem is as follows: Integration in an interpersonal situation is a process in which (1) complementary needs are resolved (or aggravated); (2) reciprocal patterns of activity are developed (or disintegrated); and (3) foresight of satisfaction (or rebuff) of similar needs is facilitated.

This theorem is an extremely general statement which, thus far in my explorations, has seemed to have no serious defects. I believe that if one studies its full implications, a great many things pertaining to the study of interpersonal relations, and pertaining to the participant observation by which the interviewer gets his data, will be clarified. In this general statement, I use the word "needs" in the broadest sense, in the generic sense. Thus, in discussing the development of personality, we speak of all the important motives, or "motors," of human behavior as *needs for satisfaction.* There is a *need* for satisfaction of various forces such as lust and hunger; and *need* in this particular sense also includes the need for a feeling of personal security in interpersonal relations, which in turn can be called a need to avoid, alleviate, or escape from anxiety, or, again, a need for self-esteem.

Now, I have stated, in the first part of the theorem, that complementary needs may be resolved, and reciprocal patterns of activity developed. For example, in the realm of security operations, the urge to reassure is complementary to the need for reassurance. Reassuring by implication, instead of by direct praise or direct reassurance, is the pattern of activity which is reciprocal to the pattern, in the other person, of discounting or inverting direct praise or appreciation. In other words, if a person must discount, disbelieve, or convert into its opposite, all direct praise, then the reciprocal pattern of activity which would appear in a simple interpersonal situation would be reassurance by implication—by saying something which would have very little to do directly with the other person's self-esteem, but would, on further elaboration, be seen to imply a favorable view or hopeful outlook. The experience of an interpersonal situation thus characterized—that is, characterized by such complementary needs and reciprocal patterns of action—tends toward its future reintegration (that is, its recurrence), on the basis of either witting or unnoted anticipation of improvement of one's self-esteem in or by the relationship.

This is a very general pattern of thinking about all interpersonal relations. Now I wish to show how this general pattern may bear on interview situations. Let us consider an interview situation in which the *interviewer* communicates—by tonal gestures, or by the pattern of his remarks, or both, which is usually the case—*his own* need for reassurance. The most common way in which interviewers show their need for reassurance is not by asking for it, but by some form of activity which is calculated to "score off," disparage, belittle, or humiliate the patient in the course of the interview. In fact, such activities, almost without exception, really express a need of the interviewer for some reassurance as to his importance, however dimly the patient may realize this. In this case, the need in the patient which would be complementary, and therefore lead to resolution, would be a somewhat curious thing: a need to be despised. As a matter of fact, there actually are situations in which it is perfectly reasonable to say that a person needs to be despised. However, this is quite a novelty in security needs, and is not likely to occur in the psychiatric interview. In fact, it could really occur in the psychiatric interview only as a complex motive addressed to a goal quite exterior to that of the ordinary interview situation. I can suggest an example of it in another situation, however: A number of our OSS agents accomplished very good work toward winning the war by supplying in their behavior a clear expression of a "need to be despised," as a result of which people in need of this type of reassurance became quite free with them, and gave away things that the agents needed to find out. But these were not interview situations, in the sense that I am discussing them. The OSS men were really the interviewers and not the interviewees, but their informants, in making them the victims of their contempt, fortunately mistook their roles. One does not expect this to happen in successful psychiatric interviews.

Now what does happen in the psychiatric interview if the interviewer expresses a need to be reassured by lording it over his victim? I have said that, by cultural definition, the patient is the client of an expert, and therefore is inferior in significant respects. Because in this situation he feels himself less capable, he must need reassurance by the performance of the interviewer. Consequently (and this follows the first part of my theorem), the need of the interviewer himself to be reassured is not met by a complementary need on the part of the interviewee, and thus the interviewee's need for security, instead of being resolved, is *aggravated*. To take up the second part of my theorem: If the interviewee is to develop a pattern of activity which is *reciprocal* to the interviewer's pattern, this must be a pattern of submissive or other interviewer-reassuring activity. Or, if he does not develop such a pattern, the communicative activity is *disintegrated*—the thing breaks up.

The development by the interviewee of this reciprocal pattern of a submissive attitude represents an unfortunate situation. If in the development of the interview relation, the interviewee gets the impression that he must have certain views to please the interviewer, and proceeds to submit to this demand, from then on the data that the interviewer gets will be practically beyond interpretation. Unless the interviewer is extremely clever at interpreting interpersonal data, he will make nothing, except what he reads into it, out of the information which the submissive informant dutifully gives him. The interviewer will get a very poor picture of the informant, in comparison with the picture that, for example, an esteemed neighbor would have of him. This is a very poor result for a psychiatric inquiry to have, and so the interviewer, if he is at all skillful at interpreting very complex situations, will not permit the interviewee to fall into one of these submissive relationships in the first place.

And finally, to apply the last part of my theorem: In this situation, the interviewee will develop an alert foresight of the rebuff of his implied need for reassurance, and this will make it certain that he will protect his self-esteem. That is, the longer such a situation goes on, the more he is governed by the foresight of any indication that there will be an aggravation of his anxiety. Since his anxieties are always detestably unpleasant and a potent driving force to get him away from that which causes them, he becomes more and more careful that none of his insecurities are advertised to the security-needing interviewer.

The Patterns of Outcome of Interpersonal Situations

The interpersonal processes making up the interview follow the general pattern of all interpersonal processes, which can be illustrated by a diagram:

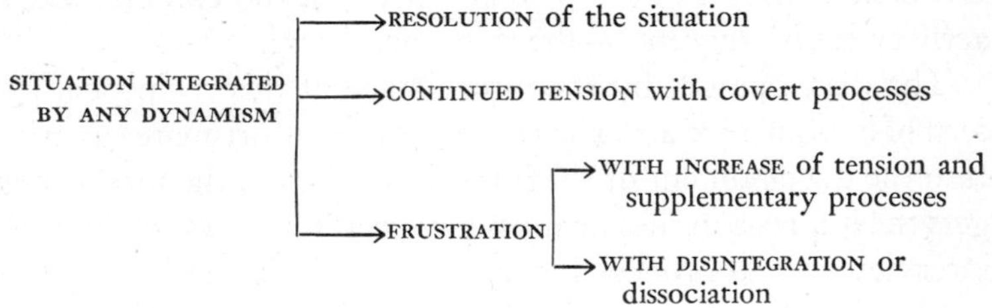

A situation integrated by any dynamism—for example, lust or the pursuit of security—manifests processes which result in one of three subsequent situations: First, there may be a resolution of the situation. For example, the waitress may say, "Do you want cherry or banana pie?" When the customer says, "Banana," that resolves the situation. And in all other situations, the simple, delightful, and final outcome of an interpersonal configuration is that it is resolved: all tension connected with it is washed up, and the thing is finished until something provokes a similar situation.

The second possibility is that a situation may be continued with tension and with covert processes. In this case the person goes on doing the same thing, more or less covertly, but he also begins *to think*, whether noted or unnoted. In other words, he begins to look around for what is wrong, to discover what can be done to effect a satisfactory resolution.

The third possibility is that the processes in the situation may lead to what we call *frustration*. There are two possible states subsequent to frustration. One is marked by an *increase of tension*, reflecting the need which was concerned, and by *supplementary processes*, which may range all the way from circus movements to exceedingly skillful ways of circumventing the obstacles, so that there is a belated resolution of the situation. Sometimes the psychiatrist must deal with situations in which he knows that any frontal attack, any direct approach, would lead to complete frustration. Thus he devises supplementary processes that will weave around the blocking anxiety, so that finally the patient, feeling reasonably secure, will arrive at a point which could never be approached frontally. The other outcome of frustration may be *disintegration of the dynamism* itself and the whole motivational system, or *dissociation*—and processes in interviews involving dissociation are very complex.

The Interviewer's Use of the Foregoing Formulations

I have now tried to set up two very general considerations: (1) that all interview situations fall under the theorem of reciprocal emotion, and (2) that the processes in interview situations follow this general pattern of all interpersonal processes. From these two relatively broad considerations, it follows that the interviewer shows his skill in his choice of a passive or active role at particular junctures in the interview. He may work successfully in a deteriorating situation *if it is not permitted to disintegrate*. Sometimes working in a deteriorating situation is unavoidable; sometimes it is desirable. In general, however, other things being equal, he secures best results most economically in a situation that is improving.

At awkward moments, the interviewer's inquiry progresses from expressed puzzlement to direct questions and, if necessary, finally to the use of "as if." For example, the psychiatrist may tell the patient that he gets the impression that the patient is acting "as if" the psychiatrist had done so-and-so; and then he sees what happens. In any case, he attends respectfully to anything that seems to be communicatively "intended" in the way of answers and comments. If he can make nothing of a remark of the patient's, or if it seems irrelevant, he seeks to recall the earlier context of the interviews, which may be what it relates to. He does not hesitate to take "time out" for this review; he may be silent for a while before pushing further. If he finds nothing from this hurried looking-back which gives what the patient has said any meaning or relevance, he pauses perhaps momentarily to decide whether it is important; there is a good deal that does not actually deserve any particular further inquiry. But if it does seem that the matter might be important, then the interviewer tries to find out about it. He may take a chance by asking some question about it, and as a result the patient may be able to correct him emphatically. As I have said before, often a great deal of real illumination is gained when the interviewer expresses something which is clearly wrong and the informant puts him right. Somehow, there is a curious relaxation when the interviewee has a chance to correct the interviewer, and at such a juncture the interviewee usually tells a good deal more than he had intended. In fact, my own experience in psychotherapy has been that the occasions when patients have been able to correct my errors—for example, about their histories or about what had moved them in some situation—have been fully as valuable as any equal space of time I have ever spent doing anything else. Sometimes, of course, it is useful for the therapist to deal with a remark that he does not understand by simply saying, "I am not sure that I follow. Will you say it another way?" In this way he avoids committing any errors in the asking of his question.

When I spoke earlier of anger, I suggested that anger is not one of the attitudes which an interviewer is permitted to experience toward the interviewee. I trust that this is an absolutely, completely, explicit statement: *anger, in either its mild or severe grades, is one of the most common masking operations for anxiety*. The interviewer may "use" signs of mild irritation or even expressions of anger, but if he is actually angry, that usually means that he himself is in need of some psychotherapeutic help, either from himself or from someone else. It is impossible for an interviewer who really loses his temper now and then with his informant to meet the very technical needs of interviewing and to obtain anything like dependable conclusions.

On the other hand, anxiety is scarcely to be avoided by any interviewer, at least in the course of some few of the interviews which make up his work. Even an interviewer with twenty-five or thirty years of experience will certainly, particularly if he interviews incipient psychotics, be very acutely anxious in his work now and then. And when the interviewer is inexperienced, it is often a question as to whether he or the interviewee has the most anxiety.

Skill in interviewing includes, as a very great part of its basis, certain *processes* for so dealing with occasions of anxiety that the work of the interview is not seriously impaired. There are two statements which I can make about these processes which save the interview situation from the anxiety which the interviewer is bound to experience now and then in his work. *First*, the interviewer should *be alert* to the minor movements of anxiety "in himself" so that he can exercise foresight with respect to the processes which follow. In almost everyone, a great deal of anxiety occurs of which the person concerned has no clear awareness. Some supplementary process such as irritation or anger is rushed onto the scene, and only the most careful retrospective search could give a hint that there was anxiety.

In the interview situation, instead of getting away from anxiety as quickly as possible, the interviewer must pay great attention to the movement as he experiences it. If he avoids it, somehow "ignores" that anxiety, he will not learn from it. By observation of those events to which the anxiety is related, the interviewer may learn, not only about himself, but also about the relationship with his patient. Anxiety is unpleasant, but since its experience is inevitable, it should not be lightly cast aside as an ally.

Second, the interviewer should attempt to *identify the seeming cause* of the anxiety. By "seeming" I imply that such "cause" may be quite simply an incipient rationalization—and it will do no harm for the interviewer to recognize this possibility. In looking for the cause, the interviewer may first consider the interviewee as a source of reflected esteem. If the therapist feels that his esteem is falling in the eyes of his patient, he then has the task of exploring whether this is so, and if it is, the reasons for this shift in position.

The next step is to consider the possibility that the anxiety arises in reference to the therapist's supposed failure to live up to what he imagines is the patient's ideal, although this ideal might scarcely be within the effective knowledge of the actual patient. Thus the therapist might "observe himself being a therapist" in comparison with what he imagines is the behavior of Dr. A, some more or less distinguished colleague. In such a comparison the therapist may feel "inferior" and suffer anxiety. Here he may ask a simple question: What is there in the relationship between the therapist and the patient that at this juncture leads the therapist to entertain daydreams concerning his supposed comparison with a colleague?

Last, in looking for the seeming cause of the anxiety, the interviewer may ask if it has some reference to a *foreseen* development—something that will or may happen. The possibilities of this suspected future event may usefully be studied, the anxiety having served a somewhat indirect but important purpose in attracting attention to the possible developments.

In any case, anxiety in the interviewer cannot be entirely avoided; it is clear indication, at least, that he is quite human. Since it will be with him at times, he might as well make use of it. That he can only do by observing it as best he can.

CHAPTER VII

The Developmental History as a Frame of Reference in the Detailed Inquiry

I HAVE SUGGESTED that it is very important indeed for the interviewer to pay attention to anxiety, particularly his own anxiety. Anxiety is of such overwhelming and all but ubiquitous significance in the understanding of interpersonal relations that it is helpful to keep in mind during the entire interview a two-part schematization of the hypothetical personality of the interviewee, which the interviewer is trying to formulate. This two-part schematization—which, like every abstract scheme, is misleading if you take it too literally—is a useful way for the interviewer to organize his thinking. According to this, the personality is divided into (1) the *self-system* and (2) *the 'rest'* of the personality.

The interviewer is always in contact with this self-system of the interviewee. If I have made any sense in my comments to you about anxiety, you must realize that whenever you are dealing with a stranger, both you and the stranger are very seriously concerned with matters of appraisal, of esteem, respect, deference, prestige, and so on, and that all of these are manifestations of the self-system. The protection of these matters is the very reason for the existence of the self-system.

Therefore the one thing you can always be sure of is that it is a rare moment indeed in an interview situation, however prolonged, in which the self-system of the interviewee is not centrally concerned.

This means that all through the development of the interview situation, however prolonged, the interviewee is showing efforts to avoid, minimize, and conceal signs of his anxiety from the interviewer and from 'himself' [1]—that is, in a certain locution, keeping himself from *knowing* that he is anxious. In other words, the concealment applies both to the interviewer and to the person interviewed. But that is to some extent a figure of speech rather than a precise statement; that is, people conceal their anxiety from themselves and others by the promptness with which they do something about it.

The interviewee's self-system is at all times, but in varying degrees, in opposition to achieving the purpose of the interview. This is an elaborate but fairly correct way of saying what might be said casually as: The self-system of the stranger is always viewing the other person as an enemy and taking due precautions against the other person on that basis. The interviewer's skill, therefore, addresses itself to circumventing the interviewee's security operations without increasing the scope or the subtlety of these operations. The amateur interviewer, in trying to circumvent the anxiety of the interviewee, may make the manifestations of the security operations more subtle so that they won't disturb him. Thus the interviewer must have skill in order to avoid this calling out of more security operations or more obscure and subtle ones. This, in effect, amounts to the interviewer's avoiding unnecessary provocation of anxiety without at the same time missing data which are needed for a reasonably correct assessment of the person with whom he is dealing.

The developmental history of the *self-system* implies the

[1] [*Editors' note:* Sullivan says in his Notebook that this use of 'himself' is "a locution that is descriptive of phenomena rather than a precise statement."]

circumstances under which the interviewee will experience anxiety—at least momentary anxiety—and sets the general patterns of the security operations which will be manifested under these circumstances. The developmental history of the *person,* which includes the developmental history of the self-system, is accessible to the interviewer only in the form of: (1) experience formulated *in* the self-system—even if it is manifested only in the form of *precautionary operations against* the clear recall and unmistakable showing of the effects of certain formative experience; and (2) data which form an adequate basis for inference about experience—and *deficiencies* in experience—of universal developmental significance. In other words, in one's dealing with an interviewee one is provided with data which are fairly clearly related to the developmental history of the interviewee's self-system, which is *manifested* in his security operations, his precautions against anxiety; and these data form a reasonably good basis for *inference* as to his deficiencies in a good, basic experience for living. In the first group, the signs are clear if the interviewer can read them; the second is always a matter of inference. It is from these considerations that the here-indicated technique for interviewing has its origin; from them comes the necessity for the interview situation to have a probable utility to the interviewee, the definition of the interviewer-interviewee relationship, or the physician-patient relation, as that of an expert and a client, and the setting up of four phases of the interview situation.

From these considerations arises also the principle that the interviewer needs to have a good grasp on some *schematization* of the way people, under the most fortunate circumstances, come to be as capable and as human as they are. Among all the schemata that have been useful to me in developing psychiatric ideas and building certain psychiatric techniques, the most useful—other than the concept that man is a highly adaptive creature and that a useful approach to a study of him lies in the observation of his interpersonal relations—has been the conception of the stages of his developmental history. I have mentioned that the interviewer must always have in mind one really pertinent question about the patient: "Who is this person and how does he come to be here?" The generic answer is that a combination of his native endowments and personal experience has brought him to this pass. I have already described how the interviewer may get a rough idea of the answer to this question in the reconnaissance. But how does he go about filling the gaps which are left in the social, statistical data? What is the thread which keeps him more or less on his course through the detailed inquiry? The best thread, so far as I know, is the developmental history. I have found the following heuristic classification of personality development to be useful: infancy, childhood, the juvenile era, preadolescence, early adolescence, late adolescence, and adulthood. I shall presently consider these eras at some length.

In addition, there are two gross categories of developmental history which seem pertinent in arriving at some plan for organizing the data: The first is the relationship between the serial maturation of ability that characterizes the earlier years—the first twenty-six or twenty-seven years of the human being after birth—and the probable opportunities for experience which the person has had. One cannot have an experience that requires ability not yet manifested; on the other hand, the fact that one has matured an ability does not in any sense guarantee him an opportunity to have experience to which the ability is peculiarly fitted. Thus there is always the problem of the coincidence of the opportunities for experience with the maturation of the abilities to have those experiences. The second category, much more complex than the first, is made up of signs of personality warp uncovered in the interview. Such signs are evidence of deficiencies in needed experience—that is, needed in the sense that every one of us must have it to grow up—and are also indications of security operations pertaining to these deficiencies, which not only reflect the deficiencies but also limit or distort the recognition of, and the profitable utilization of, subsequent opportunities for remedying the deficiencies. In the last part of this statement I refer to one of the basic truths in the understanding of personality: as the self-system develops it shows a very potent tendency to influence, if not to control, the direction of its immediate future development; thus security operations actually stand in the way of the patient's gaining the experience that would remedy those deficiencies in earlier living which initially gave rise to the security operations.

According to my outline of personality development, the first stage, *infancy*, begins at birth and ends with the appearance of articulate speech, however uncommunicative. During this brief period, the expansion of human potentialities goes on at a truly prodigious rate. The learning of speech habits—or, in certain cases, the indication that speech habits could be learned—ushers in the era of *childhood*. In childhood the velocity of development, which has already begun to slow down at the end of infancy, continues to diminish. Nevertheless, those things that are learned in childhood—speech, toilet habits, and so on—are of such spectacular importance that it still seems as if the child learns with almost lightning speed. Even though mothers are sometimes not greatly impressed by this speed, anyone who tried to teach these things to an adult who knew none of them would realize that the child is incredibly educable, and is able to catch on to new things in a positively dumbfounding way.

During infancy and childhood, a "significant adult" has appeared as a queer kind of creature not clearly comprehended but of great importance as a source of the exceedingly uncomfortable experience of anxiety. But only at the end of childhood does each of us develop a need for the "other," in the sense of someone who is like us and is quite clearly *not* a significant adult. In other words, childhood ends when the child begins to show a need for compeers—a discriminating interest in, or rather realistic fantasies of, other playmates. Now there are some infants who have what adults may call "playmates," and certainly quite a number of children *seem* to have them. But the "play" in which these people are "mates" is actually composed of the independent operations of two entities, each of whom makes some minor accommodations to the presence of the other.

The need for compeers ushers in what I call the *juvenile era.* This stage is chiefly characterized in our culture by its relationship to school and formal education. Learning at this time continues at a somewhat diminishing rate, perhaps because of the increasing complexity of that which must be learned—"complexity," in my usual sense, meaning incongruity and lack of rational principle. Up to this time, the culture has been transmitted to the child by as few as two, three, four, or five people, and of necessity it has been distorted by their particular outlooks and peculiarities. But now many of the errors in the juvenile's acculturation which have existed because of the peculiar warp of his home are corrected by contact with other juveniles who also have ideas of what is right and proper, learned in *their* homes. All of these things tend to focus in minor respects on the teacher, and the formal education tends to show the juvenile what is unquestionably wrong, and what is unquestionably right, in what he knows already.

Another learning process which appears at this time can only be carried on with compeers, and not with significant older people: the juvenile discovers that he has certain successes and failures in competition—that is, in performances in which he falls into active comparison with another, more or less similar, person. And along with this, the juvenile learns that at times it is very necessary to compromise, and that there are certain ways in which he can compromise without loss of self-respect, and without being humiliated as a weakling. And as the years of schooling go on, the juvenile learns that he gets status for being bright, or for being teacher's pet, or for being popular, or for playing football, and things of that kind.

At the end of the juvenile era, another great developmental

change appears. This may occur anywhere between the ages of eight and a half and ten, or even later, for the stages of development grow progressively less fixed in their relation to chronological age—a reflection of the influence of acculturation on maturation. The change which ends the juvenile era is rather startlingly abrupt—that is, it is a matter of weeks; however, this abruptness is apparently never noticed by the person who undergoes it. He begins to show positively adult caution in that he doesn't say very much about it until he gets used to it; as a result, his family has, at first, little awareness of the new occurrence. The change is this: One of those compeers of the same sex, who has been so useful in teaching the juvenile how to live among his fellows, begins to take on a peculiar importance. He is distinguished from others like him by the fact that his views, his needs, and his wishes seem to be really important: he begins to matter almost as much, or quite as much, as does the juvenile himself; and with this, the juvenile era ends and the phase of *preadolescence* begins. This person who becomes so important is ordinarily referred to as a *chum*, and he matters even when he isn't there, which is quite unlike anything that happened in the juvenile era.

During preadolescence, certain dramatic developments, which are probably necessary to elevate the person to really human estate, move forward with simply astounding speed. During this brief period, which may precede puberty by a matter of only weeks, or, more commonly, months, there is an acceleration of development, which, if one likes to think physiologically, may reflect the oncoming puberty change. Be that as it may, in the new-found importance of another person, there is a simply revolutionary change in the person's attitude toward the world. Thus far, regardless of his parents' fond belief in his utter devotion to them, and regardless of his ability to get along with his compeers, it is measurably correct to say that the young human has been extraordinarily self-centered. The startling change in preadolescence is that this egocentricity, this concentration on one's own satisfactions and securities and the wonderful techniques at one's disposal for obtaining them, now ceases to be the primary goal in living. The thing that seems most important now is the using of all these techniques to draw closer to another person. It is what matters to this other person, the chum, that is of the utmost importance. In other words, here is the first appearance of the need for intimacy—for living in great harmony with someone else. Because the need for intimacy makes the other fellow and living in harmony with him of such importance, a great deal of attention is paid to how he thinks and "feels," to what he likes and dislikes; and from this more careful observation of the other is gathered a great deal of data on the rest of the world. As long as Little Willie was learning his geography, giving the right answers in school, and all that sort of thing, it might be inferred that he had a very intense interest in visiting Germany or Canada, or in learning the multiplication tables, although such interests didn't hound him in his sleep. When, however, he discovers that life cannot really be complete without an increasing closeness and harmony with someone else, he begins to develop quite rapidly a personal interest in the larger world.

I believe that the best grasp on the problems of life that some people ever manifest makes its appearance in these preadolescent two-groups. Such comprehension is often horribly unlettered and in woefully undocumented form, but it includes a remarkable awareness of another person and a quite astonishing ability to reveal oneself to that other. Because our culture is so forbidding to the development of certain human expressions, the next step in personality development is frequently accompanied by a state of being more or less chronically anxious—and the chronically anxious are not apt to have very free, constructive, and philanthropic interests in their fellow men. Thus the brief epoch of preadolescence very often represents the maximum achievement of a particular person, as far as a constructive interest in the welfare of the world is concerned.

The puberty change comes along at the end of preadolescence, and for a time the course of events does not seem to be greatly disturbed by changes in the voice, the appearance of new hair, and so on. The last astonishing physiological maturation of which we know is the appearance of the orgasm, by which I mean nothing more mystical than, in the male, the simple ejaculation of semen. Some time after ejaculation is established, he (to continue using the male as our example) begins to feel that one of the girls is far more attractive than he had previously noticed, and does something about his discovery. His chumship then disintegrates rather rapidly, and the youth wanders into *early adolescence*, in which, to be very crude about a magnificent and very troubled period, he attempts to find a pattern of life which includes the satisfactory discharge of lust. Even after he has found something in the way of a technique, so to speak, to deal with this drive which appears with the puberty change—and which, if unsatisfied, is apt to be extremely troublesome—he may spend several years more, if not the rest of his life, in attempting to learn how to get other people to collaborate with him in dealing with it.

When a pattern of life is achieved which satisfies this drive, *late adolescence* has begun. It continues until, through many educative and eductive steps, the person is able, at *adulthood*, to establish a fully human or mature repertory of interpersonal relations, as permitted by available opportunity, both personal and cultural.

These are the classical developmental eras of personality; for each of these I have given a threshold point which is very rich in its implications, and which must have profound significance for the future of the person. In each of these eras of personality development there are certain experiences which are the ordinary lot of the comparatively fortunate human being; and if—perhaps because of peculiarities of the parental group to which the person is subjected—these experiences cannot be had, they show, until they are remedied, as serious deficiencies in the development of personality, with many concomitant signs and some symptoms. And it is these deficiencies which make up the principal business of the psychiatrist, as well as the business of those concerned with the adjustment of personalities to jobs. Of course, there is unquestionably some difference in what an interviewer can investigate in interviewing a person for the position of fifteenth vice-president in charge of operations of a manufacturing company, compared to what a psychiatrist can do in interviewing a patient. But while there are differences in what the interviewer can ask and what attitude he can manifest, and so on, there are no differences in the significance of the data that he must seek to obtain.

A Suggested Outline for Obtaining Data

I wish now to give some hints as to the type of approach, type of surmise, which may be useful in conjunction with the developmental history in order to learn the important details about the interviewee and how he has come to be who he is. I trust you will realize that this is not a definitive outline—there are unnumbered things which do not appear in it; but from a consideration of your own recallable past, you will see that this outline hits the high points, and you can utilize your own past to fill in many of the details.

DISORDERS IN LEARNING TOILET HABITS

One of the first things which the interviewer might obtain information about is the patient's history of learning 'toilet habits.' The establishing of such patterns is usually begun before the end of infancy, and as a result the patient's information about them is probably not formulated and would require months of investigation to bring to any state of certainty. Thus almost no one knows consciously much about his own toilet training. But often he has picked up some clues about it.

Some of the really unfortunate people of the world have been exposed to strict bowel training well before early childhood, and as a result of their parents' preternatural interest in their toilet habits (which interest is but one expression of the parents' personalities) have come to suffer rather grave disturbances of life thenceforth. In other words, the very early learning of perfectionistic toilet habits—occurring well in advance of the appearance of speech, however autistic in nature—may lead a person to show very serious warp from the average course of human development from thenceforth, unless more fortunate experience occurs later.

The very driven, obsessional parent who teaches his children to be extremely tidy before they have any chance of developing those patterns of expression which should have gone on nicely before they became tidy, is usually so proud of the achievement that he brags of it every now and then to sort of puff himself up with how good he has been. A child usually learns of all this by hearsay from the parent to whom it was terribly significant that the child be wonderfully tidy from a very early age.

The patient, however, won't think of all that in a psychiatric interview; and, even if asked directly, he may be so dashed by the scope of the inquiry—if not by the apparent irrelevance of it—that he may be intensely annoyed and quickly put an end to it. So the interviewer looks for such little signs as he may notice in this connection. Such signs are often obscure. I know nothing which is peculiarly indicative of extremely early tidiness or very belated tidiness. But I do know that disorders of toilet habits may be obscurely reflected—to the extent of a significant statistical coincidence—in personal cleanliness and in certain other things. Among these are the attention given to the dust which may have accumulated on chairs on which one is about to sit, to the keeping of clothing from any casual contact with dirt, to the careful preservation of creases in trousers, and so on. Such things are hints which suggest that it might presently be worth while for the psychiatrist, without any undue precipitateness, to make some inquiries as to the family mythology about how early the patient became tidy. In my inquiry I tend to emphasize the *estimable qualities of the abnormality*—thinking that no one need feel great shame or offense at my noting some particular neatness or carefulness in his dress. I do not wish to frighten the interviewee away by too blunt reference to a carefulness that he might consider peculiarly private or 'strange.' Parents who have produced tidy infants are usually so proud of it that the child later hears about it; and so I come to hear also.

This personal cleanliness pertains not only to whether the patient is coarsely dirty, but also to how carefully he has combed his hair, cleaned his fingernails, shaved, and all that sort of thing. Fortunately, since we know so much more than we usually get formulated—otherwise we would long since have died from exhaustion—we can fairly easily get an impression of whether a person is clean, is unkempt or unclean, is tidy, or is positively neat. The feeling that a person is ordinarily clean, and not unduly clean or unduly dirty, is the norm; that condition indicates that the patient has no preternatural interest in this field.

Disorders in learning toilet habits may also be reflected, more subtly, in the patient's attitude toward certain words, which he regards as definitely offensive and does not use. Such words are those which are ordinarily considered 'dirty' words by juveniles. Since they are not ordinarily used by psychiatric interviewers, it is a little bit difficult to get at this. But nonetheless the interviewer keeps such things in mind. A psychiatrist may gradually realize that a patient is a little restricted in his freedom to use such words as he knows. If, after the initial interview, the psychiatrist takes such a patient for intensive psychotherapy and gives him the old psychoanalytic prescription that he should lie on the couch and say every littlest thing that comes to his mind, he probably will sweat and blush, and one thing and another, for several hours, because the only thing that comes to his mind is one of these Anglo-Saxon words that he can't say. That is interesting, but it is also a poor technique for saving time.

Among the things that one may think of as related to the period of toilet training are prolonged enuresis (years past the time that most people cease to wet beds), habitual constipation, recurrent diarrhea (episodes of diarrhea so frequent that one never knows from week to week, or day to day, when the next one will come), and even an occasional soiling of the bed. Unthinking bluntness about matters such as these may only serve to block communication. It is helpful for the interviewer to have in mind the possible meaning of little hesitancies and so on. With such meanings in mind, he can find times at which he can ask, quite frankly and simply, and obviously for professional information, rather pointed and ordinarily prohibited questions. However, he can do this successfully only if he has caught on to the clues that make such questions relevant. If the interviewer asks a number of pointed questions that prove to be irrelevant, then he is not showing the skill in interpersonal relations which the client expects of him. But if he asks relevant questions at times when they are faintly apropos, the patient will probably not be at all offended and will be able to give relevant information.

DISORDERS IN LEARNING SPEECH HABITS

Since, in the more fortunate, the learning of speech habits usually collides with the learning of toilet habits, so that one or the other seems to be neglected for a little while, the interviewer next thinks, in the developmental scheme, of disorders in learning speech behavior. Such disorders may show up in faint suggestions of earlier trouble (such as hesitancy in speech), in oral overactivity, or in manneristic accompaniments of speech at times of stress.

If an interviewer is interested in such phenomena, he may notice that a patient shows a little tendency to hesitancy in speech at those times when he seems to be a little embarrassed about one thing or another. The second time this occurs, the interviewer can pause and, making a somewhat abrupt transition, say, "Tell me, did you stutter as a child?" And lo! he learns that the patient did. A great many people who have had serious speech disorders show some suggestion of an impediment in speech at times of stress for many years after they have overcome the more gross disorders. It is not so difficult to notice these signs, but there are others whose relationship to difficulties in speech development is not at first so easy to observe. There are some people, for example, who show, while talking, a good many obscurely unnecessary movements of the face around the mouth—which I call oral overactivity. There are others who display various mannerisms while talking; for example, a person may have to pause for a moment and do something, such as gesture with his hand, before he is able to speak freely.

All of these things suggest that there may be great value in developing an interest in the distortions of personality occurring as far back as the learning of speech. The signs that come to the interviewer's attention may all have some relationship to a history of disorders or deficiencies in speech habits, which the interviewer can discover by careful questioning. This history may show any of the following difficulties: (1) delay in learning to speak; (2) disturbed speech in the shape of stammering, stuttering, or lisping; (3) peculiarities of vocabulary; and (4) the continued use of autistic or frankly neologistic terms.

Delay in beginning to speak is not a disorder of learning speech behavior but a manifestation of a morbid situation in which there is no sufficient need for learning speech and, in fact, a positive premium on not learning. Lisping, which may be partly organic, has great social disadvantage and is therefore important to personality, however neurological or anatomical it may be in origin. The more obscure distortions, such as peculiarities in vocabulary, are not a disorder in acquiring speech behavior, but a defect in acquiring the knack of consensual validation—that is, the ability to move words around to the point that they convey what you mean to the person to whom you are going to speak.

Disorders in this last category are much more widespread than most people realize. As I have tried to suggest before, it is easy to believe that you understand everything said to you, and vice versa, but if you did not overlook negative instances, you would be greatly impressed with what queer things people mean by words that you use to mean something else. Sometimes the patient's use of words is extraordinary; he is apparently depending on a word to communicate something to you which it doesn't communicate at all, and you realize that he is still quite autistic in his verbal thinking and that there has been a very serious impairment of this extremely important aspect of his socialization. This reaches its positively pathological state in the use of neologisms which have meaning and existence as words only in the mind of the user. They are to be found in no dictionary, and they are not ordinarily subject to any of the philological laws. They are purely autistic, usually very highly meaningful, but utterly uncommunicative combinations of phonemes (that is, articulate sounds) which the person uses just as if they meant something to the hearer, and which cannot under any circumstances mean anything to the hearer except that they indicate the presence of a problem.

ATTITUDES TOWARD GAMES AND PARTNERS IN THEM

We now move into the juvenile era, admittedly leaving a great deal of an exceedingly rich period untouched, such as all the attitudes toward authority which have their buttresses in childhood, in the gradual domination of the parents over certain unregenerate impulses of the child, and so on. If you glance back into your school years, one of the things that may impress you immediately is that you were inducted into games which represented a certain cooperation, a certain element of competition, and often a very large element of compromise with compeers. That, I sometimes think, is the easiest approach to understanding the development of idiosyncrasies in the juvenile era. I hope that an interviewer will always get some idea of his client's attitude toward games and toward the people who are his partners in these games.

There are some wonderful eccentricities that appear here. A certain small section of Manhattan society rise from bed in the late forenoon, dress rather carefully, gather up their husbands or wives—their concessions to social necessity, as it were—and proceed to the bridge club. There they engage in an intensely concentrated performance, almost without speech or with only very highly formalized speech. After a considerable number of hours at this, they go out and retrieve their social remnant—by which I mean their mate—get something to eat, and go through a practically meaningless routine of life until the next meeting of the group. These utter devotees to bridge, thanks to the peculiarities of the Manhattan concentration of eccentricity and so on, do live a life which is all bridge; the rest is a matter so obviously of boring and tedious routine that it is very impressive. If you should feel very superior to these queer people, let me suggest that I don't find them to be very much different—except in the completeness with which they have organized their lives around what they want to do—from certain large prosperous communities which center more or less around a suburban country club. In those instances all of life which is not involved in golf and the club is treated as a boring routine that one must go through. One's husband or wife who does something for a living to facilitate this pleasant life is obviously an infrahuman creature and is treated more or less as such. Now, these are truly juvenile people, but they have found very satisfactory ways of life. The fact that a person has been so sadly distorted at a certain phase of development that he doesn't get anywhere near being an adult does not mean that he becomes horribly abnormal and passes the rest of his life in a mental hospital. Far from it! It doesn't even mean that he is likely to become a candidate for a psychiatric interview, except in wartime and at other times when his volition doesn't have so much to do with what he does.

In any case, the interviewer can learn a good deal from inquiring into people's attitudes toward games. People who have had very stressful juvenile eras very probably are not members of New York bridge circles, or suburban clubs, or things of that kind. They are likely, in fact, to have a quite restricted interest in games and a very sharply restricted interest in people with whom to play them, but that is another story.

ATTITUDES TOWARD COMPETITION AND COMPROMISE

As I have said, there are some topics which one approaches somewhat indirectly, not wishing to arouse great anxiety by too blunt an exploration of some 'dangerous' ground. But the patient's attitude toward competition is a thing about which one can ask directly, since competition enjoys, if not great social esteem, at least great tolerance. There is no particular harm in asking the person before you what his attitude toward competition is. He will always say something interesting, if only "What do you mean?" On the topic of competition such an answer is amazing. Maybe he is puzzled by what you mean by "attitude." You can then inquire what puzzles him. If you get anywhere on that, you ask, "Well, what do you think of compromise?"—that is, what does the patient think of people who compromise, would he easily compromise, would he *never* compromise, *what* would he compromise on, and so on.

As all this goes on, the interviewer observes whether the interviewee is manifestly competitive in the interview situation—has to know more about things than you do, has to beat you to what you are driving at—or, on the other hand, whether he is unduly conciliatory in an effort to give you the feeling that he agrees with even your lightest utterance. Such things are quite significant; they may be overlooked or misinterpreted unless the interviewer follows some sort of scheme for organizing his thoughts and his procedure.

AMBITION

Among the people who have been relatively, if not absolutely, arrested in the juvenile era—in other words, whose subsequent development of personality has been either rudimentary or very much delayed—are some who, from their competitive nature, you might say, develop an intense ambition. This ambition is usually rather clearly revealed by some remarkable successes. This is a culture very rewarding of competition, and within it anybody who sets his whole personality, tooth and nail, on a certain type of thing is apt to have experienced astonishing successes and failures. It is worth while to notice not only how intensely ambitious a person may be, but also the character of the goal which is the point of his ambition. The interviewer will discover a few people who are intensely ambitious about one thing after another; ambition is a characteristic of them, and the particular goal they are seeking seems to be purely a function of the situation they are in. There are many other people, more significant because they are quite apt to hold important positions in society, who have been pursuing a more or less well-defined goal for years and years, doing everything short of homicide to get to it.

INITIAL SCHOOLING

In addition to competition, compromise, games, and what not, the juvenile era is also the period of correcting the over-individualistic warp of acculturation which nearly everyone brings to the school from the home. It is particularly important to distinguish, therefore, in one's thought and perhaps in one's questions, the initial schooling. I do not refer to the first day of school, which unhappily has been so exciting that most people retain nothing but a foggy memory of it, but rather to the general period of grammar school. In the first place, everybody has been there, and in the second place, it is there that one begins so rapidly to learn social techniques to cover one's 'real' feelings that what happens thereafter is often not very revealing. The psychiatrist wants to know in general anything that will give him a notion of the way the patient felt toward grammar school. Did he have a good time? Did he learn a lot? Did he like to learn the sort of things that were offered there? Does he have the impression that some teacher was wonderful to him? And so on. In some ways this is a reflection of the happiness or unhappiness that he may have brought to school from his home.

One thing may be noticed which has a bearing on events in the juvenile era: this is simply that some people have a curious lack of facility for using the Anglo-Saxon. While it is practically impossible to talk English without using words derived from Anglo-Saxon, to some people words of Greek or Latin derivation seem to be much more attractive, more welcome, and more frequently used than their equivalents from the Anglo-Saxon. I, being one of these people, can tell you that a person may use words derived from Latin and Greek because Latin and Greek roots have been mixed up in the development of science. I started a science education very young, and was enamored of the precise reference which science had conferred on these Greek and Latin roots. That, however, doesn't explain those instances in which the use of the Anglo-Saxon becomes practically vestigial wherever a good Latin- or Greek-derived word can be used instead. If a person grows up in the home of a Latin or Greek professor, it probably isn't strange. But it is of great interest when a person has grown up in a situation in which there was no obvious reason for distrust of the Anglo-Saxon, and in which it was the prevailing form of English used, and yet goes through life thereafter using chiefly words derived from Latin and Greek. It may be that he found in the acculturation in school, and in the educational possibilities that opened to him there, something much more attractive than anything he had come to expect at home. And thus the interviewer may gain, indirectly it is true, further knowledge of how the patient felt about his home.

EXPERIENCE IN COLLEGE

If the interviewer's development of the inquiry too clearly follows the developmental eras as I have set them up, he will, as it were, be warning the interviewee of what 'should be' produced. In other words, he will be telling the interviewee what security operations to use to defeat the purpose of the interview. Therefore, as I try to pick up the data from the very last months of the juvenile era to maturity, topics are mentioned in an order which I believe discourages a too easy appreciation of just what is being driven at; yet this perhaps represents an exceedingly hurried sketch of what might, in the hands of the skillful and the diligent, be an adequate outline of a prolonged interview.

Rather abruptly, after asking something that is highly significant for the earlier years of the juvenile era, the interviewer can leap over high school to college. Such sudden transitions disturb the sets that are already beginning to develop in the patient, and therefore improve the probability that he actually refers to his recall instead of just attempting to adjust nicely to a certain type of questioning. Thus, after having learned something about the patient's experience in grammar school—for example, whether he was good in math or in English, or in both (which is rare indeed)—I ask, if I have already learned in the reconnaissance that he went to college, what was his experience there. I ask if he fitted in with the "studes"—that is, the very studious—or with the "socialites" at college. These are the two groups into which most of the student body can be classified. So far as one's future is concerned, under ordinary circumstances, it is better to be one or the other than to be the exception. And in America, unless one really has a career spreading before one, it is better to be a social success than to be a stude. In other words, the American pattern of normality is to go to college and spend your parents' money, and to avoid any information that you can elude; that is the more 'normal' pattern of development. Remember, norms are not given by God, or by you, but are the outcome of statistical nose-counting. So, the interviewer wants to know where his patient stood in college. Was he identified with the unduly studious, or the unduly frivolous, or was he not identified?

INTEREST IN BOYS' OR GIRLS' CLUBS

The interviewer also inquires whether his patient, before he became a father—or before she became a mother—showed any particular interest in leading boys' or girls' clubs, in being a "big brother" or a "big sister," for a period of years. If he did, I think it is a fairly important clue to deficiencies in his preadolescent experience.

THE PREADOLESCENT CHUM

Having reached this point in the interview, I usually inquire whether the patient had a chum in the preadolescent era. The preadolescent change has so much to do with one's social adaptability, one's actual place in at least the potential world of the future, that not to have gotten some experience along this line seems to me very unfortunate. Since there would seem to the interviewee to be little direct connection between whether he had an interest in boys' clubs and whether he had a chum, I like to have a little transition. Without any great show of abruptness, I try to indicate that everything breaks here, and we are starting on an entirely new line. Then I inquire, "Does anyone stand out in your recollection as having been especially your chum in your early school years?" If the answer is in the affirmative, I wish to learn what became of the friendship and of the friend. Are they still great friends?

There is so much looseness in speech about these relationships that a categorical question such as mine is quite necessary if, in the space of a minute or two, you are to get some useful clue. You can be wonderfully misled in this field. Many people think that they ought to have had chums, and they are glad to enumerate fifty or so that they did have. But when you say, "Does anyone stand out in your recollection?" the "anyone" means the chum is singular and indicates that the patient may have to say who, and what, and which, and why he was. Thus the patient usually pays a little serious attention to the question, rather than making an immediate social gesture to indicate his normality and so on. The further inquiry as to what became of the relationship gives the interviewer some notion as to its true character—whether it is an imaginary construct or an excerpt from life. Quite often the patient has not thought of his chum for twenty-two years, so that he is a little dashed by the question for a moment, but is able to say, "Yes, I had a chum, but I can't think of his name." If he is astonished that he can't think of the chum's name after twenty-two years of not using it, this is a strong confirmation of his having had one. Thus the outcome is often quite convincing, and after listening to what the patient has to say in response to a categorical stimulus like this, you feel pretty sure that you know what was the case; whereas any casual questions, or careless leading up to the subject, may bring conventional, obscuring responses that are likely to be quite far from the true facts.

PUBERTY

Then I often ask, "When did you undergo the puberty change?" I ask this merely to introduce a topic, because not one out of perhaps seventy or eighty people has the ghostliest idea of when he underwent the puberty change. The person was old enough to remember, but events then were so disconcerting, so much was going on at that time, that it's like the first day at school—everything is in a fog. I vividly remember the experience of one day trying to whistle and finding that I couldn't;

but I haven't any idea as to what day or year it was. So it is with most people. But it doesn't do any harm now and then in the interview for the patient not to know the answer to something asked directly.

You then inquire about certain things: when the patient's voice changed, when he began to shave, and when he had orgasm; or in the case of a woman, when she first menstruated, when she noticed changes in the breasts, and so on. On all of these things most people are extremely vague. Yet, as you enumerate them, the patient may recall something important about one of them. If the patient's puberty was very late, which may be very significant, he is likely to recall something about more than one. That is really the most significant thing about the puberty change: if it occurs two or three years after most of the people in the patient's group have undergone it, this delay may be in itself a sign of very serious warp in personality, and in turn causes further increasing warp in personality. Under those circumstances, a great deal of the misery in life is dated to the actual delay in puberty change, and about all this the patient will have a remarkable amount of information. That in turn means a great deal about the misery of life that has separated that time from now.

Once I have gone through the process of being unable to determine at what age a patient became pubescent, I am able to inquire somewhat further about these phenomena, and I try to find out whether there were any unfortunate ideas connected with them. If I then learn that there are concrete recollections —for example, a woman may say something like, "I thought that something must have gone dreadfully wrong because I never dreamed of anyone bleeding there"—I know that there was indeed unfortunate experience. However, if I were to go about it the other way and say to the woman, "Did your mother warn you about it?" or "Did you know what was going to happen?" she could only reply, "Of course Mother did" or "Of course Mother didn't." And with such answers I wouldn't know anything. First I verify the fact that the interviewee does or does not know when puberty happened, but at least knows what I am talking about, and then I learn if there were any unfortunate ideas connected with the event. With this indirect approach I may come to know something which is reasonably trustworthy.

UNFORTUNATE RELATIONSHIPS IN EARLY ADOLESCENCE

Having gone thoroughly over all the amnesias, and so on, of the puberty change, I then ask, again rather categorically, "Is anyone recalled as having been a particularly bad influence in early adolescence?" Should the patient after a moment's thought say "Yes," I use my judgment of the degree of his anxiety as to whether to proceed any further on that topic. If the answer is in the affirmative, I more generally leave the matter right there rather than inquire into it, but I try not to forget it since such data may be developed later. It is very seldom important to know all about this unfortunate relationship. The important thing is that there does seem to have been such a relationship, and in many, many instances it is well to restrain your curiosity and to confine yourself to the significant question of what became of that relationship. If it has been treasured ever since, that's interesting; if, on the other hand, it was exterminated as soon as possible, that sounds pretty healthy.

ATTITUDE TOWARD RISQUÉ TALK

The interviewer then asks about the patient's recollections of the pornographic art in the school conveniences, his memories of the types of obscenities heard in high school, and so on, and how the patient felt about them. If he is comparatively well, the patient, very vaguely and without any conviction, guesses that he didn't like them at first, which is correct. The interviewer then moves very suddenly into the present and wants to know what the patient thinks of risqué or frankly sexual talk. Does he participate in it easily? Does he find it rather repellent?

And so on. If the patient seems to you to be quite eccentric, and you are still terribly at sea, you might ask him if he feels that such sexual talk is obscene. Now, what "obscene" means to one person is probably different from what it means to another, but in this culture, "obscene" usually carries a very vigorous condemnation. Thus it is not unusual for a person to be embarrassed by risqué stories. However, when a person feels that all risqué stories are positively obscene—when they would not impress most people as such—he has probably been subjected to pretty warping influences in bygone years and hasn't escaped from them.

ATTITUDE TOWARD THE BODY

Having gotten some hints as to the freedom with which the patient can contemplate the fact that he or she has genitals, without ever having mentioned them, you may then take up a somewhat related topic: namely, does the patient's attitude toward his genitals apply also to the rest of his body? A gentle way to approach this, if you have learned nothing from the discussion of games and sports, is to ask if the patient is a member of the YMCA, an athletic club, or something of that kind, and to ask what he does in such a place. If the patient turns out to be a member of the swimming team, for example, the chances are that he is willing to have some of his skin seen in public, and you don't need to ask foolish questions about that.

If you have led up to it so that he doesn't think you have an unjustifiable curiosity of some kind, you ask him if he has any remaining objection to being seen nude by people of the same sex. If he hasn't, then you can ask him if he still feels a little modest about some parts of his body. This can be interesting. In other words, you are trying to pick up some idea of the patient's attitude toward his genitals and the rest of his body.

SEX PREFERENCE

Having led the patient to thinking a little in terms of later adolescence, you can ask whether he actually prefers men or women for companionship. If the patient shows a little increase in reserve at this point, you can always modify your question amiably by saying, "Well, it may vary with the moods that you're in. Of course you would prefer the company of women when you are retiring with a view to sexual satisfaction." If he looks suspiciously at you, you were wrong—which is information. And you can continue by asking the patient whom he likes to dine with, and so on.

Now, the preference for members of the other sex really does vary from situation to situation in most people. And yet the interviewer's general questioning should proceed in the fashion I have outlined. You can't be too precise in questions without getting the patient somewhat startled. In other words, you ask general questions fairly often merely as a method of transition, to get a topic into the open. Having accomplished this, you become specific.

ATTITUDE TOWARD SOLITUDE

The interviewer should also find out what his patient's attitude toward solitude is. There are, believe it or not, some people who regard the possibility of solitude as the better among you regard your reward in heaven—except that they find their reward now. There are other people who would really run four miles to avoid solitude. And there are many in between. If the patient either likes solitude or doesn't seem to know what it means—in other words, probably doesn't need it very often—then the interviewer can ask this rather categorical question: "Are you ever so lonely that you become restless?" (Now, this is not "Were you ever" or "Do you recall," but "*Are* you ever.") The answer is highly significant when it is in the affirmative.

USE OF ALCOHOL AND NARCOTICS

By all these techniques, I have covered the developmental history except for neglecting attitudes toward authority which I shall not attempt to cover here. And now I come to a few other topics which seem to me to require very special consideration. They are not at all as rewarding, or as basically significant, as is the notion of the developmental history, but they serve their purpose.

The first that I will mention is the relationship of the interviewee to alcohol or narcotics. A good many psychiatrists overlook the possibility of the use of narcotics, which is of course very much more restricted as an outstanding idiosyncrasy than is the use of alcohol. But don't utterly forget narcotics, because you do sometimes see a drug addict.

This business of alcoholic beverage is something which I think is revealing enough so that I seldom fail to inquire about it. I shall run very swiftly over some of the things I like to find out. When was the patient first drunk? I say "drunk" with a slight falling inflection to apologize for the idea that he could ever have been drunk. The patient usually tells me. Nearly everybody has been drunk for a first time. The really interesting thing is whether he got drunk again. After the patient has survived the shock of my thinking that he may have been drunk, I ask him if he has ever been fairly seriously injured when under the influence of alcohol, or more or less because he was intoxicated. It is remarkable what a large proportion of people have been deterred from going down the alcoholic road by suffering some rather serious injury when they were drunk, or an accident that might have had serious consequences; such people have gained certain high discretion about the blending of alcohol with dangerous activities. So it is worth knowing about that.

Then I wish to know what the patient does when he takes quite a bit of liquor. Does he become quarrelsome? Does he engage in fights? Does he develop crying spells or weep easily? Or does he become very friendly with everyone? The answer very frequently is, "I get sleepy"—which is not always true. In those cases in which the patient indicates that he shows a very disagreeable complex of behavior when drunk, but is not eager to talk about it, I don't question further. Such behavior indicates a very unhappy person who takes to alcohol when social pressure is too high and who, under the loss of inhibitions, reveals a good deal of the misery and hostility which have led him into grief with society. Quarreling and pugnacity are more or less degrees of the same thing, and are, so far as I am concerned, definitely suggestions that the personality is not excellently integrated, and has not achieved a high degree of development in late adolescence.

I then ask the patient how much he can "carry"—that is, how much alcohol can he ordinarily take with no serious inconvenience to coordination or judgment. When he has given me some kind of answer—usually rather vague, because here again I am introducing a topic more than expecting data—I want to know what circumstances provoke him to exceed this amount. I sometimes hear amazingly revealing things. In other words, many people are so distressed at their incapacity at times to avoid excessive alcohol that they have actually worked out a pretty good pattern of the situations that provoke them to do so. I then wonder if the patient has noticed anything which alters his capacity or tolerance for liquor. There are a good many people who can drink a great deal most of the time, but who at times become intoxicated on a remarkably small amount. If the patient has noted something like that, he may also have been so impressed by the risk connected with it that he has actually figured out some data on what seems to affect him.

Having gotten all this, I may ask something to determine to what extent the person is a connoisseur—that is, how insistent he is on either the variety or the quality of alcoholic beverage. There are people who, other things being unobtainable, take ethyl alcohol, with or without water; there are other people who are so unpleasant about not having what they want that their intimate friends always see that the right kind of liquor is available before having them in. That is not merely a peculiarity of the drinking habit; it is also a reflection of one's importance, both to oneself and to others, and is, from that point of view, rather interesting. People who have nothing to go on in the way of self-respect are not apt to be connoisseurs.

I then want to know just how emphatic are these matters of taste? If I find out that they are quite emphatic, I wish to learn how this great emphasis is explained or rationalized. I don't really care about the rationalization; I simply want to hear the patient talk about this emphasis on taste. His comments will give me a clue as to how seriously he takes himself, what he may have learned from experience, and many other things which appear in the rationalizing of any strong taste or insistent preference.

EATING HABITS

Next, I may inquire about matters of eating. There is no personal preference shown in my putting alcohol before eating. Alcohol is actually a much better introduction to a whole state of mind than eating would be, since everyone eats, and usually not entirely to his satisfaction. I almost always, even at Army induction centers, want to know about the state of the stomach and bowels, and I ask, "Does any food disagree with you?" And, of course, in a twenty-five-dollar-an-hour practice one asks, "Are there any food allergies?" This makes a most respectable introduction to the general topic of eating. I then ask, if I haven't been told, if there is any food that the patient dislikes—in other words, is he notional about food. If he is, this, in general, reflects a considerable interest, even if a highly pathological one, in food matters in very early years. Sometimes I hear a history to the effect that the patient once disliked this and that, but that the Army cured him of it. Such an account is interesting, because that is a type of stress that many people have never undergone. I want to know if the patient is a heavy or light eater, if he has irregular meals, if he eats late at night, and so on. Sometimes such things are quite interesting to learn—and often they seem to be drearily irrelevant. You must use some judgment as you go along.

In case of an unusual, puzzling, or quite possibly very important person, it is well to get at the question of how ceremonially he treats the meals for which he has time. Now, oddly enough, some extremely busy people have time for lunch. They enjoy the ceremony of lunching with certain people, whereas to eat dinner at home may be dully routine. Is some particular meal likely to be treated rather ceremonially? In other words, does the patient give a considerable amount of attention to arrangements, to things being right, and does he experience considerable distress if, for example, the Blue Points run out at the restaurant and he can't have what he expects? All this is an interesting reflection of the patient's attitude toward life. Even his attitude toward friends may come out in this consideration of the extent to which some meal comes to be a real occasion which he looks forward to and takes a good deal of interest in and trouble about.

SLEEP AND SLEEP FUNCTIONS

The interviewer next hints at the sleep habit and the sleep functions. If he does not lead up to this topic with some careful inquiry, he will often draw only misleading blanks. Sleep functions are known to most people only by way of their dreams. But if you think of the phenomena as *sleep* and the *sleep functions*, you will be a little safer than if you thought, in the traditional way, of just sleep.

One way to introduce this topic is to ask, "How much sleep do you seem to need?" If the patient tells you, well and good; if he doesn't, you are at least in the field and can ask further questions, such as whether he is a heavy or light sleeper, whether he sleeps well in strange beds or Pullman berths, and so on. You then ask if he ever dreams. Some people will consider that question just too naïve for words, and others will say "No" with perfect honesty, as far as they know. If the patient dreams, you ask whether he ever has nightmares. Sometimes you come upon a curious phenomenon—the person who doesn't dream but who has nightmares. I tell you, you don't know what people mean, or what your words mean to them, until you find out!

In some cases, where everything seems to be most shockingly normal, I may indicate that I am not too pleased to discover that the patient sleeps eight hours every night, never dreams, and never had a nightmare. Looking at the poor patient somewhat irritably, I say, "Did you ever have night terrors? Did anybody tell you about your having night terrors?" I suppose about half the human race doesn't know what night terrors are, but if you have had them, you do know. The recollection is usually sufficiently unpleasant that the patient gives a sign of it, no matter what he wishes to conceal. If he has had night terrors and has been a little discomposed by my irritation and my question, I ask again what he dreams when he does dream—this last, in spite of his having told me that he never dreams. The patient may start to say again, "But I don't dream!" And I say, "Oh, I mean—recall a dream. Everybody has at least two or three dreams that he can remember, and I think that would apply even to you. What do you recall having dreamed ten, twenty years ago? Tell me a little something about your dream life." If he still has no dreams, I give it up as a bad job, figuring that here I am meeting a type of resistance that indicates one of two things: either the person has a very rigid self-organization, or he is a very guarded person who, under any pressure that I feel I can apply, still maintains what is obviously a very risky attempt to carry out his plan of being 'normal.' There are people who do not know they dream. Those people have a self-organization that, under sufficiently unhappy circumstances, would probably put them in a mental hospital, but would otherwise make them pillars of the church or of almost anything else that was highly respectable with which they happened to be identified.

THE SEX LIFE

Then we come to the topic of sex. You notice that I am quite interested in people's attitudes toward their genitals and in the history of certain changes which, at least in many people's minds, tend to concentrate in the genitals. I am not prodigiously interested in what can be learned in the early phases of a psychiatric interview by questions on sex. I particularly want to emphasize that the general doctrine that sex is in some curious fashion a mirror of personality is, so far as I can discover, capable of being astoundingly wrong. Sex is important for the twenty minutes it may occupy from time to time, but it is not necessarily behind everything else that fills the rest of the time.

If an interviewer has stumbled through all these topics in somewhat the fashion which I have suggested, he can say to the patient, "Well, and what of the sex life? Are you very restrained in such things, or are you quite free? Are you promiscuous?" That happy thought at the end sometimes gets big returns. Having gotten some kind of a sputter in response to that question, I ask, "Well, how long has it been true? I don't suppose you've always been like that. Give me a notion of the history of your sexual experience. For example, when did it begin?" When you know something about the beginning of the patient's developmental history, you may know what is being discussed; but missing the beginning, you often just *think* you know what is being discussed.

Some people, in fact a remarkable number of people, recall their first sexual encounter with another person; while it may be a little hard to place in time, it is usually vividly registered some way or other. If the patient tells me a little bit of something, I am satisfied. I don't care if it is not detailed at this time, because I have gathered almost all the data I need to guess about his great problems and his probable adjustment to the set of circumstances that may be before him. I am really sparring around for something I may have missed in everything that has gone before, and am not really looking for anything more intimately sexual than how he deals with members of the opposite sex—as friends or enemies. For example, if the patient is a man, is a large number of female conquests terribly important to his prestige? Or does he avoid intimacies with women, except for a dear old friend with whom he's been having them for twenty years? All of these things have much less to do with sex, you see, than they have to do with personality as a whole.

Having led the patient to think in terms of the backward glance, I then ask him something like (with women I may use something more by way of transition): "Was there much trouble over masturbation?" God pity us! I suppose that about three quarters of the people of my age immediately bridle and go through the motions of being terribly annoyed at the idea they ever masturbated. At these I look with a fine imitation of scorn, and say, "Now please don't tell me you never did. I don't believe I could stand that at my age. But now tell me, is there still some difficulty about it?" When that question is asked of people who have been married for eighteen years and have two or three children, they usually look at me sharply to decide whether to be indignant or not, but since it is just a question, they sometimes say "Yes."

Having given this awful shock, I may ask if the patient ever had any contact with prostitutes or streetwalkers. After listening to something or other on that topic I ask him if he has had venereal disease, and how often. I want to know if prostitutes are still of some considerable interest, and so on. Curiously enough, it has become increasingly apparent to me that in questioning either old men or young adolescents about their genital behavior, the same inquiries are relevant.

In certain cases I ask if the patient has had any experience with adultery. I don't ask that when I think it would be regarded as preposterous, but if I surmise that adultery is still a terrifying word to a person, I ask if he has engaged in it, how it affected him, and so on. In cases in which adultery wouldn't be of any interest to the patient or would seem a preposterous, archaic inquiry, I wonder if he has ever been involved, or threatened with involvement, in any divorce actions.

In case my informant appears to be notoriously normal—that is, vigorously but restrainedly heterosexual—I attempt by inquiry to discover whether his heterosexual genital performances are actually autoerotic in character—that is, using the genitals of the other sex in lieu of one's hands. I also attempt to discover whether his heterosexual performances are in the nature of a security operation—in which I wish to know how his having heterosexual relations contributes to his prestige, and so on. Last, I want to learn whether the patient's heterosexual genital operations are calculated to satisfy him and his partner.

COURTSHIPS AND MARRIAGE

That is a very reasonable sort of point at which to pass to marriage and the history of courtships, plural. If the plural doesn't apply, that in itself is interesting data. If you have developed the interview somewhat after the fashion that I have previously suggested, you are already warned from the social reconnaissance of a good many things with respect to marriage, courtship, children, and so on, pertaining to your interviewee. Therefore you do not at an exceedingly late moment need to become curious as to whether the patient has consolidated the exceedingly important status performance of becoming a husband and father, or a wife and mother. That is one of the reasons for the reconnaissance. You gather all these overwhelmingly important data so that in the detailed inquiry you can proceed methodically without so much attention to the prestige necessities of the patient. In other words, the reconnaissance tells you what you will have to deal with when the proper time presents itself later in the detailed inquiry.

Next may come an assessment of interpersonal patterns, again plural, characterizing the married life—the satisfactions and dissatisfactions, and the securities and insecurities. When I use these alternatives, I refer to *every* case. I have yet to find a marriage which has only satisfactions and only securities. In other words, there may be many more satisfactions than dissatisfactions; but if a person tells me that his home life is perfect, I take off my glasses, which means I can't see him, and gaze at him, and say, "Extraordinary!" I then pass on to some other topic, but I return to this later.

I wish to know whether the mate is the person who runs things or the person who is run, or whether husband and wife happily share in their dominance over each other. And by whom outside of the marriage is the mate influenced: in-laws and so on, and particularly and never to be forgotten, the neighbors—in other words, to what extent is the mate harassed by a necessity of keeping up with the Joneses? Also, is there a sense of deep disappointment associated with the marriage relationship? Much of this you infer by the way the interviewee answers, not by asking him.

PARENTHOOD

Then we come to the mighty topic, if suitable, of parenthood. I try to assess the actual characteristics of the person as a parent, as well as his ideals of what he *should be* as a parent. And to those ends I ask such things as the awkward question: "Is there a problem child in the family?" If there is, what is the explanation considered to be? I also ask if there is a preferred child, and why that child is preferred. Has the preference had any bad effects on that child, or on any other child? If it has, are there any neutralizing influences that can be learned of from the informant? The attitude of the parent-interviewee to the school influences that are bearing on his child or children is an excellent entering wedge here, because school is somewhat impersonal. Then you want to know of grandparents, uncles, aunts, neighbors, and others who may be influencing his child or children.

There are two things to inquire about here which should not be forgotten. If you have been clever in your reconnaissance, you may already have some of these data. First, don't fail in the exploration of this area to discover if the wife has had any miscarriages and if some younger siblings died before the birth of the surviving child. In other words, you should know if such influences existed which would act to increase the importance of the surviving child, and so on. Second, inquire not only about half siblings, because there may have been a divorce on one side or the other, but also about wards or other pseudo-siblings in the family, people of approximately the same age who are looked after because for some reason there is not adequate care elsewhere. It is simply incredible how few hints you get of these things when they are significant, unless you ask about them.

VOCATIONAL HISTORY

After you get through all of these topics, you come to the vocational history. Remember that vocation in this culture usually means work, not esteem. Here again your reconnaissance in the second phase of the interview may have given you some excellent clues as to the advisability of working back with the person from his present vocation to get the history, or of starting at the very beginning of his vocational life.[2] If you decide

[2] [*Editors' note:* In a question-and-answer session at the end of the 1944 series of lectures, Sullivan was asked whether the patient's attitude toward his present job was of more significance than his attitude toward previous jobs. Sullivan discussed this point as follows, relating it to the investigation of current events in the patient's life:

"The attitude of a person toward the job that he's now working on is likely to be his attitude toward employment in general. What he reports about his attitude toward former jobs may consist of little more than the beautiful tinting effect of distance on memory. Thus I would certainly always want to

to begin at the beginning, remember that in many homes some work contribution is required of the child long before he would be regarded as in any sense a wage earner. He may have had chores to do, and you want to know to what extent he did them, what compulsion he was under, and so on. You want to know about the first paid employment, about the first full-time employment, about any full-time vacation employment, and so on. What happened to the earnings? What good did they do the person? Who used the earnings, and for what? Did they just get dissipated by the family, or were they used to buy

know a good deal about a person's attitude toward his present job. If he says he is all for it, that is interesting; and I may find out whether that really is his attitude by inquiring whether he ever had any work that he didn't particularly care for. If he says that he doesn't like his present employment, I try to find out whether this has been his general attitude toward employment, or whether there are particular circumstances surrounding his present employment which justify considerable antagonism toward the situation.

"In general, in the treatment of personality there are three fields of events which are of very great relevance. The first of these is the field of current events in the patient's life outside the treatment situation—including his current employment. The second is his current relations in the treatment situation—that is, his relations with the psychiatrist. And the third field of relevant data is the events of the patient's past.

"It is difficult for most people to be straightforward and forthright in discussing their feelings, thoughts, impulses, and so on, with respect to a person with whom they are in the peculiar relationship of patient to psychiatrist. For a fairly long time at the start of all therapeutic work, therefore, most of our field of investigation is concerned with current events outside the treatment situation. One might not think so from reading some of the popularizations of psychoanalytic history, but this is nonetheless true. It is from current events that we move into the current therapeutic relationship between doctor and patient, uncovering both the noted and unnoted emotional problems which constitute the patient's difficulties in living.

"When we locate a problem, identifying something that is impractical, inefficient, and definitely contrary to the achievement of the patient's idealized goals, we have every reason to turn to the third field of greatly relevant data—the distant past in which this particular emotional difficulty had its beginning. It is important to notice that finding out how things start often provides a great deal of information as to what they represent, whereas their more sophisticated, mature manifestations may be very obscure indeed. However, some patients, as I have already said, have a distinct tendency to alter history to suit their wishes or needs; with them, the present has the virtue of being capable of at least some investigation, whereas the past is apt to be pretty heavily colored. From this general standpoint, what is currently going on has a very special significance."]

roller skates or some other valuable thing? What training in thrift and all that sort of thing was received?

Note that in all occupational history you are actually attempting to learn about data pertaining to a job which is defined. It is simply incredible how wrong you can be if you merely assume that what a person says about his earlier jobs means what you think the words do. You attempt to discover what the interviewee did, his reasons for taking a job, his attitudes toward it, his retrospective idea of success or failure in it, and his status movement in taking it—that is, whether he dropped down or moved up in taking this job. Was the next job an upward move or a downward one? What is his retrospective attitude toward the skill-learning value of a particular job? Some people have hated some of their earlier jobs, but have thanked God for many years that they went through them because these jobs were helpful in skill-learning for some later occupation. As the interviewee looks back at it, was he encouraged or discouraged by his experiences in a job? Did the work in the job under discussion seem to have social usefulness? This is a very tricky thing because there are two approaches covered by the term "social usefulness": First, it refers to the effect of the job on the interviewee's self-respect. Self-respect is what important members of society reflect to you, so a job may improve your self-respect, or otherwise. Second, social usefulness may refer to the making of social contacts that have been useful subsequently. In other words, what was the outcome of the job with regard to the people the interviewee knew?

If you can keep track of all these criteria, you will know a great deal about a person just from investigating his vocational history.

AVOCATIONAL INTERESTS

The next thing to investigate is the avocational and recreational history. This is a very important field of data for the assessment of personality with respect to the degree of maturity of the person with whom you are dealing. Do not overlook the application of vocational criteria to avocational activities. Again, don't believe that because something sounds familiar to you, you know exactly what a person is talking about. When I finally developed the idea that I should ask two or three additional questions to find out what a person was talking about, I discovered, for instance, that the game of bowling actually means quite different things to different people.

The interviewer wants to know what is being discussed, you see, and he must take reasonable care to be sure that he knows what the thing really means to the person who is talking. This is especially important in dealing with the thoroughly immature, because their real interests in life are in their avocations, not in their vocations. Of such people you learn nothing much from the vocational history, but in a study of their avocational history you may discover something that begins to make sense. Even the most diligent people are more free in this field of avocation than the economic system permits them to be in vocational work. With this in mind, I have taken the trouble of trying to throw together a few hints of the field covered by avocational interests.

Every field of interest in avocational or recreational work has not only its own value, but also an importance as an area of contact with others. This contact with others, ranging from close to very remote, may be sharply restricted to the field of avocational interest or may show no restrictions whatever. Therefore, quite aside from the actual name of the avocation, there are always the problems of the relationship to the other people who participate in it.

There are, of course, a variety of fields of interest: the religious, the political, the social, and the scientific. It is of some importance in the organization of data about personality to distinguish among the various scientific fields—the social sciences, biological sciences, medical sciences, and human sciences.

Beyond the religious, political, social, and scientific is the aesthetic. When you come to that, look for the *fields*, because there are often more than one although one is conventionally presented. In all of these several aesthetic fields, you want to know whether the interest is manifested in passive or in active relationship. For example, does the interviewee spend hours looking at great oil paintings, or does he putter diligently making oil paintings? And in any aesthetic avocational interest, you want to know what the degree of socialization is. Is the interest something that the interviewee must share with other people who are doing it or is it something that he can do only if there is an appreciative audience that is not doing it?

Other avocational fields include the mathematical field of interest, the linguistic field, and the literary. This last divides sharply into the productive, the critical, and the consumptive. For those who read, what is the history of the books they like? Has their taste changed; or are they still devoted to detective stories as they have been since they can remember, or to mythologies as they have been for still longer; or have they gradually evolved a great interest in the classics and biographies?

The next great field of avocational interest is current history. Much more restful for some people is noncurrent history: the Civil War, medieval history, the history of pre-Hellenic culture, and so on.

In all these fields of interest there are important discriminations to be made among special aspects of larger fields. And we can learn much from the interviewee's particular avocational preoccupations, his reasons for developing these, the benefits or harm derived from them, and the role played by them in his relationships with other people. As we explore these interests, we learn to what extent the interviewee is aware of his fellow men, and of his own relationship to them and to their productions.

All of these things that I have touched on represent stresses, indices of direction of development, strong hints of persistent durable warp, and so on. Those are what we wish to learn about in the psychiatric interview. We are trying to find out who and what the person is. To do that we need to discover how he got where he is—and by what route he arrived. And the developmental history serves as a useful guide.

The Personified Self

I now wish to comment rather briefly on data to be obtained about the personified self, as contrasted with the personality as a whole. That about oneself of which one is from time to time clearly aware—that is, what one knows about oneself—makes up the data comprising the personified self. This is not the same as the self-system, for the personified self is necessarily less inclusive than is the self-system. The personified self is that "part," to use a locution, of the self-system which is reflected in statements pertaining to the subject, "I," and as such it is a source of communicated information, as contrasted with other information about the person's self-system which must necessarily be inferred. In other words, there is something of a distinction between what an informant can tell an interviewer, in contrast with what the interviewer can safely infer, and may, in fact, be able to validate by experiment, but about which the informant cannot tell him. What the informant can tell about his self-system is the content of the personified self.

I would now like to suggest a schematization of the personified self which is useful to the interviewer in this phase of the investigation:

(1) *What does the interviewee esteem and what does he disparage about himself?* It is a rare person indeed who disparages nothing about himself, but if he comes anywhere near wisdom, he is very chary about revealing what he disparages. It is, therefore, much easier to discover what a person really esteems about himself than it is to discover what he disparages. In the "perfect" psychiatric interview the interviewer discovers both what the patient esteems and what he disparages about himself.

(2) *To what experiences is the patient's self-esteem particularly, unreasonably, vulnerable?* In other words, what sort of situation puts him at an acute disadvantage against all of his reason?

(3) *What are the characteristic "righting movements"—security operations—which appear after the patient has been discomposed—made "consciously" anxious?* At this point I wish to draw attention to the distinction between these characteristic security operations at the times when the person knows that he has been made anxious, and those data which indicate the presence of security operations when the person does not notice that he has become anxious. I have already suggested that people often become annoyed, or irritated, or even angry when they have been made anxious, and never know that they have been anxious. The emotional state, the anger or hostility, has appeared so swiftly that the person is spared the realization that he has been anxious. But now I am talking about the security operations which appear in a different situation: the way that the person acts when he *knows* that he has been discomposed.

(4) *How great are the interviewee's reserves of security?* For instance: (a) *How well is the person's life justified?* How adequately, in other words, can the person state characteristics of his life which are, beyond reasonable doubt, estimable and worth while? (b) *Are there exalted purposes in his life which are demonstrated in action other than mere speech?* Speech is one form of activity in interpersonal relations. But for exalted purposes to be significant in validating the person's living and giving him a reserve of security, speech is not enough; he must have demonstrated those purposes in something other than mere statements. Speech may be terribly important in validating his living, but only if it is rigidly oriented toward a remote goal and not to the service of mere security operations. Thus the interviewer seeks to determine whether there are exalted purposes which the person has demonstrated over the years by something other than talk. (c) *Are there secret sources of shame or enduring regret?* And, if there are, what is their relation to the

person's justification of his life? Those who are really in touch with what happens to them from the cradle to the grave almost always have some enduring regrets, and they are fortunate indeed if they escape durable shame about this or that. But that does not mean that such people lack a reserve of security. Whether they have a great reserve of security depends on whether the justification of their lives as it exists in the personified self greatly outweighs their secret recriminations, shames, and regrets.

So far, I have named the four great criteria of the quality of the personified self that have proven durably useful in my experience. There may be many other criteria that would be better, but I have come to depend upon these. Now let me suggest some of the ways by which the interviewer discovers these things. In other words, I have tried to indicate what the interviewer wants to know; now I shall suggest *fields of data* which will shed some light on these major points.

Does the patient habitually seek to be regarded in a particular light? Does he seek to give the impression to most people that he is amiable, considerate, kind, and thoughtful; or—somewhat the reverse of these—does he seek to convey the impression that he is thoughtless, severe, cruel, inconsiderate, or austere? And remember that I am talking now about what the person *knows* that he seeks to convey. There are a notable number of people who go to a great deal of trouble to impress their environment with their austerity. These people may be among the most valuable citizens in the world, deeply and carefully considerate, very wise in their attempts at being kind. But I am talking about the impression on others that a person seems to be trying to convey; and that impression may vary from amiable to austere, from considerate to inconsiderate, from kind to severe or cruel, and from thoughtful to thoughtless. This merely indicates the way of showing himself to others which the person has consciously organized. It is significant as such, as the way he has found suitable for dealing with most life situations, and not as a product of the interview situation. And remember in this connection that I am discussing the data which arise from the standpoint of the accessible, or personified, aspects of the interviewee's self-system.

In this same inquiry, the interviewer wants to know what is the usual attitude manifested by the patient toward servants, and after some considerable digression, what attitude he manifests toward animals, meaning inferior creatures, domesticated or otherwise.

The interviewer may also usefully find out what are the characteristics of the person's attitude toward others in relatively unaccustomed contacts. That is, how does his attitude in *unaccustomed* contacts with certain groups differ from his attitude in *accustomed* contacts with them? Among such groups, I might name, first, those definitely superior, more fortunate, or wealthier. Second, I would mention people belonging to a different culture complex, such as those he encounters in a foreign country. A disturbance of attitude is particularly noticeable when the person is visiting in a country where there is a very considerable language barrier. In other words, this criterion of the personified self is more apparent in an American when he is on the Continent than when he is in England, for the English may seem quite natural to him, and even if they seem somewhat "odd," at least he can discuss their oddity with them. But when an American goes, for example, to France, Germany, Sweden, Spain, Italy, or Eastern Europe, then the element of foreignness is far more conspicuous to him, and the manifestations of his personified self become more striking. Also of interest are the characteristic attitudes in unaccustomed contacts with the definitely inferior, the less fortunate, or the less well-to-do.

It is important to note that the data that may be obtained pertaining to the *relatively unaccustomed* contacts may be quite different from those which are displayed in *recurrent* or *habitual* situations. A person may, in the course of making his living, have some contact with others who are definitely superior, more fortunate, wealthier, or more powerful, who fall in the general category of "bosses." He may be accustomed to participating in conference situations with people of much greater gifts than his own, to dealing with wealthy clients or with very poor clients, or to meeting those extraordinary people to whom one is likely to be introduced at cocktail parties. There are also many people, particularly those engaged in social work, who deal with clients whose background is, in a measurable sense, foreign to their own. And we all have certain contacts with people who are definitely inferior, less fortunate, and less well-to-do than we are. But such situations, if they are recurrent or habitual, are definitely less significant in the data they yield about the personified self than are parallel situations to which the person is really unaccustomed.

In addition to these things, the interviewer always hopes to get an impression in the interview situation of how greatly the patient is gifted with real humor, with the capacity for maintaining a sense of proportion as to his place in the tapestry of life. This again pertains more to the personified self than to anything else. There are many things that are called humor by the careless, but I define it quite rigidly as the capacity for maintaining a sense of proportion as to one's importance in the life situations in which one finds oneself.

And lastly, how dearly does the interviewee actually value his life, and how steadfastly, and for how long, has he so valued it? Here I refer to a sense of proportion which is perhaps even broader than the life-saving real sense of humor. What does the person consider to be worth more than himself? For what would he really sacrifice his life? When did that come to be the case? How unalterable is it? How much of it is a matter of mood? As I have said, all of these data bear on a consideration of the personified self of the interviewee, in contrast with all the other data that the interviewer may pick up in an interview.

CHAPTER

VIII

Diagnostic Signs and Patterns of Mental Disorder, Mild and Severe

BEFORE GIVING you a list of diagnostic signs—which is anything but a definitive list—I would like to point out that while almost every one of these signs can be found in one or another of the classical mental disorder states, these signs may also appear in any of us. That is, there is nothing unique about any mental disorder except its pattern, and perhaps the emphasis laid on various of its manifestations. Thus we all show everything that any mental patient shows, except for the pattern, the accents, and so on.

Diagnostic Signs with Associated Symptoms

The psychiatrist can make diagnostic observations on the basis of *signs* as they are verified by *symptoms* reported by the patient. It is well to keep in mind that signs are phenomena which the psychiatrist can observe more or less objectively, while symptoms must be reported by the patient; in other words, only the patient experiences the symptoms. When the interviewer observes a sign, he must then make certain inquiries to determine whether there are corresponding symptoms which are experienced by the interviewee. Otherwise, some facial appearance of the patient's which is genetically determined may lead the observer into gross errors as to what the prevailing mood of the patient is. There are some people who have been so heavily accursed by heredity that they cannot avoid looking supercilious. Their expression, however, may not have much relation to the way they feel toward others. When there is a coincidence between what the observer recognizes as signs and what the interviewee experiences, the observer has found an area which warrants further investigation. These diagnostic signs do not mean that the person under consideration has a certain disease, or anything of that kind. They are instead terms fairly rich in useful meaning to the psychiatrist; in other words, they help him orient himself as to what he is up against in the interview and what he has to do. Some of these signs are more apt to appear in the early, more formal phase of the interview, because the patient is not at that time moving with as much self-consciousness as he may be when the psychiatrist really gets down to detailed interrogation. Some signs, on the other hand, are definitely more likely to show up in the more elaborate descriptions of things which take place in the detailed part of the interview.

The first of these signs with associated symptoms is *apathy*. Apathy is a curious state; as nearly as I can discover, it is a way used to survive defeats without material damage, although if it endures too long one is damaged by the passage of time. Apathy seems to me to be a miracle of protection by which personality in utter fiasco rests until it can do something else. An apathetic patient shows no particular interest in the procedure of the psychiatric interview or in anything else. This lack of interest might be described as a certain absence of the presenting aspects of practically any emotion that a person can have. Nothing much in the way of living is going on in such a person. Naturally, many of the interviewer's best efforts to get information prove very disappointing under these circumstances, for the effort of the apathetic person is directed toward simply getting done with things. Of course, if the patient is profoundly apathetic he does nothing; he doesn't talk. But I am referring here to the patient who is just about at the bottom of the ambulatory states of apathy; in such a case the psychiatrist finds that whatever slight response he manages to get is quite clearly an attempt to be civilized rather than any evidence of the patient's feeling that anything can be done in this situation. The patient is simply there, and he goes through certain motions without any expectation of their making sense to the psychiatrist or to himself. Fortunately, we don't see many such people in ordinary times in this country. In certain branches of the military service, and in certain large areas of war-torn countries, there is an excellent opportunity to become acquainted with apathy of all degrees and grades.

Much more common in ordinary experience are states of *sadness* and *depression*. There is just about as much difference between sadness and depression as there is between any two things that pertain to people, but the initial impression does not clearly differentiate them. Depressed people look and sound sad; and if a person looks and sounds sad, the perceived sign is that of sadness. Whether the apparent sadness is a sign of depression—which is a very much more serious and quite different state—will gradually become evident. Sorrow can always be explained. That is, if the person feels willing and free to tell the interviewer what he feels grieved by, the account will be meaningful; there is an adequate explanation for his feeling pretty low in spirit. But the depressed person's explanation for his sadness—if he is able to come out of his depression long enough to make an explanation—puts him in a class with all the great martyrs of history; it is the unpardonable sin, or some such thing, that has brought him down—and this is a mental state somewhat different from sadness. The procedure in interview for these two states is very different. Sadness is quite apt to change during an interview; even a person who has suffered a great bereavement is apt to cheer up somewhat in the process of giving statistical data, and so on. But the psychiatrist who attempts to change depression has a very difficult task.

Practically the opposite of sadness is *elation,* in which one has extraordinarily high spirits. The difference between having extraordinarily high spirits because of a great success, for instance, and being elated, lies in whether or not the person has an adequate explanation for his high spirits. Somewhat in the same direction is *ecstatic absorption,* which an interviewer is seldom able to observe, no matter how skillful he is. In such a state the patient believes that he literally has the ear of God, or indeed that he is a victim of apotheosis so that he has become God. At such times the person is so profoundly occupied with the signal distinctions and the transcendental importance that have descended upon him that he has little time for the mere trifles of living, such as food, drink, income, deference, and so on. *Mercurial change* is a term which describes those who pass in a comparatively short period of time from a lowering to a heightening of mood, without any apparently reasonable basis for the change. Such people can usually be led to manifest these mercurial mood swings during the course of the interview.

Another sign is what I would describe as *overdramatic extravagance* about matters of fact, quite often literally going to the point at which there are no simple adjectives used, but only the comparative or the superlative form of adjectival terms, and so on. The person has had a "wonderful" childhood, a "marvelous" father and mother, and a "perfect" marital partner; he lives a life of the "most beautiful" joy, and so on. Everything is "wonderful." And, since it works both ways, "terrible" things have happened to him too; he had the most "appalling" experience day before yesterday, which may mean, when you come down to earth, that somebody spoke unpleasantly to him. This behavior when it is patterned may characterize what I shall later discuss as hysteria.

Another of these diagnostic signs, that appears even in taking the social history, is *hesitancy* or *indecisiveness*. In such a person the operations seem to be missing by which another person "makes up his mind" and becomes relatively sure that the probability is strongly in favor of one side or the other. To a great many questions such a person replies quite honestly that he doesn't know, that he is not "sure," although he says enough to make another person quite sure. I assure you this is no pose; it is a frightful nuisance to the sufferer; it is no more a pose than the extravagance of many hysteroid people is a pose with them. The indecisive and the hysterics just live that way—the lilies need a little operation on them before they are quite good enough.

A more positive aspect of this indecisiveness, this doubt as to whether one has gotten the thing straight, is *habitual qualifying*, the routine correction of all statements. A person who qualifies everything he says acts as if no simple statement is sufficient; a few clauses must be added to be sure that there is no misleading of the interviewer. If the latter, in a wise effort to save time, says, "Well, did perhaps so-and-so happen?" with astonishing frequency the answer is, "Well, not quite." After five minutes the interviewer may learn that one of the words which he used wasn't quite the ideal word, and that the patient felt that the interviewer would be misled if he said, "Yes."

The next signs and related symptoms which I would like to mention pertain to the extremely important matter of *tenseness*—that is, the manifestation of tensions which do not seem to be conventionally justified by the situation. One sign of tenseness appears in vocalization. All of us have known from very early in our lives how people sound when they are anxious, when they are tense, in contrast to how they sound when they are perfectly at peace as to their prestige and so on. Without this knowledge we would not do very well in our attempts to communicate. But we may not realize how much we know, and so the interviewer must look for the meaningful changes in tone and so on that occur, in which case he will notice them. Although he probably began to notice such signs in the cradle, perhaps no one has ever talked about them specifically, and so he has no particular frames of reference into which to fit his observations about them. But such frames must be built. Most of the changes in tension during the interview are shown by changes in the voice; even if tension shifts are so gross that anybody could observe them—that is, are shown by bodily movements, by actual blocking, or something of the sort—they are foreshadowed by changes in the voice. In other words, of all our behavior equipment, the voice is probably the most exquisitely sensitive to movements of anxiety. A second, and much more gross, of these signs of tension is tenseness in posture, which, as I have already suggested, is much easier for the inexperienced observer to be certain of. This may show in an abrupt roughness in movement, or in recurrent episodes of real trembling.

Beyond this is what I describe as *gross anxiety*, in which the person shows not only tension, but also various symptoms more or less pertaining to the common pattern of fear, such as sweating even when the room is cold, serious disturbance of vocalization, and general tremor.

A sign which is in quite a different category is what I call *psychopathic fluency*. The patient is very fluent, and seems to have a most estimable past and quite a good future. All of his statements are plausible in their immediate context; they all fit in beautifully with what is being said. With such people the interviewer must be alert not only to changes in the voice, or something of that sort, but also to the improbability that all the things reported by the patient in the course of a fairly long interview could be true of one person. Only when the interviewer raises his eyes from the plausible individual statements to look at the interview as a whole does he realize that astonishingly contradictory statements have been alleged to be equally true of the person. And even when the interviewer questions these fluent contradictory statements, he is unable to bring anything into what I call life relevancy. Instead, everything stays at this plausible, easygoing, conversational level, in which it is very hard for the interviewer to get any test made in terms of "But such and such contradicts this, does it not?" Instead of saying, "Well, I guess it does," the patient provides another burst of plausible utterance—these test situations make no particular impression on him. That is what I mean by psychopathic fluency.

Another group of signs are the *fatigue phenomena.* These are encountered every now and then in many interview situations, and may appear as a gross change during the interview, when the procedure seems to be tiring the patient almost visibly. The phenomena that are of particular concern are loss of perspective as to the relative importance of things, and distinct incapacity to move from one topic to another. For example, the interviewer may have arranged a transition so that anybody should ordinarily be capable of following him easily and be all ready for the new topic; but the fatigued person either is at first somewhat puzzled and mildly annoyed, and then gradually catches up, or he doesn't notice that there has been a transition, and tries to go on with the former topic in some approximation to the interviewer's question. This relative immobility of attention, and the very serious impairment of a sense of the number of things that are important, is striking; in fact, I know of nothing else that is particularly like it. It is important for the interviewer to notice this, because there isn't very much sense in trying to conduct a detailed inquiry of considerable scope when the interviewee is in a state of severe fatigue. The information one gets at such times is almost certain to be seriously misleading, since it will suffer from this relative immobility which restricts the awakening of more important things.

The last two categories in my list of signs, which should have associated symptoms, relate to very much more profound phenomena. The first is *disturbance of verbal communication* with the interviewer, and the second is *disturbance in the gestural components of communication.* By disturbances of verbal communication, I refer to phenomena which no ingenuity of the interviewer can relate directly to felt or avoided anxiety in the interviewee—that is, which cannot be explained on the basis of security operations, in the ordinary sense. The interviewee may have not the faintest notion of what has happened, and certainly has no capacity to realize that he has been made anxious by something.

These phenomena are obscure, puzzling, in some cases bizarre, disturbances of the flow of information by speech. I have sometimes called these the *autistic disturbances*. The term "autistic" pertains to the predecessors of communicative behavior, to the stage of development in which the child has learned something, such as a word, but has not yet attached to it a meaning making it useful for communication. The child may use the word, may play with it, and may attach private meanings to it which make it perfectly significant to him, but it is no good for interpersonal communication. In adulthood, the intrusion into communicative situations of very private meanings and symbols—autistic phenomena—often has a peculiarly estranging effect on things. It is not always estranging, simply because we have all quite probably had considerable experience with this sort of thing without noticing it. When we do notice it, we feel rather weirdly at a loss; apparently something has happened that we don't grasp at all.[1] One sign of an autistic process which

[1] [*Editors' note:* The text here is taken from a 1945 lecture. In his 1944 lecture on the same topic, Sullivan made the following comments on autistic phenomena in the interview:

"A commonplace parallel to the appearance of autistic phenomena in the interview sometimes occurs in the conversation of the people of the Old South—all of them now very elderly—who still reflect the 'Polysyllabics Period' in Negro education, as a professor at Fisk once described it. The state of these people was so unhappy that when they got a chance to learn something that might be helpful to them, it was a real joy merely to use words with a lot of syllables. When you converse with one of these old people, sometimes one of these words, which is tossed in simply to decorate speech, connects with meaning in your mind; but the meaning doesn't quite fit the sentence, and so you are a little dashed. And so it is with autistic phenomena. They appear and they have a somewhat dashing effect. The word

almost anyone can notice, however, is the *absence* of something happening.

First, I might mention what can be described as '*loss of thought*'; the person suffers an ablation, a complete loss of any recollection of what in the world he was talking about; in the midst of something or other, he just draws a blank. Sometimes one is able to discover that a very markedly autistic process swept in and dominated attention, with the result that what was there before is gone really completely. Although such a vanished thought apparently leaves no trace by which it can be recalled, occasionally it can be recaptured by repeating the situation which preceded its loss. A more severe manifestation of much the same thing is 'blocking'; the person is telling something, but then stops suddenly, obviously is somewhat dashed,

---

that is used couldn't mean what it ordinarily does; it couldn't describe what happened.

"Incidentally, let me say here that there are few things more disastrous to the therapeutic hopes of an interview than for the interviewer to be surprised at what occurs. Surprise and astonishment on the part of the interviewer are useful only when forged—when done for effect. When spontaneously expressed, surprise always has a most disconcerting effect on the patient, even when he was trying to surprise the interviewer; it invariably disturbs the situation in a markedly unfavorable fashion. Thus when these autistic events occur, the interviewer should pause a moment before he blurts out, '*What was that?*' For one thing, he may simply have misunderstood. And he might also consider the possibility that the autistic process was in himself. But if it was autistic on the part of the patient, that should be carefully confirmed, because it is of very great importance. If there are frequent autistic interferences in an interview, that almost certainly means that the patient is either in or near a schizophrenic state. Such people, if they get bad results from one interview because of the interviewer's surprise at what they say, will probably not return for another interview.

"Thus, without showing astonishment, the interviewer should try to find out what is really meant. He may be told things which, according to all ordinary grasp on the universe, could not be so—as in the case of the woman I have mentioned who said that her breasts were tampered with at night by her sister who lived a quarter of the way across the United States. In this particular case, when I asked a further question or two, I found that the woman meant just what she had said. But it is possible that a patient who made such a statement might, on being asked further about it, go on to say, 'I mean my sister *used* to live out there. She sleeps with me every night now, you see.' Thus it would have been unfortunate to assume immediately that this statement indicated a paranoid delusion."]

and by no use of ingenuity can get the topic finished, or take up anything else. He is just sort of stymied, and he is in an extremely distressing, very puzzled mental state in which it looks as if nothing went on, except that he is obviously very uncomfortable about it—and in fact the interviewer is too, usually.

More subtle are *peculiar misunderstandings* or *mistaken interpretations* of the interviewer's questions or remarks, as if autochthonous ideas or actual hallucinations had intruded into the communication. Autochthonous ideas are thoughts which suddenly burst into awareness as if they were terribly important, often as if they had come from "outside" in some fashion. A more spectacular instance of the same thing is the hallucination, in which the person hears, feels, or sees something to which no one else could agree, but the reality of which is not open to any doubt whatsoever by the person who experiences it. As I have said, these things are manifested in the interview situation by peculiar misunderstandings and mistakes—for example, the person may hear something which the interviewer has not said, and has not meant to say. Related to these are obscure *emotional disturbances* which the interviewee cannot explain, but which are unquestionably very impressive.

Much less conspicuous, but also falling in this group of disturbances of communication, are *stereotyped verbal expressions* which are simply not communicative. I am not referring here to the people we have all suffered who seem to have a peculiar poverty of expression, so that they use certain hackneyed phrases to cover a great many differences. Some of these people are simply underprivileged, although not all of them are. I am reminded of the young lady whom I admired a great deal when I was a boy; one evening she came along in her sables and jewels with her obviously prosperous escort and looked into the sunset—one of the most moving experiences I believe that many such people ever get on this old globe of ours—and said, after taking a deep breath, "My God, how cute!" I'm not talking about that sort of thing. I'm talking about the situation in which a person uses certain recurrent tags of expression which are not at all simply communicative, they're just things; they obviously mean something to the speaker which they fail to evoke in any way in you. You can find no clue in your experience with the underprivileged or with anyone else that will make these recurrent, stereotyped verbal expressions relevant to the situations in which they are used.

The last of these disturbances in verbal communication is the indication by the interviewee that he feels there are *secret understandings* between you and him, that there is some kind of unknown agreement, that you are with him in some queer kind of unstable conspiracy to ignore certain facts, and so on. He sometimes grows very cute and evasive, and you haven't the ghostliest notion of what he thinks the situation is.

My last grand division of these signs which should be accompanied by symptoms is *disturbances in the gestural aspects of communication*. Here there are three major divisions. The first is *stereotyped gestures;* the person recurrently makes the same movement in the most incongruous situations. You soon come to realize that this gesture is important, even though it often seems peculiarly poorly related to what is going on. It is as if the movement had broken loose completely from any real communicative purpose and instead was serving some very obscure purpose in the interpersonal situation, some end which is very difficult to interpret. The next among these signs are *mannerisms*—peculiar bodily movements which are not the usual accompaniments of certain thoughts and so on. In fact, usually they seem not to have any particular relation to the thought which is being expressed, but go on more or less routinely exterior to the verbal performances of the person, in a quite highly ritualized fashion, so much so that some people have thought that they were automatic and resulted from some irritation in the central nervous system—which is a futile explanation. And last among these disturbances in gestural communication are the *tics*, in which certain groups of muscles seem, as it were, to perform with complete disregard to everything else that's going on. They may range from an extensive contortion of the face, which isn't very strikingly suggestive of behavior, to a momentary start at a smile, a vigorous blinking of one of the eyelids and so on. But in every case they are fragmented communicative gestures, which are apparently grossly unrelated to what is going on. The person is very often unaware of their occurrence, and the only thing that accompanies them as a symptom is that if you can get the person to know when they happen, then you discover that they seem to be more abundant when he feels insecure and so on than when things seem to be going fine. Thus while they usually occur in exceedingly obscure relationship to mental processes, their timing, in particular situations and in the neighborhood of particular topics, may be of some considerable use to the interviewer in directing his attention to certain areas of inquiry.

One difference between tics and stereotyped gestures is that the latter have a much nearer simple connection with meaning, although they are still a fairly long distance away from it. While many people do not know, or only now and then know, when they are showing a tic, they often are aware of, or can easily be led to recognize, their stereotyped gestures, and sometimes they have a pretty good idea of just why they make them at some particular time. More generally, the person doesn't know why he makes a particular gesture, because that is lost in the distance of early childhood; no one at that time told him what it was for, and nobody subsequently has found out. These habitual gestures are rather interesting reliefs, one might say, to various nuisances that one is encountering in living. Sometimes I begin scratching my head, partly because I am sweating, and partly because I am tired; in this way I notice the irritation, and it is pleasant to at least give myself the relief of scratching the place where I am tired. But the way I do it—ah, that's something else again.

Any of these gestural disturbances, particularly when it

constitutes a change—when, for example, a tic breaks out in a person who previously has had a comparatively undisturbed facies—may be looked upon as a sort of red flag, indicating that the current topic seems to be of some importance to the person who shows the disturbance.

As I said at the beginning of this discussion almost every one of these diagnostic signs I have mentioned may appear in one of the mental-disorder states, but they may also appear in any of us. Thus the presence of these signs in an interviewee in no sense means that he necessarily has a fully developed mental disorder, either mild or severe. These things appear in everyone now and then, but fortunately they don't always become fixed parts of the person.

But in some people certain processes of living are conspicuously misapplied. In other words, behavior that might be useful for something or other is used by these people to meet problems for which it is singularly ineffective, if not positively the wrong thing. Other people do something that every one of us does at some time during the day, but they do it almost all the time, and thereby seem very eccentric indeed. In such ways disorder patterns are built up from the general repertory of human adaptive performance. Some of these patterns are encountered often enough to get formally named, and the psychiatrist becomes familiar enough with them so that when he sees a part of one of these patterns he expects the rest. He comes to know a good deal about what may be done concerning such patterns and what may have been causal in their formation.

Patterns of Mental Disorder

I shall now present a very brief and quite sketchy outline of some patterns of mental disorder and related personality types. To put this another way, I shall discuss *recurrent eccentricities in interpersonal relations of or pertaining to the so-called mentally deviant, the mentally deficient, and the mentally disordered.*

My first term, the "mentally deviant," is a broad one; if one groups people, in terms of their contact with social reality, their 'intelligence,' or their other characteristics, as the superior, the oh-so-average, and the deficient, both the superior and the deficient may be considered *deviant*. It is important for the interviewer to know whether a particular interviewee is superior, average, or deficient in various respects, but this is not always easy to determine immediately. This difficulty arises in part because the principal medium in the interview is verbal communication, and because of the effect of education on verbal communication. The same difficulty used to arise in trying to determine intelligence quotients: for a good many years, intelligence quotients chiefly measured verbal fluency instead of what they were presumed to measure.

Therefore, it will help the interviewer, in trying to assess the interviewee in terms of whether he is superior, average, or deficient in various respects, to think in terms of a fivefold grouping: the overeducated, the well-educated, the educated, the poorly educated, and the uneducated. He must keep in mind the fact that when he encounters an uneducated person in a single, rather hurried interview, he will have little way of knowing that this person is a superior deviant. And there may not be many clues to the fact that another person is an overeducated mental deficient. Nevertheless, these are important discriminations, because the difference between the outlook of the uneducated superior person and the outlook of the overeducated deficient person is simply enormous.

With these considerations in mind, the first type of deviant I would like to mention—and one which is hard to define very clearly—is the *psychopathic personality*, or, which is the term I prefer, the *sociopath*. Here the interviewer is dealing with factors bearing on the person's habitual contact with reality, which is extraordinarily broad in the superior and extraordinarily restricted in the deficient, and which is intensely restricted, particularly regarding social reality, in the sociopath. In the interview situation, in which the interviewer does not have any too good access to the actual history of the interviewee as many people have seen it, but instead must deal with communication, it is sometimes very difficult indeed to decide whether or not one is dealing with a profound deviation of the sociopathic type, which seems literally to be a matter of incapacity to evaluate matters of interpersonal relations. There are certainly some psychopaths who can realistically read a compass and have just as firm convictions of direction as I have, but what they think of as possible in the realm of interpersonal relations can be looked upon only as fantastic.

I have already mentioned psychopathic fluency as a sign which one may encounter in the interview situation—and which is the sign that suggests to the interviewer that he is dealing with a psychopathic or sociopathic personality. The person is very fluent and plausible in recounting both the glorious and the heartbreaking events of his past. But if the interviewer can shake the facts out of him by any device, it may develop that this glorious past was glorious only in the speed with which he moved from one failure to the next, or took in one victim after another in a sort of witting or unwitting confidence game. And while some of the hard luck stories wring the heart, no one person could have had the remarkable assembly of experiences which he recounts with such convincing fluency. What comes to his mind in a conversational situation is apt to be well adjusted for conversation, but there is no necessary connection between what has happened and what he says about it, any more than there is any necessary connection between what he does and what he very carefully plans to do. Thus his relation with reality is nebulous. Such people have suffered a grave miscarriage of development of personality, occurring after they have become greatly impressed with the utility of speech behavior, with which they almost invariably have a remarkable facility. But while they usually talk very well, they don't realize that some of the things that it is convenient to recall could scarcely have happened if certain others did.

The most difficult problem in deciding whether or not a person is a sociopath lies in distinguishing him from people who are *habitually inadequate and unresisting*—who seem never to rise to any real opportunity, who have no particular capacity to resist any not very useful influence that may bear upon them, and who, like the sociopath, seem to have a restricted habitual contact with social reality. Superficially they are easily confused with the psychopathic or sociopathic personality, but there is at least one rather significant difference: the habitually inadequate and unresisting can, theoretically at least, be benefited by intensive psychotherapy. I have yet to be greatly impressed with that probability in the case of the sociopath.

I now come to a group in which such deficiencies in the contact with reality are only episodic. Among these we find the *epileptics*, and also the people who are what is ordinarily called '*pathologically*' *addicted* to powerful depressants, hypnotics, narcotics, or other drugs. The lives of these people are strongly colored by utterly inexplicable, or all too painfully explicable, suspensions of their contact with significant events of current reality. With the aid of drugs, the pathologically addicted develop states having some bearing on the characteristic patterns of their life, and very practical bearing on their usefulness for certain types of occupation, and so on.

Next, I would mention *those handicapped by persistent distress or disorder of the somatic physiology*. In this class I would include, first, the *gravely tired*, whose condition is actually tragic, but who sometimes seem comic to others. These people are so profoundly fatigued that they are incapable of those processes which in the more mildly fatigued lead automatically to rectification of the condition. A second subgroup are the *hypothyroid*, who have a deficiency in the endocrine substance secreted by the thyroid gland, as a result of which their capacities for emergency expenditures of energy may be fair, but their capacity for the expenditures required by the routines of life are grossly inadequate. Consequently, these people live in a curiously low key, as it were; even if they do not feel tired, they perform in many connections as if they were. Their difficulty is not fatigue, but a very low metabolic rate, and anything which is beyond that rate, unless it calls out crisis responses elsewhere, doesn't get met. Another group among those handicapped by distress or disorder of the somatic physiology are the *anergic*, without thyroid deficiency. These are the people who have an obscure, but rather grave, deficiency of energy; some of them also have very low blood pressure, although one cannot translate a reading of blood pressure into terms of the energy supply of the person. Many of these people are able to accomplish almost anything in the way of exertion, but are "ruined" when the job is done. In other words, the various emergency resources of the body take care of many things in a sufficiently critical situation, but the general effect—a picture of chronic exhaustion and debilitation year after year—is very conspicuous. The opposite of these, one might say, are the *hypertensive*, who eventually have manifest evidences of the consequences of high blood pressure in the shape of changes in elasticity of the blood vessels—the arteriosclerotic changes—which have a rather profoundly significant effect on the person's living when they involve the blood supply of the central nervous system. So much for those handicapped by conditions effecting disorder of the somatic physiology.

Another major group, which is nearer the realm of the purely psychiatric, is the *demoralized*. While in peacetime such cases are not very conspicuous, in certain disasters of war they are very conspicuous; and they are at all times an important group to recognize. Most people can endure only a certain number of disasters at a certain rate of speed before they pass into a state of demoralization, in which they are practically incapable of initiating anything, although they are able to keep walking, to maintain routines, and to carry on customary tasks. They may not carry these on very intelligently, however.

A somewhat related class are the so-called *deteriorated* people. To illustrate what this means, I shall say that if you were removed from almost all contact with life for five years, with nothing stimulating happening to your mind or your body during that time, and if you were then returned to an active life with others, you would impress other people as being seriously deteriorated. You would have lost touch with the current of life, and unless you were a very remarkable person, or were given much help, you would never regain that touch. In such case you might be said to have "deteriorated" as a result of your experience.

Earlier, in discussing signs which the interviewer may note, I mentioned mercurial change, the sign which suggests the *cyclothymic* type of person. I shall comment briefly here on the cyclothymic people only to give them some place in this outline, and not because I know much about them; I don't. In fact, I suppose I know less about them than about almost any other variety of the human race. These are the people who have profound mood swings; when they are "up" nothing can get them down, and when they are "down" nothing can get them up. When elation (which I also mentioned as a sign) reaches the frankly hypomanic state, the person, even though he may look frightened, acts as if he were feeling fine; he is very gay, and he wants to cheer you up—and now and then he probably pulls some most inopportune wisecracks to do so. It is hard to keep him on the topic long enough to find out anything that carries conviction; and in fact he must get up quite often, and fumble with and admire some of the objects on your desk—and I always feel that next he will have to muss my hair to show how good he feels. It is very much like having the office full of jumping beans. This elated mood is not apt to change during the interview except that it will get worse if you make the patient more anxious. And depression, which looks like a profound state of sadness without an adequate explanation for it, is, as I said before, also very difficult to change in the interview situation.

The behavior of cyclothymic people may be looked upon as an obscure expression of movements away from the experience of anxiety—depression or an unhappy manic state being more tolerable than anxiety itself. The anxiety is apparently rarely felt as such, and it is extraordinarily difficult to isolate the event which threatens to expose the anxiety and in turn sets up the patterns known as manic and depressive. So involved does the observer become in the symptoms and signs, the defensive operations, that the person displaying these remains most remarkably obscure and unknown.

I come finally to a group of mental disorders which are probably of most intense interest to the psychiatrist who is concerned with the theory and practice of psychotherapy. The older nosology in this field is undergoing dissolution, and one may hope that something much better will arise out of the disappearance of ancient errors. I think, however, that the following rubrics still represent important distinctions: (1) those who suffer *anxiety attacks;* (2) the *hysterical;* (3) the *obsessional;* (4) the *hypochondriacal;* (5) the *schizophrenic;* and (6) the *paranoid.* I would like to emphasize again that the people to whom such rubrics refer manifest nothing which is not known in the personal life of each one of you. It is not their manifestations of these processes which is novel, but the misapplication of these processes to things for which they are not particularly suited. It is this which leads to gross embarrassments of others with whom these people are integrated. Thus we come to say that these people are characterized by the misuse of human dynamisms. These characteristic misuses of dynamisms are apt to be relatively durable. There are certain exceptions, however, for they may change under extraordinary stresses. And a frequent instance of change appears in people who have very severe eruptions of schizophrenic processes in lieu of healthy adjustment, for they are likely to move in one of two directions: toward a paranoid development—a misuse of still other processes—or toward the hebephrenic change, which amounts to the deterioration of which I spoke earlier, a shrinking of interest to very primitive, very early levels, separating them strikingly from all the affairs of life.

I shall now discuss each of these rubrics in somewhat more detail. The first of these refers to those people whose outstanding difficulty is their disability by *attacks of anxiety* of the most major character, in which they manifest practically all the symptoms of the most acute fear. These attacks are patterns of fear erupting in interpersonal situations to the point of completely disordering everything except the suffering of the symptoms.

In discussing signs which the interviewer may notice, I mentioned overdramatic extravagance. This is likely to be the sign of the *hysteric*, for it is a rather outstanding trait of the hysteric that no lily is good enough; it must always get a little extra verbal paint. While one may find hysterics who do not show this need to gild everything, when it is conspicuous one may immediately wonder whether or not the person is a hysteric, and by further inquiry can confirm or correct the impression.

Hysterics get themselves disliked with remarkable frequency. For example, occasionally in the pressure of the war I had to work at such high speed that I was not anywhere near par in alertness. I would notice that I was getting terribly annoyed with an interviewee, and begin to wonder what was getting under my skin. Not infrequently I would realize that I had just been listening to one of these conversations in which only superlatives were used, and that I probably had a hysteric before me. One reason why the hysteric is annoying is that the interviewer is quite badly misled for a while if he fails to look beneath the lush, overdramatized, overemphasized picture of things that the hysteric usually presents. Then when the interviewer gradually comes to realize that he has been misled—for hysterics are not so skillful that he can fail indefinitely to recognize it—he is often very angry about it, which is too bad. I think that any interviewee is entitled to be quite skeptical of the skill of a psychiatrist who loses his temper during an interview, or becomes offended by the patient, for this is a very poor demonstration of skill in handling interpersonal relations. This is quite different from the psychiatrist's being very unpleasant for a purpose concerning which he is perfectly clear, in which case his temper is so sufficiently under control that he can turn it on and off very precisely for a desired result. Hysterics annoy me to the point that I realize they are hysterics; in this way my annoyance can at least be turned to good use.

Another reason why hysterics are disliked is that they are not uncommonly believed by others to be deliberate malingerers; for example, they may be accused of being sick for a purpose, which is really quite stupid of the accusers. At the same time, there is in the structure of the hysteric pattern a close approximation to what another person would do who was engaged in deliberate fraud, particularly as to the unfavorable state of his health. In fact, anybody frequently may do just about what the hysteric does; this is a peculiarly obvious example of the fact that these patterns of "mental disorder" are made up of things which certainly everybody can do, and literally does do at times.

In this day and age the much more abundant disorder pattern —which, like the others I have named, is more common as a marked tendency in this direction than as a disabling mental disorder—is the *obsessional* state, or, as some people would say, the *compulsive* state. Obsessional people, when only mildly affected and when employed at types of work which require a great deal of care about little details, are sometimes really advantaged by their trouble. The great general principle of the obsessional state is that the person is so frightfully busy living that he doesn't have time to suffer some of the greatest pains of life. Thus, if he can be fearfully concerned about getting every figure in the ledger precisely correct, and all the sums right, and so on, going over them eight or nine times so that he then has the greatest difficulty in catching the bus, he does not have time to wonder what his wife will throw at him when he gets home. There is no shadowy vestige of conscious fraud about all this, and no deliberate purpose in it. In some cases the obsessional behavior literally penetrates everything, and these people become exhausted with the problem of getting everything right. For example, the obsessional person may develop the most laborious way of putting on a shoe, and the technique may be so elaborate that fatigue, or the dog barking outside, or something of the sort, will cause him to forget one little step, whereupon he must take the cursed shoe off and do it all over again. It may take over forty-five minutes to get a shoe on, and there's nothing funny about that.

If the patient manifests a rather striking predominance of obsessional traits, it is well for the interviewer to be very much aware of this, so that in the earlier interviews he can keep to what he has to know, which is going to be hard enough to do. If, on the other hand, the interviewer, without being aware of the patient's obsessional traits, tries to get anything like a well-rounded picture of him, Heaven help us! he'll be at it forever. It can't be done. We psychiatrists have a flip way of saying, "It's terribly important to the obsessional not to be clear on the most problematic and insecurity-provoking aspects of life," and, if we know what we mean by that, it is so. In other words, when the obsessional person is on the verge of seeing through something that looks pretty disastrous to him, he gets so busy that he doesn't come to see it, and any efforts to lead him to it will, if attempted early in the interview situation, be quite futile, and likely only to lead the interviewer to the grave. Thus it is quite important for the interviewer to spot the signs of obsessional traits in the first interview, and not to wander from the things he must know.

The obsessional states are sometimes related to the schizophrenic conditions by a sort of bridge; and when the bridge isn't there, the relationship is even closer. Such a bridge is composed of a group of troubles which is atrociously named, at the moment, the *psychosomatic* states. The interviewer is not likely to observe signs of the psychosomatic conditions during the recital of social history. However, since they are related to the obsessional and schizophrenic states, if the interviewer in the reconnaissance sees signs of obsessionalism, or encounters autistic interruptions, and so on, it is ordinary common sense for him to inquire about certain parts of the body which are notoriously apt to suffer (be "diseased," as some doctors would put it) as a result of the type of personality problems the person has encountered. Notorious in this field at the moment are the gastric-ulcer syndrome, so called, certain disturbances of lower bowel function, some cases of asthma and hay fever, a few cardiac disorders, and so on. I literally cannot tell you whether certain disturbances of the genital area represent a psychosomatic difficulty or schizophrenia purely and simply. Most surely many of these disturbances in the young are disastrous precipitates of life problems, and often—in part because they are so horribly handled by uninformed physicians, and in part because it is a rather grave business anyway—they represent the earlier signs of severe schizophrenic disturbance.

Thus the field of the psychosomatic disorders should rise to an interviewer's mind when he runs onto a distinctly obsessional person or when he comes across an odd, detached, queer duck—which is, I suppose, the way the schizoid person would ordinarily be described. There is a way of making inquiries about psychosomatic disorders with a minimum of risk. The interviewer may first ask rather casually about the stomach and bowels, as if he were immediately going on to the usually more innocuous subject of the hands and feet. If there is a distinct response, then, of course, the interviewer is interested, but not overly active in pursuing the subject. There are times when you don't try to get a live specimen by setting off a bomb, for to do so might destroy the specimen.

The term *schizophrenia* covers profoundly odd events which are known to most of us only through what happens in our sleep; in our earlier years of life, a great part of our living was schizophrenic, but we have been carefully schooled to forget all that happened then. When a person is driven by the insoluble character of his life situation to have recourse in waking later life to the types of referential operations which characterized his very early life, he is said to be in a schizophrenic state. People who come to be called schizophrenic are remarkably shy, low in their self-esteem, and rather convinced that they are not highly appreciated by others. They are faced by the possibility of panic related to their feelings of inferiority, loneliness, and failure in living. But in all this I see no reason to believe that schizophrenics are startlingly different from anybody else.

The catatonic schizophrenic, who is often mute and engages in practically none of the communication by gesture on which we ordinarily depend, seems to many of us very strange and very inaccessible. However, many years of intense interest have taught me that the patient is rather closely in touch with events, even though for a variety of reasons he cannot communicate. In other words, although there is very little coming out, there are very decidedly things going in. In such situations I proceed with the business of the interview under the restrictions that are imposed by operating with an almost purely hypothetical other person. I am denied what I insist is necessary—any news of who the person is; I must proceed with only the knowledge that he is a person who has a profound disturbance of interpersonal relations which manifests itself in a way that I am by now somewhat familiar with. Because of the extreme handicap on any real interchange with this person, there is a very great possibility of the most serious error in his understanding me, and there is also a strong possibility that a great deal of what I might be inclined to guess or to say to him will be profoundly irrelevant. Therefore, I reduce my attempted communication to certain things which seem to me so very highly probable that the chances of their being irrelevant are small. I then talk slowly and carefully, perhaps saying the same thing several ways, not necessarily in succession, but still trying to cover the ground from various angles. If the patient is "in touch," if I guess correctly what is profoundly important to him at the time, and if I express it in language that is meaningful to him and that connects in his mind with the correct implications, rather than with some very highly autistic content, then I have achieved the objective of the interview. That objective is not primarily my obtaining information, but the patient's receiving some durable benefit. The durable benefit, at this stage, is simply that the patient gets the idea that I am really interested in him, that I take a lot of trouble over him, that I know something about what has probably happened to him, and that I deal with urgent matters of real importance. This is what I have gathered from patients who recovered and later talked about what they recalled of their experience. It was not that after coming out of the dark regions of catatonic stupor they recalled having felt, "That psychiatrist was wonderful! He understood everything!" It was merely that they had gotten the impression that I knew something about what ailed them and that I was interested in them; that was what they needed at that stage, and it meant that they were at least willing to see me again. In other words, if I urgently attempt to keep to those things which are very probably significant, and if I go to a lot of trouble to avoid misunderstanding about what I am trying to communicate, it does have an effect even on these least communicative of people.

It is true, of course, that any psychiatrist who deals with mute patients will find his sense of accomplishment undergoing grave stress. It is very sad indeed to be confronted with fifty minutes of an utterly uncommunicative patient, when you have only one or two ideas that seem to meet the criterion of being highly probable. Long ago I realized that it was not how much time I spent that counted, but the seriousness of my attempt to avoid any possible misunderstanding in communicating what I had to say, and the keenness of my interest in what had happened to the patient. When I have done my best in these respects, and before I am discouraged, I am through, and I leave. It is not useful for the therapist to keep on until he gets annoyed and pushes, for the catatonic can resist this for the rest of time; nor is it useful for the therapist to indicate discouragement and frustration, which the catatonic may recognize as such. I don't believe the catatonic has the feeblest interest in frustrating the psychiatrist; but he has been frustrated so much that he is an expert on frustration. If his psychiatric Statue of Liberty suffers badly from the frustration of his muteness, he may not want to come to America. He may decide it isn't safe. So I suggest that you don't try to continue after you have run out of gas. When you have done your best, depart. It will be no surprise to the patient.

Hypochondriacal preoccupations, as we ordinarily refer to them, shift the sufferer's interest from disturbing aspects of the outer world to gloomy ruminations about the state of his health, impending developments of cancer, and one thing and another *within himself*. Such preoccupations gradually take precedence over all profitable interests in how to pay his income tax, and so on. The hypochondriacal preoccupations, curiously enough, are very apt to skid at times. They are unequal to certain stresses, in which case the patient progresses to the next rubric, the *paranoid state*, in which he makes a massive transfer of blame out of himself onto others. Thus he becomes "blameless" and comfortable, because "not *I*, but *they*" are to blame for those things which are lamentable in his life performances.

CHAPTER

IX

The Termination of the Interview

An important part of every interview situation is its *termination* or *interruption*. In terminating the interview, or in interrupting it for any length of time, the important thing is to consolidate whatever progress has been made. This progress is represented, not by the interpretations that have been made by the interviewer, but by the degree to which the purpose—the interviewee's expectation of some durable gain from the experience—has been realized. Even if the interview is with a person seeking a job for which he is unqualified, it is the interviewer's business, insofar as he uses the psychiatric method, to see that the person gets something out of the interview. In fact, the interviewer's data are valid only to the extent that he has a lively interest in seeing that the interviewee gets something constructive out of the interview.

The consolidating of the interview's purpose is done, grossly, by the following four steps: (1) the interviewer makes a *final statement* to the interviewee summarizing what he has learned during the course of the interview; (2) the interviewer gives the interviewee a *prescription of action* in which the interviewee is now to engage; (3) the interviewer makes a *final assessment* of the probable effects on the life-course of the interviewee which may reasonably be expected from the statement and prescription; and (4) there is the *formal leave-taking* between the interviewer and the interviewee.

The Final Statement

I don't believe that there is a person in the world who doesn't get something positively constructive from a careful review, by someone who has some judgment of what really does matter in life, of what has been accomplished in, say, an hour and a half's serious interview. Thus the first step in the final termination of an interview or a series of interviews is in the form of a statement; that is, the interviewer makes a succinct survey of what he has learned. As I have suggested elsewhere, this kind of summary statement is useful at various times during an interview or series of interviews. That is, it is useful for the interviewer to repeatedly test the events noted in the interview by stating his impressions of these to the interviewee for his reaction and possible correction. In this final statement, therefore, the interviewer is—insofar as the interview or series of interviews has been successful—stating things which are not open to any ready contradiction or emendation. He is presenting the gross conclusions of which he is by now quite sure. If by chance the interviewee's immediate reaction indicates that these conclusions are inadequate and this seems a valid reaction, the interviewer should take more time and make his summation adequate. But this same reaction may merely relate to the fact that this is a person who must engage in all kinds of hesitating, doubting, qualifying, and so on, in which case the interviewer should merely go ahead as if nothing had happened, having already recognized that it is necessary for this person to qualify everything to the point of uselessness.

In a good many interviews there are things which are heard and inferred about the patient which are not included in the summary. For example, if the interviewer feels that the interviewee has an unfavorable prognosis, he almost never mentions it in a final summary. In other words, the interviewer attempts to avoid destroying what chance the person has. All of these unfavorable things are related to matters which can be summarized, and thus the interviewer can avoid disturbing a patient deeply, and at the same time can review with profit a good deal of what has been observed. For instance, if I were interviewing a person for a highly technical position for which he was unsuited, I would rather carefully omit from the summary any incapacities which seemed to close the door to practically any gainful employment. I might take considerable trouble to emphasize things which made this particular employment potentially undesirable, without, however, making the interviewee feel hopeless or discredited. I have sometimes found it quite useful to propound riddles of this general type to the interviewee who has a poor employment record, a poor study record, and so on: "Well, have you ever thought of a career of such-and-such?"—picking something which seems to be fully as well within his grasp as what he has been considering. Having said something like this, I am inclined to listen, for the interviewee may get started on something. Quite often there is the best reason in the world why such a career is not open to him. But anyway, I may learn more by listening to that than by pointing out all the reasons why he may be a failure. And the patient does not suffer a loss in self-esteem and does not become anxious—and that may be useful for his later progress in other situations. My point is that I try never to close all doors to a person; the person should go away with hope and with an improved grasp on what has been the trouble.

The Prescription of Action

The second step in consolidating the results of the interview is by a prescription of action in which the interviewee is now to engage. The interviewer should offer such a prescription whether he plans a subsequent contact with the interviewee or whether this is presumably his final interview with him.

When the interview is interrupted, however briefly, the

prescription which the interviewer offers for the interval is in the nature of homework, as a setting for the next session. For example, I may at the end of an interview mention some point which I am puzzled about because the patient has been unable to recall the details. I may say, "The business of how so-and-so came about is obscure. Well, maybe it will come back to you by next time." In this way, the interviewer can give the patient something to do; whether or not the interviewer suggests homework, the patient will do some before the next session, and the interviewer may have somewhat better judgment about what might be useful than the patient has.

If the interviewer does not plan to see the interviewee again, he may prescribe that the interviewee is to find someone with whom to do intensive psychotherapy, or, in the case of an employment interview, that he is to look for a kind of job different from the one he came to get, and so on. In other words, the interviewer indicates a course of events in which the interviewee might engage and which, in the interviewer's opinion, in view of the data accumulated, would improve his chances of success and satisfaction in life.[1]

[1] [*Editors' note:* The text here is from a 1945 lecture. In his 1944 lecture on the same topic, Sullivan made the following distinction between the "prescription of action" and the usual giving of advice:

"When patients want my advice, I am usually given to some sort of feeble witticism such as, 'Why pick on me? You can ask anybody, anywhere, for advice, and get it. Now why in the world waste your time with a psychiatrist by asking for advice?' If a psychiatrist advises on very adequate grounds, then he is often insulting the intelligence of the person advised. If he advises without grounds, then he is just talking for his own amusement. Therefore, if one is to advise—and certainly the psychiatrist has very often to do this—it is really a clearing of the field for the exercise of foresight, and one usually takes care to do it quite indirectly.

"As I have mentioned earlier, I once gave some advice which was extremely unwelcome, but was perhaps in keeping with an adequate discharge of my professional function. On that occasion I told a psychotic woman that I had no objection to her having a psychosis, which she certainly had in abundance, but that if she ever felt like doing anything to any of the 'troublesome' people with whom she worked, I should advise her to go first to Bellevue Hospital. This advice was very harsh indeed, and it promptly terminated the interview; but I think that in that situation I was doing what had to be done. I was saying that the only time at which it becomes really dangerous to have

The Final Assessment

The third step in the termination is the final assessment by the interviewer of what he has told the interviewee in the final survey and prescription of action, and what the effects of this on the life-course of the interviewee are likely to be. In other

---

a psychosis is when the behavior may lead to an invasion of the affairs of others in a hostile, punitive fashion. At that time the person is better off in a mental hospital where he is protected from making mistakes.

"Although a person may come to a psychiatrist for help, he may have very real doubts that any such help actually exists. In handling the referral for this kind of patient I may be able to outline the general area and characteristics of some very serious problem with some certainty that the patient can be helped; but I may realize at the same time that the ease or difficulty of his being helped is dependent to some extent upon the skill of the therapist to whom he goes. It is seldom wise to bluntly advise the patient to go to a particular therapist. Instead I formulate the problem as I see it, and discuss the general character of an attack on such a problem and the ways in which a cure could probably be brought about; I then suggest a person who is, to my knowledge, thoroughly familiar with this type of problem and this type of treatment, winding up with a suggestion that an attempt be made to see if this therapist has any free time. When I have done this, I can then strongly advise that the patient get treatment. Thus the advice comes in at the very end to round out the obvious. As a psychiatrist, you see, I sometimes have to round out the obvious because there are people, notoriously obsessionals, who are very unwilling indeed to draw a conclusion—and therefore the psychiatrist gives them the conclusion. Actually, the 'advice' is for the most part an overwhelming display of the factors relevant to the problem, plus a clear statement by the psychiatrist of what he firmly believes can be done about them.

"There are occasions on which one definitely *disadvises*—with force. Occasionally a patient says that he is going to do something, which it is apparent will almost certainly be disastrous. There are several ways of handling this matter, depending on the clarity with which the psychiatrist perceives the irrational character of the act. If it is not clear why the patient is committed to this disastrous course, then I suppose that the way to give advice is to say, 'Why, how did you ever decide upon that?'—and then listen. If the irrational nature of the impulse is quite clear and quite certain disaster lies ahead, it has been my policy to say, 'No!' in quite an emphatic fashion as a way of interrupting the person. I then follow this up by saying, 'Merciful God! Let us consider what will follow that!' Then I try to do that which is really my 'disadvising.' I depict the probable course of events as I expect them to unfold. When I am finished, I turn to the patient and ask, 'Wherein have I done any more than expect the obvious?' If he can show wherein I have been unduly pessimistic, or wrong, I am glad to hear it. If he can't do this, then the situation stands with clear foresight of disaster, and very few people will go ahead with their plans under such circumstances.

"In those cases in which I am not sure that the proposed action is strongly,

words, this is a matter of the interviewer's giving some thought to how the interviewee is going to take what he has been offered in this final interview. If the effects of the final statement and prescription of action are not likely to be constructive—if, to take an extreme instance, they have been so discouraging that the patient's prompt self-destruction would be the logical outcome—then there has been some serious deficiency in them, and it is the responsibility of the interviewer to mend this deficiency. As the interviewer grows more skillful, he learns to direct his final statement and prescription of action in such a way that they point to a reasonably constructive picture from the standpoint of the patient. But in any event, the interviewer

---

conspicuously irrational in its motivation, I inquire further, 'Why in the world do you think that?'—with the strong suggestion that I think it's strikingly curious and undesirable. Again I listen. When finally I perceive that the matter is anything but a normal ingredient of a self-furthering plan, I attempt to depict its probable consequences, attempting to call in enough security motives and so on to choke off any direct expression of the impulse. Of course, that does not cure the possibility of irrational acts. I attempt it only when something impends which the patient will clearly regret at his leisure.

"The difficulty which psychiatrists get into by rash advice is often quite simply pathetic. There are few things that I think are so harrowing as the occasional psychiatrist who knows a great deal about right and wrong, how things should be done, what is good taste, and so on and so forth. Such a psychiatrist often feels a missionary spirit so that he wants to pass his own values on to his patients. Not only is this hard on the patient but it also makes things difficult for any other psychiatrist who wants to get something useful done. I think that the psychiatrist's role is to discover the origin of views of indecency and decency, goodness and badness, and so on, except for fields in which there is practically no question. Even when the psychiatrist is quite sure there is no question, it is still always worth while for him to keep a wee crack open in his mind to the possibility of a question existing. I, for example, am bitterly opposed to violence—so opposed, in fact, that I try to suppress it in the puppies that grow up around me. Yet there are today on the face of the earth a great many situations in which I recognize that violence is quite the indicated activity. I suppose that years of intense interest in what went on on a particular ward in the mental hospital where I was working has done a good deal to accentuate my intolerance of physical violence around me, for violence on the wards of a mental hospital has far-reaching evil consequences on people other than those directly subjected to it. Yet in spite of my attitude about violence, in general I discourage the practice of giving advice on this subject, or on any ultimate things, great social problems, and so on."]

will do well to assess what this picture is; and if it is not a constructive one, he must realize that he has not yet accomplished his aim—the consolidation of some gain for the interviewee.

The Formal Leave-Taking

There then comes the fourth step, which can really do a good deal of damage if it's done badly—the formal leave-taking. Just as the formal inception of the interview situation is very important, so it is also very important that the interviewer should, as soon as he can, find a way of detaching himself from the interview situation without awkwardness and without prejudicing the work that has been done. In actual fact, much good work in psychiatric interviews is horribly garbled or completely destroyed in the last few minutes.

This is just as true of the leave-taking at the end of one interview in a series of interviews as it is of the leave-taking in a situation when the psychiatrist will not see the patient again. As a matter of fact, in dealing with a certain kind of obsessional patient, I have found that the leave-taking for each interview in a series may present a real problem, so much so that for years I have contemplated having two suites of offices. At the end of such interviews, having said my say, I would arise suddenly, step through a door behind my chair, and go to work at my next interview, leaving to the nurse or the secretary the business of escorting my ex-interviewee out, just to avoid the fearful turmoil that such a patient produces in his attempt to get more of something. Just what this 'more of something' is, never becomes really clear to me. These people won't let you be through if they can help it. After you have formulated with the greatest care some really profoundly important truths, and have risen and looked at the door, hoping that the patient will move toward it, such a person may say, "Tell me, Doctor, have we got anywhere today?" or something like that. All of these frantic reachings for some kind of reassurance, or for the Great Formula, have the general effect of confusing all issues that have previously been clarified with so much effort. And so—and I am not attempting to amuse you in the least—the interviewer will be very wise to learn how to rapidly exclude a patient when the interview has come to its end. This takes skill sometimes, but it is very important. In other words, the psychiatrist should not go over things: he should not explain that which is now clearer than it ever will be if he repeats it. The psychiatrist is the expert and he should be expert enough to be done when he is through. Otherwise, much of the benefit of the work can be quite literally wiped out.

So it is in the final leave-taking also. There are way of getting done with people; and there are ways—it seems to me much more commonly manifested—of having a terrible time disentangling oneself, so that anything accomplished in the final attempt to consolidate the benefits of the interview is confused or exhausted by the efforts of the poor victim and the interviewer to shake each other off. That isn't a good technique. There is no reason why one should have an exhausting turmoil in trying to say good-bye to an interviewee. There should not be all sorts of damnable questions that have long since been answered or never will be answered; there should be a clean-cut, respectful finish that does not confuse that which has been done.

CHAPTER

X

Problems of Communication in the Interview [1]

IN DEALING with people, one must realize that there are always reservations in communication—things that all of us are taught from the cradle onward as dangerous to even think about, much less to communicate freely about. Thus the interviewer recognizes automatically, and as a preliminary to all communication, that no one will be simply 'frank'; such a phenomenon is purely of the language—it does not describe interpersonal relations.

The chief handicap to communication is anxiety. There are times when anxiety on the part of the interviewee is unavoidable or even necessary, but in general an important part of the psychiatrist's work is his use of skill to avoid unnecessary anxiety. There are two important aspects to this "handling" of anxiety: first, one attempts to avoid arousing anxiety; and second, one acts to restrain its development. Reassurance might be termed a third technique for handling anxiety when it refers to a purposive, skillful therapeutic move in interpersonal relations. However, I am not talking here about the use of reassuring ver-

1 [*Editors' note:* Unlike the other chapters in this book, this chapter does not represent a lecture as delivered by Sullivan, nor did he include this topic in his outline for his lecture series. This chapter brings together comments which Sullivan made at various times throughout these lectures—sometimes as digressions, sometimes as answers to questions from students—on the problems of communication in the interview, and, in particular, on anxiety considered from a clinical viewpoint.]

balisms, which merely represents an attempt by the therapist to do magic with language, and is usually a matter of the therapist's reassuring himself rather than the patient. I shall say a few words about this later.

The problems presented in handling anxiety are, it seems to me, vastly clearer if, whatever your initial predilections or previous training, you come to accept my definition of anxiety. As I use the term, anxiety is a sign that one's self-esteem, one's self-regard, is endangered. This is a sign which occurs with a strikingly prospective quality—that is, anxiety is often a sign of *foreseen* lowering of self-esteem. In this sense, anxiety is very smooth-working, and usually not very disturbing, for it usually precedes that which would disturb self-regard, indicating by its appearance that a change must be made in the progression of activity—even if only in the progression of thought—in order to insure the maintenance of an appropriate regard for the self. In other words, anxiety is a signal of danger to self-respect, to one's standing in the eyes of the significant persons present, even if they are only ideal figures from childhood; and this signal, other things being equal, leads to a change in the situation.

In the psychiatric interview, where the therapist is presumably relatively beyond the power of the patient, this change often consists of the patient's doing something to disorder the situation. What he most frequently does, I think, is to become angry, for most people, when even faintly anxious in a relationship with a comparative stranger, get angry, and some do so with their most intimate friends. Next to anger, the most frequent move made to avoid anxiety is to develop "misunderstanding," in which case the person begins talking about something else. This misunderstanding is of such a peculiar nature that I refer to it by the special term "selective inattention," by which I mean that one overlooks, or is inattentive to, that which has provoked anxiety, and shifts to some other topic. If these moves fail, and none of the many others of their kind are effective, the person may experience severe anxiety, in which case

he is incapable of any constructive or useful communicative performance.

Perhaps I should comment here on the concept of "resistance" as it may be related to anxiety. Disregarding for our present purpose the derivation of the term and its earlier definitions, I would say that in general it has come to mean *something that opposes what was presumed to be helpful*. I have no great quarrel with the idea that anxiety may be regarded as "resistance." Anxiety is always a handicap to adjustment, and a block to communication, in the therapeutic situation or anywhere else. Any concept that carries, along with its other qualities, some hint that it will reflect unfavorably on the therapist's esteem of the patient will rouse anxiety in the patient and provoke "resistance." That is, following the introduction of the threatening subject, things don't go so well or so simply. The patient begins to use all manner of devices to avoid any foursquare collision with the disturbing topic, and the instrumentalities available to the human for doing just this are often exceedingly impressive. But it is of such things as these that the practice of psychiatry is composed. They can be no more than subject matter for further observation and study. They are data.

This sort of thing is not restricted to the psychiatric interview. Even beloved friends—who actually every now and then startle each other by finding out that they have been thinking along the same lines prior to any verbal communication on a given subject—know well that there are some things that one is very careful about communicating to the other; certain things might disturb the other person and possibly threaten the friendship. So it is everywhere. There are always reservations, attempts at clever compromise, smooth evasion, and so on. Thus their appearance in the psychiatric interview is in no sense a reflection on the psychiatrist or his skill; they do not represent the patient's conclusion that the doctor is feeble-minded and can be "taken in." They are necessary, for they are ingrained in the personality. To the extent that the interviewer recognizes them as such, skillfully picking his way between that which is inevitably the case with the patient, and that which is exquisitely adjusted to the interviewer, he can rapidly cut off the illusions of the patient as to what he can get away with, or, to put it another way, what will go unnoticed. If the psychiatrist stumbles in this, regarding as offensive some evasion that is utterly natural to this patient—an evasion that his parents spent a long time engraining in him—the psychiatrist obviously is not an expert in interpersonal relations; his irritation with the patient's evasion miscarries and actually reduces the possibility of a good result.

The first way to "handle" anxiety which I have mentioned is to avoid arousing it unnecessarily, and in the interview this is often a question of progression and transition. Insofar as the work permits, the psychiatrist should try to proceed with simple clarity, so that the patient can follow his direction of thought, for if the patient hasn't any idea of what the psychiatrist is driving at, the psychiatrist, pathetically enough, is not apt to have much of an idea of what the patient means. So it pays, unless there is clear reason for being a bit subtle and obscure, to be quite simply direct and clear. In your personal experience you have no doubt encountered people whose minds leap in such a fashion from topic to topic that every second thing they say astonishes you. With time and enough peace of mind you might figure out how various remarks arose out of what was being said or what had been asked, but by and large you merely have the feeling: "Well, that's a queer kind of person." There are other people to whom it is so very easy to talk that you say a good deal more than you ever intended to say, and if you stop to consider why, you will usually find that each topic grew "naturally" out of that which preceded. Or if events did not proceed in the most "natural" way, then there was very probably a quite careful attention to transitions, so that you were never surprised. The questions which were asked seemed to be the right, sensible ones, and the other person seemed always to show a rather sensitive comprehension of what you were attempting to evoke in his mind; and so it was very easy to go on and on.

In the same way, the competent interviewer usually introduces each new topic with certain conversational gestures which conclude the current subject and open the mind to something new. If he presents a new point of view or a difference of opinion, he does it in such a way as to clearly indicate that there is no reflection on the interviewee's standing as a personality. Any patient who comes to a psychiatrist is apt to be insecure, and this insecurity will considerably increase whenever the patient must stop and think, "Now what is the doctor getting at? What does this lead to?" Such an increase in insecurity is almost certain to play a good deal of hob with the interview.

I would like to say a few words here about "blocking." This is a term of rather indeterminate meaning, but commonly refers to a state in which the progression of approaching speech through awareness—the preparation of things to say—is very seriously disturbed by contradictory impulses, one of which does not predominate. In other words, the impulses have practically equal importance, as a result of which the patient says nothing, and feels very awkward. He is not likely to be aware of the contradictory impulses; at some point of "disagreement" or "misunderstanding," he simply draws a blank.

Most of the things that we say are reviewed before they are spoken. This is a very swift process, for there is a great deal to be reviewed. A person who is reasonably sure of what he is attempting to do, and reasonably sure that a very large number of errors and inaccuracies are bound to happen, will often say things which need to be modified after having been said. That is, even as he passes from the initial review, which is extremely hurried, to hearing it as the other person has heard it, he realizes that it is inadequate and in need of correction. If all of this procedure is blocked at the moment that one gets ready to speak, it is easy to understand why very little comes to be said.

The extent to which a person will be free of blocking is to a large degree the result of the ease and freedom with which he can say what occurs to him, and so the simple and easy progression of inquiry will often avoid the precipitation of blocking. For example, asking a direct question will sometimes result in a kind of blocking. However, you may not even notice it, for we have all, in the process of growing up, become skillful at accommodating to what amounts to a lack of communication with the person with whom we are talking; and so you may assume that something has been communicated which has not. The indirect question, composed of running comment, additions, corrections, and so on, which imply what you want to know, or suggest the information desired, is possibly the ideal way of getting information in such a way that you can be reasonably certain of what is being communicated.

Thus, in general, it is wise to avoid disconcerting cessations of communication, and to proceed by steps that are within the grasp of the other person, so that he feels that he knows what you're driving at, and therefore knows what he's talking about. This is what I have earlier referred to as the "smooth transition" in the interview.

A consideration that may lead to your *not* being so simple and obvious in the train of your questioning is again that of avoiding arousing anxiety—that is, guarding against any unnecessary discomposure of the patient. There are some areas in the inquiry in which you do not permit the patient to follow your thought—when it is desirable for the patient to be, as it were, out of touch for a moment, in order to avoid his having too troublesome a train of thought. You don't plunge gaily into things that are going to make him horribly tense and uncertain as to how you will respond to what he says. Furthermore, when the intervention of anxiety makes it impossible for the patient to go any further in a particular direction—when you see that his tension is increasing to the point of interfering with communication—you will find it wise to move emphatically out of the particular topic which is being discussed into another. Perhaps you can come back to it later. As a matter of fact, most topics of human living are so interlocked that you can approach the same thing from six or seven different directions. It sometimes happens that something which provoked considerable anxiety when it first came up is much less intimidating to the patient when it is later investigated from another approach. Because people are often unable to communicate anything when they get very anxious, you should not go out of your way to discompose a patient unnecessarily—in fact, you can show your skill by avoiding that.

I make one of these emphatic moves out of one topic into another—"abrupt transitions," as I call them—when I foresee that there will not be, in the particular interview, enough time to get the patient's anxiety down to reasonable proportions. Certainly, in the earlier stages of psychiatric work, it is very risky to let a person get intensely anxious and then cut off the interview because the clock has gotten to a certain point; that is a way of intimidating patients on the whole subject of psychotherapy, which may delay almost intolerably their really getting deeply to work—and it is also a way of increasing the rate of suicides and admissions to mental hospitals. One of the heaviest responsibilities of the psychotherapist is to try to get the patient on the downgrade of anxiety before the end of a session, instead of in a state where he is becoming increasingly anxious. When the patient's anxiety is mounting, this abrupt transition, in which you simply rip apart the communicative situation and present another—where there is a sudden change of topic at your behest—usually comes as a very distinct relief to the patient, and it can have a distinct educative influence also. For example, in the earlier phases of the interview, before what I would call a dependable situation has been established, if I see a patient getting pretty tense about something in the last part of the session, I often turn around to face him fully, or in some other way indicate alertness, and say, "You're getting quite anxious, aren't you? Well, what's the hurry about this? We can drop it and go on about so-and-so, can't we?" Now, that is what I would call a very abrupt transition. The educative element is in what I say about anxiety; I want the patient to understand why I broke in, but I don't want to give him a dissertation.

Incidentally, dissertations—these fine, windy explanations by the analyst of what he is doing and what he thinks, and so on—are very, very apt to miscarry in the earlier stages of the detailed inquiry; some of my colleagues have worked with very gifted analysts, but heard almost nothing that the analysts said to them for the first year or two. They knew it was terribly important, but somehow they just didn't quite follow it—it didn't leave much of any trace. I think the development of psychiatric skill consists in very considerable measure of doing a lot with very little—making a rather precise move which has a high probability of achieving what you're attempting to achieve, with a minimum of time and words. If you realize the importance of the transitional effect in a communicative situation, you will find that you can spare the patient extensive discourses, which in the early stages of psychotherapy almost never communicate what you suppose you've said, even though you may say it beautifully. Often the patient doesn't hear any of it; an authority is speaking, and he feels that all he has to do is maintain an attitude of reverence and be ready to do something when the authority stops.

Another grave limitation to the smooth and easy progression of inquiry appears when you have become so involved with the patient's self-system that you are being sold an extended piece of goods—that is, being misinformed by the minute, which is very expensive to the patient. In this case, an easy progression of inquiry will merely keep up an unforunate motion. I use an accented transition to suppress these security operations. I may not change the subject, but I do change the communication by showing traces—or sometimes very glaring amounts—of satire, boredom, restlessness, annoyance, or something of the sort. Now, I don't recommend that to others; each psychotherapist brings to his work his own equipment which he uses every day with other people, some of it for good and some for ill. The problem for every psychotherapist is to sort out the things he does well with others and try to build up his psychotherapeutic armament out of those.

So far, I have been discussing chiefly the techniques of progression and transition in the interview as ways to avoid arousing anxiety and to restrain its development. Incidentally, it is the latter problem which most people have in mind when they say, "How do you *handle* anxiety?" In other words, they are not referring to anxiety as a rather smooth-working advance warning of danger to one's self-esteem, but to the very severe loss of euphoria when the person feels that his security actually *has* diminished, when his self-regard, or his estimate of another person's regard for him, actually is greatly reduced. When the interviewee suffers such a gross loss of euphoria, it is sometimes possible for the interviewer, moving very swiftly after the signs of anxiety appear, to restrain its development by some means other than transition, or sometimes to reassure the patient—provided, as I said before, this is not merely a matter of using reassuring verbalisms. For instance, sometimes the interviewer may ask a question which leads the interviewee to make what he feels is a most damaging admission, so that he then becomes intensely anxious—although he may cover the anxiety by equally intense feelings of anger or other emotion. The remedy lies in the interviewer's then asking a question about the "damaging admission"; for example, he may ask, "Well, am I supposed to think very badly of you because of that?" Now this may seem like a strange kind of operation, but its value is that it puts into words the content of the interviewee's signs of anxiety. The answer is ordinarily "Yes," and the next step is to ask,

"Well, how come? What is so lamentable about such a thing?" Without waiting for an answer, the interviewer explains that while the interviewee may regard the event concerned as something to be greatly ashamed of, and so on, such happenings are quite the universal experience of human beings; while the informant may not know this, the interviewer can scarcely avoid knowing it, and so he is not very much impressed with this "damaging" data. That completes that process. The interviewer can then inquire where in the world the interviewee got the impression that this particular thing which has caused anxiety is so deplorable. In all of this, if the interviewer moves smoothly, naturally, and in a manner unstudied enough to carry conviction—instead of giving the impression of merely being very clever in the technical sense—he may discover something of real importance in the person, a vulnerability in the organization of the self which is especially related to some particularly pestilential moral censure in the past.

The reassurance of schizophrenic adolescents seems to consist almost entirely of this sort of thing—trying to discover just what in the world is supposed to be so terrible, and what in the world is terrible about it. One thing that used to be terrible in male adolescence was masturbation; I don't know how it is now, but in my earlier years this "practice," as it was called, carried a heavy load of moral censure. Sometimes when I was interviewing a male adolescent I would say, after prodding around for a while and drawing blanks, "Well, I suppose you're another of the people who has been ruined by masturbation. Is that it?" The patient often would nod to indicate that such was the dreary truth. I think that my asking this question was usually in itself extremely reassuring to the patient, for it introduced the idea that many people regarded themselves as ruined by masturbation, but that I had other views about this matter. Having thus created the impression that this was by no means the first time that I had heard this sad and somewhat erroneous story, I would say, "Now tell me, how much did you masturbate to accomplish this ruin?"—I would endeavor to get across some faint satire by this repetition of "ruin." I would usually find that the person masturbated once in a fortnight, or something like that, and then I would want to know how long this had been going on. And as I prodded away at this topic, I would seem to be struggling against an all-encompassing boredom, and that too was often reassuring, for it showed that I was not at all excited about this supposedly terrible business. After I had found that the young man had had a frightful struggle for the past two and a half years, swearing off repeatedly, only to fall back into the miserable habit, or something of the sort, I would rouse myself from almost a stupor, and say, "Yes, I see. Now tell me, how did the ruin appear? How did things begin to go wrong?" At this I would begin to get an account of his relationships with people, and I would get more and more interested as that went on. Perhaps an hour later I would say, "Now why is it you connect masturbation with all this? How do they get mixed up together in your mind?" If by that time I had been successful, the person was apt to say, "Well, aren't they connected?" I would say, "Yes, by the fact that you experienced all of these things, but I don't know how otherwise." With this I might feel that I had done a fairly good job.

The point is that there is no use trying to reassure an adolescent—or anyone else—if you don't know what you are reassuring him about. And you ordinarily don't know what to reassure him about, aside from a few good bets such as masturbation used to be—and even in that case, you still had to be told about it before you could do anything about it. You cannot do magic with reassuring language. The magic occurs in the interpersonal relations, and the real magic is done by the patient, not by the therapist. The therapist's skill and art lie in keeping things simple enough so that something can happen; in other words, he clears the field for favorable change, and then tries to avoid getting in the way of its development.

Some patients show the ways in which they are distressingly

insecure by displaying a marked need for reassurance. For example, upon being asked in the reconnaissance if he married his first love, a patient may hesitantly reply that he didn't, and then begin to wonder if that is all right. He wants to be told whether he should or should not have married his first love; there is almost a clutching for agreement that he is all right, that he may go on living, that there is nothing to be ashamed of. All of this grinds up a lot of time. Yet the insecurity which the patient is showing is a very important aspect of his problem, and something that is quite worth finding out about.

Some such people try to make a hash of everything without knowing it by groping for some magical reassurance at the end of the interview. This may happen at the end of a first interview, with a patient you are undertaking to treat, or one whom you are sending to someone else for treatment; or it may occur during the course of intensive psychotherapy. In any case, you should not attempt any private miracles at the end of the interview. There is no justification other than your own insecurity—which is no justification at all from the patient's standpoint—for any attempt to reassure unless you are in a position to document what you say. I am not suggesting that the interviewer should curtly throw out the person who suddenly says at the end of the interview, "Tell me, Doctor, have we gotten anywhere?" But in this situation I do try by my response to make the patient aware of the extreme irrelevance of his final performance, and yet leave him integrated enough to be able to think over the interview. Thus I may look at him with surprise and chagrin and mutter to myself, "For God's sake!"—and let him make what he can of that; I hope to invite his attention to the preposterous nature of his attempt to pull that kind of a rabbit out of the bag.

Some interviewers, particularly those who are inexperienced, feel called upon to pour some healing balm on the victim at the finish of an interview, as if finding out what the trouble is were not in itself a life-size job. Such therapists tell a patient that although they are not quite clear on what the trouble is, they are very sure that they can find out what it is, and that it can be fixed—which, so far as I am concerned, is utterly gratuitous magic. In fact, it may disturb the patient when he thinks it over, for I don't believe that it is particularly good for a patient to realize how much distance has yet to be covered before the expert knows much of anything about what is going on.

Occasionally a patient asks fairly urgently at the last moment if he can see the doctor on the next day, looking as if he were having violent anxiety, and were preparing to do something about it. My suggestion in such a case is to indicate a time on the next day when the patient can call to find out if you have time for a session. There will probably be a lucid interval, perhaps when he is on his way home, or when he is going to bed that night, during which he can take stock of what has happened. If, after this stock-taking, he still wants to see you next day, he can always call up and find out if it is possible. But if he actually feels greatly reassured as a result of the lucid interval, and you have already agreed to his request, he may feel somewhat like a fool; and, incidentally, since it is unpleasant to feel like a fool, he may wonder whether you, the expert, may not be a bit of a fool too, or whether you have nothing to do except run in emergency appointments next day.

All in all, when you can't reassure a person except by magic, the sensible thing is not to try. When you don't know anything in particular to say, don't say it. Yet you need not resort to curt refusals when the patient wants reassurance at the end of an interview. Instead, you need only realize that the interview, so far as you are concerned, is done; and so far as the patient is concerned, the phase which is perhaps most important is only about to begin—the retrospective appraisal of what he has undergone. Try to leave things so that that will happen, because it can be very valuable.

I mentioned earlier that a common manifestation of anxiety is talking about everything but the problem. Then, people sometimes ask, how do you find out what the problem is, and how do you get the person to talk about it? The rule, so far as I can formulate one at the moment, is this: If you know how you arrived at the point at which anxiety put in its appearance, you can often guess what seemed to be ahead from the standpoint of the interviewee. If you follow closely what is discussed, trying to promote easy communication and to keep things moving, you will observe the patient veering off from certain topics in a fashion which strongly suggests the general area of the problem. If you approach this area, you notice that the patient more or less skillfully shifts to talking about something else before arriving at it. But notice that the failure to arrive after just *one* approach doesn't prove anything beyond the simple fact that you didn't arrive; in such a case you do not know wherein the difficulty lies. However, if you try two or three times, coming in from rather different angles toward much the same topic, each time without success, you are then in a position to say quite simply, "I notice that you haven't had anything to say about so-and-so. Obviously it is difficult to discuss it." And putting the obvious into words often markedly improves things. Then the patient can say with considerable force, "Yes! I don't like to talk about that." Then I can be amazed, and my amazement means, "Well! I don't see that that follows at all. What's so difficult about it? How come you dislike it? Is it supposed not to be respectable or something?"

I would now like to mention a communicative situation which arises when the patient loses some of his caution, exerts less effort to maintain distance from the interviewer, and feels more free to say what is in his mind. He will then begin to experience more keenly the significant people of his past. There will be times when the patient will so distort the psychiatrist because of the situation that has been revived in the patient that a *parataxic situation* exists. In such a situation there are actually three people: the *'imaginary' psychiatrist* to whom the patient is addressing his behavior and words; the *patient* who is reacting to this 'imaginary' third person; and the *psychiatrist* who is observing and trying to get some clue as to what this imago to whom the patient is reacting might be like. If the psychiatrist identifies this role and fits it long enough to become a perfectly convincing illusion or delusion to the patient, he is in a position to inquire of the patient, "Is it possible that you think I am actually thus and so?" Whereupon the patient may say, "Why, of course." The psychiatrist can then say, "When did you begin to think that?" Having discovered when all this began, the psychiatrist says, "But isn't this curious? You recall that I said so-and-so and several other things that are incongruent with this imaginary person." The patient may say, "Yes, it is curious." At this point, the psychiatrist says, "Well, now, tell me—there must have been someone in your past, very significant indeed, who acted like that. Who occurs to you?" Whereupon the psychiatrist may discover who the really significant person was in the patient's past—that is, the person with whom the patient has been in an inferior position, whether the relationship was one of tenderness or otherwise.

Such intrusions of past people do not appear until after the patient begins to feel safe in saying various things to the interviewer which ordinarily he would not say. After that point is reached, the wise interviewer notices whether things begin to be a little bit strange in some way or other; he tries to learn what this strangeness consists of by inquiring about it, and thereby learns about certain people in the patient's past, the great significance of whom may never have been clear to the patient.

A special instance of the avoidance of anxiety is found in the problem of relating to the paranoid person in the interview. The anxiety of the paranoid person is intensified by any impulse to draw close to another person. If anything occurs which makes the paranoid person feel that someone is being kind to him, is loving to him, wants to make him feel friendly, and so on, he experiences anxiety. As he experiences it, this anxiety is a sign, a warning, that he has overlooked something, and that the "friendly" person is endangering him. Therefore he usually reacts hostilely, although his reaction may be delayed. In many cases the therapist discovers that because he has been quite nice to a paranoid person, this person is put to the necessity of inventing a more or less delusional idea of what the therapist is trying to put over on him.

Thus it becomes almost a first principle for the therapist to be distant in dealing with paranoid people. He may, in fact, often be rather forbidding. I am sure that I have received a great deal of information from some paranoid people because they felt I was a thoroughly disagreeable person. I asked unpleasant questions unpleasantly—and got some answers. If I had asked unpleasant questions in a friendly way, these people would probably have gotten all tied up in knots about what I was trying to get at, and what I was trying to convict them of. But when all that they ordinarily supplied to a social situation—unpleasantness—was provided by me, there was no danger of their feeling friendly toward me, and therefore becoming anxious and suspicious.

Thus, while the therapist ordinarily should try to make things run rather smoothly, with the paranoid person he should go to some trouble to make all implications, especially the unpleasant ones, very clear. For instance, I have suggested that, in dealing with the adolescent schizophrenic, it is very useful if the conversation proceeds so smoothly from here to there that the person feels amazingly comfortable and gets to talking about things he had no intention of talking about, and so on. But with the paranoid person—to take the same sort of instance I have just discussed—if I say, "Oh! and I suppose you figure that masturbation destroys you, eh?" I make it sound very cold and almost insulting. That is the trick, for if he feels that I am possibly a little bit tough, the greatest problem a paranoid person has—people who act "friendly" toward him—does not arise. Such people give him a feeling of acute disadvantage. That is what anxiety is; it is a warning of impending disadvantage, and immediately calls out suspicions and various "righting movements."

Unless the proper precautions are taken—and with experience the taking of these becomes almost automatic—the interviewer may get involved in some very serious delusional misinterpretation. There is a way of handling such a misadventure. If you have a certain mental agility and a clarity of focus on what is currently happening, you can put into words the nature of the misinterpretation, saying something like, "Do I understand that such-and-such is the case?" The patient may say, somewhat guardedly, "Yes." Then you say, "And pray, out of what was that built?" You then review all the data which may have been twisted to fit into such a picture. As you hit on a particular event that was woven into it, the patient usually gives some sort of sign—an increase of muscular tension or something of the sort—and then you rather sardonically tear up the suspicious character of that innocent event. In this way you rip up the whole thing piece by piece. And you can wind up with some semblance of being outraged at having your time wasted by such misinterpretations. You may find that *he* is outraged at the discovery that you have "shown him up." You must overlook that; and the only way that you can do this is by seeming to be annoyed at how things have been misinterpreted. Then, as a final move, you say, "And how often do you suppose that kind of misunderstanding comes up in your ordinary life?" That question makes sense. The problem is no longer localized in the relationship of you and the patient. You have suddenly become a competent psychiatrist; you have uncovered his difficulty, and have verified the natural history of a particular instance of it. At this the patient will usually mutter something like, "Well, it's possible that it happens now and then"—whereupon it's my practice, however unpleasant, to say, "Yes, I surmise at least that frequently," and we are on our way again.

If I seem to be suggesting that you insult paranoids, I have failed to make my meaning clear. I don't know what would happen if you insulted such people; the results might be exciting. But in any event don't, for the sake of all concerned, try to befriend them. I *do* know what happens then, and it is exciting, but very unpleasant. What is important in these relationships is to maintain distance, a rather unkind, but actually very careful, reserve. By that locution, "unkind but very careful," I mean that you administer no wounds that do not heal. Taking falls out of people is no part of the psychiatric interview, unless it is necessary to open the mind to something that must be dealt with. The interviewer can be quite unpleasant, if he is sure that he isn't unpleasant at a point, or in a way, that leaves an open wound. Anything which makes a person feel "small," if you please—a really excellent figure of speech—is apt to leave a long-enduring wound, and to be anything but a help in the further development of the interview. The interviewer tries very carefully not to belittle or humiliate people; he can be remarkably unpleasant and distant, without actually humiliating in any way other than by interpretation. Humiliation or belittling that requires interpretation before it is experienced may be interpreted in retrospect in a different way, and thus is not so lastingly hurtful.

I hope I have made it clear that the psychiatrist should avoid giving tacit consent to delusion or to very serious errors on the part of the patient. Let us say that you are a young psychiatrist, and that the scion of a very wealthy family, who has been referred to you for treatment, comes in and tells you something, the probability of which impresses you as being very near nil. It may seem the most natural thing in the world to say, "Oh, yes, yes! Is that so?"—and to go on with something else. But you pay for such things at your leisure, and gradually learn to do better, because the patient in such cases doesn't stay with you a very long time. The patient probably doesn't stay very long, either, with the psychiatrist who brashly and firmly asserts, "I can't believe it!"

In these cases, you should first confirm, by asking the most natural questions that would follow, that the patient intended to say what he did, and that there was no misunderstanding on your part. Having made sure that the patient's statement was as bad as it sounded—that he is entertaining an idea which is not only wrong, but also, in a sense, does violence to the possibility of his living in a social situation among others—you do not then say, "Oh, yes, yes. How interesting!" You rather say, "I can scarcely believe it. What on earth gives you that impression?" You note a marked exception.

That is all you need to do, in my experience, in order to go on with the interview. If something seems terribly off the beam, you register your amazement and ask about it; even if you don't get much information, at least you note your exception, and do not agree tacitly. Often I merely shake my head as if it were just a bit beyond me, conveying a rather strong negation. The patient is often quite grateful that I am not willing to go along at once with a marked misapprehension about something; although he may not be able to say it to me directly at the time, he, too, would like to get rid of these troublesome distortions. Always remember that no matter how sick a person is, the chances are that he is still more like you than he is different.

Curiously enough, the fact that the psychiatrist doesn't start a holy war about the patient's delusions, but at the same time isn't agreeing with them, often gives the patient the impression that the psychiatrist may be sane and is not in any plot against him—and therefore something may come of it. If, however, the psychiatrist says, "Oh, yes, yes. Very interesting. And now tell me about so-and-so," changing the subject, the patient may get the idea that the psychiatrist is a fool, poorly trained, or part of a plot—no one of which ideas is particularly helpful to therapeutic progress.

I wish now to comment on a rather commonly asked question: What is it that brings about favorable change in a person? How do patterns of living undergo significant alteration for the better?

The thing that keeps people from favorable change, from profitable return on certain of their experiences, is that they do not learn anything from those experiences, or, if they learn anything, it is not enough to produce much benefit. It may be surmised that something specifically stands in the way of such learning. But if one assumes that man is as highly adaptive as I always try to suggest that he is, the great question is: Why does a given person not overcome the handicap to learning? Why is he not moving forward? The answer lies in the fact that at some time in his past it became dangerous for him to inquire into certain aspects of what happened to him. That is, such inquiry became so fraught with anxiety that he goes on year after year feeling threatened by experience in some particular field. That experience may be anything from telling a superior what he really thinks about something, to approaching apparently genial members of the other sex with an idea of perfecting his acquaintance with them by genital behavior. Whatever it is, he has been taught by early experience to shy off, to permit no tests, to make no adventures in this dangerous field. When the field concerns lust, or some other very powerful motive, he may make ventures in it, but only after surrounding them with such precautions that they are practically useless.

An example of such precautions is provided by the person who is quite promiscuous but never has sexual relations except when seriously intoxicated. Incidentally, it has been very well stated by some one of my colleagues that alcohol is that material by which one tests the ideals of a personality, ideals being notoriously soluble in alcohol. The sort of person I am describing is afraid to do certain things, and yet is seriously driven by his motivational system to do them; thus he has hit upon the happy idea of so divesting himself of his more complex capacities that he can engage in this behavior with considerable vagueness as to whether it was *his* wish to do so, or *somebody else's*, whether it *did* or *did not* happen, and so on. Under these circumstances, unhappily, experience is very seriously garbled by the impairment of the person's ability to maintain clear contact with the environment.

What I am driving at is this: When a person comes to an interviewer with a problem, the assumption is that this person has been *restrained from using the totality of his abilities*. The problem of the psychiatrist in treatment is to discover what the *handicaps* to the use of his abilities are. I believe that this is quite profoundly and generally true. Let me illustrate as follows.

After certain oddly confusing motions by a patient which I have learned usually mean that a "Great Problem" is about to be revealed, and considerable delay at which I finally show some slight impatience, he may say: "Well, I have a sexual problem." Since I suspect that at this rate we'll get nowhere in an hour and a half, I may say, "And doubtless a homosexual problem." The patient then says, "Yes, Doctor, that's it." Then I may learn that my patient has often had sexual relations with a member of his own sex, or that he has been unable to think of having relations with a member of the other sex, or *something*. That's what this "homosexual problem" means to me—just "something." The *real* problem which I hope finally to uncover, to my patient's satisfaction and with his clear insight, is *what stands in the way* of his making the conventional, and therefore the comparatively simple, adjustment which is regarded as normal. In other words, I don't treat any alleged entities such as homosexuality. I have come to recognize homosexuality as a developmental mistake, dictated by the culture as substitutive behavior in those instances in which the person cannot do what is the simplest thing to do. Thus I try to find out why he *can't* do the simplest thing, and in such investigation may come to solve the problem.

Consider again the question: By what dynamisms does one

change? Invariably one changes by the removal of obstacles to perceiving where one is and what the situation that confronts one is, and why it has been so difficult to perceive these things. In some ways that is the great problem of the interview itself: what is the patient's situation, how can the interviewer discover it, and to what extent can the patient accompany the interviewer in discovering it? Thus when you encounter a person with a "homosexual problem" (in quotation marks, for homosexual is only a name), what counts is what you discover about the person—what particular terrors, menaces, and risks other people hold for him. Quite often that leads you back into the very early years of his life, and through their study change comes about. In problems which bear upon such important things as relative security with members of one's own or the opposite sex, change cannot be brought about in a few interviews. Nor will change occur quickly when the problem reflects years of effort on the part of the parents to indicate to the person that he is unable to get along by himself. There are a great many other things that cannot be changed quickly, simply because the anxiety which the patient undergoes in presenting the relevant facts is so great, and because nothing can be learned by him until that anxiety is lessened. In other words, a person must feel fairly safe in order to make use of anywhere near 100 per cent of his abilities. If he feels extremely insecure, he will be unable to present adequately the simplest proposition, and unable to benefit from its discussion.

Thus we try to proceed along the general lines of getting some notion of what stands in the way of successful living for the person, quite certain that if we can clear away the obstacles, everything else will take care of itself. So true is that, that in well over twenty-five years—aside from my forgotten mistakes in the first few of them—I have never found myself called upon to "cure" anybody. The patients took care of that, once I had done the necessary brush-clearing, and so on. It is almost uncanny how things fade out of the picture when their *raison d'être* is revealed. The brute fact is that man is so extraordinarily adaptive that, given any chance of making a reasonably adequate analysis of the situation, he is quite likely to stumble into a series of experiments which will gradually approximate more successful living.

Sometimes a patient asks: "Doctor, how can I do better at what it is vital to me to do?" And sometimes a therapist asks: "What do I do to be of help in all this?" The answer to both questions is this: work toward uncovering those factors which are concerned in the person's recurrent mistakes, and which lead to his taking ineffective and inappropriate action. There is no necessity to do more.

Conclusion

WHAT I HAVE said in these lectures is intended to pertain to the practical work of interviewing in the psychiatric manner, which was defined as that type of relationship with the interviewee that would produce dependable data on something important about him and bring him benefit. That is what makes it "psychiatric," you might say, in contradistinction to all the other types of cross-examination, and what not, to which people are subjected.

You may feel that all this has been very impractical, in that you could not possibly in the next five or ten years get to the point of covering all that has been touched on in this very sketchy, skeletonized outline. My aim has not been to be pleasant and discursive, or provocative, but to present schemes for organizing one's thought, outlines of approaches, and the type of data that would be relevant in such approaches. I do this with two things in mind: first, that you will get an idea of the general framework that must exist in the psychiatric interview, and an idea of practical ways of setting up this minimal framework; and second, that you will then devise the outlines, schematizations, and so on, best suited to you, which will encompass the essential data and make best use of the interview time. I have given you not a definitive plan, not a carefully thoroughgoing detailed outline of any particular phase or aspect of the interview, but a suggestion of what the outstandingly significant data are.

Until an interviewer has opened his mind to the rather intimidating complexity of interpersonal relations and of those hypothetical things, "personalities," which enter into them, and until he has organized a rather systematic way of keeping all these data in mind, he invariably overlooks a great many events. This is all the more so since all conversation between two people is directed by attempts to avoid insecurity on the part of both of those engaged in the verbal intercourse. Many of the people whom the interviewer sees have developed quite subtle ways of maintaining security, and unless he has a fairly organized notion of what are likely to be the relevant data and how extensive they may be, and has a great many schematizations handy in his mind, he may be led into blind and unprofitable alleys, and may be very successfully deflected from important areas by the unwitting skill of his interviewee. It is for that reason, chiefly, that it has seemed to me important to present, not a definitive statement in each of these fields, which I could never adequately formulate, but a large number of the high spots characteristic of each. Let me say very simply that I never expect anybody to have all the information about any interviewee that I have suggested as being obtainable and important. For instance, if one is interviewing someone fourteen years of age for the position of office boy, with a view to his emptying wastebaskets before the office force arrives, and seeing that there is ink in the inkwells, and so on, it is not really profoundly important that one know his outlook toward life. As a matter of fact, I would expect the outlook toward life of a fourteen-year-old to be quite a transitional phenomenon, subject to remarkable changes in the course of his employment in any stable office. Thus there are many things that may have no particularly high relevance to a certain situation. But it is nevertheless important that we, as interviewers, have a rather clear idea of what is significant or not in the behavior of humans. It is, at least in part, through our ability to observe events and to evaluate their significance in the life of the interviewee that we may come to serve some useful purpose to him.

Throughout this discussion of the interview situation, the interviewer has been considered as an expert in interpersonal relations. That is, the interviewer is alert to interpersonal phenomena not only in terms of the interviewee's behavior but also in terms of what happens in his own behavior and in his covert processes. He is careful in dealing with the interviewee's anxiety as evidenced in multiple reservations and attempts at deception. He checks adequately any important parataxic distortions which seem to be present. He notes where information seems to be lacking and in some cases supplies it. And finally, he never ignores the limitations of his own experience and the restrictions which are imposed upon him by his role as an expert in the observation and interpretation of interpersonal phenomena.

The course of the interview situation proceeds on the basic assumption that the interviewee can derive at least some durable benefit from his contact with expert skill, but that this can occur only in the measure that a valid relationship comes into being. Thus the interviewer must handle himself like an expert in interpersonal relations from his first meeting with the patient, through every detail of the formal inception of the desired situation, through the reconnaissance into the social identity of the client, through the detailed inquiry into all that is highly relevant to the success of the interview, and finally in the carefully organized termination or interruption of the contact. In this expert role, the interviewer is seriously interested in the problem presented by the interviewee; he is careful to avoid misunderstandings and unintentional erroneous impressions; he is ready to be corrected, yet chary of repetitive, circumstantial, or inconsequential details; he foregoes the satisfaction of any curiosity about matters into which there is no clear technical need to inquire; he eschews all procedure chiefly calculated to impress the client with the interviewer's clairvoyance or omniscience; he avoids all impractical meaningless comment, the clouding of issues, or tacit consent to dangerous delusion or error that will be difficult or embarrassing subsequently in the interview; he proceeds in general with such simple clarity that the interviewee can follow the direction of the inquiry; and from time to time, he offers his impressions for correction or discussion by the interviewee. And finally, the interviewer as an expert makes sure that the interviewee 'knows himself' the better for the experience.

Index